NURSING TODAY

Transition and Trends

FIFTH EDITION

ELSEVIER

evolve

To access your Learning Resources, visit:

http://evolve.elsevier.com/Zerwekh/nsgtoday/

Evolve Learning Resources for **Zerwekh/Claborn: Nursing Today: Transition and Trends, fifth edition,** offers the following features:

- **Sample NCLEX Test Tutorial**
  Provides access to a computerized test tutorial that simulates the NCLEX test-taking experience through similar questions and methods for selecting answers.
- **Sample NCLEX Questions**
  Includes over 20 questions to demonstrate how a broad range of nursing content may be tested, as well as introduce students to the types of questions they will encounter on the NCLEX exam.
- **Sample Memory Notecards**
  Provide a variety of learning techniques to encourage retention and understanding of fluids and electrolytes and pharmacology in preparation for the NCLEX.
- **Resume Maker**
  Provides access to templates that help to create a professional resume and cover letter that match current career level, background and career objectives.
- **Case Studies**
  Involves case scenarios designed to help students apply their knowledge and to stimulate critical thinking.
- **Weblinks**
  An exciting resource that lets you link to hundreds of websites carefully chosen to supplement the content of the textbook. The WebLinks are regularly updated, with new ones added as they develop.

http://evolve.elsevier.com/Zerwekh/nsgtoday/

FIFTH EDITION

NURSING TODAY

Transition and Trends

JOANN ZERWEKH, EDD, RN, FNP, APRN, BC
EXECUTIVE DIRECTOR
NURSING EDUCATION CONSULTANTS
INGRAM, TEXAS
NURSING FACULTY—ONLINE CAMPUS
UNIVERSITY OF PHOENIX
PHOENIX, ARIZONA

JO CAROL CLABORN, MS, RN, CNS
EXECUTIVE DIRECTOR
NURSING EDUCATION CONSULTANTS
INGRAM, TEXAS

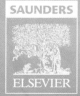

SAUNDERS
ELSEVIER

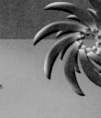

SAUNDERS
ELSEVIER

11830 Westline Industrial Drive
St. Louis, Missouri 63146

NURSING TODAY: TRANSITION AND TRENDS
ISBN-13: 978-1-4160-2313-5
ISBN-10: 1-4160-2313-5

ISBN-13: 978-1-4160-2313-5
ISBN-10: 1-4160-2313-5

Senior Editor: Yvonne Alexopoulos
Senior Developmental Editor: Lisa P. Newton
Publishing Services Manager: Jeff Patterson
Project Manager: Clay S. Broeker
Designer: Jyotika Shroff

Printed in Canada
Last digit is the print number: 9 8 7 6 5 4 3

To the loving memory of my mother,
Hazel L. Cooper,
for her love and support
of my endeavors in nursing

Jo Carol Claborn

Contributors

Susan Lynne Ahrens, RN, Ph.D.
Director, Surgical Trauma ICU
Parkview Hospital
Fort Wayne, Indiana
Workplace Issues

Jo Carol Claborn, MS, RN, CNS
Executive Director
Nursing Education Consultants
Ingram, Texas
Reality Shock; NCLEX-RN and the New Graduate

Sharon Decker, RN, CS, MSN, CCRN
Professor and Director of Clinical Simulations
Texas Tech University Health Sciences Center
Lubbock, Texas
Time Management

Valerie S. Eschiti, RN, MSN, CHTP, AHN-BC
Assistant Professor
Midwestern State University
Wilson School of Nursing
Wichita Falls, Texas
Cultural and Spiritual Awareness

Michael L. Evans, PhD, RN, CNAA, FACHE
Vice President, The Center for Learning
Texas Health Resources
Arlington, Texas
Political Action in Nursing

Mary E. Foley, RN, MS
Associate Director, Center for Research and Innovation in Patient Care
University of California School of Nursing
San Francisco, California
Immediate Past—President
American Nurses Association
Washington, DC
Collective Bargaining

Tom Gaglione, RN, MSN
Nursing Faculty
Nursing Education Consultants
Ingram, Texas
Effective Communication and Team Building

Ruth Hansten, RN, PhD, MBA, BSN, FACHE
Principal, Hansten Healthcare PLLC
Port Ludlow, Washington
Delegation in the Clinical Setting

Marilynn Jackson, PhD, MA, BSN
Intuitive Options
Kasilof, Alaska
Delegation in the Clinical Setting

Ela-Joy Lehrman, MS, MAEd, PhD, RN, CNM
Chair, Nursing & Health Administration for Southern Arizona
University of Phoenix
Tucson, Arizona
Using Nursing Research in Practice

Janet M. McLellan, RN, MSN, BC, NSA
Nursing and Health Sciences Faculty, University of Phoenix
Phoenix, Arizona
Business Consulting Services, Healthlink, an IBM company
Houston, Texas
Nursing Informatics

Barbara J. Michaels, EdD, LMFT, RN
Faculty (retired)
Dallas, Texas
Self-Care Strategies

Mary Ellen Murray, PhD, RN
Associate Professor
University of Wisconsin-Madison
School of Nursing
Madison, Wisconsin
Economics in the Health Care Delivery System

Tess Pape, PhD, RN, CNOR
Assistant Professor
Patty Hanks Shelton School of Nursing
Consortium of Abilene Christian, Hardin Simmons and McMurray Universities
Abilene, Texas
Quality Patient Care

Alice B. Pappas, PhD, RN
Director for Education and Nursing Research
Children's Medical Center
Dallas, Texas
Employment Considerations: Opportunities, Resumes, and Interviewing

Robin L. Perin, RN, BS, JD
General Counsel for University Physicians Healthcare
Tucson, Arizona
Legal Issues

Susan Sportsman, RN, PhD
Dean, College of Health Sciences and Human Services
Minnie Rhea Wood Professor of Nursing
Midwestern State University
Wichita Falls, Texas
The Health Care Organization and Patterns of Nursing Care Delivery

Linda Stevenson, PhD, RN
Assistant Professor
Baylor University
Louise Herrington School of Nursing
Dallas, Texas
Image of Nursing: Influences of the Present

Anne Sullivan, RN, MSN
University of Phoenix Faculty
Phoenix, Arizona
Nursing Theory

Gayle Varnell, PhD, RN, CPNP
Associate Professor
Associate Dean for Advanced Practice
The University of Texas at Tyler
College of Nursing and Health Sciences
Tyler, Texas
Nursing Education

Joann Wilcox, RN, MSN
University of Phoenix Online Faculty
Phoenix, Arizona
Challenges of Nursing Management

Kathleen O. Williams, RN, PhD
Associate Professor
Jefferson College of Health Science
Roanoke, Virginia
Collective Bargaining

Ashley Zerwekh, RN, BA
Telemetry Unit at Chandler Regional Hospital
Chandler, Arizona
MSN Graduate Student in Rural Health Education
Northern Arizona University
Flagstaff, Arizona
Mentoring and Preceptorship

JoAnn Zerwekh, EdD, RN, FNP, APRN, BC
Executive Director
Nursing Education Consultants
Ingram, Texas
Nursing Faculty—Online Campus
University of Phoenix
Phoenix, Arizona
Reality Shock; Mentoring and Preceptorship; Historical Perspectives: Influences of the Past; Conflict Management

Reviewers

Lori Jo Bork, RN, MS, CCRN
Instructor of Nursing
Dakota Wesleyan University
Mitchell, South Dakota

Nancy Harms, RN, PhD
Chair, Nursing Division
Midland Lutheran College
Freemont, Nebraska

Karen Kelly, EdD, RN, CNAA, BC
Associate Professor
School of Nursing
Southern Illinois University at Edwardsville
Edwardsville, Illinois

Polly Gerber Zimmermann, RN, MS, MBA-CEN
Assistant Professor
Henry S. Truman College
Chicago, Illinois

PREFACE

Nursing Today: Transition and Trends evolved out of the authors' experiences with the nursing student in his or her final semester and the student's transition into the realities of nursing practice. There is an increasing need for the graduating nurse to become aware of the challenges of the transition process before graduation. Nursing education and the transition process is experiencing a tremendous impact from changes in the health care delivery system. We have responded to these changes by adding information in areas that nursing faculty specifically requested. In this fifth edition, we have continued to provide the graduate nurse with information on delegation and management, and we have added chapters on Mentoring and Preceptorship, Nursing Theory, Cultural and Spiritual Awareness, Quality Patient Care, and Workplace Issues. We have also combined chapter information to make topics easier to find and make for easier reading with less repetition. We kept the same easy reading style to present timely information along with information on nursing management, leadership, and delegation in both hospital and community settings. One of our goals with this book is to provide the graduating nurse with practical guidelines that can be implemented in his or her transition from nursing student to effective nursing practice at entry level.

The classic findings and experience of Marlene Kramer and her research on reality shock, as well as Patricia Benner's work on performance characteristics of beginning and expert nurses, continue to impact the need for transition courses in the school curriculum. These courses focus on trends and issues to assist the new graduate to be better prepared to practice nursing in today's world. With the increased demands and realities of the health care system, it is necessary for the new graduate to rapidly make the transition to an independent role. We have written this book to be used in these transition-type courses, as well as by individual students to assist them in anticipating encounters in a rapidly changing, technologically oriented work environment.

We have revised and updated each chapter regarding the changes in the health care delivery system. We have continued the increased focus on the use of the Internet as a resource for the transitioning graduate. We have maintained the cartoons drawn by CJ Miller, RN. We feel they add a smile and perhaps make the difficult information a little easier. Each chapter begins with student objectives and a quote as an introduction to the content of the chapter. Within each chapter, there is a practical application of the concepts discussed. Critical Thinking boxes in the text highlight information to facilitate the critical thinking process. Using a question approach, material is presented in a logical, easy-to-read manner. There are also opportunities to respond to thought-provoking questions and student exercises to facilitate self-evaluation.

The student is given an overall view of the nursing profession from past historical events that influenced nursing to the present day image, as well as the legal, ethical, political, and on-the-job issues confronting today's nurse. Communication in the workplace, time management, how to write an effective resume, interviewing tips, employee benefits, and self-care strategies are among the sound career advancement tools provided.

FOR NURSING FACULTY

Our key goal in developing this book has been timely information that is applicable to current practice and fun to read. An Instructor's Manual, which is web-based, is available from the publisher to assist faculty in planning and promoting a positive transition experience. This valuable website contains suggestions for classroom and clinically based student activities.

At the request of nursing faculty using our book, we have provided a secure, updated web-based Test Bank and have expanded the content within Evolve, which supports the textbook. The Evolve website will continue to provide updated information as new trends and issues affect the practice of nursing.

Please consult your local Elsevier representative for more details.

JoAnn Zerwekh
Jo Carol Claborn

Acknowledgments

The success of previous editions of this book is due to the contributions and efforts of our chapter contributors, who provided their expertise and knowledge. This new edition is no exception. We thank the staff at Elsevier: Yvonne Alexopoulos, Senior Nursing Editor, for her expertise and advice, and Lisa Newton, Senior Developmental Editor, who we have worked most closely with in this revision process. Their creativity and guidance have provided a new look for this fifth edition, and we are grateful for their ability to quickly smooth out the wrinkles that often occur in the production of a book. A big thank you also goes to Clay Boeker, who monitored the production of this book and another one of our books simultaneously, kept us on schedule, and was not *too* overworked.

Last, but certainly not least, we want to thank our adult children for their continued support in our writing endeavors—Tyler, Ashley, Jaelyn, Mike, and Kimberley. We also thank Tom Gaglione and Robert Claborn for their unending support, patience, and sense of humor. We love you all!

Contents

Unit I Professional Growth and Transitions

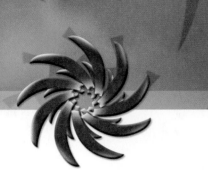

UNIT II CAREER DEVELOPMENT

UNIT VI CONTEMPORARY NURSING PRACTICE

UNIT I

Professional Growth and Transitions

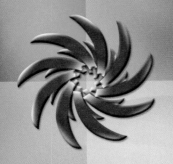

CHAPTER 1

Reality Shock

JOANN ZERWEKH, EdD, RN, FNP, APRN, BC
JO CAROL CLABORN, MS, RN, CNS

If only dreams and reality were not so far apart.
—Miguel de Cervantes

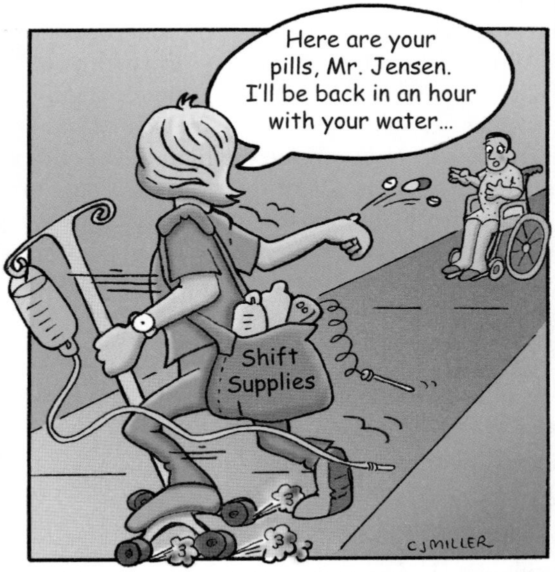
Here are your pills, Mr. Jensen. I'll be back in an hour with your water...
Shift Supplies
CJMILLER

Role transition can be a complex experience.

After completing this chapter, you should be able to:

- Discuss the concept of transitions.
- Identify the characteristics of reality shock.
- Compare and contrast the phases of reality shock.
- Identify times in your life when you have experienced a reality shock or role transition.
- Describe methods to promote a successful transition.

Welcome to the world of nursing! This book is written for nursing students who are in the midst of transitions in their life. As a new student, you are beginning the transition to becoming indoctrinated into nursing, and sometimes it is not an easy transition. For those of you who are in the middle of nursing school, do you wonder if life even exists outside of nursing school? To the student who will soon graduate, hang on; you are almost there! For whatever transition period you are encountering, our goal is to help make your life easier during the transition period as you begin to adjust both personally and professionally to either being a nursing student or anticipating graduation from nursing school and the beginning of your first job as a professional nurse. We have designed this book to help you keep your feet on the ground and your head out of the clouds as well as to boost your spirits when the going gets rough. We offer many down-to-earth tips that will save you time and energy.

As you thumb through this book, you will notice that there are cartoons and critical-thinking questions that encourage your participation. Do not be alarmed; we know you have been overloaded with "critical thinking" during nursing school! These critical-thinking questions are not meant to be graded; instead, their purpose is to encourage you to begin thinking about your transition, either into nursing school or into practice, and to guide you through the book in a practical, participative manner. Our intention is to add a little humor here and there while giving information on topics we feel will impact your transition. For the beginning, or even advanced student, topics on conflict management, finding and using a mentor, time management, testing strategies, and effective communication will offer some insight into how to handle some difficult situations while still in school. Topics such as reality shock, the job search, selecting a mentor, nursing education programs, nursing management skills, ethical and legal issues, career planning, and burnout prevention, are designed for the student who has graduation in sight. We want you to be informed about the controversial issues affecting nursing today. After all, the future of nursing rests with **you**!

Are you ready to begin? Then let's start with the real stuff. You are beginning to experience transitions—for some of you, just getting into nursing school has been a long struggle—and you are there! For others, you can see the light at the end of the tunnel, as graduation becomes a reality. Nursing is one of the most rewarding professions you can pursue. However, it can also be one of the most frustrating. As with marriage, raising children, and the pursuit of happiness, there are ups and downs. We seldom find the world or our specific situation the exact way we thought it would or should be. Often your fantasy of what nursing should be is not what you will find nursing to be.

You will cry, but you will also laugh.

You will share with people their darkest hours of pain and suffering, but

You will also share with them their hope, healing, and recovery.

You will be there as life begins and ends.

You will experience great challenges that lead to success.

You will experience failure and disappointment.

You will never cease to be amazed at the resilience of the human body and spirit.

TRANSITIONS

WHAT ARE TRANSITIONS?

Transitions are passages or changes from one situation, condition, or state to another that occur over time. They have been classified into the following four major types: developmental (e.g., becoming a parent, mid-life crisis), situational (e.g., graduating from a nursing program, career change, divorce), health/illness (e.g., dealing with a chronic illness), and organizational (e.g., change in leadership, new staffing patterns) (Schumacher and Meleis, 1994).

Transitions are complex processes, and a lot of transitions occur at the same time.

WHAT ARE IMPORTANT FACTORS INFLUENCING TRANSITIONS?

Understanding the transition experience from the perspective of the person who is experiencing it is important because the meaning of the experience may be positive, negative, or neutral. The transition may be desired (e.g., starting school, successfully finishing school, passing NCLEX) or undesirable (e.g., the death of a family member, after which you have to assume a new role in your family). Expectation about the transition process may or may not be realistic.

Often, when you know what to expect, the stress associated with the change or transition is reduced.

Another factor in the transition process is the new level of knowledge and skill required, as is the availability of needed resources within the environment.

Your control over the basic conditions of your school and work life is usually limited, but your ability and skill in creating the experiences can be unlimited. Therein is the key to your successful role transition. Transitions are a part of life and certainly a part of nursing. Although the following discussions on role transition and reality shock focus on the graduate nurse experience, there are many applicable points for the new student as well. As you learn more about transitions, reality shock, and the graduate nurse experience, think about how this information may also apply to your transition experience into and through nursing school (Critical Thinking Box 1-1).

CRITICAL THINKING BOX 1-1

What is your greatest concern about your transition from school to practice?

Looking back, what transitions have you experienced? What transitions are occurring in your life now? Has your entry into, as well as progress through, nursing school caused transitions in your personal life? Has your anticipated graduation and job search caused transitions in your professional as well as personal life?

TRANSITIONS IN NURSING

The paradox of nursing will become obvious to you early in your nursing career. This realization may occur during nursing school, but it frequently becomes most obvious during the first 6 months of your first job.

Health care organizations are very concerned about your transition experience and job satisfaction during that first 6 months of employment. Have you been hearing about "evidence-based practice"? Well, it is working for you now! During the first 6 months of employment, new graduates need a period of time to develop their skills in a supportive environment. Employee retention and job satisfaction are key issues with the hospital; confidence in perfoming skills and procedures, peer and preceptor relationships, and independence versus independence are key graduate nurse issues driving this research. The well-being of the graduate nurse and the ability to deliver quality nursing care during the transition period has sparked research to validate the need for special considerations of the graduate nurse experiencing transition. (Casey et al, 2004; Godinez et al, 1999; Steinmiller, Levonian, & Lengetti, 2003; Lavoie-Tremblay et al, 2002). With identification of the basic problems encountered by new graduates during this first 6 months, there is a concerted effort to begin to meet the special needs of the graduate nurse.

The role-transition process that occurs on entry into nursing school and the process from student to graduate nurse does not take place automatically. Having the optimal experience during role transition requires lots of attention, planning, and determination on your part. How you perceive and handle the transition will determine how well you progress through the process. It is important that you keep a positive attitude. Emotions, clinicals, tests, as well as work situations are going to be up and down, but that is okay. It is expected, and you are going to be able to deal with it effectively. The wide range of emotions experienced during the transition process can often affect your *emotional and physical well being;* check out the discussion of self-care strategies in Chapter 2.

So, let's get started. Reality shock is often one of the first hurdles of transition to conquer in your new role as a graduate nurse or registered nurse (RN, or Real Nurse☺).

REALITY SHOCK

WHAT IS REALITY SHOCK?

Reality shock is a term often used to describe the reaction experienced when one moves into the work force after several years of educational preparation. The recent graduate is caught in the situation of moving from a familiar, comfortable, educational environment into a new role in the work force in which the expectations are not clearly defined or may not even be realistic. For example, as a student you were taught to consider the patient in a holistic framework, but in practice you often do not have the time to consider the psychosocial or teaching needs of the patient, even though they must be attended to and documented.

The recent graduate in the workplace is expected to be a capable, competent nurse. That sounds fine. However, sometimes there is a hidden expectation that graduate nurses should function as though they have 5 years of nursing experience. With the current nursing shortage, along with the increasing acuity level of patients, this is not an uncommon problem for the new graduate. This situation may leave the graduate with feelings of powerlessness, depression, and insecurity because of an apparent lack of effectiveness in the work environment. There are positive ways to deal with the problems. You are not alone! The process of reality shock and transition is not unique to nursing. It is present in many professions as the graduate moves from the world of academia to the world of work and begins to adjust to the expectations and values of the work force.

WHAT ARE THE PHASES OF REALITY SHOCK?

Kramer (1974) described the process of reality shock as it applies to nursing (Table 1-1). Although she identified this process in 1974, these phases of reality shock remain a classic in understanding the implications, as well as successful progression through reality shock. In our current world of nursing, we are still dealing with this same process. Adjustments begin to take place as the graduate nurse adapts to the reality of the practice of nursing. The first phase of adjustment is the honeymoon phase (Figure 1-1). The recent graduate is thrilled with completing school and accepting a first job. Life is a bed of roses because everyone knows nursing school is much harder than nursing practice. There is no more creating concept care maps, or writing nursing care plans deep into the night, or burning the midnight oil for the next day's examination. No one is watching over your shoulder while you insert a catheter or give an intravenous medication. You are not a "student" anymore; now you're a nurse! During this exciting phase, your perception of the situation may feel unreal and distorted, and you may not be able to understand the overall picture.

I just can't believe how wonderful everything is! Imagine getting a paycheck—money, at last! It's all great. Really, it is.

The honeymoon phase is frequently short-lived as the graduate begins to identify the conflicts between the way she or he was taught and the reality of what is done.

TABLE 1-1

Phases of Reality Shock

Honeymoon	Shock and Rejection	Recovery
Sees the world of nursing looking quite rosy Often fascinated with the thrill of "arriving" in the profession	Has excessive mistrust Experiences increased concern over minor pains and illness Experiences decrease in energy, and feels excessive fatigue Feels like a failure, and blames self for every mistake Bands together and depends on people who hold the same values Has a hypercritical attitude Feels moral outrage	Beginning to have sense of humor is first sign Decrease in tension Increase in ability to be objective

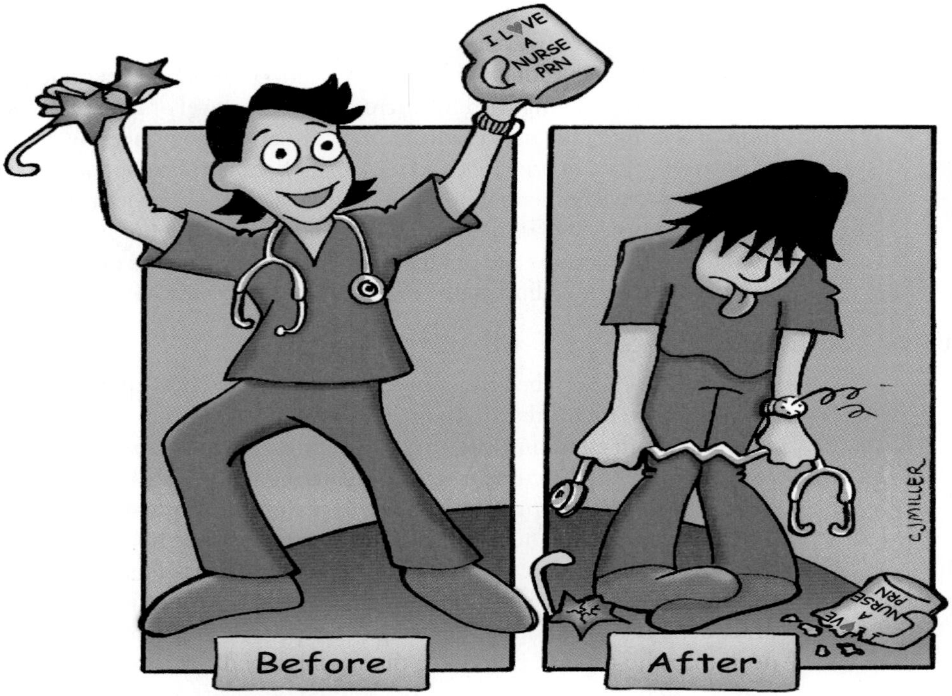

FIGURE 1-1
Reality shock. The honeymoon's over.

Every graduate nurse will have a unique way of coping with the situations; however, some common responses have been identified. The graduate may cope with this conflict by withdrawing or rejecting the values learned during nursing school. This may mark the end of the honeymoon phase of transition. The phrase "going native" was used by Kramer and Schmalenberg (1977) to describe recent graduates as they begin to cope and identify with the reality of the situation by rejecting the values from nursing school and beginning to function as everyone else does.

Mary was assigned 10 patients for the morning. There were numerous medications to be administered. It was difficult to carry all of the medication administration records to each room for patient identification. Because she "knew the patients," and the other experienced nurses did not check identification, she decided she no longer needed to check a patient's identification before administering medication. Later in the day, she gave insulin to Mrs. James, a patient she "knew"; unfortunately, the insulin was for Mrs. Phillips, another patient she "knew."

With experiences such as this during transition, the graduate may begin to feel like a failure, and taking the blame for every mistake. Moral outrage may occur at having been put in such a position. When the bad days begin to outnumber the good days, the graduate nurse may experience frustration, fatigue, and anger and may consequently develop a hypercritical attitude toward nursing. Some graduates become very disillusioned and drop out of nursing altogether. This is the period of shock and rejection.

> I had just completed orientation in the hospital where I had wanted to work since I started nursing school. I immediately discovered that the care there was so bad that I did not want to be a part of it. At night, I went home very frustrated that the care I had given was not as I was taught to do it. I cried every night and hated to go to work in the morning. I did not like anyone with whom I was working. My stomach hurt, my head throbbed, and I had difficulty sleeping. It was hard not to work a double shift because I was worried about who would take care of those patients if I were not there.

A successfully managed transition period begins when the graduate nurse is able to evaluate the work situation objectively and to effectively predict the actions and reactions of the staff. Prioritization, conflict management, time management, and support groups (peer, preceptors, and mentors) can make a significant difference in promoting a successfully managed transition period.

Nurturing the ability to see humor in a situation may be the first step. As the graduate begins to laugh at some of the situations encountered, the tension decreases and the perception increases. It is during this critical period of recovery that conflict resolution occurs. If this resolution occurs in a positive manner, it enables the graduate nurse to grow more fully as a person. This growth also enables the graduate to meet the work expectations to a greater degree and to see that she or he has the capacity to change a situation. If the conflict is resolved in a less-positive manner, however, the graduate's potential to learn and grow is limited.

Kramer (1974) described four groups of graduate nurses and the steps they took to resolve reality shock. The graduates who were considered to be most successful at adaptation were those who "made a lot of waves" within both their job setting and their professional organizations. Accordingly, they were not content with the present state of nursing but worked to affect a better system. This group of graduates was able to take worthwhile values learned during school and integrate them into the work setting. Often they returned to school—but not too quickly.

> I am really glad that I became a nurse. Sure, there are plenty of hassles, but the opportunities are there. Now that I am more confident of my skills, I am willing to take risks to improve patient care. Why, last week my head nurse, who often says jokingly, "You're a thorn in my side," appointed me to the Nursing Standards Committee. I feel really good about this recognition.

Another group limited their involvement with nursing by just putting in the usual workday. Persons in this group seldom belonged to professional organizations and cited as their reasons for working "to provide for my family," "to buy extra things for the house," and "to support myself." Typically, this type of conflict resolution leads to burnout, during which time the conflict would be turned inward, leading to constant griping and complaining about the work setting.

> I was so happy, at first. Gee, I was able to buy my son all those toys he wanted. Things here always seem to be the same—too many patients, not enough help. I get so upset with the staff, especially the nursing assistants, and the care that is given to patients. I wonder whether I will ever get the opportunity to practice nursing as I was taught. Well, I'll hang on 'till my husband finishes graduate school, then I'll quit this awful job!

Another group of graduates seemed to have found their niche and were content within the hospital setting. However, their positive attitude toward the job did not extend to nursing as a profession; in fact, it was the opposite. Rather than leave the organization during conflict, these "organization nurses" would change units or shifts—anything to avoid increasing demands for professional performance.

During those first few months as I was just getting started, I sure had a tough time. It was difficult learning how to delegate tasks to the aides and practical nurses. But now that I have started working for Dr. Travis, everything is under my control. I just might go back to school someday.

The last group of graduates frequently changed jobs. After a short-lived career in hospital nursing, this group would pirouette off to graduate school, where they could "do something else in nursing" (i.e., "I can't nurse the way I've been taught, so I might as well teach others how to do things right."). Achieving a high profile in professional nursing organizations was common for these graduates, along with seeking a safer, more idealistically structured environment in which the values learned in school prevail.

Finally, I got so frustrated with my head nurse that I just resigned. What did she expect from a recent graduate?! I couldn't do everything! Cost containment; early discharge; no time for teaching; rush, rush, rush, all the time. Well, I've made up my mind to look into going back to school to further my career.

The job expectations of the hospital administration or the employing community agency and the educational preparation of the graduate nurse are not always the same. This discrepancy is considered to be the basis of reality shock. Relationships among the staff, nursing professionalism, job satisfaction, and employee alienation were studied by Roche and colleagues (2004), Casey and colleagues (2004), and Godinez and colleagues (1999). What is interesting is that the issues of reality shock and role transition described by Kramer in the early 1970s are still around. We (nursing) have entered the 21st century with many of the same issues we had in the 20th century. Much of this problem may be related to the fact that clinical instructors often focus on the needs of the patient rather than the needs of the student (Polifroni et al, 1995). We need to search for a way out of this situation (Critical Thinking Box 1-2).

It might seem to you right now, after reading all of this information, that reality shock is a life-threatening situation. Be assured, it is not. You may, however, experience some physical and psychologic symptoms in varying degrees of intensity. For example, you may feel stressed out or have headaches, insomnia, gastrointestinal upset, or a bout of poststudent blues. Just remember that it takes time to adjust to a new routine and that sometimes, even after you have gotten used to it, you still may feel overwhelmed, confused, or anxious. The good news is that there are various ways to get through this critical phase of your career while establishing a firm foundation for future professional growth and career mobility. Try the assessment exercise in Critical Thinking Box 1-3.

CRITICAL THINKING BOX 1-2

What is your greatest concern about your transition? Is it personal or work transitions because you are a student nurse, or is it your transition from school to practice?

CRITICAL THINKING BOX 1-3

REALITY SHOCK INVENTORY

All students, as well as new graduates, experience reality shock to some extent or another. The purpose of this exercise is to make you aware of how you feel about yourself and your particular life situation.

Directions: To evaluate your views and determine your self-evaluation of your particular life situation, respond to the statements with the appropriate number.

1 Strongly agree	4 Slightly disagree
2 Agree	5 Disagree
3 Slightly agree	6 Strongly disagree

1. ☐ I am still finding new challenges and interests in my work.
2. ☐ I think often about what I want from life.
3. ☐ My own personal future seems promising.
4. ☐ Nursing school and/or my work has brought stresses for which I was unprepared.
5. ☐ I would like the opportunity to start anew knowing what I know now.
6. ☐ I drink more than I should.
7. ☐ I often feel that I still belong in the place where I grew up.
8. ☐ Much of the time my mind is not as clear as it used to be.
9. ☐ I have no sense of regret concerning my major life decision of becoming a nurse.
10. ☐ My views on nursing are as positive as they ever were.
11. ☐ I have a strong sense of my own worth.
12. ☐ I am experiencing what would be called a crisis in my personal or work setting.
13. ☐ I cannot see myself as a nurse.
14. ☐ I must remain loyal to commitments even if they have not proven as rewarding as I had expected.
15. ☐ I wish I were different in many ways.
16. ☐ The way I present myself to the world is not the way I really am.
17. ☐ I often feel agitated or restless.
18. ☐ I have become more aware of my inadequacies and faults.
19. ☐ My sex life is as satisfactory as it has ever been.
20. ☐ I often think about students and/or friends who have dropped out of school or work.

To compute your score, reverse the number you assigned to statements 1, 3, 9, 10, 11, and 19. For example, 1 would become a 6, 2 would become a 5, 3 would become a 4, 4 would become a 3, 5 would become a 2, and 6 would become a 1. Total the number. The higher the score, the better your attitude. The range is 20 to 120.

Modified from White E: Doctoral dissertation, *Chronicle of Higher Education*, April 23, 1986, p 28. Reprinted with permission.

ROLE TRANSFORMATION

Remember when you first started nursing school? The war stories everybody told you? The changes that occurred in your family as a result of your starting nursing school? Are you in the midst of that now, or does it seem like a long time ago? Can you really believe where you are now and where you were when you first began nursing school, those first nursing courses, and clinicals? There has been lots of work and sacrifice to get to where you are now. Believe it or not, you have already experienced a role transition—you successfully transitioned to a student nurse. Now, as you draw nearer to the successful completion of that experience, you are ready to embark on a new one. Take a minute to read the thoughts of one of your peers about her transition into nursing. I'm sure you will smile at her satire (Critical Thinking Box 1-4).

CRITICAL THINKING BOX 1-4

SURVIVAL TECHNIQUES FROM ONE WHO HAS SURVIVED

You finally did it; you have decided nursing is what you want to do for the rest of your life. After all, who would go through all this anguish if you only wanted to do this as a pasttime? If you are taking this like everyone else, you are probably going to do this by trial and error, "war" stories, or by helpful hints from the nursing staff.

You need to prioritize your time. This is a familiar and much used term that you will hear often. It is also easier said than done. If you are single, you have an advantage—maybe. You can decide right now that single is "where it's at" and stay that way for the duration. Of course this means literally living the "single" life. There are no "dinners-for-two," no telephone conversations, no movies at the cinema (rarely any TV)—in other words, no physical contact with the opposite sex. I know you were not thinking about it anyway, but in case you are studying anatomy and physiology, and hormonal thoughts pervade your consciousness, dismiss them.

If you are married, I am not suggesting divorce, just abstinence. Hopefully, you kissed your spouse good-bye when you came to school for your first day of class because your next chance will be on your breaks or when you graduate.

If you happen to be a parent, do as I did. I put pictures of myself in all rooms of my house when I started to school so that kids would not forget me. My children, in return, helped me by plastering their faces in my fridge (they know I'll look there) or on my mirror (another sure spot). I have acquired a son-in-law, a daughter-in-law, and five grandchildren in the past 2½ years, and I usually do not recognize them if I run into them on the rare occasions when I go to the store for essentials (like food) or out to pay our

Continued

CRITICAL THINKING BOX 1-4—cont'd

utility bills. Christmas is fun, though, because each year I get to spend a few days getting to know the family again. But we all must wear name tags for the first day!

If your children are small, buy them the Fisher Price Kitchen and teach them how to "cook" nourishing "hot" cereal on the stove that does not heat up. For the infant, hang a TPN (hint: Total Parental Nutrition) of Similac with iron at 40 cc/hr that the baby can control by sound! Crying should do it! Instead of a needle, use a nipple....

Diapers—what would we do without those disposable diapers that stay dry for 2 weeks at a time? You can even buy the kind that you touch the waistband, and Mickey Mouse and his friends jump off to entertain your baby.

Some of you may feel guilty about not fixing those delicious meals your family once enjoyed. Do not! We get two "breaks" a year, and during that time, fix barrels of nourishing liquid (you can add a few veggies). When your family gets hungry, just take out enough to keep fluids and lytes balanced. Remind them that this is only going to last another year or two.

Have I covered everything? Oh I forgot dust.... Dust used to bother me, but not anymore. I use it to write notes to my 17-year-old, to let him know what time I am going to be in the house, so he will not mistake me for a burglar, and to say "I Love You."

On a serious note, each semester you will get regrouped with new classmates. They will become your family, your support group. You will form a chain, and everyone is a strong link. This is a group effort. These are people who will laugh with you and cry with you. You will form friendships that will last a lifetime. Take advantage of these opportunities.

On a closing note, do not listen to all the "war stories" that go around—just to the credible ones like mine!

From Beagle B: Survival techniques, *AD Clinical Care*, May/June, 1990, p 17. Reprinted with permission.

Give yourself a well-deserved pat on the back for what you have accomplished thus far. It is important to learn early in your practice of nursing to take time to reflect on your accomplishments. Now, back to the present. Let's look at the current role-transition process at hand, from student to graduate nurse RN (real nurse).

WHEN DOES THE ROLE TRANSITION TO GRADUATE NURSE BEGIN?

Does the transition begin at graduation? No. It started when you began to move into the novice role while in your first nursing course (Table 1-2). According to Benner (1984, p. 20):

TABLE 1-2

From Novice to Expert

Stage	Characteristics
Novice Nursing student Experienced nurse in a new setting	• No clinical experience in situation expected to perform • Needs rules to guide performance • Experiences difficulty in applying theoretical concepts to patient care
Advanced Beginner Last-semester nursing student Graduate nurse	• Demonstrates ability to deliver marginally acceptable care • Requires previous experience in an actual situation to recognize it • Begins to understand the principles that dictate nursing interventions • Continues to concentrate on the rules, and takes in minimum information regarding a situation
Competent 2-3 years' clinical experience	• Conscientious, deliberate planning • Begins to see nursing actions in light of clients' long-term plans • Demonstrates ability to cope with and manage different and unexpected situations that occur
Proficient Nurse clinicians Nursing faculty	• Ability to recognize and understand the situation as a whole • Demonstrates ability to anticipate events in a given situation • Holistic understanding enhances decision-making
Expert Advanced practice nurse clinicians and faculty	• Demonstrates an understanding of the situation and is able to focus on the specific area of the problem • Operates from an in-depth understanding of the total situation • Demonstrates highly skilled analytical ability in problem solving, performance becomes masterful

Modified from Benner P: The Dreyfus Model of Skill Acquisition applied to nursing. In *From novice to expert*, 1984, Addison-Wesley. Reprinted with permission.

> Beginners have no experience of the situation in which they are expected to perform. To get them into these situations and allow them to gain experience also necessary for skill development, they are taught about the situation in terms of objective attributes, such as weight, intake/output, temperature, blood pressure, pulse, and other objectifiable, measurable parameters of a patient's conditions—features of the task world that can be recognized without situational experience.

For example, the instructor gives the novice or student nurse specific directions on how to listen for bowel sounds. There are specific rules on how to guide their actions—rules that are very limited and fairly inflexible. Remember your first clinical nursing experiences? Your nursing instructor was your shadow for patient care. As nursing students enter a clinical area as novices, they have little understanding of the meaning and application of recently learned textbook terms and concepts. Students are not the only novices; any nurse may assume the novice role on entering a clinical setting in which he or she is not comfortable functioning or has no practical experience.

Consider an experienced medical-surgical nurse who floats to the postpartum unit; she would be a little uncomfortable in that clinical setting.

By graduation, most nursing students are at the level of advanced beginner. According to Benner (1984, p. 22):

> Advanced beginners are ones who can demonstrate marginally accepted performance, ones who have coped with enough real situations to note (or to have pointed out to them by a mentor) the recurring meaningful situation components...

To be able to recognize characteristics that can be identified only through experience is the signifying trait of the advanced beginner. Thus, when directed to perform the procedure of checking bowel sounds, the students at this level are learning how to discriminate bowel sounds and understand their meaning. They do not need to be told specifically how to perform the procedure.

Let's look at what you and your nursing instructors can do to promote your well-being and success during the role-transition experience. These activities reinforce your progress and movement along the continuum from advanced-beginner to competent nurse (see Table 1-2).

HOW CAN I PREPARE MYSELF FOR THIS TRANSITION PROCESS?

During the last semester of nursing school, it is very advantageous to have as much clinical experience as possible. The most productive area for experience is a general medical-surgical unit. This will help you ground your assessment and communication skills, as well as help you to apply prinicples that are most often tested on NCLEX. This is also the area in which you will most likely be able to obtain some much needed experince with basic nursing skills.

No More "Mama Management." It is time to have your nursing instructor cut the umbilical cord and allow you to function more independently during the last semester of clinical training.

More Realistic Patient-Care Assignments. Start taking care of increasing numbers of patients to help you with time management and work organization. Evaluate the nursing staff's assignments to determine what is a realistic workload for a recent graduate.

Clinical Hours That Represent Realistic Shift Hours. Obtain experience in receiving shift reports, closing charts, completing patient care, and communicating with the oncoming staff. As a recent graduate, you will be in for a rude awakening if you have never had the opportunity to work a full shift.

Perform Nursing Procedures Instead of Observing. Take an inventory of your nursing skills. If there are nursing skills you lack or procedures you are uncomfortable with, take this opportunity while you are still in school to gain the experience. Identify your clinical objectives to meet your personal needs. Request opportunities to practice from your instructor and staff nurses. Casey and colleagues (2004) identified skills that were challenging for the graduate nurses in the first year of practice. These skills included: code blues, chest tubes, intravenous skills, central lines, blood administration, and patient-controlled analgesia (PCA). Make an effort to gain experience in these areas while you are still in school; you will be more comfortable in your nursing care as a graduate.

More Truth About the Real Work-Setting Experience. Identify resource people with whom you can objectively discuss the dilemmas of the workplace. Talk to graduates: Ask them what they know now that they wish they had known the last semester of school.

Look for Opportunities to Problem-Solve and Practice Critical Thinking. No more "spoon-feeding" from instructors who tell you what to do and how to do it. Now is the time to stand on your own two feet while there is still a backup—your instructor—available.

Request Constructive Feedback from Staff and Instructors. Stop avoiding evaluation and constructive criticism. Find out now how you can improve your nursing care. Evaluate your progress on a periodic basis. The consequences may be less severe now than later with your new employer.

Request Clinical Experience in an Area or Hospital of Interest. If you have some idea of where you would like to work, it is very beneficial to have some clinical experiences in that facility the last semester of school. This gives you the opportunity to become involved with staff nurses, identify workload on the unit, evaluate resources and support people. It also gives the employing institution an opportunity to evaluate you—Are you someone that institution would like to have work for them?

HOW CAN I PREPARE MYSELF FOR A TRANSITION?

> Attitude is the latitude between success and failure.

Think Positively! Be prepared for the reality of the workplace environment, including both its positives and negatives. You may have encountered by now the "ole' battle-ax" who has a grudge against new nursing graduates.

> **I do not know why you ever decided to be a nurse. Nobody respects you. It's all work, low pay. I guess as long as you've got a good back and strong legs, you'll make it. Boy, do you have a lot to learn! I wouldn't do it over again for anything!**

When you find these nurses, tune them out and steer out of their way! They have their own agenda, and it does not include providing supportive assistance to you. Eventually, you will learn how to work with this type of individual (see Chapter 12), but for now, you should concentrate on identifying nurses who share your philosophy and are still smiling.

> Surround yourself with nurses who have a positive attitude and are supportive in your learning and growing transition.

Another way to keep a positive perspective is to focus on the good things that have happened during the shift rather than on the frustrating events. When you feel yourself climbing onto the proverbial "pity pot," ask yourself "Who's driving this bus?" and turn it around! Review the job duties of the nurse from the year 1887 (Figure 1-2)—and be grateful!

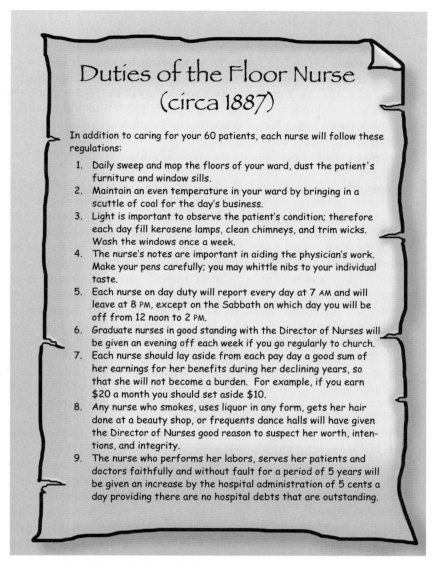

Duties of the Floor Nurse (circa 1887)

In addition to caring for your 60 patients, each nurse will follow these regulations:

1. Daily sweep and mop the floors of your ward, dust the patient's furniture and window sills.
2. Maintain an even temperature in your ward by bringing in a scuttle of coal for the day's business.
3. Light is important to observe the patient's condition; therefore each day fill kerosene lamps, clean chimneys, and trim wicks. Wash the windows once a week.
4. The nurse's notes are important in aiding the physician's work. Make your pens carefully; you may whittle nibs to your individual taste.
5. Each nurse on day duty will report every day at 7 AM and will leave at 8 PM, except on the Sabbath on which day you will be off from 12 noon to 2 PM.
6. Graduate nurses in good standing with the Director of Nurses will be given an evening off each week if you go regularly to church.
7. Each nurse should lay aside from each pay day a good sum of her earnings for her benefits during her declining years, so that she will not become a burden. For example, if you earn $20 a month you should set aside $10.
8. Any nurse who smokes, uses liquor in any form, gets her hair done at a beauty shop, or frequents dance halls will have given the Director of Nurses good reason to suspect her worth, intentions, and integrity.
9. The nurse who performs her labors, serves her patients and doctors faithfully and without fault for a period of 5 years will be given an increase by the hospital administration of 5 cents a day providing there are no hospital debts that are outstanding.

FIGURE 1-2
The duties of a floor nurse in 1887.

Anticipate small irritations and disappointments, and keep them in perspective. Do not let them mushroom into major problems. Turn disappointments and unpleasant situations into learning experiences. Once you have encountered an unpleasant situation, the next time it occurs you will recognize it sooner, anticipate the chain of events, and be better able to handle it.

Do not major in a minor activity.

Be Flexible! Procedures, policies, and nursing supervisors are not going to be the same as those experienced in school. Be prepared to do things differently than you learned as a student. You do not have to give up all the values you learned in school, but you will need to reexamine them in light of the reality of the workplace setting.

School-learned ideal: Never prepare a medication ahead of time; always prepare it immediately before administration.

Workplace reality: Staff nurses set up medications for the entire 3 PM to 11 PM shift at 4 PM.

Compromise: Your value system does not allow you to feel comfortable about setting up medications this early in the shift. However, your time-organization skills tell you the necessity of planning ahead to complete medications on time. Therefore, in light of the reality of the workplace, you compromise by preparing medications at 3:30 PM for the 4 PM and 6 PM medications and at 7:30 PM for the 8 PM and 10 PM medications. Your primary objective is to administer medications according to the Five Rights. You have appropriately and effectively adapted your value system to meet the challenges of the workplace without losing sight of your values.

School-learned ideal: Sit down with the patient before surgery, and provide preoperative teaching.

Workplace reality: One of your home-care patients is receiving daily wound care for an extensive burn. You receive a pager message that the patient has been scheduled for grafting in the outpatient surgery department and is to be a direct admit at 6 AM the next morning. You have two more home visits to make: one to hang an intravenous preparation of vancomycin and the other a new hospice admission, which you know will take considerable time.

Compromise: You delegate to one of the home-care practical nurses to take the preoperative teaching and admission instructions to your patient. Later on, you make a telephone call to your preoperative patient and go over the preoperative-care teaching information from the home-care practical nurse. You make arrangements to meet this patient at home immediately after the grafting procedure is complete.

Get Organized! Does your personal life seem organized or chaotic, calm or frantic? Sit back and take a quick inventory of your personal life. How do you expect to get your professional life in order when your personal life is in turmoil? For some helpful tips on organizing your personal life, review the 10 suggestions for getting organized in Figure 1-3. How many do you currently use? Check out the time management chapter (see Chapter 13).

Stay Healthy! Have you become a "couch potato" while in school? Are you too tired, or do you lack the time to exercise when you get home from work? Candy bars during breaks, pepperoni pizza at midnight, and Twinkies PRN? How have your eating habits changed during your time in school? Your routine should include exercise, relaxation, and good nutrition. Becoming aware of the negative habits that can have detrimental effects on your state of mind and overall physical health is important in developing a healthy lifestyle.

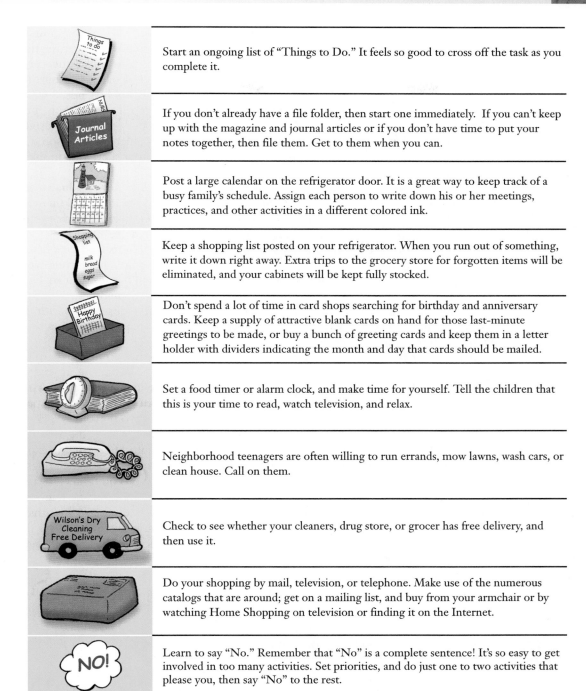

Start an ongoing list of "Things to Do." It feels so good to cross off the task as you complete it.

If you don't already have a file folder, then start one immediately. If you can't keep up with the magazine and journal articles or if you don't have time to put your notes together, then file them. Get to them when you can.

Post a large calendar on the refrigerator door. It is a great way to keep track of a busy family's schedule. Assign each person to write down his or her meetings, practices, and other activities in a different colored ink.

Keep a shopping list posted on your refrigerator. When you run out of something, write it down right away. Extra trips to the grocery store for forgotten items will be eliminated, and your cabinets will be kept fully stocked.

Don't spend a lot of time in card shops searching for birthday and anniversary cards. Keep a supply of attractive blank cards on hand for those last-minute greetings to be made, or buy a bunch of greeting cards and keep them in a letter holder with dividers indicating the month and day that cards should be mailed.

Set a food timer or alarm clock, and make time for yourself. Tell the children that this is your time to read, watch television, and relax.

Neighborhood teenagers are often willing to run errands, mow lawns, wash cars, or clean house. Call on them.

Check to see whether your cleaners, drug store, or grocer has free delivery, and then use it.

Do your shopping by mail, television, or telephone. Make use of the numerous catalogs that are around; get on a mailing list, and buy from your armchair or by watching Home Shopping on television or finding it on the Internet.

Learn to say "No." Remember that "No" is a complete sentence! It's so easy to get involved in too many activities. Set priorities, and do just one to two activities that please you, then say "No" to the rest.

FIGURE 1-3
Ten suggestions for organizing yourself.

Find a Mentor! Negotiating this critical transition as you begin your nursing career should not be done in isolation. Evidence suggests that close support relationships, mentors and preceptors are key, if not essential, ingredients in the career development of a successful, happy graduate (Casey et al, 2004; Roche, Lamoureaux, & Teehan, 2004). In addition to your family and close nursing-school friends, it will be important to develop professional support relationships. Keep in touch with nurse recruiters. Recruiters will know where all the recent graduates are in the hospital. They may be able to put you in touch with another recent graduate or with someone who would be a great mentor. Finding a mentor will be an important step in taking care of yourself during your transition process.

Find Other New Graduates! Frequently, there are several new graduates who are hired at the same time. Some of them may even be your classmates. Find them and establish a peer support group. Sharing experiences and problems, knowing that someone else is experiencing the same feelings you are is frequently a great relief!

Have Some Fun! Do something that makes you feel good. This is life, not a funeral service! Nursing has opportunities for laughter and for sharing life's humorous events with patients and coworkers. Surround yourself with people and friends who are lighthearted and merry and who bring those feelings out in you. Remember: the return of humor is one of the first signs of a healthy role transition. Loosen up a little bit. Go ahead, have some fun! Check out the information in Chapter 4 for more on selection of mentors and preceptors.

Know What to Expect! Plan ahead. Plan your employment interviews; ask to talk to nurses on the units, and find out how nursing care is delivered in the institution. The length of orientation, staffing patterns, opportunity for internship, areas where positions are open, and resources for new graduates are all important to establish prior to employment. This helps you know what to expect when you go to work. Work satisfaction is a positive predictor of a successful role transition during the first year (Roche, 2004). Know what is expected of you on your work unit. How can you expect to do a job correctly if you do not know what the expectations are? Learn the "rules of the road" early. This may be in the hospital, doctor's office, or community setting. While still in school, you may find it helpful to interview nurse managers to determine their perspectives on the role of the graduate nurse during her first 6 months of employment. This will give you a base of reference when you interview for your first job. How do you measure up to some of the common expectations nurse managers may be looking for in a graduate nurse?

Are you:

- Excited and sincere about nursing?
- Open-minded and willing to learn new ideas and skills?
- Comfortable with your basic nursing skills?
- Able to keep a good sense of humor?
- Receptive to constructive criticism?
- Able to express your thoughts and feelings?
- Able to evaluate your performance and request assistance?
- Comfortable talking with your patients regarding their individual needs?

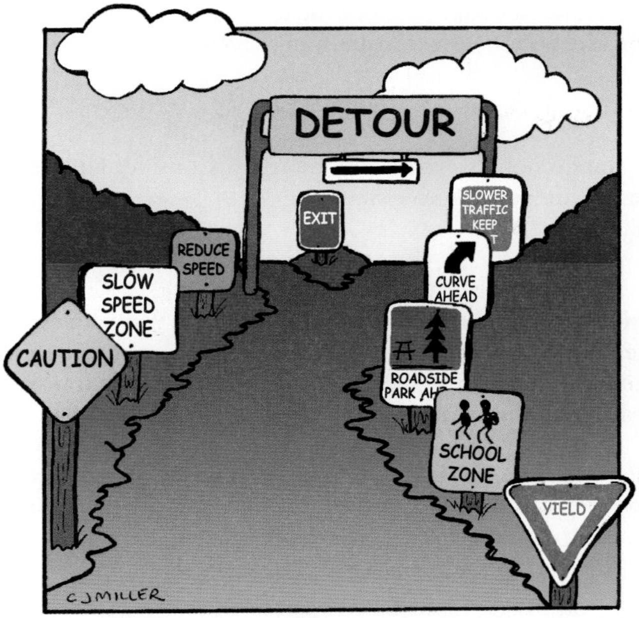

FIGURE 1-4
"Rules of the road" for transition.

CONCLUSION

To summarize, the "rules of the road" for role-transition can be likened to a stoplight. There is the *green light* for *GO*—move ahead, you are going in the right direction. The *yellow light* denotes *CAUTION*—proceed slowly, be sure to look around. The *red light* means *STOP*—do not proceed; your career direction may need to come to a screeching halt. The following are helpful tips (i.e., "rules of the road"; Figure 1-4; also see Figure 1-5) contributed by graduates who have successfully made the transition.

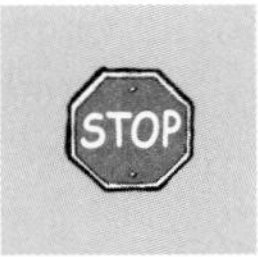

Stop: Take care of yourself. Take time to plan your transition. Get involved with other recent graduates; they can help you. Do not be afraid to ask questions, and do not be afraid to ask for help.

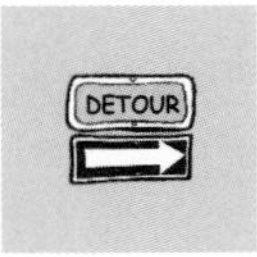

Detour: You will make mistakes. Recognize them, learn from them, and put them in the past as you move forward. Regardless of how well you plan for change, there are always detours ahead. Detours take you on an alternate route. They can be scenic, swampy, or desolate, or they can bog you down in heavy traffic. Do not forget to look for the positive aspects—the detour may open your eyes to new horizons and new career directions.

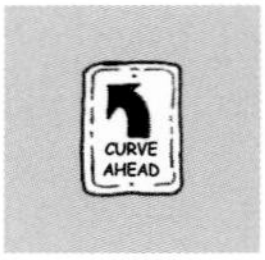

Curve ahead: Get your personal life in order. Anticipate changes in your schedule. Be adaptable, because the transition process is not predictable.

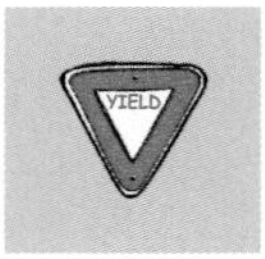

Yield: You do not always have to be right. Consider alternatives, and make compromises within your value system.

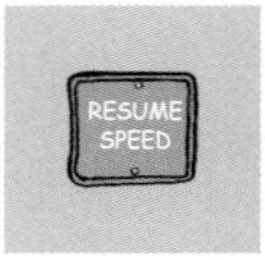

Resume speed: Maintain a positive attitude. As you gain experience, you will become better organized and begin to really enjoy nursing. Be aware; sometimes as you resume speed, you may be experiencing another role transition as your career moves in a different direction.

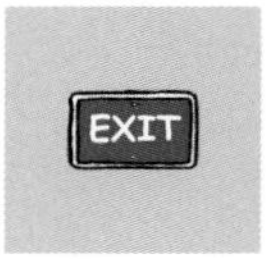

Exit: Pay attention to your road signs, and do not take an exit you do not really want. Before you exit your job, critically evaluate the job situation. "Look before you leap" by making sure the change will improve your work situation.

Slow traffic, keep right: You may be more comfortable in the slower-traffic lane with respect to your career direction. Take all the time you need; it is okay for each person to travel at a different speed. Do not get run over in the fast lane.

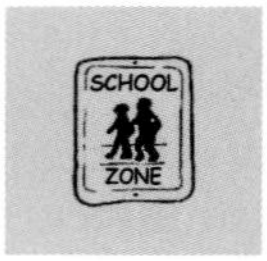

School zone: Plan for continuing education, whether it is an advanced degree program or one to maintain your clinical skills or license. Allow yourself sufficient time in your new job before you jump back into the role of full-time student.

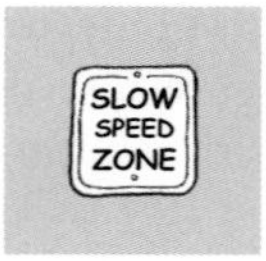

Slow speed zone: Take time to get organized before you resume full speed! Have a daily organizational sheet that fits your needs and works for you both in your job and your personal life.

Caution: Do not commit to anything with which you are not professionally or personally comfortable. Think before you act. Do not react. Do not panic. If in doubt, check with another nurse.

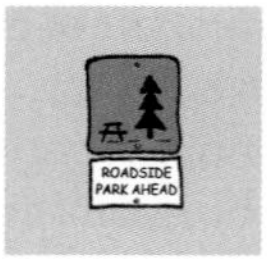

Roadside park ahead: Take a break, whether it is 15 minutes or 30 minutes a day, to indulge yourself, or a week to do something you really want to do.

Look for the humor in each day, and take time to laugh. You will be surprised by how good it makes you feel!

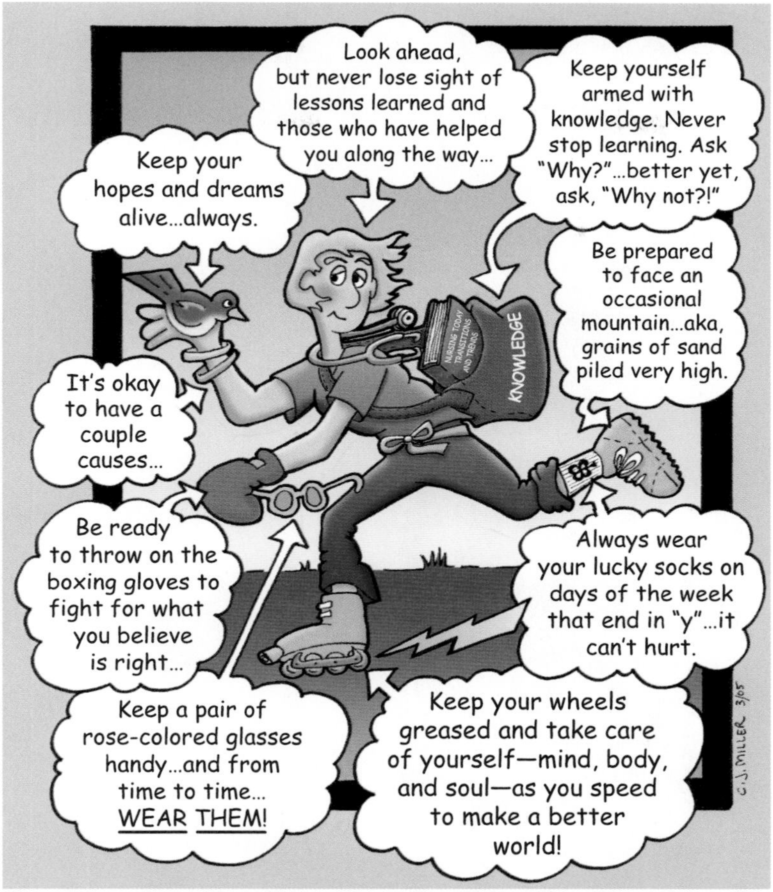
Look ahead, but never lose sight of lessons learned and those who have helped you along the way...
Keep yourself armed with knowledge. Never stop learning. Ask "Why?"...better yet, ask, "Why not?!"
Keep your hopes and dreams alive...always.
Be prepared to face an occasional mountain...aka, grains of sand piled very high.
KNOWLEDGE
It's okay to have a couple causes...
Be ready to throw on the boxing gloves to fight for what you believe is right...
Always wear your lucky socks on days of the week that end in "y"...it can't hurt.
Keep a pair of rose-colored glasses handy...and from time to time... WEAR THEM!
Keep your wheels greased and take care of yourself—mind, body, and soul—as you speed to make a better world!
C.J. MILLER 3/05

FIGURE 1-5
Advice for the new grad.

REFERENCES

Benner P: *From novice to expert*, Menlo Park, Calif, 1984, Addison-Wesley.

Casey K, et al: The graduate nurse experience, *JONA* 34(6):303-311, 2004.

Godinez G et al: Role transition from graduate to staff nurse: a qualitative analysis. *J Nurse Staff Dev* 15:97-110, 1999.

Kramer M: *Reality shock*, St. Louis, 1974, Mosby.

Kramer M, Schmalenberg C: *Path to biculturalism*, Rockville, MD, 1977, Aspen.

Lavoie-Tremblay M, et al: How to facilitate the orientation of new nurses into the workplace, *Journal for Nurses in Staff Development* 18(2), 2004.

Myrick F: Preceptorship: a viable alternative clinical teaching strategy, *J Adv Nurs* 13:588-591, 1988.

Polifroni C, et al: Activities and interaction of baccalaureate nursing students in clinical practice, *J Prof Nurs* 11:161-169, 1995.

Roche J, Lamoureux E, Teehan T: A partnership between nursing education and practice, *JONA* 34(1):26-32, 2004.

Schumacher KL, Meleis AI: Transitions: a central concept in nursing, *Image* 26:119-127, 1994.

Steinmiller E, Levonian C, Lengetti E: Rx for success, *American Journal of Nursing* 103(11):64A-66A, 2003.

CHAPTER 2

SELF-CARE STRATEGIES

BARBARA J. MICHAELS, EdD, LMFT, RN

I will use words which emanate power, strong words to guide me. My words today will be strong and powerful. I will choose words that convey a sense of mastery, competence, and ability: I can. I will. I am. I do…

—*Rochelle Lerner, 1985*

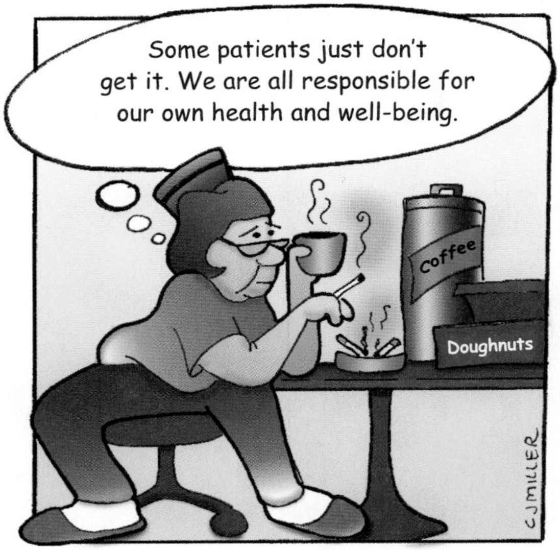
Some patients just don't get it. We are all responsible for our own health and well-being.
coffee
Doughnuts
CJMILLER

How do I take care of my physical self?

After completing this chapter, you should be able to:

- Discuss how burnout affects nurses.
- Describe early signs of burnout.
- Discuss the importance of caring for yourself.
- Identify strategies for self-care.
- Formulate a plan of care for yourself that is based on identified deficits in self-care.

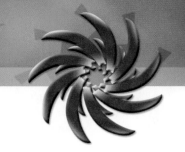

For nurses to effectively take care of their patients, they must first take care of themselves. As a new graduate in your first year of practice, you need to make "taking care of yourself" a top priority. The work environment will be demanding; you will be exposed to learning opportunities and be introduced to a whole new area of professional responsibilities. How you perceive yourself often determines how effective you are as a nurse. The way you feel about yourself will be influenced by your values, actions, successes, and failures during your first year after graduation. Self-care is the foundation that will assist you in thriving in nursing instead of just surviving.

IS BURNOUT INEVITABLE FOR NURSES?

Much has been written about the concept of burnout in nurses. In early research, burnout was thought to be a problem within a nurse or a problem inherent in the nursing profession. However, the stressors in the current workplace caused by restructuring, increased use of unlicensed personnel, and staffing shortages have increased the potential for burnout among nurses employed in hospitals or in other types of health care delivery systems. Over the years, nurses have learned to recognize and manage burnout related to caring too much for their patients. What nurses are currently struggling with is that they are working in toxic environments that are not congruent with their personal philosophies of nursing care.

Burnout associated with job stress can leave nurses vulnerable to depression, physical illness, and alcohol and drug abuse. Symptoms include a loss of energy, weariness, gloominess, dissatisfaction, increased illness, decreased efficiency, absenteeism, and self-doubt. Burnout typically progresses through five stages that are particularly notable within the work setting: initially a feeling of enthusiasm for the job, followed by a loss of enthusiasm, continuous deterioration, crisis, and finally devastation and the inability to work effectively. Box 2-1 lists early warning signs of burnout.

The concepts of managed care, capitation, cost containment, and shortened hospital stays are often not compatible with the emphasis on quality care and customer service.

BOX 2-1 Early Warning Signs of Burnout

Irritability
Weight changes
Frequent headaches and gastrointestinal disturbances
Chronic fatigue
Insomnia
Depression
Feeling of helplessness
Negativity
Cynicism
Angry outbursts
Self-critical

Brace ourselves—strengths and weaknesses alike—and acknowledge

These opposing philosophies create conflict for nurses and lead to burnout that is not as easily remedied as burnout caused by internal factors. Hospital restructuring can be very stressful for those involved in the changed institutional philosophy. Cross training and changes in job description and staffing structure contribute to burnout.

It is important to recognize clearly the mission of the hospital or corporation when you apply for your first job. Is their mission similar to yours? Will you be able to give the quality care that you want to deliver, or will you be required to compromise your values to fit into the system?

There are many strategies designed to combat burnout, and many of them are detailed in this chapter on self-care. However, nurses today will need to determine whether their burnout is caused by internal or external factors. In some cases it may be necessary for the nurse to change to a place of employment that is more in line with her or his belief system.

EMPOWERMENT AND SELF-CARE

Learning about self-care is really about empowerment. The word power comes from the French word *pouvoir*, which means "to be able." To empower means to enable—enable self and others to reach their greatest potential for health and well-being. However, the concept of enabling is seen in a negative light because it refers to doing things for others that they can do for themselves. Actually, preventing friends and loved ones from dealing with the consequences of their behavior is very disempowering.

With empowerment comes a feeling of well-being and effectiveness. There are times and situations in our lives when we feel more or less powerful. Examples of occasions when one feels powerful or powerless are given in Box 2-2. You may find as you read through the list that there are some situations in your life in which you do feel powerful and some in which you do not. Self-assessment of our sense of well-being and self-esteem helps us to know where to begin. Because change is a constant, and all

BOX 2-2 Examples of Times When One Feels Powerless or Powerful

I FEEL POWERLESS WHEN

- ☐ I'm ignored.
- ☐ I get assigned to a new hospital unit.
- ☐ I can't make a decision.
- ☐ I'm exhausted.
- ☐ I'm being evaluated by my instructor.
- ☐ I have no choices.
- ☐ I'm being controlled or manipulated.
- ☐ I have pent-up anger.
- ☐ I don't think or react quickly.
- ☐ I don't speak loudly enough.
- ☐ I don't have control over my time.

Continued

BOX 2-2 Examples of Times When One Feels Powerless or Powerful—cont'd

I FEEL POWERFUL WHEN

- ☐ I'm energetic.
- ☐ I get positive feedback.
- ☐ I know I look good.
- ☐ I tell people I'm a nurse.
- ☐ I have clear goals for my career.
- ☐ I stick to decisions.
- ☐ I speak out against injustice.
- ☐ I allow myself to be selfish without feeling guilty.
- ☐ I tell a good joke.
- ☐ I work with supportive people.
- ☐ I'm told by a patient or family that I did a good job.

Adapted from Josefowitz N: *Paths to power*, Menlo Park, Calif, 1980, Addison-Wesley, p 7. Reprinted with permission.

of us are in varying states of emotional, physical, and mental change at any given time, it is important to assess ourselves on a regular basis. As a matter of fact, knowing one's self is the very first step in learning to care for one's self. Empowerment in all spheres of our being is very important. Examine the Holistic Self-Assessment Tool (Critical Thinking Box 2-1), which includes measures of our emotional, mental, physical, social, spiritual, and choice potentials.

Emotional wholeness is about our ability to feel. The ability to express a wide range of emotions is indicative of good mental health. Nurses are often very good at helping their patients "feel" their feelings but often have a difficult time feeling and expressing their own.

Experiencing mental wholeness implies that we maintain our childlike ability to dream and fantasize about the future. Nurses frequently have an overabundance of

CRITICAL THINKING BOX 2-1

HOLISTIC SELF-ASSESSMENT TOOL

EMOTIONAL POTENTIAL

______ I push my thoughts and feelings out of conscious awareness (denial).
______ I feel I have to be in control.
______ I am unable to express basic feelings of sadness, joy, anger, and fear.
______ I see myself as a victim.
______ I feel guilty and ashamed a lot of the time.
______ I frequently take things personally.

Continued

CRITICAL THINKING BOX 2-1—cont'd

SOCIAL POTENTIAL

______ I am overcommitted to the point of having no time for recreation.
______ I am unable to be honest and open with others.
______ I am unable to admit vulnerability to others.
______ I am attracted to needy people.
______ I feel overwhelmingly responsible for others' happiness.
______ My only friends are nurses.

PHYSICAL POTENTIAL

______ I neglect myself physically—overweight/underweight, lack of adequate rest and exercise.
______ I feel tired and lack energy.
______ I am not interested in sex.
______ I do not engage in regular physical and dental check-ups.
______ I have seen a doctor in the past six months for any of the following conditions: migraine headaches, backaches, gastrointestinal problems, hypertension, or cancer.
______ I am a workaholic—work is all-important to me.

SPIRITUAL POTENTIAL

______ I see that events that occur in my life are controlled by external choices.
______ I find the world a basically hostile place.
______ I lack a spiritual base for working through daily problems.
______ I live in the past or the future.
______ I have no sense of power greater than myself.

MENTAL POTENTIAL

______ I read mostly professional literature.
______ I spend most waking hours obsessing over people, places, or things.
______ I am no longer able to dream or fantasize about my future.
______ I can't remember much of my childhood.
______ I can't see much change happening for myself, either personally or professionally.

CHOICE POTENTIAL

______ I have difficulty making decisions, I am prone to procrastination and am frequently late for personal and professional appointments.
______ I find it difficult to say no.
______ I find myself unwilling to take reasonable risks.
______ I find it difficult to take responsibility for myself.

From Zerwekh J, Michaels B: Co-dependency: assessment and recovery, *Nurs Clin North Am* 24(1):109-120, 1989.

concrete knowledge of the practice of nursing. We appreciate the challenge of a difficult patient. However, because of the mental and physical demands of the nursing profession, we often do not take time out to learn other disciplines.

Nurses frequently neglect their physical health. We make certain that our patients receive excellent health education and discharge instructions and worry when they are noncompliant. As nurses, however, we do not always follow through when it comes to such things as physical examinations, mammograms, and dental health for ourselves. We work long hours and do not plan adequate time for physical recuperation.

Because our profession is such a demanding one, we often do not take the time to cultivate our social potential. When we do spend time with friends, it is because they "need" us. When we get together with friends who are nurses, we spend the time together talking about work.

Spiritual potential simply means that we have a daily awareness that there is something more to living than mere human existence. The lives of nurses with spiritual potential have meaning and direction.

The ability to know that we have choices in life is the final area of the assessment tool. Nurses without "choice power" see life as black and white, with little gray in the middle. Awareness of our choices eliminates the black and white extremes and enables us to act rather than react in situations. Nurses with choice power are able to make decisions and take risks, and feel good about it.

Remember to use this tool not only to assess the negatives in your life, but also to assess areas in which you are experiencing growth. You cannot survive nursing school, for example, and not experience growth in all areas.

SUGGESTED STRATEGIES FOR SELF-CARE THAT ARE BASED ON THE HOLISTIC SELF-ASSESSMENT TOOL

Not having our life in a state of balance and not having a vision for the future often reflect a state of poor self-esteem. Nathaniel Branden (Branden, 1992), often referred to as the father of the self-esteem movement, has identified several factors found in individuals with healthy self-esteem. These include the following:

- A face, manner, and way of talking and moving that project the pleasure one takes in being alive.
- Ease in talking of accomplishments or shortcomings with directness and honesty.
- An attitude of openness to and curiosity about new ideas, new experiences, and new possibilities of life.
- Openness to criticism and comfortable about acknowledging mistakes because one's self-esteem is not tied to an image of perfection.
- An ability to enjoy the humorous aspects of life in one's self and others (Branden, 1992, p. 43).

The key to developing healthy self-esteem is to become aware of the areas that need the most repair and work on them. However, it is essential to maintain a sense of balance; going overboard in one or two areas is counterproductive. For example, a nurse who exercises five times a week, follows a healthy diet, and sleeps well but is emotionally numb and does not have a clear vision for her future is out of balance. It is a good idea to use this tool (see Critical Thinking Box 2-1) every 6 months to a year, similar to taking an inventory at home or in a business.

AM I EMOTIONALLY HEALTHY/EMOTIONALLY INTELLIGENT?

Being emotionally healthy means that you are aware of your feelings and are able to acknowledge them in a healthy way. In the best-selling book *Emotional Intelligence*, Goleman (1995) states that emotional intelligence consists of the following five domains: knowing one's emotions, managing emotions, motivating one's self, recognizing emotions in others, and handling relationships. It is certainly best when the basics of emotional intelligence are taught by parents who are good emotional coaches. However, it is never too late to learn.

Nurses who have good emotional health know when they are feeling fearful, angry, sad, ashamed, happy, guilty, or lonely, and they are able to distinguish these feelings. They have found appropriate ways to express their feelings without offending others. When feelings are not expressed or at least acknowledged, they frequently build up, which results in emotional binging. Sometimes our bodies take the brunt of unacknowledged feelings in the form of headaches, gastrointestinal problems, anxiety attacks, and so on.

Feelings or emotions are neither good nor bad. They are indications of some of our self-truths, our desires, and our needs. Critical Thinking Box 2-2 is an exercise to help access and acknowledge feelings.

WHAT ABOUT FRIENDS AND FUN? HOW DO I FIND THE TIME?

An occupational hazard of nurses is overcommitting, both personally and professionally. As a result, they frequently have difficulty in meeting their social potential.

Student nurses often say they do not engage in recreational activities because they cost money and that all their money goes into living expenses. First of all, it is important to include some money in your monthly budget for fun. Depriving yourself of time for recreation on a regular basis may lead to impulsive recreational spending such as a shopping binge with credit cards or money allotted for something else. Second, there are many things to do and places to go that are pleasurable and do not cost a lot of money. Several examples are found in Box 2-3.

Another area in the social arena in which many nurses have difficulty is forming relationships outside of nursing. If you spend all your free time with nurses, chances

CRITICAL THINKING BOX 2-2

EXERCISE TO HELP ACCESS AND ACKNOWLEDGE FEELINGS

1. Turn your attention to how you are feeling. What part of your body feels what?
2. Recognize to yourself that this is how you are feeling, and give it a name. If you hear an inner criticism for feeling this way, just set it aside. Any feeling is acceptable.
3. Let yourself experience the sensations you are having. Separate these feelings from having to do anything about them.
4. Ask yourself whether you want to express your feelings now or some other time. Do you want to take some other action now or later? Remind yourself that you have choices.

BOX 2-3 Some Pleasurable Activities

Go on a picnic with friends.
Invite friends over for a potluck dinner.
Go to a movie.
Plan celebrations after exams or completion of a project.
Introduce yourself to three new people.
Visit a museum.
Call an old friend.
Play with your children.
Borrow someone else's children for play.
Volunteer for a worthwhile project.
Get involved in religious or spiritual activities.
Spend some time people-watching.
Take up a new hobby.
Invite humor into your life.

are that you will "talk shop." Nursing curricula are very science-intensive because there is so much to learn in such a short period of time. Cultivate some friends who have a liberal arts or fine arts background. Choose friends who have different political opinions or come from a different part of town, a different culture, or a different socioeconomic class.

SELF-CARE

HOW DO I TAKE CARE OF MY PHYSICAL SELF?

Nurses are great when it comes to patient education. As a matter of fact, it is one of nursing's strengths as a profession. Sometimes we have difficulty applying this information to ourselves. Taking care of ourselves physically is very important. Our profession is both mentally and physically challenging. Taking care of ourselves physically entails getting proper nutrition, maintaining a healthy weight, obtaining adequate sleep, quitting smoking, limiting alcohol consumption to one drink daily, and exercising on a regular basis (Critical Thinking Box 2-3).

The U.S. Department of Health and Human Services Agency for Healthcare Research and Quality recommends the following for eating the right foods:

Fats and cholesterol: Select low-fat/low-cholesterol foods such as lean meat, fish, poultry, and low-fat products. Avoid butter, deep-fried foods, marbled meats, and processed cheeses. Limit saturated fat, palm and coconut oils, and lard.

CRITICAL THINKING BOX 2-3

What am I doing that interferes with my health and well-being?

Complex carbohydrates and fiber: Choose whole-grain bread and cereal products, pastas, vegetables (dark-green leafy and deep-yellow, such as spinach and carrots), and fruits naturally high in complex carbohydrates. Avoid desserts and canned fruits that contain refined sugars.

Sodium: Select foods naturally low in salt and cut down the amount of salt added during food preparation and at the table. Reduce intake of foods such as ham, bacon, salted snacks, and other highly processed foods.

Alcohol: Consume no more than two drinks a day (if male) and one drink per day (if female); alcohol contains only empty calories. One drink equals a 12-ounce bottle of beer or wine cooler, a 5-ounce glass of wine, or 1.5 ounces of 80-proof distilled spirits, such as gin, whiskey, or rum.

Exercise: Incorporate 30 minutes or more of moderate-intensity physical activity, such as walking, into your schedule (preferably daily).

A good exercise program is one that includes activities that foster aerobic activity, flexibility, and strength. A very important part of an exercise program is that it be a regular habit. To be effective, the program should take 3 to 6 hours a week. And it does not have to cost money. You do not need to belong to a gym or invest in exercise equipment. Aerobic activities include walking, jogging, swimming, bicycling, and dancing. Minimal fitness consists of raising your heart rate to 100 beats/min and keeping it there for 30 minutes (Figure 2-1).

STRATEGIES TO FOSTER MY SPIRITUAL SELF: DOES MY LIFE HAVE MEANING?

People who have a sense of spiritual well-being find their lives to be positive experiences, have relationships with a power greater than themselves, feel good about the future, and believe there is some real purpose in life. If we find that our lives lack meaning and our spiritual health is lacking, how do we go about finding spiritual well-being?

Daily prayer and meditation are very important in maintaining a spiritual self. M. Scott Peck (1978) states that the process of spiritual growth is an effortful and difficult one because it is conducted against a natural resistance, a natural inclination to keep things the way they were, to cling to the old maps and old ways of doing things, to take the easy path. Reading religious or philosophical material and studying the great religions are two examples of ways to foster spiritual growth. There are also many spiritual books, enough reading for a lifetime.

In addition to reading what others have written about the subject, many people access their spiritual selves with the practice of meditation. Meditating allows us time to become quiet, heal our thoughts and bodies, and be grateful. A sample meditation on gratitude and healing is included in Box 2-4.

HOW DO I INCREASE MY MENTAL POTENTIAL? IS IT OKAY TO DAYDREAM?

Nursing students get considerable opportunity to exercise their mental potential while they are in nursing school. This activity, however, is primarily in the form of formal education. There are many other ways to exercise this potential. One of the

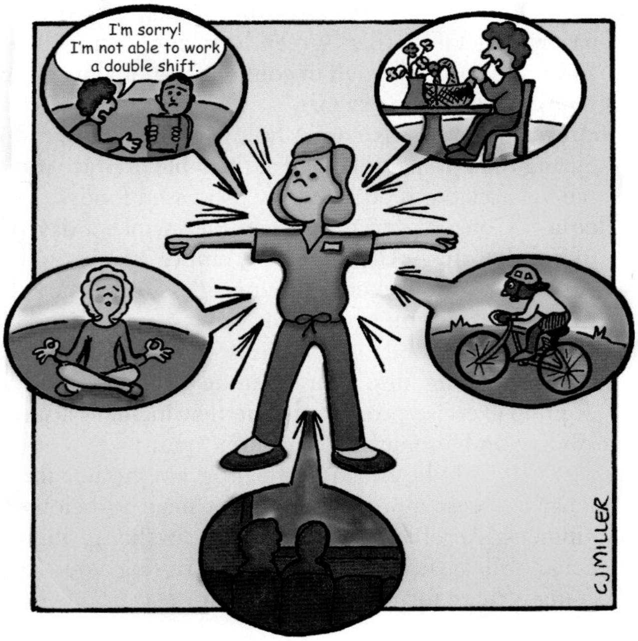

FIGURE 2-1
Learn to take care of yourself.

BOX 2-4 A Meditation on Gratitude and Healing

Take a deep breath and gently close your eyes. Give a few big sighs ... sighs of relief ... and see if your body wants to stretch a little ... or yawn ... (pause).

Now pay attention to the rhythm of your breathing ... Feel your body rise gently as you breathe in, and relax as you breathe out ... (pause for several breaths) ... every outbreath is an opportunity to let go ... to feel the pleasant warmth and heaviness of your body ... a little more on each outbreath ... (pause).

Now, as you breathe in, imagine your breath as a stream of warm, loving light entering through the top of your head. Let it fill your forehead and eyes ... your brain ... your ears ... and nose ... feel the light warm and relax your tongue, your jaw, and your throat. Let your whole head float in an ocean of warm light ... growing brighter and brighter with each breath ... (pause) ... Thank your eyes for the miracle of sight ... your nose for the fragrance of roses and hot coffee on cold mornings (or whatever you like) ... your ears for the richness that sound is ... your tongue for the pleasure of taste ... and let the light fill and heal every cell of your senses ....

Continued

BOX 2-4 A Meditation on Gratitude and Healing—cont'd

Breathe the light into your neck … let it expand gently into your shoulders … and breathe it down your arms … and into your hands … right to the tips of your fingers …. Thank your arms and hands for all you have created and touched with your life … All the people you have hugged and held to your heart … Rest in the warmth and love of the light … light that grows brighter with every breath ….

And breathe the warm light into your lungs and your heart … feeling it penetrate your entire chest, filling every organ, every cell with love. As you breathe, send gratitude to your lungs for bringing in the energy of life—and to your heart for sending life to all the cells of your body, for serving you so well for all these years … rest in the gratitude and love … in the light that continues to grow brighter with each breath … (pause).

And breathe the light into your belly, feeling it penetrate deeply into your center, into the organs of digestion and reproduction … and sense the miracle of your body … the mystery of procreation and of the ability to beget life … let the light expand through your torso and down into your buttocks … growing warmest and brighter … balancing and healing all the cells of your body ….

Breathe the light into your thighs … into bone and muscle, nerve and skin, alive with the energy of light … comforted in your caring and your love … and let the light expand into your calves … and your feet … right to the soles of your feet … feeling gratitude for the gift of walking … letting the lovelight grow brighter and brighter ….

Rest in the fullness of the light … enjoying the lifeforce … and, if there is any place in your body that needs to relax or to heal, direct the light there and hold that part of yourself with the same love you would give to a hurt child … (pause).

Now, as you breathe, sense how the light radiates out from your body … just as a light shines in the darkness, surrounding you in a cocoon of love … and you can sense that cocoon extending all around your body, above and below you, and to all sides, for about three feet … like a giant cocoon … a place of complete safety where you can recharge your body and your mind … (pause).

And you can imagine the light around other people … surrounding them with the same radiance of love, gratitude, and healing … see your loved ones in the light … see those whom you think of as your enemies in the light … then let the light expand until you can imagine the entire world as an orb of light … (pause) … amidst a universe of light … (pause) … all connected … all at peace … and feel the wonder and majesty of creation … (pause).

Now for a minute or two just rest … just breathe … returning to the warm, comfortable feelings within you … (long pause).

Begin fading out the music now, and then read the instructions for reorientation.

And now, begin to reorient yourself to the room … slowly and at your own pace … bringing the peace and gratitude back with you.

From Borysenko J: *Minding the body, mending the mind*, Menlo Park, Calif, 1987, Addison-Wesley. Reprinted with permission.

first ways is to concentrate on removing negative thoughts or self-defeating beliefs from our minds. Examples of statements that nursing students frequently make are:

- "I must make *A*s in nursing school."
- "I must have approval from everyone, and if I don't, I feel horrible and depressed."
- "If I fail at something, the results will be catastrophic."
- "Others must always treat me fairly."
- "If I'm not liked by everyone, I am a failure."
- "Because all my miseries are caused by others, I will have no control over my life until they change."

If you relate to any of these statements, you have some work to do on your belief system. You are setting yourself up for failure by having extremely high expectations of yourself. You are also giving other people power over your own destiny. Remember, you cannot change others. The only person you can change is yourself.

One way that we can change these internal beliefs is to learn how to give ourselves daily affirmations (Figure 2-2). Simply put, affirmations are powerful, positive statements concerning the ways in which we would like to think, feel, and behave. Some examples are "I am a worthwhile person"; "I am human and capable of making mistakes"; and "I am able to freely express my emotions." Always begin affirmative statements with "I" rather than "you." This practice keeps the focus on self rather than others and encourages the development of inner self-worth.

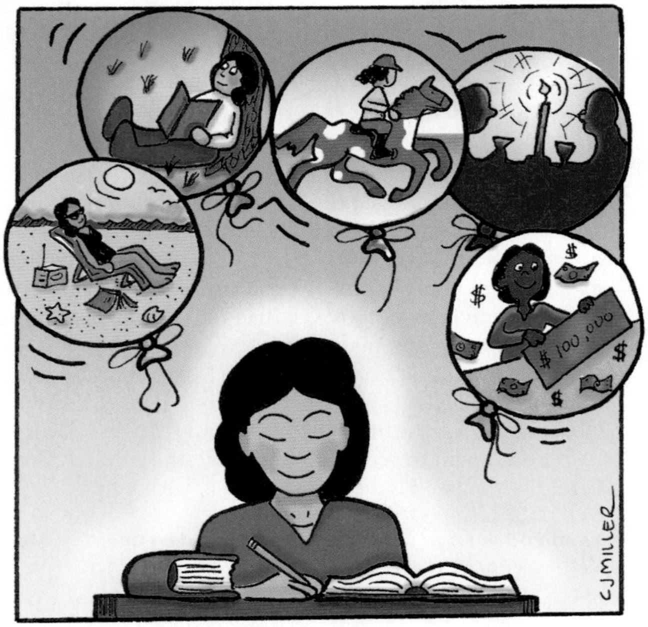

FIGURE 2-2
Daydream: Send up your brain balloons!

BOX 2-5 Affirmations

- ☐ I am a worthwhile person.
- ☐ I am a child of God.
- ☐ I am willing to accept love.
- ☐ I am willing to give love.
- ☐ I can openly express my feelings.
- ☐ I deserve love, peace, and serenity.
- ☐ I am capable of changing.
- ☐ I can take care of myself without feeling guilty.
- ☐ I can say no and not feel guilty.
- ☐ I am beautiful inside and out.
- ☐ I can be spontaneous and whimsical.
- ☐ I am human and capable of making mistakes.
- ☐ I can recognize shame and work through it.
- ☐ I forgive myself for hurting myself and others.
- ☐ I freely accept nurturing from others.
- ☐ I can be vulnerable with trusted others.
- ☐ I am peaceful with life.
- ☐ I trust the process with life.
- ☐ I am free to be the best me I can.
- ☐ I love and comfort myself in ways that are pleasing to me.
- ☐ I am automatically and joyfully focusing on the positive.
- ☐ I am giving myself permission to live, love, and laugh.
- ☐ I am creating and singing affirmations to create a joyful, abundant, fulfilling life.

The power of affirmation exercises lies in consistency—repetition encourages ultimate belief in what is being said.

Begin each day with some affirmations. Try some of the examples in Box 2-5. These enable us to feel better about ourselves and consequently raise our self-esteem. Stand in front of a mirror and tell yourself that you are a special person and worthy of self-love and the love of others. Another suggestion is to record some positive affirmations on your telephone answering machine and call your telephone number in the middle of the day or when you are having a slump or attack of self-pity; hearing you own voice say you are okay can have a very positive effect. For example, “Hello—Glad you’re having a great day, please leave a message.” Also consider signing up to receive a daily affirmation from the website *www.rutts.com*. When you sign up for this free service, you receive a daily affirmation in an e-mail message (Critical Thinking Box 2-4).

CRITICAL THINKING BOX 2-4

What are some positive affirmations that work for you, and how can you increase the effectiveness of these affirmations?

BOX 2-6 Examples of Reactive and Proactive

There's nothing I can do.	Let's look at our alternatives.
That's just the way I am.	I can choose a different approach.
He makes me so mad.	I control my own feelings.
They won't allow that.	I can create an effective presentation.
I have to do that.	I will choose an appropriate response.
I can't.	I choose.
I must.	I prefer.
If only.	I will.

WHAT ARE MY CHOICES, AND HOW DO I EXERCISE THEM?

Many of us negotiate our way through life never realizing that we have many choices. We remain victims, waiting for life to happen, rather than taking a proactive stance. In his best-selling book *Seven Habits of Highly Effective People*, Stephen Covey (1989) states that the very first habit we must develop is to be proactive. We stop thinking in black and white and come to realize that in every arena of our lives, we have choices about how to respond and react. Covey differentiates between people who are proactive and people who are reactive. Examples of proactive versus reactive language are included in Box 2-6. Pay attention to your own language patterns for the next few weeks. Are there times when you could say "I choose?" You can choose to respond to people and situations rather than react. Exercising our choice potential also entails that we act responsibly toward others. We recognize that other people have the right to choose for themselves and to be accountable for their own behavior.

CONCLUSION

Before we can act responsibly toward others, we must first act responsibly toward ourselves. This involves self-acceptance and self-love. In his book *Born for Love: Reflections on Loving*, Leo Buscaglia (1992) states this very eloquently:

> Being who we are, people who feel good about themselves are not easily threatened by the future. They enthusiastically maintain a secure image whether everything is falling apart or going their way. They hold a firm base of personal assuredness and self-respect that remains constant. Though they are concerned about what others think of them, it is a healthy concern. They find external forces more challenging than threatening.
>
> Perhaps the greatest sign of maturity is to reach the point in life when we embrace ourselves—strengths and weaknesses alike—and acknowledge that we are all that we have; that we have a right to a happy and productive life and the power to change ourselves and our environment within realistic limitations. In short, we are, each of us, entitled to be who we are and become what we choose (p. 177).

REFERENCES

Borysenko J: *Minding the body, mending the mind*, Menlo Park, Calif, 1987, Addison-Wesley.

Branden N: *The power of self-esteem*, Deerfield, Fla, 1992, Health Communications.

Buscaglia L: *Born for love: reflections on loving*, Thorofare, NJ, 1992, Random House.

Covey S: *Seven habits of highly effective people*, New York, 1989, Simon & Schuster.

Goleman D: *Emotional intelligence*, New York, 1995, Bantam Books.

Josefowitz N: *Paths to power*, Menlo Park, Calif, 1980, Addison-Wesley.

Peck MS: *The road less traveled*, New York, 1978, Simon & Schuster.

Lerner R: *Daily affirmations*, Pompano Beach, Fla, 1985, Health Communications.

The pocket guide to good health for adults, 2003, US Department of Health and Human Services Agency for Healthcare Research and Quality, *www.ahrq.gov/ppip/adguide/adguide.pdf*.

UNIT II

CAREER DEVELOPMENT

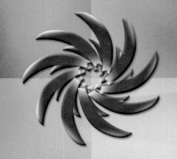

CHAPTER 3

Employment Considerations: Opportunities, Resumes, and Interviewing

ALICE B. PAPPAS, PhD, RN
JO CAROL CLABORN, MS, RN, CNS

School is almost over and I will soon be able to get paid as an RN (Real Nurse)!

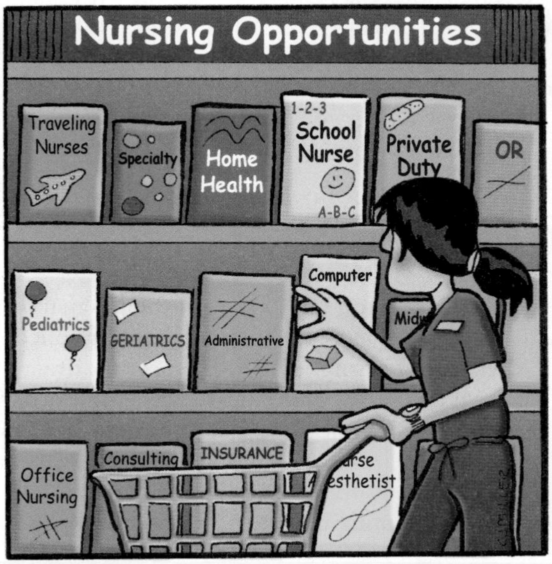

There is a smorgasbord of opportunities in nursing. You can always go back and make another selection.

After completing this chapter, you should be able to:

- Assess trends in the job market.
- Review the primary aspects of obtaining employment.
- Describe the important parts of a resume.
- Describe the essential steps involved in the interviewing process.
- Discuss the typical questions asked by interviewers.
- Analyze your own priorities and needs in a job.
- Identify short-term career goals.

With graduation in sight, you are excited but probably a little anxious about moving into the workplace, looking for the perfect match to your hard-earned degree. As you consider possible employment opportunities, prepare for the upcoming job search as you would any graded class assignment: Do your homework! Careful preparation is the key to finding a job you really want. Very few worthwhile job offers happen to someone who just walks into the human resource department. The continued expansion of the health care field and the growing nursing shortage has created a vast array of opportunities for recent graduates. You have developed marketable skills that are in demand, but to sell yourself successfully to prospective employers, and get the job you really want, you must do some "homework."

Plan your campaign each step of the way to enhance your chances for success!

Give yourself plenty of time to consider what type of position you want and need, in addition to the possibilities and limitations of the job market under consideration. You can compare the process with the selection of a marriage partner, car, home, or any other major life choice. Your first professional position will help define who you are and influence your career path. Become informed and selective in the process. Too often, recent graduates accept their first job without sufficient knowledge of their own needs or the organizations they select. Days or weeks into the job, surprise and disappointment set in as the reality of the situation becomes obvious: "I'm not happy in this position," "I can't believe I took a job like this," or "They never said anything about this during the interview." Although there is no guarantee that a job will be a perfect fit, career dissatisfaction and turnover can be decreased if careful consideration is given to possible job selection before the resume and before the interview.

This chapter provides some guidelines to a thorough background preparation for your job search. Critical Thinking Box 3-1 will help you identify your clinical interests and the possible reasons for these preferences. Hint: This will also help you answer interview questions about your choices.

WHAT IS HAPPENING IN THE JOB MARKET?

During the past 10 years, there have been many ups and downs in the job market for nurses. In the mid-1990s, there was downsizing, increased employment of unlicensed assistive personnel, and a tight job market for nursing. This was especially true of the job market for the recent graduate. Late in the 1990s, there were again signs of change. The twenty-first century ushers in another nursing shortage. The federal goverenment has estimated that, with the aging population, there will be a 40% increase in the demand for registered nurses over the next 20 years. The problem is further compounded by the fact that by 2010 the number of older nurses coming into the workforce will peak, and there will be a large number of nurses starting to retire.

The changing picture of nursing employment was very aptly described by Lucille A. Joel in an editorial in the *American Journal of Nursing* in 1997.

CRITICAL THINKING BOX 3-1

ASSESS YOUR WANTS AND DESIRES, LIKES AND DISLIKES

Identify your interests and the possible reasons for them.

Interests	Reasons
1. I prefer to work with clients whose age is ______	______
2. I prefer to work in a small hospital versus a large medical center ______	______
3. I prefer rotating shifts versus straight shifts ______	______
4. I prefer an internship versus general orientation ______	______
5. I prefer to have a set routine or a constantly changing environment ______	______
6. I prefer these areas (e.g., geriatrics, pediatrics, community, health, medical) ______	______
7. Which of my religious beliefs or values might have an impact on where I work? ______	______

> **The mental image of shifting sands suggests a loss of control, an absence of stability, impermanence in the presence of permanence. Nursing's on-again, off-again courtship with surpluses and shortages is suited to that metaphor.**
>
> **Our forte has been to adapt, sometimes grudgingly, sometimes with panache for the victor, ameliorating the symptoms but avoiding the challenge of coming to terms with the underlying problem (Joel, 1997).**

The "baby boomers" of the late 1940s are now graying and are going to begin to need more health care. The graying of the American population is going to have a tremendous impact on the health care industry. There has been and will continue to be a substantial increase in the number of older patients, and they will also have

CRITICAL THINKING BOX 3-2

What changes have you observed as a result of the nursing shortage? What impact has the shortage had on salaries and staffing in your community? If the signs of a nursing shortage were beginning to surface in 1997, why are we (nursing, education, hospitals, and government) just now responding to the problem?

increased multilevel health care needs (CBS News, 2003). By the year 2025, those individuals older than 65 years old will represent 20% of the population. Not only is there a significant graying of the population, there is also a graying of the nursing workforce. The experts indicate that in the year 2000, the average age of a nurse in the United States was somewhere between 45 to 48 years old; 31.7% of the nurses were younger than age 40. At this rate, half of the nurses in practice today will be at retirement age within 15 years (Nursing Facts, 2005).

What is going to happen with nursing employment, the job market, and health care when a large percentage of nurses become part of the older generation? Will hospitals focus on retention of the older nurse? Who will mentor the new nurses? What will the job market be for the graduate nurse during the next 5 years? What changes will be forced on nursing and health care? There is only one thing for sure—it is going to continue to change (Critical Thinking Box 3-2).

SELF-ASSESSMENT

WHAT ARE MY CLINICAL INTERESTS?

Next, start writing down possible settings where you could pursue your areas of clinical interests. For example, if you thrive in a fast-paced environment with high-acuity patients, a critical care unit or emergency department may be for you. Within this category, however, are many specialties. Do you enjoy the medical or the surgical aspects more? Cardiac or general medicine? Depending on your interests, there will be a number of possible paths to pursue (Figure 3-1).

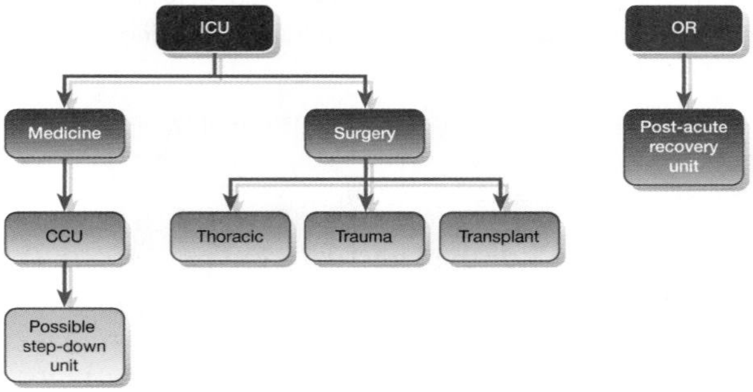

FIGURE 3-1
The environment in which I would like to work. *CCU*, Critical care unit; *ICU*, intensive care unit.

As you identify areas of clinical interest, try to prioritize them. This step may seem like a nonissue if you "eat, sleep, and drink" one specific specialty, but many people have two or more strong interests, and this step helps to outline some possibilities. Believe it or not, some graduating students confess to liking every clinical rotation and feel pulled in multiple directions when they consider where to begin a job search. If that description fits you, hang in there—you are not alone! Thanks to a phenomenal job market, there are tremendous opportunities for both new and experienced nurses. You may have to sample a few areas in your first years of work before you find the one that really fits your needs on a long-term basis. That is a major advantage of nursing as a health career choice—if you get into an area you do not like, you have the option to make a lateral change. Keep in mind that all nursing experiences, both negative and positive, can contribute to your career in a productive way. The more areas you sample, the broader your knowledge base. Recruiters like flexibility in new graduates, but let's try and narrow your professional interests just a bit prior to the job search. Perhaps you can identify what you liked about each clinical rotation and then prioritize possible interests or identify common experiences.

Peds: Enjoyed the children and opportunity to teach families.

Med/Surg: Diabetic patients were challenging, staff was friendly, opportunities for teaching postoperative patients existed.

Gerontology: Enjoyed opportunities to get to know patients, liked being able to have continuity with long-term care patients.

Psych: Increased communication skills and self-confidence.

OB: Teaching opportunities, enjoyed challenge of caring for both young families and high-risk OB population.

Intensive care unit (ICU): Increased technical skills and learned to prioritize, opportunity to work with complex patients, supportive environment with staff.

Community: Working with families, opportunity to be more autonomous and identify outside resources.

From this example, you can see that teaching, communication skills, working with families, challenging environments, and supportive staffs are common themes. Remember these characteristics; they are important starting points for identifying your areas of interest. Depending on how you prioritize them, they can be applied in a variety of settings. The specific job market you are looking at may then narrow your interest to a more manageable list. For example, communication skills and family teaching may be your priority. As a result, community health may be a strong interest, but job inquiries reveal that staff positions usually require at least 1 year's experience in an acute-care setting. Knowing this fact eliminates a possible nonproductive search; it may also be useful information for later career planning. Where could you work in the immediate future to gain the experience that will make you marketable in a community health setting in the future?

WHAT ARE MY LIKES AND DISLIKES?

Another way to approach self-assessment involves identification of your likes and dislikes. This is related to interests, but on a more personal level. The job you eventually

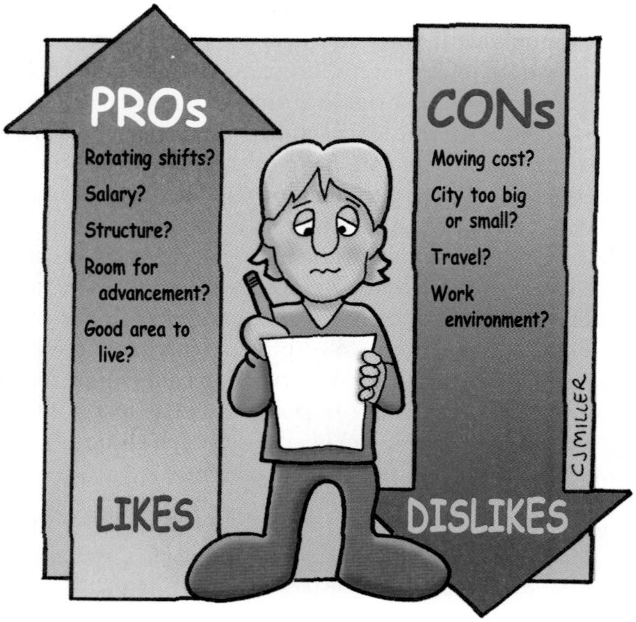
PROs
Rotating shifts?
Salary?
Structure?
Room for advancement?
Good area to live?
LIKES
CONs
Moving cost?
City too big or small?
Travel?
Work environment?
DISLIKES
CJMILLER

FIGURE 3-2
Assessing personal needs and interests. Is the job a good fit?

select may have some drawbacks, but it should meet many more of your likes than dislikes to be a good "fit" (Figure 3-2).

Write out your responses to the following questions:

1. Do you enjoy an environment that provides a great deal of patient interaction, or do you thrive in a technically oriented routine? Think back to your clinical rotations, and see if you can find a pattern to what was most enjoyable or disagreeable.
   - I liked opportunities for using many technical skills.
   - I was uncomfortable with slower-paced routines (e.g., postpartum, nursery).
   - I liked to see the results of care as soon as possible (e.g., postoperative recovery).
   - I disliked the constant turnover of patients every day.
2. Do you enjoy working closely with other staff or prefer a more autonomous role in patient care? This question may influence a setting with primary care or team nursing. Why did you like or dislike one type or the other? Talk over your responses with some friends who may have had other experiences and get their opinions as well. Remember that the current trend for interdisciplinary care approaches is decreasing options for "autonomous" practice. Interviewers value job candidates who can work and thrive in a "team" atmosphere.
3. Do you learn best in a highly structured environment or in more informal on-the-job training? Knowing your learning style can guide your interest in and selection of an internship or orientation program. For example, internships range from formal classes with lengthy preceptorships to more informal orientations of fairly short duration. Remember that a program that meets your needs may not be the answer for

your best friend. Write down what you would like from an orientation or internship program. Look over your list and prioritize what you need and want most.

4. Do you feel comfortable functioning with a significant degree of autonomy or do you want and need more direction and supervision at this point in your professional development? You will shortly have completed nursing school, backed up by employment in an ICU throughout your senior year. Are you ready to be a 3 to 11 PM charge nurse in a small rural hospital, or do you want a slower transition to such responsibility? If this situation were offered, would you be flattered, frightened, or flabbergasted? Write down your reaction and consider how you would respond to the recruiter who offers you such a position.
5. How much physical energy are you able and willing to expend at work? Running 8 to 12 hours a day may or may not act as a tonic. Think back to the pace of your clinical rotations, and consider how your body reacted (minus the anxiety associated with instructor supervision, if you can!). Would you prefer a unit that has some predictable periods of frenzy and pause, or do you thrive on the unpredictable?
6. Are you a day, evening, or night person? In other words, are there certain times of the day when you are at your best? How about your worst? Be honest and realistic with your answers. Very few people are equally efficient and effective 24 hours a day. If your body shuts down at 10 PM, or you resist all efforts to wake up before 9 AM, a certain shift may need to be eliminated. However, if the job market is tight in your area of interest, the available positions may be on a less-desirable shift and you may need to make adjustments in other areas of your life to temporarily acclimate better to a professional position.
7. Do you like rotating shifts, or, perhaps more realistically, can you work rotating shifts? One aspect of reality shock for some new graduates is the realization that straight days may have ended with the last clinical rotation in school. Hospital and long-term care staffing is 24 hours a day, 7 days a week. In other words, it is a "24-7 profession"—a possibly unpleasant aspect of nursing, but a real one nonetheless. Assess your ability to work certain shifts, and try to strike a flexible approach before you speak with nurse recruitment. The increased trend of 12-hour shifts (7 AM-7 PM or 7 PM-7 AM) can be very demanding for the days assigned, but is very popular with many nurses because of the increased days off.

   Consider the impact of these choices on your family, social, and recreational needs. If there are certain shifts you must rule out, recognize that this may limit your job choices and plan accordingly. Giving some thought to your flexibility ahead of time will help you avoid committing to any and all shifts during an interview and will facilitate your job hunt. On the other hand, it is probably not realistic to request a Monday through Friday schedule in an acute care setting unless the organization has a separate weekend staff or a high level of personnel who request to work only weekends.
8. Can you work long hours (e.g., 12-hour shifts) without too much tension and fatigue? The 12-hour staffing option offers flexibility (e.g., six 12-hour days of work in an 80-hour pay period) but leaves some people exhausted and irritable. Consider your personal needs outside of work when you respond to this item. Can you climb into bed or put your feet up after a nonstop 12-hour shift, or do you need to pick up family responsibilities when you walk in the door? The 4 days off may well compensate for 3 days of fatigue, but map out your needs before you begin your job search.

9. Do you like making decisions quickly or generally favor a more relaxed approach to clinical problems? In general, ICU and stepdown units require more immediate reactions than adolescent psychology and orthopedics. Does the ICU environment excite or overwhelm you? Would you prefer a slower pace? Do not criticize yourself for your likes or dislikes. Slower-paced units require different strengths, not less knowledge. You have nothing to gain by working in an ICU if you dislike the setting. Meet your own needs, not someone else's.
10. What do you need in a job to be happy? This question does not mean money or benefits, but rather the sense that the job is worth getting excited about. Think about past employment you have had, whether health care–related or not. What did you like or dislike about the job? What made you stay? Possible answers include opportunities for growth, advancement, working with people you respect, or collegiality. Remember, your answers should include things that are important to you. These are the kind of issues that make you eager to go to work or to help you work through difficult clinical days. You may want to compare your answers with those of others whose opinions you value to gain a broader perspective.

WHAT ARE MY PERSONAL NEEDS AND INTERESTS?

A third aspect of self-assessment focuses on personal needs and interests. How much time and effort are you willing and able to give to your career at this point in time? Will work be a number one priority in your life, or does family or continued education take precedence?

Is relocation a possibility? If you are considering relocation, decide how you will gather information on possible job opportunities in the area or areas under consideration. Include newspapers, Internet websites, professional journals, as well as professional and family contacts as possible sources of information. If this is a voluntary move, develop a list of pros and cons for each location under consideration. Include your personal interests in the decision (e.g., cost of living, possible relocation allowance, access to recreational activities, opportunities for advanced education, and clinical opportunities).

How much are you willing to commute? The job opportunity may be terrific, but can you live with a 1-hour commute each way? Find out the probable commuting time for the hours and days you want to work, and add this piece of information to your collection of facts about various institutions. If you are remaining in the same locale, this may be common knowledge, but if you are relocating, this will determine the need for housing arrangements.

What salary range are you willing to consider? Although starting salary for new graduates is generally nonnegotiable, differentials for evenings, nights, and weekends create a range of salary possibilities. If you want an extended internship, a lower starting salary may be offered. Are you willing and able to trade this off for the benefits of an extended internship? The quality of the internship may be worth a temporary lower salary because of later advancement opportunities. Some areas of the country offer considerably higher salaries than others, but factor in the cost of living before you move out of town. You may be unpleasantly surprised by a monthly rent that swallows up a significant percentage of your salary.

Is overtime desirable in your life? Can it be reasonably juggled with other interests and time demands? The extra money may sound great and look impressive on your paycheck, but do not put unreasonable demands on your physical and emotional well-being. Staffing needs create overtime in many settings, but give some thought to what kind of overtime you can and cannot do when the question is asked. As the nursing shortage worsens, there has been increasing concern regarding mandatory overtime. Mandatory overtime has been such a hot issue that states are now passing laws prohibiting it. The pressure and the adverse effects of mandatory overtime have been repeatedly cited as major reasons for nursing job change. Make sure you have a clear understanding of the overtime policy at your institution of interest before you agree to a position.

WHAT ARE MY CAREER GOALS?

The final step of your self-assessment is the development of career goals. Yes, you really do need to have some goals! You are the architect of your professional future, so take pen to paper or fingers to the keyboard and start designing. Consider your answers to the following questions.

What do you want from your first nursing position? Possible answers might include developing confidence in decision-making, more proficiency with technical skills, and increased organizational abilities.

What are your professional goals for the first year? Third year? Fifth year? If you cannot imagine your life, let alone your career, beyond 1 to 2 years, relax. Many people feel uncertain planning beyond their initial position and first paid vacation. Close your eyes and try to imagine yourself 1 year out of school. Compare yourself with recent graduates you have seen during your rotations, and try to imagine the roles they are developing. The following are possible answers:

- First-year goal
  - Becoming a competent staff nurse in pediatrics or ICU.
- Third-year goal
  - Achieving certification in your specialty area.
  - Joining a professional organization.
  - Possibly moving into a charge position on your unit.
  - Returning to school for advanced education.
- Fifth-year goal
  - Completing an advanced degree and moving into a leadership position within your specialty area of practice.

If you honestly do not think you will return to school at this point in your life, do not feel as though you should fake your answer to impress someone. Develop a comfortable response to a question regarding your goals for the first year, and consider what you might want to be doing after that time. Remember, it is far easier to gauge how your career is progressing if you have established some benchmark goals to which you can refer. This is also a favorite question posed during interviews, so spend some time thinking about it! Recruiters are interested in nurses with a plan. They are encouraged to "hire for attitude and provide training for skills." Prepare to have an enthusiastic attitude toward your future as a professional.

RESEARCHING PROSPECTIVE EMPLOYERS

WHAT EMPLOYMENT OPPORTUNITIES ARE AVAILABLE?

You have a world of nursing to choose from; there are incredible opportunities available to begin your practice as a graduate nurse. The largest employers are hospitals or acute-care facilities. In hospitals, there are a wide variety of positions, although, often recent graduates are placed in staff nurse positions. If it is a general hospital, you need to choose what areas interest you most. Your first position may not be exactly what you want, but remember, it is the first step toward your career goal. As you build your competence and self-esteem, you may find just the position you want. In many hospitals, staff positions represent many different levels and areas, especially if the hospital participates in clinical or career ladders (Figure 3-3).

The staff nurse position is one of the most challenging, in addition to providing an "incubator" to begin your nursing practice.

Charge positions may involve responsibility for a particular staff or a particular day or they may involve managing staff for an entire unit. There are a variety of opportunities in management as your experience level increases and you continue your education. Many institutions now refer to the person charged with the management of all of nursing as vice president: these persons usually have a master's or doctoral degree in nursing. Exact job titles depend on the organizational structure of the institution. It is

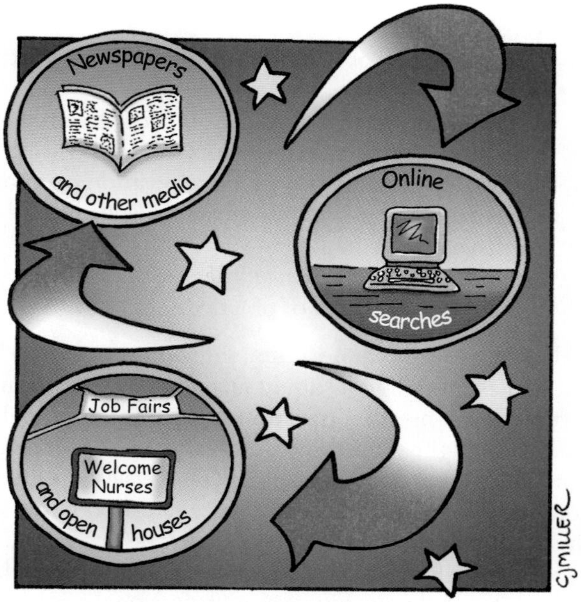
Newspapers
and other media
Online
searches
Job Fairs
Welcome Nurses
and open houses
CJMILLER

FIGURE 3-3
Ways to research prospective employers.

very important in your first few years of nursing to watch the trends in nursing, realize what opportunities are available, know where your interests are, and understand what it will take (experience and education) to get you where you want to be.

Entry-level positions in the hospital are usually staff nurse positions. In the current nursing crisis, the staff nurse positions are the areas of critical need. Staff nurse positions in medical-surgical nursing are some of the most demanding—and rewarding—positions. Frequently, nurses begin their careers here with the intention to move on to greener pastures; however, the rewards and challenges more than fulfill their needs. It is important that your first position offers you an opportunity to further develop your nursing skills. Whether it is working in the emergency department, day surgery, specialty units, or medical-surgical units, staff nurse positions give you a very valuable opportunity to polish your time management, patient care organization, and nursing skills (Figure 3-4). Once you are confident with skills, procedures, and the overall practice of nursing, you may be ready to move on to new challenges. This may be 6 months for some recent graduates; for others, it may take a year or more. Take the time to reinforce your nursing competencies; it will prepare you for your future practice in nursing. Other areas in which nurses may also find employment include community health, home health care, and nursing agencies. Working in the community in such positions as occupational health, school health, and the military often requires a bachelor's degree in nursing and at least 1 year of hospital nursing, or both.

WHAT ABOUT ADVANCED DEGREES IN NURSING?

There are many advantages to advanced degrees in nursing. Review Chapter 6 for the different choices regarding an advanced degree. One of the most important aspects of

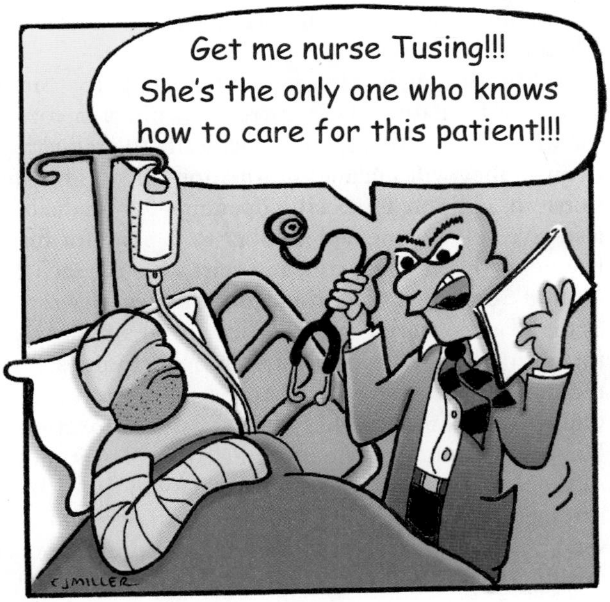
Get me nurse Tusing!!!
She's the only one who knows
how to care for this patient!!!
CJMILLER

FIGURE 3-4
Being competent has its rewards.

obtaining an advanced degree is your experience as a nurse that helps you to determine what direction you want to go. Do not expect this to come early in your career; it may take a little time as you sample different areas of practice to determine whether you want an advanced degree and in which area to focus. If you are an associate-degree graduate, you might want to consider the basic requirements for your bachelor's degree, including what schools are available and what their requirements are. This is an area you can begin to work on immediately after graduation. Remember, you can do this a little at a time without having to declare an area of special interest. Although an advanced degree is important to some nurses, others may prefer special education programs that do not lead to an advanced degree, but to expertise in a specialty practice area. Keep an open mind as you begin to investigate this great world of nursing.

HOW DO I GO ABOUT RESEARCHING PROSPECTIVE EMPLOYERS?

EMPLOYMENT CONSIDERATIONS: HOW DO YOU DECIDE ON AN EMPLOYER?

In 1980, the American Academy of Nursing identified criteria for what was designated as "magnet hospitals." This designation recognized hospitals for their lower turnover rates, visionary leaders, value they placed on education, and ability to maintain open lines of communication. To identify magnet hospitals in your area, check the website *www.nursingworld.org.ancc* (Valentino, 2002). In your search for a job, it is important to look for institutions/hospitals that create a work environment that supports professional nursing practice. In the current job market, locating magnet hospitals in your community would be an important consideration in your job search.

Media Information

Newspapers. It is time to start reading the Sunday employment section to get specific information about current openings in your area. Scan the advertisements to see whether any are targeted specifically to graduating seniors. Focus on these initially because they will include information on possible internships or specialized orientations, in addition to specific openings for graduate nurses. The advertisements will also give you a name and number to contact for further information. Clip the advertisements that interest you, and start a file for each potential employer.

Online Searches. Electronic job searches have replaced newspapers for many people as the place to start a search. They are so popular because you can access information for both local and distant nursing opportunities with the ease of a few clicks. Some recruiters find their website to be more cost-effective than newspaper advertising. Online/electronic searches may reveal websites for specific hospitals and institutions. You may then review the positions available within that one institution. If you intend to use this method to follow-up on a job posting, be prepared to submit your flawless resume electronically and spell-check all of your correspondence before you click the send button. Many institutions are now requiring electronic applications, occasionally raising issues of software compatibility for applicants, but be prepared to comply with Human Resources requirements. Patience in the application process is essential for your professional success.

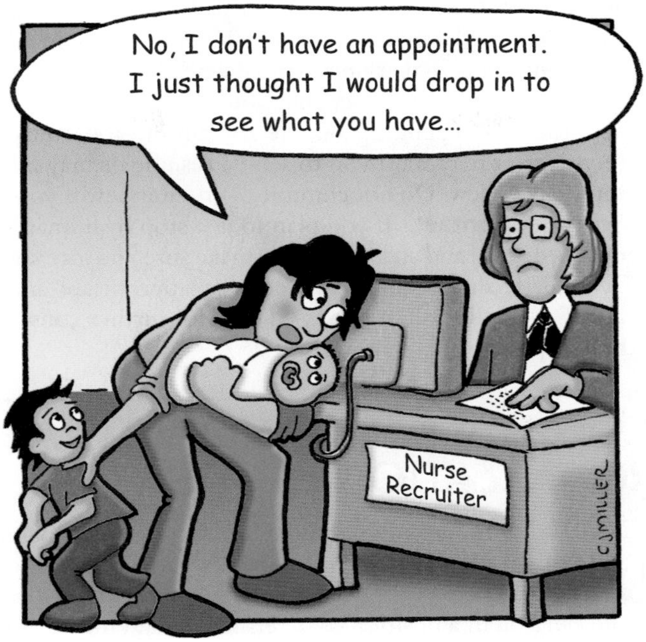
No, I don't have an appointment. I just thought I would drop in to see what you have...
Nurse Recruiter
CJMILLER

FIGURE 3-5
The first impression is a lasting one, so make it count for you, not against you.

Job Fairs/Open Houses. You may have the opportunity to attend a nursing job fair or hospital open house as a soon-to-be graduate nurse. Take advantage of this opportunity to collect information about specific employers and possibly make initial contacts for later interviews. Leave your jeans and tennis shoes at home on these occasions, however. Take some time with your appearance, because first impressions are important! (Figure 3-5)

If you plan to formally interview at the institution in the future, take home their brochure and become familiar with the information it contains. Recruiters appreciate applicants who know some basic facts about their institution. It will also help you respond to one of their favorite lines of questioning: "Why do you want to work for our institution?" or "In what ways do you feel you can contribute to our organization?"

Employee Contacts. If you have a friend or family member—or simply know someone—who works at an institution you are considering for employment, make an effort to speak with him or her about the job environment. As insiders, they may be able to provide you with a perspective about the employer that the advertisement, recruiter, or interview cannot. Possible questions you may want to ask them include "Why do they enjoy working there?" "What was orientation like?" and "How is employee morale?"

Personnel/Recruitment Contacts

Letter-Writing Campaign. Plan to send your resume with a cover letter, and triple-check both for grammatical errors. Your resume and cover letter are the first impression you will make with a prospective employer.

Telephone Contact. Before you pick up the telephone, get out your calendar and start planning likely dates for possible interviews, in addition to the approximate date you want to begin working. Armed with this information, you can comfortably answer questions beyond the fact that you would like them to send you a brochure and an application. Depending on the institution you contact, human resources or nurse recruitment may want you to send a resume or may ask you to set up an appointment for an interview. Do not commit to an interview if you are not ready.

Personal Contact. If you plan to just stop by human resources or nurse recruitment for a brochure and an application, make sure you give some thought to your appearance. Tee shirts, shorts, and jeans are not appropriate and have caused otherwise well-qualified applicants to be passed over for further consideration. Again, remember that first impression!

WHAT DO I NEED TO KNOW TO ASSESS THE ORGANIZATION?

Now that you have described yourself and have thought about the kind of setting in which you work best, continue these exercises on a consistent basis. This ongoing analysis will help you make decisions about the kind of organization that is best for you and put you in a position to determine what kind of organization fits you.

HOW DO YOU GO ABOUT ASSESSING AN ORGANIZATION TO FIND WHAT YOU WANT?

Talk to People in the Organization. One obvious answer is to ask the people who work in that organization. When you interview for a position, you can meet people who work in the specific setting in which you are interested. Ask questions that will help you learn about certain situations. Think of questions to present to staff to determine their reactions to situations. How people handle these questions will give you great insight into the way the organization works. If they feel uncomfortable with your approach, you will know that this kind of approach is not usual for them. If they rise to the occasion and very openly and candidly discuss their reactions, this will give you a different perspective on their viewpoints. Take some time to think about questions and situations you would like to present when you talk to people in various facilities.

Read and Analyze the Recruitment Materials. Organizations also present themselves to you through their documents. When organizations send recruitment materials to you or advertise online, they are telling you the things they want you to know about them. Organizations spend a good deal of time and money on material that they believe presents their philosophy and attitude toward patients and staff. What an organization chooses to highlight tells you about the organization. Carefully analyze the materials presented to you. This is another way of determining the values the organization lives by and deems important. All of these materials are intended to make a statement to you about who they are.

Is There a Mission or Philosophy Statement? There are other written documents to examine. For example, a specific nursing unit may have a mission statement that tells you who they are and what they are about. The department of nursing will

CRITICAL THINKING BOX 3-3

What are some observations that you may have during your interview process that would cause you to have second thoughts about accepting a position at the institution?

have a philosophy statement that should be the organizing framework around which the members structure themselves in delivering nursing care. In some organizations, the staff knows what this mission statement says and how it provides direction to them. In other organizations, the staff will be unfamiliar with the statement of philosophy and may react with confusion when you ask them. All of these written materials should send a message to you about the organization. Do your observations during the interview process support the organization mission/philosophy statements? (Critical Thinking Box 3-3).

Evaluate the Reputation of the Leadership. Organizations are guided by people at the top and take on the characteristics these people support. What do you know about the chief executive officer? This person sets the stage and the direction for the organization. You can gather information about the chief executive officer by asking people during the interview what this person is like. People in the community will also be familiar with this person and will give you insight into the values and characteristics that this person represents. If there has been stability in the top-level executive team over a period of years, there is a high likelihood of stabilty in the staffing. If there has been considerable change in upper management, some degree of organizational instabilty is likely. Neither of these situations is inherently good or bad because change, while very possibly innovative, is also unsettling for many staff.

The same can be said for the chief nursing officer. This person sets the direction for the nursing organization, either by active design or benign neglect, and sets into motion an organization that structures the beliefs about patients, staff, and nursing. It is very important to talk with nurses who are working with this person and determine how they feel about the management in their organization. Has he or she had a successful tenure? Is this person well respected? Can people point to a strategic direction and philosophy this person has given to the organization?

Is a Nursing Theory or Philosophy Used? Some nursing divisions organize themselves around a nursing theorist or a philosophy of care. Orem's self-care theory, Neuman's systems model, and King's theory of goal attainment are examples of organizing frameworks that nursing organizations have adopted (see Chapter 8). If an organization does not have a nursing theorist, it often adopts a philosophy or model according to which it operates. The organizing framework that is adopted will determine how the organization is developed. From the organizing framework will come the goals and objectives of the department of nursing. These goals and objectives will provide you with a long-range view of the direction of this organization. Individual nursing units occasionally have such an organizing framework on which to base their direction of care. It is appropriate to find out information like this so you know if you can agree with the organization's direction or philosophy. The more you know about an organization upfront, the more likely you are to select the "best fit" for your talents and goals.

RESUME WRITING

HOW DO I WRITE AN EFFECTIVE RESUME?

Design your resume by using the KISS principle: Keep It Simple, Sincerely! (That is, use concise wording, and make it easy-to-read, informational, and simple.)

Nurses are not famous for exceptional skills in putting together their own resumes! Most nurses would rather be taking care of patients and families. However, all nurses should keep a current resume handy. It helps you keep track of where you have been and what you have done. You do not have to be a computer wizard. You can do this.

Your resume is the first introduction a prospective employer will have to you. It will give the employer a basic idea of who you are professionally and what your objectives are for your nursing career. While defining your strengths, it is important not to overstate your skills. Most employers in this economic time are willing to train you on all or some of the components of the position you are applying for. A resume is a concise, factual presentation of your educational and professional history (Box 3-1). Do not be surprised if a recruiter suggests other areas to you than what you have initially indicated on your resume or in your interview. Be open to suggestions; they may have some ideas or considerations you have not even thought about.

BOX 3-1 Resume Guidelines

- Catch all typos and grammatical errors. Have someone proofread your resume.
- Present a clear objective that emphasizes your skills and strengths.
- A good first impression is critical, so if written, your resume should be neat, appearing on white or off-white paper.
- Avoid using the "I" or "me" words in your resume.
- Keep the information concise, preferably limited to one or two pages.
- Rule of thumb on work experience is to show most current work experience. This is generally the last 10 to 15 years unless there is something in your background that is critical to note.
- Do not try to impress anyone with big words. Jargon for the profession is okay if everyone knows what it is.
- Do not inquire about salary or benefits in your resume. It is not the right time or place for that.
- Do not exaggerate about what you can and cannot do because the potential employer will check it out.
- Present yourself in a positive light.
- Your resume should be neat and visually appealing.
- Do not list all of your references. Be prepared to provide them with a list when asked. You may want to have different references for different types of positions.

WHAT INFORMATION IS NECESSARY FOR A RESUME?

Here are the components of a resume. Be sure to proofread what you write for spelling and grammar. Do not forget that this is the first impression someone may have of you.

Demographic Data: Who Are You? Your name, address, telephone number, and e-mail address should be at the top of the page. Be sure to give correct, current information so that the employer can easily contact you. If you need to give an alternate telephone number or e-mail address, please note their name and advise that person that a prospective employer may be calling for you. Keep in mind that you never put personal information such as your social security number, marital status, number of children, or your picture on a resume.

Professional Objective: What Position Are You Applying for? There is a wide variety of ways to address this aspect. However, it is very important that you describe the position you are applying for and in what department/area of nursing you are interested. With the widespread use of the Internet, it has become increasingly easy to view job openings and be more educated and decisive about what you are looking for. You can identify several areas (if you have more than one area of preference). This ultimately is your short-term goal. You may also state a long-term goal (e.g., administration, quality assurance, case management, transplant team).

Education: Where Did You Receive Your Education, High School to Present? List your education in chronological order, beginning with high school. List the month/year of graduation and what degree was received, if any. If you have degrees other than nursing, you also want to include these in the chronological order in which you received them. This section will contain certifications or special training you have received, where you received it, and the date you completed it. If you are currently enrolled in school, be sure to include that as well.

Professional Experience: What Do You Know How to Do? "Easy to read" is the goal. It is very important to put this section in chronological order beginning with the present. You want the prospective employer to see what you have been doing most recently. List your current or previous employer, position held, dates from and to, and a brief description of your responsibilities. This is a good place to highlight special skills that you feel may be important to your prospective employer. This section will be different for an experienced nurse than for a recent graduate nurse. Nevertheless, it is important to list your employment history through the past 7 years. Include those areas of employment that may not be associated with nursing or the health care field. Whatever experience you have as an "employee" is necessary to demonstrate your ability to work with people, handle stress, be flexible, and so forth. It is not necessary to list clinical rotations you have completed during nursing school, most of those rotations are standardized. If you have not had any experience and this will be your first job, state that also. It is important for managers and staff educators to be aware of the levels of experience of the recent graduates.

Licensure: What Can You Do and Where Can You Do It? This is a very important area of information for nurses. With the implementation of the Multi-State Licensure Compact (see Chapters 5 and 20), you may only have to be licensed in one state. It is your responsibility to know which states will honor your license and which ones will require you to obtain a separate license. As a general rule, you will be required to be licensed in the state of your residence, then possibly in another state of practice, depending on the licensure compact of the states involved. List the state your license was issued and the expiration date. For security reasons, do not list your license number.

Professional Organizations: What Do You Belong to? You may list organizations in which you are a member or have held an office. It is good to list professional and community groups. This section is optional.

Honors and Awards: What Did You Receive Recognition for? If you have received recognition for special skills or volunteer work, you may want to include it here. You may also include any scholarships you have received. This is also an optional section.

References: Who Knows About You? A simple line at the bottom of the resume "References provided on request" will suffice. Be prepared with a separate typed sheet that lists at least three references. Provide the names and telephone numbers of two professionals with whom you have worked and one personal reference. Always notify your references that you have listed them and that they may receive a telephone call about you. Look at the example of a resume (Figure 3-6), and adapt it

Linda Smith

123 Any Street

Dallas, TX 77777

972-555-5555

E-mail: lsmith@hotmail.com

Objective:

To obtain a staff nurse position in Hematology-Oncology.

Education:

Memorial High School, Dallas, Texas, graduated 05/1998.

El Centro College, Dallas, Texas

ADN, awarded June 2002

Experience:

10/2000 to present–Baylor Hospital, Dallas, Texas–nurse tech, part-time

02/1997 to 06/1999–Kroger's Supermarkets, cashier

Licensure:

Eligible for NCLEX May 2002 (Texas)

Certifications: CPR expires 03/2002

Professional Organizations:

Texas Nursing Students Association

References: on Request

FIGURE 3-6
Resume.

to what works best for you. It is preferable to keep your resume on one page, but this is not always possible. If you need further examples of resumes or formats, check the Internet for samples *(http://resume.monster.com)*. Several of the popular word-processing programs also have resume formats in the section for office forms.

WHAT ELSE SHOULD I SUBMIT WITH MY RESUME?

Along with your resume, you should enclose a cover letter that gives a brief introduction (see Box 3-2 and Figure 3-7). Summarize your important strengths or give information regarding change of specialty, but remember that this letter should be about one page, not more than two (Feery, 2002). If you have talked with a recruiter and have a specific name, then send it to them. You do not have to address it to a specific person; it will be distributed to the recruiter who handles the units where you have indicated an interest. Simply addressing it to "Nurse Recruitment" will usually get it to the right person.

WHAT ARE THE METHODS FOR SUBMITTING RESUMES?

There are a variety of ways to submit a resume: hand-carry it, submit it electronically by means of e-mail or the hospital website, or mail it through the post office. You will probably want to send it to the nurse recruitment department of your favorite medical institution. One of the most popular methods for nurses to send resumes is through the website of the medical institution where they are interested in obtaining an interview. This is an excellent way to submit your resume, but remember to follow up with a telephone call if you have not heard from a recruiter within 1 week. You can also directly e-mail your resume to a recruiter. E-mail addresses are readily available through business cards, websites, and word of mouth. Beware: Your e-mail first page will be the cover letter when you submit your resume by using e-mail. The same resume-writing principles apply to all electronically submitted resumes because your resume will be printed for review. There are also many large job-search websites available on the Internet. You can post your resume on any of these by using their specific formats, but remember that businesses must pay a fee to search for applicants. It is important to remember that not all of the institutions belong to every job-search website. Use discretion regarding where you want to post your resume; if you are interested in a specific institution, it is best to review their website for positions available and guidelines for submitting resumes.

Now that you have your resume ready to submit, you will need to identify prospective employers. Remember, one of the first things you can do is network. Networking is

BOX 3-2 Reminders for Cover Letters

- 8½ × 11-inch paper, white, off-white, light blue
- Typed, with no mistakes
- No smudges
- 1½- to 2-inch margin on all sides
- Signed, usually with black ink
- No abbreviations
- Business letter format

Linda Smith
111 Anyplace Blvd.
Boise, ID 30203
(712) 555-5555

Nurse Recruiter
Medical Center of Texas
222 Medical Way
Dallas, TX 77777

Dear Nurse Recruiter:

There is a Diabetic Educator position posted on your Web site. I would like to apply for the position and have attached my résumé for your review. I currently have 1 year of experience in this role in a 220-bed hospital. Before that I worked for 2 years on a medical/surgical unit with a large population of new and established diabetic patients.

I will be relocating to the Dallas area in 2 months and will be in Dallas September 10 and 11 for interviews. Please let me know if this would be a convenient time to schedule an interview. I have voice mail on my phone, so you may leave me a message. I look forward to meeting with you. Please feel free to contact me.

Sincerely,

Linda Smith

FIGURE 3-7
Cover letter.

contacting everyone you know and even some people you do not know to get information about their specific organization or institution. Places that you can network are at your facility during clinical, at student organization programs, at career days at colleges, and at career opportunity fairs. Attend local chapter meetings of nursing organizations. Read nursing journal employment sections. When you have identified the institutions where you would like to discuss possible employment, send them your resume. If you have not heard from them within 7 to 10 days, give them a call to make sure your resume was received and to schedule an interview. Keep track of all this information on your record of contacts and resumes sent so that you will have easy access to the information (Figure 3-8). It will be important to document your follow-up actions and results—do not forget to keep copies of correspondence and notes on any conversations with potential employers. Remember to date all entries—briefly put information received, interviews requested and granted, resumes sent, and job offers received. Box 3-3 presents a summary of the steps to finding the job you want.

Employer Address and Phone Number	Interviewer and Title	Date Résumé Sent	Date and Time of Interview	Inquiry of Application Letter	Application Submitted	Thank You Letter Sent After Interview	Job Offer Received	Confirmation of "No Thank You" Letter Sent	Comments or Notes

FIGURE 3-8
Record of employer contacts and resumes sent.

BOX 3-3 Your Checklist for Finding a Job

- Define your goals.
- Develop your resume.
- Identify potential employers.
- Send your resume and cover letter.
- Return a follow-up phone call.
- Schedule an interview.
- Send a follow-up letter.
- Keep record of employer contacts (see Figure 3-8).
- Make an informed decision where to work.

WHAT IS THE DIFFERENCE BETWEEN A RESUME AND A CURRICULUM VITAE?

A curriculum vitae (CV) is a summary of your educational and academic background and is similar to a resume. Unlike the resume, however, your CV grows longer as you become more accomplished. You may want to include your continuing-education experiences and any publications (e.g., book chapters, journal articles). Most CVs run two to four pages or more. As with a resume, you may need several different CVs emphasizing different skills and experiences, depending on the positions or activities for which you are applying.

THE INTERVIEW PROCESS

HOW DO I PLAN MY INTERVIEW CAMPAIGN?

Set up Your Schedule. Keep the following points in mind:

- Agencies usually have specific dates for orientations, internships, and preceptorships.
- Identify when you want to begin employment, and mark your calendar.
- Work backward from this date to plan dates and times for interviews.
- Plan no more than two interviews in one day. If you do, beware of information overload and the risk of being late for at least one interview. Have two or three possible dates available on your calendar before you call the human resources office or nurse recruitment. Advance planning will keep you from fumbling on the telephone when they tell you that your first choice is unavailable!

While you are on the telephone, ask some questions about their interview process. How much time should you plan for the interview? It may range from under 1 hour to a half day. Ask about the job description on the telephone if you have not seen it in the newspaper or online. Becoming familiar with both the job description and the prospective employer are critical to interview success.

What does the interview process involve? It may involve tours and multiple interviews including human resources, nurse recruitment, one or more clinical managers, and, possibly, staff. If you are applying for an internship, it is not unusual to be interviewed by a panel of three or four people. Knowing this ahead of time may increase your anxiety, but it is less stressful than being surprised by this fact at the door.

Will more than one interview be required? Some institutions will use the first interview as a screening mechanism. You may be asked to come back for a follow-up interview.

How do you get to the human resources or nurse recruitment office? Ask for directions ahead of time if you are unfamiliar with the area. Have a good idea of the time involved for travel. Arriving late for an interview may create a very poor initial impression.

Will you be able to meet with clinical managers from different areas on the same day? Are there new graduates in the area with whom you can talk? This is important if you are interested in more than one clinical area.

Will a tour of the unit be included? If this is not a standard part of the interview process, express interest in having one so you can get a more realistic idea of the setting and possibly meet some of the staff.

Prepare to Show Your Best Side. Develop your responses to probable interview questions. If you do not plan possible responses, you run the risk of looking wide-eyed as you fumble for an answer or ramble on around the subject. Despite the reality of a severe nursing shortage, organizations still give considerable weight to the interview, and an employment offer is far from automatic to any one who walks in the door with a diploma or license in hand.

In Critical Thinking Box 3-4 are examples of interview questions with which you should be familiar. How would you answer these questions?

Rehearse the Interview. If you role-play a possible interview, it will probably increase your comfort level for the real thing. Following are some suggestions for a rehearsal:

CRITICAL THINKING BOX 3-4

SAMPLE OF INTERVIEW QUESTIONS

The following is a sampling of interview questions you should be familiar with. Prepare your responses.

1. What area or areas of nursing are you interested in and why?
2. Tell me about your clinical experiences. Which rotations did you enjoy the most? Why?
3. What is the biggest mistake you ever made and how was the problem resolved?
4. Tell me about yourself. What are your strengths? Why?
5. How about your weaknesses? Why?
6. What is your philosphy of nursing?
7. What qualifications do you have that make you believe that you will be successful in this staff position?
8. What skills do you feel you have gained from your past work experiences that may help you in this position?
9. Tell me a little about yourself. How would others describe you?
10. What are your future career plans? Where do you expect to be in 2 or 3 years? Five years?
11. We do not have any openings at the present time in the areas in which you have indicated an interest. Would you be willing to accept a position in another area?
12. How do you handle stress in the work setting? *(Spend some time looking over your answers. Do they describe you accurately? Rework your answers until you feel comfortable with them, but do not try to memorize the words. They should serve as a guide for the upcoming interview.)*
13. Tell me about a time when you went out of your way to assist a family or client when you really did not have the time.

- Dress for the part. It will add some authenticity to the situation.
- Choose a supportive friend or family member to role-play the interviewer.
- Practice your verbal responses to sample questions.
- Ask for constructive feedback regarding your appearance, body language, and responses.

Many applicants say they have no questions at the end of the interview. This may be true, or it may reflect the urge to end the interview and relax! Some words of advice: Prepare a few questions! This will be your opportunity to gather important details and possibly impress the interviewer with your interest. The following is a sampling of possible questions:

- What are your expectations of recent graduates?
- What is your evaluation process like?
- Who will evaluate me, and how will I get feedback about my performance?
- I'd like some more information about your preceptorship program. How long will I have a preceptor, and what can I expect from the preceptor?
- What is the nurse-to-patient ratio on each of the shifts I may be working?
- What is your policy regarding weekend coverage?
- What opportunities are there for professional development?

Look over the recruitment brochures for additional ideas on questions. This shows that you are interested in the institution and have done your homework.

STRATEGIES FOR INTERVIEW SUCCESS

One of the most important strategies for successful interviewing is to dress for success (Box 3-4). Watch your interviewing etiquette; your parents taught you to mind your manners, and this is an opportunity to put that education to good use. Also, make sure you know the name and title of the individual who is scheduled to meet with you.

BOX 3-4 The *Dos* and *Don'ts* of Dressing for Interviews

DO

- Look over your wardrobe and select a conservative outfit. Ladies, if you own a suit, consider wearing it, but do not blow your budget buying an outfit you will never wear again. Other acceptable outfits include a business-type dress or skirt with coordinated top. The tried-and-true rule for job interview attire is: Dress conservatively and professionally. Although a nursing shortage may loosen the rules a bit, the impression you convey by your outfit is likely to be remembered.
- Be conservative with makeup and hairdo.
- Wear minimal jewelry; you do not want to jingle and rattle with every move.
- Wear hose with a skirt or a dress; bare legs may be fashionable, but not for a professional interview.
- Consider a suit or jacket with coordinated slacks, shirt, and tie for men.
- Take a few minutes to look yourself over in the mirror.

Continued

BOX 3-4 The *Dos* and *Don'ts* of Dressing for Interviews—cont'd

DON'T

- Wear casual clothes such as tee shirts, jeans, tennis shoes, or sandals. They may reflect the "real" you, but this is not the place to show that aspect of your personality.
- Be guilty of poor grooming or hygiene.
- Wear brand-new shoes, which may turn your day into a "painful" experience.
- Bring your children with you. You should leave them at home. Do not expect the staff to act as babysitters.
- Wear wrinkled or revealing clothing. This is not a date, and a bare midsection, though attractive in a casual setting, is inappropriate for a job interview.

CRITICAL FIRST 5 MINUTES!

The decision to hire is usually made within the first 60 seconds. You will need to put your best foot forward from the start. Show up at least 10 to 15 minutes early. Smile at everyone you meet, and shake hands firmly (Restifo, 2002).

Arriving early may give you a chance to look over additional information about the institution or possibly give you more time for your interview. If you are delayed or cannot keep the appointment, call the interviewer to reschedule. Under no circumstances should you present yourself for an interview with your children in tow. They do not belong at a job interview and will create a negative impression with the interviewer. Human resources cannot provide babysitting services, and the presence of children in the waiting area is a safety concern without adult supervision. If you experience a childcare emergency, call and reschedule the interview.

Be aware of your body language; that is, establish eye contact with the interviewer and maintain reasonable eye contact during the interview (Croteau, 2004). Try to avoid or minimize distracting nervous mannerisms. Keep your hands poised in your lap or in some other comfortable position. If you "talk with your hands," try not to do this continually. If you cross your legs, do not shake your foot. If offered coffee or another drink, decide whether this will relax you or complicate your body language. Show enthusiasm in your voice and body language. Do not chew gum or have anything in your mouth. Give a winning smile when you are introduced, and offer to shake hands.

Women sometimes have a problem with shaking hands. Practice it at home to become more comfortable. Demonstrate interest in what the interviewer has to say. Do not argue with or contradict the interviewer! Wait to ask about salary and benefits until all other aspects of the interview have been completed, including your other questions! Salary and benefits are important aspects, but they should not dominate your conversation. If the salary offer is lower than you expected, do not argue with the interviewer. You may point out that another institution is offering a higher starting salary, but do not try to use this information as a form of harassment or coercion. If you want to take some notes during the interview, ask the interviewer if he or she minds. This is generally quite acceptable. Bring along your list of questions, and if you cannot recall them when given the chance, ask to take out your list. Do not check off information during the interview as if you were grocery shopping!

PHASES OF THE INTERVIEW

The interview is generally divided into three areas, each of which serves a particular purpose. The first few minutes constitute the introduction. This is a lightweight section that is designed to help put you somewhat at ease (Croteau, 2004). Some effort to "break the ice" will be made, and the communication may focus on the traffic, the weather, or the excitement you probably feel about your upcoming graduation. Take some slow, deep breaths and make a conscious effort to relax. Remember that you are making an initial impression with your verbal and nonverbal behavior.

The second phase involves fact-finding. Depending on the skill and style of the interviewer, you may be unaware of the subtle change in conversation, but questions about you will most likely now be asked. Remember the answers you rehearsed, and make an effort to use that information. Your resume may be used as a source of questions, so make sure you can speak about its contents and that every item on the resume can be verified. Studies have shown that up to 35% of all job applicants have some inaccurate or misleading information on their resumes. The information that you provide on the resume will be verified, and deliberate and "accidental" inaccuracies could cost you the job. Be prepared to offer your references and possibly explain why you have selected these particular individuals. If you have a tendency to give short responses or avoid answering questions, a skilled interviewer will reword the question or possibly note that you do not answer questions well. Interviewers strive to have the applicant talk about 90% of the time, so consider this your audition. They are really interested in getting to know you as a prospective "fit" with their institution, so you should be both enthusiastic and honest. Although many institutions offer a prolonged internship or preceptorship to increase both your confidence level and practical skill set, the interviewer is looking for prospective employees who are capable of being assertive team players. Telling a recruiter that you are uncomfortable and a misfit in the clinical setting does not create a positive impression. Remember that this is a time to portray your best assets as a future employee.

Some institutions are asking students or recent graduates to bring in a portfolio reflecting their school experiences. Included in this portfolio might be your skills checkoff sheet. This is particularly beneficial if it is signed by the faculty with occasional positive comments. Include in the portfolio some of your best nursing care plans. If you have been in a variety of clinical agencies, it is appropriate to include a list that also indicates the type of experience (e.g., Memorial Hospital—obstetrics). The portfolio should reflect your best schoolwork and present you in a positive light. If the interviewer does not ask for a portfolio, then you may offer it for their review.

The closing is the last phase of the interview process. The interviewer may summarize what has been discussed and give you some ideas about the next step in the process (e.g., a tour, a meeting with clinical managers, or a follow-up interview). This is your time to ask questions. However, if you feel full of facts and unable to ask any questions at this time, leave the door open to future contacts by saying "I believe you answered all my questions at this time, but may I contact you if I have some questions later on?"

After the initial interview, you may tour the area in which you will work. Show interest when this tour is offered, and use it as an opportunity to observe the surroundings for such things as professional behaviors and organizational and environmental factors. If you have the chance, interact with the staff, especially with recent graduates. Ask what they enjoy about their unit and job position. Before leaving, make sure you thank the interviewer for his or her time and interest.

HOW DO I HANDLE UNEXPECTED QUESTIONS OR SITUATIONS?

So, you did your homework and you are prepared for anything, but out of the blue you are asked a question you never expected. What should you do? Saying "No fair" is not a good answer! Take a deep breath, pause, and consider saying something like this: "That's an interesting question. I'd like to think about my answer for a minute if you don't mind. Can we come back to that subject later in the interview?" Given a temporary break, you will have time to develop your thoughts on the subject. Do not ignore the question, however, because the interviewer will most likely bring it up again. Suppose you answer the question but feel your response was incomplete or off the mark. Look for an opportunity at the end of the interview to bring up the subject again, saying something like "I've had some time to think about an earlier question and want to add some additional information if you don't mind" (Box 3-5).

BOX 3-5 Key Points to Remember About Your Responses During an Interview

- Answer honestly.
- Do not brag or gloat about your achievements, but do show yourself in a positive light.
- Remember that you are your best salesperson!
- Do not criticize past employers or instructors. It is more likely to reflect unfavorably on you than on them.
- Do not dwell on your shortcomings. Turn them into areas for future development: "I need to improve my organizational skills. Managing a group of patients will be a challenge, but I am looking forward to it."
- Demonstrate flexibility and a willingness to begin work in an area of second or third choice if the job market is limited in the area in which you are applying.

NOW CAN WE TALK ABOUT BENEFITS?

Sometime during the interview process the person you are interviewing will open the discussion on salary and the benefits the hospital has to offer. Salary, job responsibilities, and facility location are not the only major considerations in choosing an employer; do not forget to consider the total compensation package (that is, your benefits). Often, benefits are overlooked because their cost is less visible than the exciting new salary that you will be receiving. Some organizations spend as much as 40% of their total employee payroll to provide this extra compensation. You should consider them your "hidden paycheck" (Box 3-6).

Sign-on Bonuses. This has become a marketing tool of some institutions. Be cautious: carefully read and evaluate what is connected with the sign-on bonus. How long will you have to work to receive any of the bonus, and when will it be paid? How long do you have to work for the institution? For example, half of the sign-on bonus may be paid after 6 months of employment, but the remaining amount may not be paid until after 2 or 3 years of employment. Is the sign-on bonus in any way tied to the area in which you will be working? If you originally wanted to work in an intensive care unit but decided after 6 months that was not the area for you, can you transfer to another unit without losing your sign-on bonus?

Most employers offer similar types of benefits in their total compensation packages. For example, most employers have some type of specific traditional plan. Some may even have a flexible plan that offers a number of options from which to choose (Table 3-1).

Take a few minutes to look at some of the basic benefits that you will need to decide on.

Health, Dental, and Vision Insurance. Health insurance may be contracted through companies such as Blue Cross/Blue Shield, Prudential, Metropolitan Life, and Mutual of Omaha, to name just a few. With these plans, often you select your physician and health care facility from a list of "preferred providers" (or preferred provider organization [PPO]). You may also choose your own physician, but if he/she

BOX 3-6 Benefit Package Options

- Health and life insurance
- Accidental death and dismemberment coverage
- Sick or short-term disability pay
- Vacation pay
- Profit-sharing and retirement plan
- Long-term disability leave
- Dental and/or vision care
- Parking
- Tuition reimbursement
- Loan programs
- Dependent care programs
- Health and wellness programs

TABLE 3-1

Health Insurance Terms You Need to Know

Term	Definition
Coinsurance	The portion of your medical bills that you are responsible for paying after you have met the deductible. A ratio of 80/20 is standard, with you paying 20%.
Exclusions	Specific items not covered under your policy. Some policies exclude physical examinations, and health carriers can now legally exclude the treatment of AIDS.
First-dollar coverage	This policy pays all medical bills without a deductible. Almost impossible to find because coverage is so expensive.
Precertification	Some carriers require preapproval for receiving nonemergency treatments. These carriers may not cover certain treatments or will pay only partial benefits if precertification is not acquired. Your physician should be aware of this when choosing treatment methods for you.
Preexisting condition	An illness or condition you have before your policy is issued. Some preexisting conditions are never covered. Most companies will not pay for the treatment of a preexisting condition for at least a year after your policy is effective.
PPO	Under a PPO system, the list of health care providers from whom you can choose is limited. Your physician may not be included on that list.
Reasonable and customary	The rates generally charged for specific treatments in your area. If a physician's fees are considerably higher than the fees charged by most physicians, your insurance company may cover only partial fees.
Waiting period	The period of time at the start of your coverage during which your carrier will not pay for certain treatments.

is not part of the hospital's insurance plan, you will pay more for services. Check to see what the co-payments are and if the insurance companies pay for well visits or physical examinations. Coverage with some health plans begins on the first day of employment, but not always. Waiting periods may be as long as 3 to 6 months. Also check to see if there is a prescription drug plan included. All of these are subject to the conditions of each individual plan.

Other plans give you the opportunity to go to health maintenance organizations. In this situation, your family must go to a specified group of physicians or other health care professionals to get benefit coverage for the service. These services are covered on a prepaid basis. Usually your out-of-pocket expenses with health maintenance organizations are less. Table 3-1 provides a description of various health insurance terms that you need to know to objectively evaluate the types of insurance coverage offered.

Vision plans and dental plans may cover regular examinations and provide for corrective lenses or preventive dental work. Most often these are offered for an additional rate and are not covered under your general health insurance.

Whatever plan you choose, be sure to determine whether or not you want to arrange coverage for your dependents or spouse. After you terminate your employment at that facility, do not forget that the institution is required by law to offer you continued coverage (COBRA) at your expense for your health insurance for a specified period of time.

Life Insurance and Death and Dismemberment. Check to see what type of basic life insurance is offered by your employer. The amount of the coverage could be fixed at an amount or it might be based on a percentage of your salary. Often, this life insurance is available upon employment and may not cost you a penny. Take advantage of this. This is a smart decision. Here's a tip: It is certainly easier and often less expensive to purchase life insurance when you are just starting your career.

Disability Coverage. Short-term and long-term disability coverage becomes effective if you are unable to work, either temporarily or permanently. This is helpful to you because you can collect a major percentage of your salary while disabled.

Vacation and Sick Leave. Time off, in days or hours, is accrued during pay periods. These plans often give you a certain number of days based on your length of employment. Determine at what point after employment you will begin to accrue vacation time and sick leave. Some institutions may give you a percentage of pay or a dollar amount if you do not use your accrued or allocated leave.

Education Assistance. Employers often offer incentives for you to go back to school, ranging from the provision of a flexible work schedule to tuition reimbursement for continuing-education credits or degree completion. Check to see if the employer you are interviewing offers this benefit.

Pensions, Tax Deferments, Annuities, and Savings Plans. You are never too young to think about retirement. Usually a percentage of your paycheck is automatically deducted and placed into your retirement fund each pay period. The deduction may be a contribution to Medicare, to social security, or to a tax-sheltered optional retirement program.

Some of the tax-sheltered optional retirement programs allow taxes to be deferred until you make a withdrawal from these funds.

Reimbursement Accounts ("Cafeteria Plans"). These are reimbursement spending accounts that operate under Section 125 of the Internal Revenue Service Code. Employers may offer employees two different types of reimbursement accounts: health care and dependent day care. Each item is paid for with pretax dollars. This may translate into a big savings for you. Pension plans may require an even longer time before an employee is eligible to participate or at least be "vested." Vested means that the money that the institution invests in your retirement fund actually belongs to you after a specified period of time.

Dependent Care for Children and Elderly Family Members. Be sure to check with your employer to see what kind of on-site care or financial assistance may be available to your children or elderly family members.

Health-Wellness Programs. You may wish to participate in a health-wellness program, which might include instruction in smoking cessation, weight reduction, and fitness in addition to employee assistance programs. These may be available to promote a healthy lifestyle, which reduces employee absence and increases productivity.

When doing your job search, reviewing benefits is a major part of your decision. Therefore, as a new graduate, be sure to familiarize yourself with all the options that are available to you. The human resources department of the hospital or institution will be able to answer your questions. The decisions you make soon after graduation as well as in the early months of employment will have a far-reaching effect on your future.

JOB OFFERS AND POSSIBLE REJECTION

Let us consider a positive outcome first. If you are offered a position during or at the end of the interview, three possible reactions are likely:

- You are not ready to say yes or no. This is your first interview, and you have two more interviews scheduled.
- You would like very much to work here. The job offer is just what you are looking for.
- You do not want the position. It is not what you thought it would be, or something about the institution has created a negative impression.

Whichever decision you make about the job offer, the following are helpful tips for your response:

1. Be honest. If you have other interviews to complete, say so. Be prepared to tell the interviewer when you will make your decision about the job offer.
2. Avoid being pressured to say "yes" if you are not ready to commit to the job or feel that the position does not meet your needs.
3. Be polite. Ask for some time to consider the offer if you are unsure of what you want to do at present.
4. If you know the offer does not interest you, decline the offer graciously and express appreciation for the company's interest in you.
5. Accept the offer and smile!

Suppose you receive a rejection or no job offer for the position, despite your interest and preparation. Before you leave in a state of dejection, find the courage to ask for a possible explanation if it has not been made clear at this point. If you do not find out about the rejection until later, consider calling the interviewer for this information. Check the following list for common reasons an institution may not offer you a job. See if any of these factors might apply to you:

Lack of opening for your interests and skills. They liked you but could not find a spot right now, or a more qualified candidate was selected for the position.

Poor personal appearance, including inappropriate clothes. You stopped by for the interview on your way to work out.

Lack of preparation for the interview. You were unable to answer questions intelligently or showed lack of knowledge of, or interest in, the employer.

Your answers were superficial or filled with "I don't know."

Poor attitude, dominated by "What's in this for me?" instead of "How can I contribute to the organization?" Your first question focused on salary and perks.

Answers and behavior reflected conceit, arrogance, poor self-confidence, or lack of manners or poise. They should hire you just because you showed up! Or a resume and responses that did not reflect initiative, achievements, or reliable work history.

You have no goals or future orientation. After all, you just want a job, and they should hire you because there is a nursing shortage.

Perceived lack of leadership potential. You like being a follower in all situations and do not want to make decisions. If this scenario sounds like you, rethink your approach.

All nurses are expected to be a leader whether in a formal or informal role. In your next interview, ask the interviewer how the organization supports the development of leadership in new graduates.

Poor academic record without a reasonable explanation. You worked as hard as you could in school, but the teachers did not like you; you lacked appropriate references; or your references were not available or did not reflect favorably on you. All experiences provide us with an opportunity for growth, especially the negative ones. Avoid blaming others for your shortcomings, and look for ways to grow from the experience.

Lack of flexibility. Unwilling to begin work in an area that is not your first or second choice. Consider how rigid you can afford to be at this particular point in time or at this institution.

If at first you don't succeed, try, try again.

POSTINTERVIEW PROCESS

Now that the interview is over, you may want to relax, celebrate, or jump in your car to make your next interview appointment. Stop for a few minutes, and jot down some notes about the interview. This is particularly important if you have another interview the same day. Critique the interview. Consider the following questions:

1. What do you think were your strengths and weaknesses?
2. Is there anything you wish you had or had not said? Why?
3. Were there any surprises?
4. How do you feel you handled the situation?
5. What can you do differently the next time?

Be sure to write down details about the job, which will help you decide on its relative merits and drawbacks. If you do not do this, you may not be able to distinguish job A from job B by the time the interviews are finished. You may experience information overload after a number of interviews, but if you have taken notes about each, the sorting-out process will be easier (see Figure 3-7).

After the interviews are over, rank your job offers against your personal list of priorities to make an informed choice. This may be an unnecessary step for you if you were sold on a particular interview. However, it is a good idea to consider interviewing with at least two institutions, if only to strengthen your decision about the first interview. It will help eliminate possible doubts about your choice later on. If there is a job you think you are really interested in, do a couple of other interviews first. This will give you some experience in interviewing. You may then be able to conduct a more positive interview for the position in which you are really interested. More interviews may also open your eyes to other possibilities.

FOLLOW-UP COMMUNICATION

Remember how nice it is to get a thank-you note in the mail or a telephone call of appreciation? Well, the same idea carries over to the work world: Write those letters!

Follow-up Letter. Take a few minutes to write a note of thanks to the interviewer for the time and interest spent on your behalf (Hawke, 2004). You may want to include additional information in the note: your continuing interest in the position if you hope an offer will be made, the date you will be making your job decision, additional thanks for any special efforts extended to you (lunch, individualized tour), and any change in telephone numbers and appropriate times when they may be able to contact you. Use plain thank-you note cards, not frilly or cute. This is a situation where a handwritten note is certainly acceptable, just make sure it is legible and neat. Recruiters frequently comment on the positive aspect of a follow-up letter, and it may serve to keep your name at the top of the list because of your attention to interpersonal communication. It also helps to "separate you from the pack of applicants."

Letters of Rejection. As soon as you make up your mind regarding job offers, notify other prospective employers of your decision. Decline their job offer graciously, and include an expression of appreciation for their interest in you. The format for this letter should follow the standard rules of business letters. Remember, you have accepted a position elsewhere, but your career could take a turn in the future that may bring you back to the institution you are now declining. Leave a positive impression with human resources and recruitment.

Telephone Follow-up. On the basis of the interview, you should have a pretty clear idea of the "how" and "when" of further contact. A telephone call may be appropriate when you have not heard from a recruiter by an agreed-upon date. You can contact a recruiter or interviewer by telephone to decline a job offer, but a personal letter is preferable to leaving a telephone message. Remember to be unfailingly polite to everyone you speak to on the telephone. Secretaries and other support personnel will remember and pass on unfavorable impressions to their superiors. Recruiters do not want to hire staff that is rude or impatient. They know that this behavior is likely to be shown toward patients and families as well.

WHAT IF I DO NOT LIKE MY FIRST POSITION?

It is not uncommon to experience frustrations during your first work experience. Go back to Chapter 1 on transitions and reality shock, and review it for some suggestions on how to handle your situation. You also need to keep in touch with the nurse recruiter who hired you. Nurse recruiters can offer further support and assistance. Recruiters know where other recent graduates are working in the institution and may provide you with a network of individuals who can offer suggestions and support to improve your situation. In addition, recruiters also know the staffing needs of other areas in the hospital and may suggest transferring. A good way to get an idea of other areas where you may be interested in working is to "shadow" a staff nurse in that area. This means you would spend a day "shadowing" this staff nurse as they perform their job. This provides you with a good insight as to what the job requires and the working conditions of that area. When you take your first position, plan on staying there for at least a year. You want to avoid "job hopping," or changing jobs whenever you do not like what is going on with your current position. Remember, other positions have their benefits and problems; the grass may not be greener on the other side of the fence.

Don't trade one set of problems for another set that may be even more difficult.

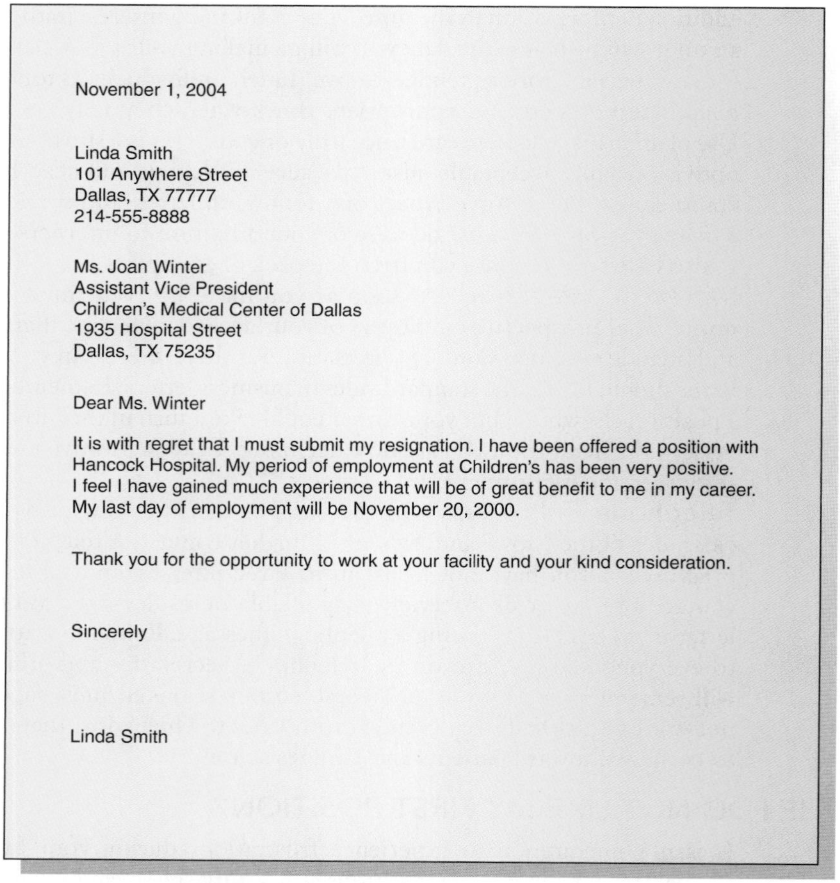

November 1, 2004

Linda Smith
101 Anywhere Street
Dallas, TX 77777
214-555-8888

Ms. Joan Winter
Assistant Vice President
Children's Medical Center of Dallas
1935 Hospital Street
Dallas, TX 75235

Dear Ms. Winter

It is with regret that I must submit my resignation. I have been offered a position with Hancock Hospital. My period of employment at Children's has been very positive. I feel I have gained much experience that will be of great benefit to me in my career. My last day of employment will be November 20, 2000.

Thank you for the opportunity to work at your facility and your kind consideration.

Sincerely

Linda Smith

FIGURE 3-9
Letter of resignation.

WHAT IF IT IS TIME FOR ME TO CHANGE POSITIONS?

If you think it is time to change positions or explore other options, it is important to submit a letter of resignation (Figure 3-9). Give at least 2 weeks notice. Check your contract to see if you agreed to give more than 2 weeks notice, and, if possible, give 4 weeks notice. If you are leaving on less than amicable terms, do not express this in your resignation letter. You can always take grievances to the personnel or human resources department.

CONCLUSION

Searching for and finding your niche in the workplace can sometimes be overwhelming. Take the plunge and start looking. Keep a positive outlook because just the job you are looking for is out there. This is one of those situations in which a little preparation and investigation goes a long way in finding what you want. Get your resume together and start investigaing what is out there for you. A basic understanding of the process of job hunting can go a long way to minimize the frustrations and promote a positive first-job experience. Good luck with your job search.

Success lies not in achieving what you aim at, but in aiming at what you want to achieve.

REFERENCES

CBS News: *Nursing shortage in critical stage*, January 17, 2003, *www.cbsnews.com/stories/2003/01/17/60 minutes/main536999.shtml.*

Croteau L: Tips for successful interviewing, *Nursing Spectrum*, 2004, *http://community.nursingspectrum. com/magazine articles/article.cfm?AID=7971.*

Feery B, Tierney C: How to create a job winning resume, *NSNA/Imprint*, January 2002, pp 51-55.

Hawke M: Ten killer interview tips, *Nursing Spectrum*, 2004, *http://communitynursingspectrum.com/magazine articles/article.cfm?AID=10637.*

Joel LA: Shifting sands, *Am J Nurs* 97(9):7, 1997.

Nursing Facts: *Todays registered nurse-numbers and demographics*, 2005, American Nurses Association, *www.nursingworld.org/readroom/fsdemogrpt/.htm.*

Restifo V: The successful interview, *NSNA/Imprint*, January 2002, p 40.

Valentino LM: Future employment trends in nursing. The nursing shortage has struck just about everywhere in the United States and there's no relief in sight—but its effects vary by region and specialty. *Am J Nurs* 102(suppl 1):248, 2002.

CHAPTER 4

Mentoring and Preceptorship

JOANN ZERWEKH, EdD, RN, FNP, APRN, BC
ASHLEY MARIE ZERWEKH, BA, RN

It is one of the most beautiful compensations of life—that no man can sincerely try to help another without helping himself.
—Ralph Waldo Emerson

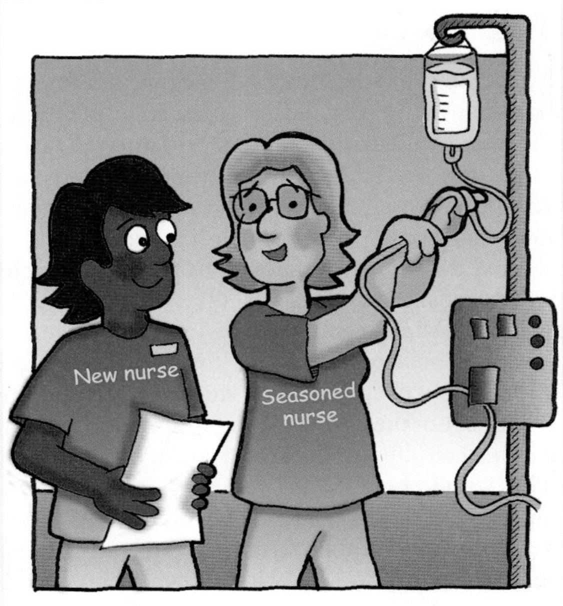

Mentoring is one of the broadest methods of encouraging human growth and potential.

After completing this chapter, you should be able to:

- Describe the difference between mentoring, coaching, and precepting.
- Identify characteristics of effective mentors and mentees.
- Discuss the types of mentoring relationships.

It was my first day as a nurse extern in a busy medical intensive care unit. As I walked into my new place of work, I saw nurses on the phones, talking with doctors and running in and out of patient's rooms with stern looks on their faces. So many questions were going through my head. Which one of these nurses was my preceptor? What would my preceptor expect from me? Would he or she be receptive to helping me develop into my role as a nurse? I entered the room where the nurses receive report from the night staff. It was there that I had my first encounter with Julie, who would become my preceptor, nursing role-model, and mentor in the months ahead.—Ashley

HISTORICAL BACKGROUND

Did you ever wonder where the word *mentor* originated? It originated from Greek mythology. Mentor was the name of a wise and faithful advisor to Odysseus. When Odysseus (or Ulysses, as the Romans called him) left for his long voyage during the Trojan War, he entrusted the direction and teaching of his son, Telemachus, to Mentor. According to mythology, through Mentor's guidance, Telemachus became an effective and beloved ruler (Shea, 1999). "Mentoring is a fundamental form of development where one person invests time, energy, and personal know-how in assisting the growth and ability of another person" (Brown, 2003). Mentor's job was not merely to raise Telemachus, but to develop him for the responsibilities he was to assume in his lifetime. Mentoring is one of the broadest methods for encouraging human growth and potential.

WHAT MENTORING IS AND IS NOT

Mentoring is often confused with coaching or precepting. Coaching is a somewhat new approach to assisting individuals to grow by partnering with a colleague or individual, who is an equal, where one person focuses on the unique and internal qualities observed within the other person that may not be recognized or appreciated. In the business world, executives are referring to themselves as coaches rather than managers, which fosters a team and collaboration approach. Coaches help individuals find new ways to solve problems, reach goals, and design plans of action to motivate people to perform at the "top of their game." According to Guest (1999), "…the strength of mentoring lies in the mentor's specific knowledge and wisdom, in coaching it lies in the facilitation and development of personal qualities. The coach brings different skills and experience and offers a fresh perspective, a different viewpoint. In both cases one-to-one attention is the key." Based on these definitions, "A good coach will mentor; and, a good mentor will coach, according to the situation. In considering the best fit, therefore, the two approaches should be regarded as synergistic and complementary, rather than mutually exclusive" (Guest, 1999).

What about preceptors? The term *preceptor* simply means "tutor," and generally refers to a more formal arrangement that pairs a novice with an experienced person for a set period of time, with a focus on policies, procedures, and skill development. Preceptors serve as role models and precept during their regularly scheduled work hours, which is part of their work assignment, in contrast with mentors, who are chosen, not assigned, and focus on fostering the mentee's individual growth and

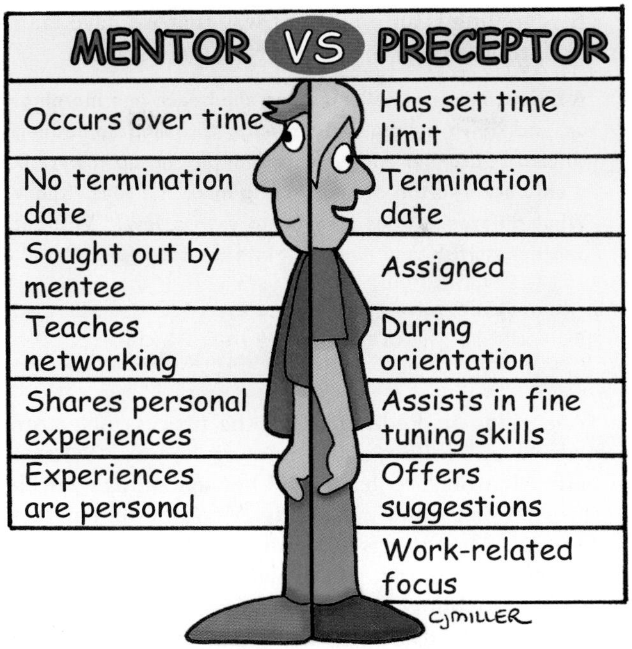
MENTOR VS PRECEPTOR
Occurs over time
Has set time limit
No termination date
Termination date
Sought out by mentee
Assigned
Teaches networking
During orientation
Shares personal experiences
Assists in fine tuning skills
Experiences are personal
Offers suggestions
Work-related focus
CJMILLER

FIGURE 4-1
Mentor versus preceptor.

development over an extended period of time. Mentors develop a professionally based, nurturing relationship, which generally occurs during personal time (Figure 4-1).

When I was in nursing school, I thought that preceptor was just a fancy term for mentor. However, I found out these two terms are very different from each other.—Ashley

In nursing, the word mentor has become synonymous with trusted advisor, friend, teacher, guide, and wise person. There have been many attempts at deriving a single definition of mentoring. Gibbons (2004) provides a detailed listing of 16 (yes, 16!) different mentor definitions. Why is mentoring so different and "special" and more encompassing than precepting and coaching?

- Mentoring requires a primary focus on the needs of the mentee and an effort to fulfill the most critical of these needs.
- Mentoring requires going the extra mile for someone else. The rewards of mentoring are enormous: a sense of personal achievement, mentee appreciation, and a sense of building a better organization.
- Mentoring is a partnership created between two people; the mentor possesses the educational degree to which the mentee aspires (Shea, 1999).

As you read through this chapter, try to develop your own definition of a mentor.

Storytelling is an important way that we have taught one another since the beginning of time. Following is a story about a starfish:

> A beachcomber is walking along the beach one morning when he sees a young man running up and down by the water's edge throwing something into the water. Curious, he walks toward the runner and watches him picking up the starfish stranded by the tide and tossing them back into the ocean. "Young man," he says, "there are so many starfish on the beach. What difference does it make to save a few?" Without pausing, the young man picks up another starfish, and flinging it into the sea replies, "It made a difference for this one."

That is what mentors do. They make a difference for one person at a time.

According to Peddy (1998), the process of mentoring can be described in eight words, "Lead, follow, and get out of the way." What does this mean?

Lead: Mentors are leaders. They encourage another's growth and development, professionally and personally. Mentors help and inspire mentees by acting as role models. The focus is on wisdom and judgment. The mentor plays a very active role: teaching, coaching, and explaining, while supporting and shaping critical thinking skills, providing invaluable advice when asked, and introducing the mentee to committees, advancements, and honors.

Follow: This is where mentees need to "get their feet wet." This is where the mentor and mentee walk the path together. At this stage, the advisor (mentor) assumes a more passive role. It is now up to the learner (mentee) to seek the advice or listening ear of the mentor.

Get out of the way: This means knowing when it is time to let go. If you have ever taught a child to swim or ride a bike, you know how hard it is to "let go" and let the child soar on their own. A helping relationship is a freeing relationship. This does not have to be a terminal relationship; you share common values and beliefs in lifelong learning.

This dynamic process of mentoring is not static. A mentor's task of self-development, learning, and mastery is never done. Each person in the mentoring process has a role. Mentors generally have more experience and are dedicated to helping mentees advance in their careers, especially in work/life skill issues. Mentoring is a two-way street, a partnership, with both parties freely contributing to the relationship as equals working together, based on mutual respect.

> On a personal note, when I think about mentors that I have had, one person comes to mind: Satora. She was my first mentor when I started working in the ICU after graduating with my diploma in nursing. She personified all that a new graduate would want in a mentor. She was understanding, patient, and compassionate, and she possessed extensive experience. She made an important, long-lasting impact on my nursing career. She nurtured me and encouraged me to reach within myself to become the nurse that I am today. I will never forget her.
>
> Approximately 25 years after I left the ICU, I had the opportunity to talk with Satora by phone. It was one of those coincidences or synchronistic moments in which I was able, via a mutual friend, to find out where she was working. I had lost contact with her over the years and in the several moves that I had made to different places. She was so surprised that I had

called, and I shared with her how important our mentoring relationship had been to me. It made me feel good to pass along my gratitude for her willingness to mentor me.—JoAnn

HOW TO FIND A MENTOR

The key to finding a mentor is having an open-mind, being flexible, and remaining optimistic. As you finish nursing school and while you are in school, write down the goals you feel a mentor will help you achieve. Keep this list of goals with you while you are working, and try to get a feel for the different personality types that you will see as a nurse among your coworkers.

When I was in my orientation program after I received my RN, my mentor Julie shared with me a saying that I will share with you, "Always remember the patient comes first." This stuck with me because it helped me realize that our jobs as nurses are not only valuable but powerful in the sense that we make an impact in people's lives everyday.—Ashley

As you progress through your nursing program, you should consider establishing a mentoring relationship. Having the feeling of comfort and building trust with this person is crucial to the process of mentoring. Here are some ideas/strategies to think about:

- Look for common background in either nursing education or an area of expertise/practice or interest.
- Tell the person about yourself. When you disclose something about yourself, it is especially helpful if you can laugh about yourself in a given situation. This sets the tone of the interaction. It is helpful to keep it light and friendly.
- Ask broad, open-ended questions such as, "How are things going?" that stimulate open discussion rather than direct questions such as, "How do you like working here?" or "What kind of problems are you having?" that make the other person feel vulnerable.
- By starting out with these basic questions, you can begin to determine a level of comfort about the person. Next, let us examine the characteristics of a typical mentor.

WHAT ARE THE CHARACTERISTICS OF A SUCCESSFUL MENTOR?

When I think about the desired characteristics or competencies of a successful mentor, the following comes to mind:

- A mentor communicates **high expectations**. Mentors push mentees and provide avenues and opportunities for them to grow. They allow the mentees to learn through many of their own failures. The mentee grows and develops through active listening, role modeling, and open communication with the mentor. When mentors act as sources of intellectual stimulation and encouragement, they encourage their mentees to trust their own abilities and skills. Mentors open doors and encourage their mentees to search out and seek professional avenues that mentees might not have known about or would have taken longer to discover their own. Rather than being the "sage on the stage," the mentor is the "guide on the side."
- A mentor is also a **good listener**. Mentors provide the nonjudgmental, listening ear, without taking on the mentees' problems, giving advice, or joining them in an "ain't it awful" game, which can serve as a powerful aid to a mentee. Many mentors believe that respectful listening is the premier mentoring act. When two people really listen to each other, a wonderful sense of synergy is created.

- A mentor has **empathy**. A mentor has a degree of sensitivity and perception as to the needs of the mentee and has an ability to teach others in an unselfish, respectful way that does not blame, but stays neutral. Mentors know what it is like to be the "new kid on the block."
- A mentor offers **encouragement**. By providing subtle guidance and reassurance of decisions made by the mentee, the mentor values the mentee's experience, ideas, knowledge of how things work, and special insights into problems. Mentors strive to promote independence with their mentees by offering suggestions, but not pushing, as growth depends on the mentee solving their own problems.
- A mentor is **generous**. Mentors are willing to share their time and knowledge with others. Much of what the mentor offers is personal learning or insight (Shea, 1999).

Wilson (2001) describes character traits of a good mentor. These include such traits as "humorous, honest, dedicated, empathetic, compassionate, genuine, patient, nonsexist, flexible, and loyal." Wilson further identifies four core values that are essential to the mentoring relationship and include integrity, courage, caring, and trust. These character traits make the mentor approachable and desirable as a role model as well as a facilitator of the mentor/mentee relationship (Critical Thinking Box 4-1 and Figure 4-2).

WHAT IS A MENTORING MOMENT?

Have you ever experienced a flash of insight or a revelation? Peddy (2001) calls this a "mentoring moment." How do you know when that moment arrives? Someone once said, "When the student is ready, the teacher appears" (Peddy, 2001). According to Peddy, mentoring is often built on a just-in-time principle whereby the mentor offers the right help at the right time. A potential mentor must recognize when the mentee feels free to expose a deep-felt need, thereby enabling the mentor to provide the right help at the right time to the best of the mentor's ability.

WHEN DO WE NEED MENTORS?

A mentor is an established professional (selected by you) who takes a long-term personal interest in your nursing career. The mentor not only serves as a role model or counselor for you but also actively advises, guides, and promotes you in your career. A mentor can be any successful, experienced nurse who is committed to a professional career and to being a key figure in your life for a number of years while you are going through school, as well as when you graduate. Mentors should have your best interest at heart and bolster your self-confidence. Mentors should be able to give feedback in a highly constructive, supportive atmosphere. As a result, trust and caring are hallmarks of the bonding that occurs between mentor and mentee. In short, a mentor is "a wise and trusted adviser," who can serve you well as you progress through school (Figure 4-3).

CRITICAL THINKING BOX 4-1

Which of these traits appeal to you the most? Which ones would be the most important for your mentor to have?

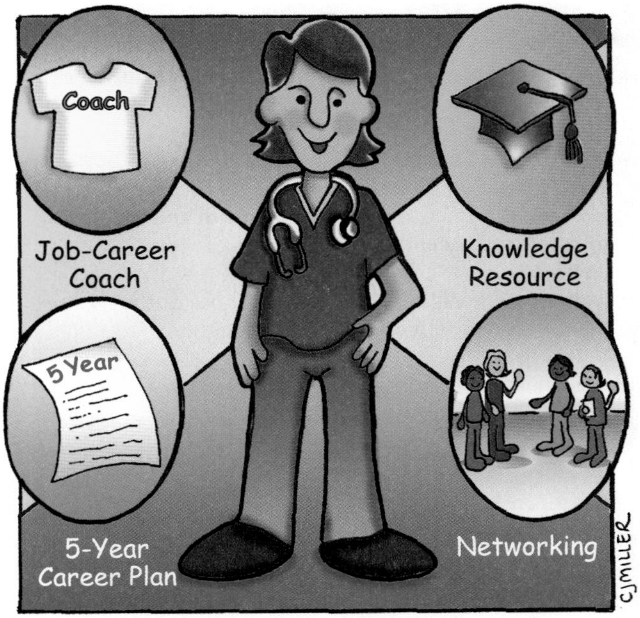

FIGURE 4-2
Expectations of a mentor.

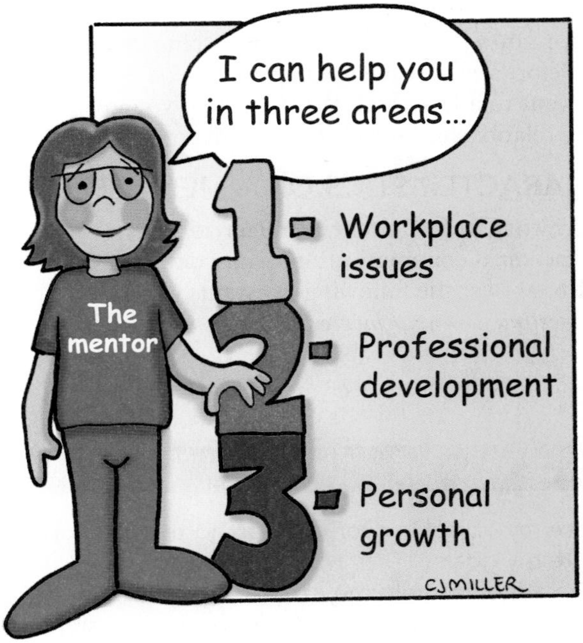
I can help you in three areas...
The mentor
1
Workplace issues
2
Professional development
3
Personal growth
CJMILLER

FIGURE 4-3
The mentor role.

BOX 4-1 Characteristics of Successful Mentors

- Make a personal commitment to be involved with mentee for an extended period of time
- Are trustworthy and sincere
- Show mutual respect
- Are not in a position of authority over the mentee
- Promote an easy, give-and-take relationship and are flexible and open
- Able to listen and accept different points of view
- Are experienced
- Have values and goals compatible with those of the mentee
- Are able to empathize with mentee's struggles
- Are nurturing
- Have a good sense of humor and enjoy nursing!

A mentoring relationship is an evolving, personal experience for both mentor and mentee. It involves a personal investment of the mentor in the direction of the mentee's professional development. The mentor also benefits from the association by gaining an awareness and perspective of the recent mentee's role in nursing. Take note of the characteristics of successful mentors in Box 4-1.

WHAT IS THE ROLE OF THE MENTEE?

As a mentee, you will be learning and absorbing the useful information that the mentor provides. Before seeking a mentor in your new job establishment, there are a few questions you may want to ask yourself that may help you get exactly what you need from the mentoring relationship (see Critical Thinking Box 4-2) (Shea, 1999).

WHAT ARE THE CHARACTERISTICS OF A MENTEE?

Just exactly what are important characteristics that you, as a mentee, should project in your interpersonal communications with your mentor? Use the following checklist in Table 4-1 to answer the following questions.

When meeting with your mentor, do you …

CRITICAL THINKING BOX 4-2

What are my objectives for developing this mentoring relationship?
What are my goals?
How can a mentor help me achieve my goals?
What is the best way for me to approach a possible mentor to gain his or her interest in developing a mentoring relationship?

TABLE 4-1

Mentor Checklist

	Always	Frequently	Usually	Seldom	Never	Score
Communicate clearly						
Welcome your mentor's input (express appreciation or tell him or her how it will benefit you)						
Accept constructive feedback						
Practice openness and sincerity						
Take initiative to maintain the relationship with your mentor						
Actively explore options with your mentor						
Share results with your mentor						
Listen for the whole message, including mentor's feelings						
Be alert for mentor's nonverbal communication, and use it as data						

Score yourself as follows: Always = 10; frequently = 8; usually = 6; seldom = 4; never =2. According to Shea, a score of 80 or better means you are among the limited group of individuals who have good mentee interaction skills (Shea, 1999, p 46).
Adapted from Shea GF: *Making the most of being mentored: how to grow from a mentoring relationship*, Lanham, Md, 1999, Crisp Publications.

How did you score? Are there areas that you need to improve in your interpersonal skills to make you a better mentee?

WHAT ARE THE TYPES OF MENTORING RELATIONSHIPS?

There are several types of mentoring relationships that you may experience when you develop an active mentoring relationship with your mentor (Table 4-2). Formal, informal, and situational mentoring relationships are three types that are commonly encountered (Shea, 1999).

MENTORING THROUGH REALITY SHOCK

The hospital setting is the largest setting where nurses work. Formal preceptorship programs have been initiated, and a mentoring environment is fostered for the new

TABLE 4-2

Types of Mentoring Relationships

	Formal	Informal	Situational
Structure	Traditional/structured	Voluntary/very flexible	Brief contact/often casual
Characteristic	Driven by organizational needs	Mutual acceptance of roles	A one-time event
Effectiveness	Results measured by organization frequently	Periodic check-ups by supervisors	Results assessed later

Adapted from: Shea GF: *Making the most of being mentored: how to grow from a mentoring partnership*, Lanham, Md, 1999, Crisp Publications, pp 73-75.

graduate to address the issues of reality shock. This type of mentoring setting appeals to many new graduates, because you have support from other health care team members. Remember Kramer's phases of reality shock in Chapter 1? Let us see how an effective mentorship relationship could address each of the phases.

Honeymoon phase: The mentor can be supportive by listening and understanding when the mentee shares the excitement of starting their new position and passing NCLEX. The mentor can act as an intermediary with other staff members and as a role model.

Shock or rejection phase: Mentors can encourage mentees to discuss their feelings of disillusionment and frustration, as well as share their own personal transition process through this phase. Asking the mentee to write down their feelings (keep a reflection journal) or discuss ideas to make changes to the situation can be helpful in mitigating the feelings associated with this phase.

Recovery phase: The mentor's role during this phase, as mentees begin to accept the reality of the situation and put issues in perspective, is to maintain an open channel of communication and encouraging them to "step outside their comfort zone" and try new things.

Resolution phase: Mentors are very instrumental during this phase to reinforce positive qualities that the mentee possesses and to encourage the mentee in problem-solving any issues relating to the desire to either change nursing positions or to stay put. *It is important to remember that any nurse may experience reality shock throughout her/his career when she/he enters a new work area.* (Brunt, 2005)

WHAT DOES THE FUTURE HOLD?

The future of mentoring programs is changing. Due to the technological advancement with offering nursing programs online, there is a new wave of mentoring known as e-mentoring. The term *e-mentoring* has been coined to mean, "the mentoring that takes place over a distance, usually by electronic communication facilitation" (Knight, 2004). According to Knight, relationships that are more personal are possible to develop through electronic communications (e-mail), and without face-to-face meetings, but the individual must be comfortable with nonvisual forms of communication.

Peer mentoring programs are developing in campuses in the Midwest region of the United States. These programs allow senior-level nursing students to mentor entering freshman nursing students. According to Sprengel (2004), "The peer mentoring teaching strategy was designed to lessen freshmen anxiety associated with their initial clinical experience and to introduce them to the role of the student nurse in the clinical setting."

CONCLUSION

Here is one final note about mentorship: There is a short anecdotal story about "Everybody, Somebody, Anybody, and Nobody" that has become part of Internet lore. I think you will understand that Everybody has to realize the importance of advancing the field of nursing through mentorship; your task will be to find that Somebody willing to extend a hand to guide you through the process.

> **There was an important job to be done, and Everybody was sure that Somebody would do it. Anybody could have done it, but Nobody did it. Somebody got angry about that, because it was Everybody's job. Everybody thought Anybody could do it, but Nobody realized that Everybody wouldn't do it. It ended up that Everybody blamed Somebody, when Nobody did what Anybody could have.**

Mentoring is a complex, interpersonal, emotional relationship. All parties involved in a mentoring relationship benefit from a mutual exchange of information, life experiences, and diversity. Mentoring is defined as a developmental, empowering, and nurturing relationship that extends over time (Vance & Olson, 1998). It involves mutual sharing, learning, and growth that occur in an atmosphere of respect and affirmation (Bower, 2000). A mentor has been described as a role model and guide who encourages and inspires. We leave you with this thought…

There are two ways of spreading light: to be the candle or the mirror that receives it.

—Edith Wharton

REFERENCES

Bower E: Mentoring others. In Bower EL (Ed.): *Nurses taking the lead,* Philadelphia, 2000, Saunders, pp 11-14.

Brown M: *Mentoring/coaching module.* Retrieved June 30, 2003, from the Department of Information and Library Science Southern Connecticut State University website at *www.southernct.edu/~brownm/mentoring.html.*

Brunt B: *Beyond precepting: developing mentor skills.* Retrieved April 30, 2005, from *www.nursce.com/courses/1067/1067.htm.*

Coach and mentor definitions, The Coaching and Mentoring Network. Retrieved April 30, 2005, from *www.coachingnetwork.org.uk/ResourceCentre/WhatAreCoachingAndMentoring.htm.*

Gibbons A: *Mentoring definitions.* Retrieved April 14, 2004, from *www.coachingnetwork.org.uk/ResourceCentre/Articles/ViewArticle.asp?artId=54.*

Guest AB: A coach, a mentor… a what?, *Success Now* 13, 1999.

Knight D: *Mentoring an online toolkit: what is E-mentoring?* Retrieved April 14, 2004, from the Industry

Canada SchoolNet website at *www.schoolnet.ca/nis-rei/e/mentoring_WEBSITE/primer2.html#6*.

Peddy S: *The art of mentoring*, Houston, 1998, Bullion Books.

Shea G: *Making the most of being mentored: how to grow from a mentoring relationship*, Lanham, Md, 1999, Crisp Publications.

Shea G: *Mentoring: how to develop successful mentor behaviors*, Lanham, Md, 2002, Crisp Publications.

Sprengel A: Reducing student anxiety by using clinical peer mentoring with beginning nursing students, *Nurse Educator* 29(6):246-250, 2004.

Starcevich MM: *Coach, mentor: is there a difference?* Retrieved April 30, 2005, from *www.coachingandmentoring.com/Articles/mentoring.html.*

Vance C: Discovering the riches in mentor connections, *Reflections on nursing leadership: Sigma Theta Tau International Honor Society of Nursing* 26(3): 24-25. Retrieved June 30, 2003, from the EBSCO-host database.

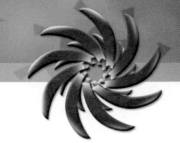

CHAPTER 5

NCLEX-RN AND THE NEW GRADUATE

JO CAROL CLABORN, MS, RN, CNS

The way I see it, if you want the rainbow, you gotta put up with the rain.
—*Dolly Parton*

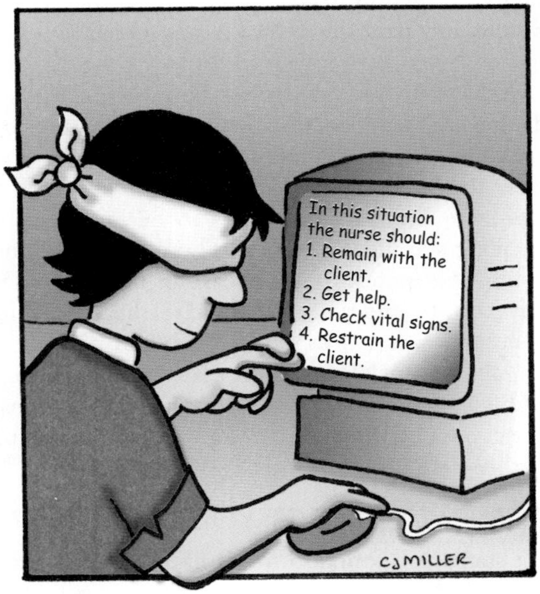
In this situation
the nurse should:
1. Remain with the client.
2. Get help.
3. Check vital signs.
4. Restrain the client.
CJ MILLER

Do not take any chances. Understand the NCLEX process.

After completing this chapter, you should be able to:

- Discuss the role of the National Council of State Boards of Nursing.
- Discuss the implications of computer adaptive testing.
- Identify the process and steps for preparing to take the National Council Licensure Examination for Registered Nurses (NCLEX-RN).
- Identify criteria for selecting a review book and a review course.

The National Council Licensure Examination for Registered Nurses (NCLEX-RN)—this is the really big test you have been preparing for since you entered nursing school. Your opportunity is getting closer! Consider the opportunity to take the NCLEX-RN a privilege; it took a lot of hard work to achieve this level, and there are a lot of people who never get there! Your passage through the "NCLEX Gate" will begin your transition into professional nursing. As with other aspects of transition, planning begins early, before you graduate. Planning ahead will help you to develop a comprehensive plan on how you want to attack that mountain of material to review. When you plan ahead and know what is expected, it will help decrease your anxiety about the examination. Being prepared and knowing what to expect will help you to maintain a positive attitude.

THE NCLEX-RN

WHO PREPARES IT, AND WHY DO WE HAVE TO HAVE IT?

The National Council of State Boards of Nursing (NCSBN) is the governing body for the committee that prepares the licensure examination. Each member board or state determines the application process and deadlines in their state, in addition to the mechanics of administering the examination. The NCLEX is used to regulate entry into nursing practice in the United States. The NCLEX represents a national examination with standardized scoring. All candidates in every state are presented with questions based on the same test plan. Every state requires the same passing level or standard. There is no discrepancy in passing scores from one state to another. In other words, you cannot go to another state and pass the NCLEX any easier (NCSBN, *NCLEX candidate bulletin*, 2005).

According to the NCSBN, the NCLEX is designed to test "knowledge, skills and abilities essential to the safe and effective practice of nursing at the entry level" (NCSBN, *NCLEX candidate bulletin*, 2005). Upon successful completion of the examination, you will be granted a license to practice nursing in the state in which you applied for licensure. The status of state licensure continues to be in a transition process of its own. It is still experiencing significant change. There are many nurses who maintain a current license in multiple states. The increase in nursing practice across state lines, the growth of managed care, and the advances in telehealth medicine prompted an in-depth research project that was conducted by the NCSBN in the late 1990s. As a result of that research, the Mutual Recognition Model for Multistate Regulation has been implemented. This is frequently referred to as the Nurse Licensure Compact. As of May 2002, the compact has been enacted through the state legislatures of 18 states (NCSBN, *Nurse licensure compact*, 2005).

HOW WILL THE NURSE LICENSURE COMPACT AFFECT YOUR LICENSE?

The nursing license in the compact states will function much like a driver's license. The individual will hold one license issued in the state of residence but will also be responsible for the laws of the state in which they are driving. The individual nurse may practice in another state; however, the nurse must comply with the Nurse Practice Act of the state in which he or she practices. The transition process has begun;

CRITICAL THINKING BOX 5-1

What is the status of the Nurse Licensure Compact in your state?

how fast it is implemented will depend on individual states. The Nurse Licensure Compact must be passed by the state legislature in each participating state. Watch your state nursing organization and Board of Nursing newsletters, or check the website for the NCSBN (*www.ncsbn.org*) to see where your state is in the process of implementing the Interstate Compact on Nurse Licensure (Critical Thinking Box 5-1).

Before the Nurse Licensure Compact is implemented, the respective states will continue to require the nurse to be licensed in the individual state of practice. Transfer of nursing licenses between states is a process called "licensure by endorsement." If you wish to practice in a state in which you are not currently licensed, you must contact the State Board of Nursing in the state in which you wish to practice. The State Board of Nursing will advise you of the process to become licensed in that state (see Appendix B, State Boards of Nursing). Transferring your license to practice from one state to another does not change your successful completion of the NCLEX, nor do you have to take the examination again. All states recognize the successful completion of the NCLEX, regardless of the state in which you took the examination or where your license was issued.

WHAT IS THE NCLEX-RN TEST PLAN?

The content of the NCLEX is based on a test blueprint that is determined by the National Council. The blueprint reflects entry-level nursing practice as identified by research and the Job Analysis Study of Newly Licensed Registered Nurses. This research study is conducted by the National Council every 3 years. The job analysis research in 2003 indicated that the majority of new graduates were continuing to work in a general medical–surgical environment. Most entry-level nurses indicated that they cared for acutely ill patients. The majority of entry-level nurses indicated they cared for adult and geriatric patients who were acutely ill, as well as adults and geriatric clients with stable and unstable chronic conditions. The majority of the new graduates surveyed also indicated their primary responsibility was in the delivery of direct patient care. The hospital and long-term care facilities were the primary employers of the new graduate. A significant number of new graduates indicated that they have administrative responsibilities. The test plan in this chapter was implemented in April 2003 and will be used until April 2006. A new test plan is implemented every 3 years. This represents the time required to conduct the research, analyze the data, and implement a new test plan on NCLEX (Smith, 2003).

The examination is constructed from questions that are designed to test the candidate's ability to apply the nursing process and to determine appropriate nursing responses and interventions to provide safe nursing care. The test plan is organized around client needs. Each of the five phases of the nursing process has equal importance and is equally represented in the test bank. There are four levels of client needs identified in the Job Analysis Study (Wendt, 2003). Each level of client need is assigned a percentage that reflects the weight of that category of client need on the NCLEX-RN. The approximate percentages of each area are:

Safe, Effective Care Environment	
Management of care	13%-19%
Safety and infection control	8%-14%
Health Promotion and Maintenance	6%-12%
Psychosocial Integrity	6%-12%
Physiological Integrity	
Basic care and comfort	6%-12%
Pharmacologic and parenteral therapies	13%-19%
Reduction of risk potential	13%-19%
Physiologic adaptation	11%-17% (Wendt, 2003)

In April 1994, the NCSBN implemented computer adaptive testing (CAT) for the NCLEX for both practical/vocational nurses (NCLEX-PN/VN) and registered nurses (NCLEX-RN). This represented a major advance in the implementation and administration of the examination. The information presented here is a brief introduction to the NCLEX-RN CAT. It is important that you carefully follow the information and instructions you receive in your *NCLEX Candidate Bulletin*, in addition to information from your state board of nursing.

Pearson VUE is the company contracted by the NCSBN to schedule candidates, administer the NCLEX examination, and score the examination. The NCSBN is responsible for the content and development of the test questions, the test plan, policies, and requirements for eligibility for the NCLEX. Pearson VUE will assist you in scheduling your examination and will provide a location and equipment for the administration of the examination.

WHAT DOES CAT MEAN?

With CAT, each candidate receives a different set of questions via the computer. The questions are assembled interactively as the candidate progresses through the examination. The computer develops an examination based on the test plan and selects questions to be presented on the basis of the candidates' responses to the previous question. The number of questions each candidate receives and the testing time for each candidate will vary. As candidates answer questions correctly, the questions will get progressively more difficult. When candidates miss questions, the computer will select an easier question to present. All of the questions presented will reflect the categories of the NCLEX test plan (NCSBN, *NCLEX candidate bulletin*, 2005).

"Pre-test" questions have been integrated into the examination in the past and will continue to be integrated into the current examination. The NCSBN Examination Committee evaluates the statistical information from each of these "pretest" questions to determine if the question is valid and to identify the level of difficulty of the test item (NCSBN, *NCLEX candidate bulletin*, 2005). Do not be alarmed—these questions are not counted in the grading of your examination, and time has been allocated for you to answer these questions. It is impossible to determine which questions are "pretest" questions and which ones are "scored" test questions, so it is important that you answer every question to the very best of your ability.

What Is the Application Process for the NCLEX CAT? In the beginning of the semester in which you will graduate, your school of nursing will have each student complete an application form and send it to the state board of nurse examiners. Upon completion of the nursing program, the school will verify the graduate's status with the board of nursing. The student now becomes a candidate for the NCLEX. After the forms have been processed, each candidate will then receive an Authorization to Test (ATT) with instructions regarding how to schedule your examination. Read your instruction packet and your *Candidate Bulletin* carefully. Keep track of your Authorization to Test. It will be required for scheduling your testing date and for admission into the testing center. Your ATT will contain your authorization number, candidate ID number, and an expiration date. The expiration date cannot be extended for any reason; *you must test within the dates on the ATT*. It is to your advantage to schedule your examination time shortly after receiving your ATT—even if you do not plan to take the test for several weeks. If you need application forms for the examination, they may be obtained by contacting the respective board of nurse examiners. All candidates will be thumb-printed and photographed at the testing location (NCSBN, *NCLEX candidate bulletin*, 2005).

Where Do I Take the Test? There are testing sites in every state. A candidate may take the test at any of the testing sites in the United States; however, license to practice will be issued only in the state where the candidate's application was submitted. Information regarding the location of the centers can be found at the candidate area on the National Council website, as well as in the ATT. There will be several testing stations at each center.

When Do I Take the Test? After receiving the ATT, a candidate may contact the NCLEX Candidate Services at the phone number on the inside cover of the *Candidate Bulletin*, or go online at the NCLEX Candidate website *(www.pearsonvue.com/nclex)* to schedule the examination. The location and telephone numbers of the testing centers and/or the website for scheduling will be included in the information from the NCSBN. Plan to receive your ATT approximately 2 to 3 weeks after you finish school. Remember, you must test within the dates on your ATT. You may schedule your examination as soon as you receive the ATT; this means that you may receive the ATT on Wednesday, call or go online to the location of your choice, and, if you want to, take the examination the next day, if there is space available. Or, call and/or go online and schedule your examination date within the next 3 to 4 weeks.

During the last 2 months of school, begin to make plans for when you would like to take the examination. The examination should be taken within approximately 4 to 6 weeks of graduation. Take into consideration some study time and whether a formal review course is available. It is important that you take the examination soon after graduation. If you wait too long, your level of comprehension of critical information will be decreased. Finish school, take a review course if you would like, get your ATT, and go take the examination. This is not a good time to plan a vacation, bring your mother to live with you, get married, or engage in other activities that cause a crisis in your life (Critical Thinking Box 5-2).

How Much Time Do I Have, and How Many Questions Are There? Each candidate is scheduled for a 6-hour time slot. You should plan to be at the site for 6 hours. Each candidate must answer at least 75 questions. Within those first

CRITICAL THINKING BOX 5-2

When do you want to take your NCLEX? Review Boxes 5-1 through 5-3 to help you get started on thinking about this process.

75 questions, there are 15 pretest items that are not scored on your examination. Whether you answer 76 or 200 questions, or you take the test for 1 hour or 6 hours, there is no indication of whether you will receive a pass or fail score. The length of your examination depends on how you answered the questions. When the computer indicates you are finished, regardless of how long you have been testing or how far past 75 questions you have gone, it just means you have "turned your test in," and your test is completed. The examination will end when the student:

- Measures at a level of competence above or below the standard and at least 75 questions have been answered.
- Completes a maximum of 265 questions.
- Has been testing for the maximum time of 6 hours (NCSBN, *NCLEX candidate bulletin*, 2005).

Do I Have to Be Computer-Literate? It is not necessary to study from a computer, nor is it necessary that you be "computer literate." Research has demonstrated that candidates who were not accustomed to working on a computer did as well as those who were very comfortable with the computer. So, previous computer experience is not a prerequisite to passing the NCLEX!

How Will I Keep the Computer Keys Straight and Deal With a Mouse? At the testing site, each candidate is given an orientation to the computer as well as a practice session. This tutorial will introduce you to the computer, demonstrate how to use the keyboard and the calculator, as well as how to use the mouse to record your answers (Figure 5-1). It will also explain to you how to record the answers for the alternate format items (more about this later). If you need assistance with the computer after the examination starts, a test administrator will be available. Every effort is made to make sure that you understand and are comfortable with the testing procedure and equipment.

There will be only one question on the screen at a time. You will read the question and select an answer. After the answer is selected, the computer will ask you to confirm the answer. When you confirm an answer, the computer screen automatically progresses to the next question. Previously answered questions are not available for review. There is an onscreen optional calculator built into the computer. The tutorial program will demonstrate the use of the calculator in calculating numeric answers.

What Is the Passing Score? Every state has the same passing criteria. Specific individual scores will not be available to you, your school, or your place of employment. You cannot obtain your results from the testing center. Your score will be reported directly to you as pass or fail. A composite of student results will be mailed to the respective schools of nursing. There is no specific published score or number that represents passing.

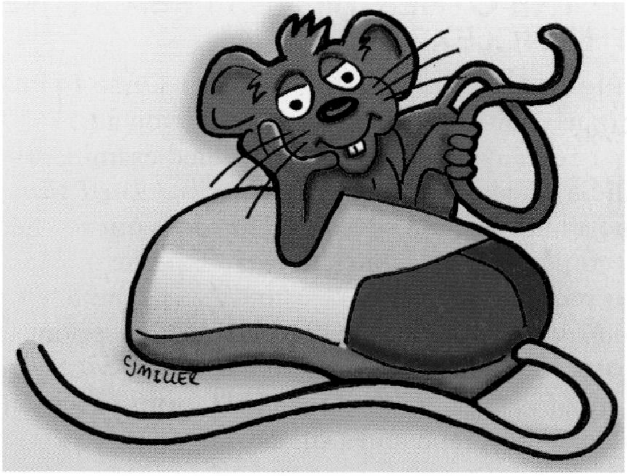

FIGURE 5-1
As of 2002, the use of the computer mouse makes navigating the CAT easier.

How Will I Know I Have Passed? The examination scores are compiled at the Pearson VUE center and transmitted directly to state boards of nursing. Most boards of nursing can advise the candidates in writing of their results within 3 to 4 weeks of taking the examination. Check your *Candidate Bulletin*, as well as the information from your state, regarding the availability of results online or from an automated telephone verification system. Do not call the state board of nursing to inquire about your pass or fail status; they cannot release information on the telephone.

WHAT KIND OF QUESTIONS WILL BE ON THE NCLEX?

Most of the questions are multiple choice, with four options. Each question will stand alone and will not require information from previous questions to determine the correct answer. All of the information for the question will be available on the computer screen. You will be provided a dry erase board for notes or calculations you would like to make. You may not take calculators into the examination; the "drop down" calculator will be available on the screen for math calculations. Everyone will be tested according to the same test plan, but candidates will receive different questions. There is only one answer to each question; you do not get any partial credit for another answer—it is either right or wrong. All questions must be answered, even if you have to make a wild guess. The computer selects the next question on the basis of the response to the previous question. (You do not get another question until the one on the screen is answered.) You will not be able to go back to a previous question once that question is removed from the screen. (You cannot go back and change your answer to the wrong one!) There will be an optional 10-minute rest period after 2 hours of testing. If you need to take a break before the 2 hours, notify one of the testing center administrators. The tutorial, and all breaks, are considered part of the 6 hours allowed for testing (NCSBN, *NCLEX candidate bulletin*, 2005).

There is not much storage space at the testing sites. There are some small lockers for your personal items. Therefore, do not take your textbooks, all your notes from school, your lucky stuffed bear, or any other materials you have been carrying around in that pack for the past 2 years!

WHAT ARE SOME OF THE OTHER THINGS I REALLY NEED TO KNOW ABOUT THE NCLEX?

What If I Need to Change the Time or Date I Have Already Scheduled?

You can change your testing date and time if you advise NCLEX Candidate Services 24 hours or 1 full day prior to your scheduled examination appointment. The phone number will be listed in the front of your *Candidate Bulletin*. You can then reschedule the test at no additional cost. If a candidate does not reschedule within this time frame or does not come at the scheduled testing time, the ATT is invalidated, and the candidate will be required to re-register and re-pay the $200 registration fee (NCSBN, *NCLEX candidate bulletin*, 2005). There are no exceptions to this policy.

What About Identification at the Testing Site? You will be required to provide one form of identification. Acceptable forms of identification (must be valid, not expired, with a photograph and a signature):

- Driver's license, state issued identification, passport (After January 2007, *these three forms of indentification will only be acceptable*, NCLEX Invitational Conference, September 11, 2006).
- United States military identification
- National identification card (in English) (NCSBN, *NCLEX candidate bulletin*, 2005)

What Are the Advantages of CAT for the Candidate? The environment is quiet and conducive to testing. The work surface is large enough to accommodate both right-handed and left-handed people, with adequate room for the computer. The time frame is much more relaxed—there is a total of 6 hours. Each candidate can work at his or her own pace. Each person has her own testing station or cubicle. There should be a minimal amount of distraction, if any, by the other candidates who are testing at the same time. If a candidate has to retake the examination, the parameters for retesting are established by the respective state board of nursing. The National Council requires the candidate to wait at least 45 days prior to rescheduling the examination. Some individual boards of nursing, require 90 days after the first examination before scheduling a second time. Candidates who take the examination again will not be given the same questions (NCSBN, *NCLEX candidate bulletin*, 2005).

What About Security? A digital fingerprint, signature, and photograph will be taken at the examination site. You will have to request permission to leave the testing area for a break, you will be required to enter your fingerprint again to be readmitted to the area.

PREPARING FOR THE NCLEX-RN

WHERE AND WHEN SHOULD I START?

Six Months Before the NCLEX

Make sure you know the dates and deadlines in the state in which you are applying for licensure. Your school will advise you of the specific dates the forms are due to the state office. If you are registering individually, contact the state board of nursing in your state of residence, or where you wish to file for licensure, and find out the filing deadlines. Make sure you follow the directions exactly. State boards of nursing do not respond favorably to applications that are not submitted on time or are submitted in an incorrect format. A listing of the state boards of nursing can be found in Appendix A. If you plan to apply for licensure in another state, it is your responsibility to contact the board of nursing in that state to obtain your papers for application. Plan early (at least 6 months) to investigate the feasibility of taking the examination in another state.

Investigate review courses. Review courses can assist you in organizing your study materials and identifying areas in which you need to focus your study time. Understanding the NCLEX-RN Test Plan will help you to prioritize your studying.

Plan an expense account for the end of school and for the NCLEX. Frequently, students are caught at the end of school with unexpected expenses, one of which may be the fees for the NCLEX. Start a small savings plan—maybe $5 a week—to help defray these expenses. For family and friends who want to "give you something for graduation," you might tell them of your "wish list," including those expenses incurred at graduation (Box 5-1).

BOX 5-1 Budget for the End of School and the NCLEX: How Much Is It Going to Cost Me to Get out of School?

REQUIRED EXPENSES

Graduating fees from college or university ____________________
Application fees for NCLEX-RN ____________________
Passport-type picture (may be required for state application) ____________________

EXPENSES TO TAKE NCLEX-RN

Travel (e.g., car, bus, airfare) ____________________
Hotel accommodations at NCLEX testing site ____________________
Miscellaneous (e.g., food, transportation to site) ____________________

OPTIONAL EXPENSES

School pin ____________________
Uniform or cap and gown for graduation ____________________
Graduation expenses passed on to graduate ____________________
Graduation pictures (class or individual) ____________________
Graduation invitations ____________________
Commercial exit testing ____________________
NCLEX-RN review course (need to plan this before school is out) ____________________
NCLEX-RN review books (get these early, as they really help with the last year of nursing school!) ____________________

EXPENSES AFTER GRADUATION (IT'S NOT OVER YET!)

Professional organizations (most organizations will give a discount on new membership to the graduate nurse) ____________________
Professional journals ____________________
Uniform, scrub suits, and shoes to begin new job ____________________
Professional liability insurance (check with the school regarding transfer from school policy to individual policy) ____________________

Two Months Before the NCLEX: What Do I Need to Do Now?

If you have a job, discuss your anticipated NCLEX-RN test date with your supervisor. You can project your test date by checking your graduation date, then determine from previous students or nursing faculty the estimated time to receive the ATT in your state, think about review courses, study time, and where that puts your scheduling. Remember, you can change your testing appointment, without penalty, as long as you do it within 24 hours of your scheduled appointment and within the dates on the ATT. Submit your request for days off in writing as soon as your test date is confirmed. This is something you want to make sure that your manager understands. Supervisors may not be aware that each candidate can schedule his or her own testing date. Plan to take off the day or two before the examination and, if possible, the day after as well. This will allow you time to relax and, if necessary, travel to and from the testing site.

Decide how you are going to get to the test site and if it will be necessary for you to stay overnight. If the closest testing site is not easily accessible, is more than a 1-hour drive away, or involves driving through a heavily congested traffic area, you may want to consider staying overnight in a hotel room close to the site. For some graduates, this will prevent unnecessary hassle and increased anxiety on the day of the examination.

Are you going with a group or by yourself? How will you feel if the group is finished and you are still working on your examination? Will you feel rushed because everyone is waiting for you? Do not create a situation to increase your anxiety at one of the most important times of your nursing career. If you are okay with the group waiting for you, and everyone understands the situation, then it may be a source of support for you. If a group of graduates are traveling together, and everyone is able to schedule the examination on the same day, consideration should be given to planning the hotel accommodations. Do not have a crowd in your room. Plan to have your own bed. Five people in a room designed for two or four will not be conducive to sleep the night before the examination. If you are rooming with another person, select someone you like and can tolerate in close quarters for a short period of time. Surround yourself with people who have a positive attitude; you do not need complainers and negative thinkers.

Develop a plan for studying. Do you need to study alone, or do you benefit from group study time? Set yourself a study schedule that you can realistically achieve. About 2 to 3 hours a day for 2 or 3 days a week is realistic; 8 hours a day on your days off does not work. If you take a formal review course, plan your study time to gain the most from the course. A review course is not meant to be your only study time. When you finish a review course, you should have a much better idea regarding what is going to be tested, how it will be tested, and where you need to focus some study time. Priority areas to study are those you are the weakest in; focus on those first.

The Day Before the BIG DAY

Make sure you have all of the papers required for admission. Read your information packet again. The ATT that you received from the testing service will be required at the testing site. The information packet that you receive should have all of the necessary information and directions needed for the test site. Check to see if there is anything else you will need to take with you to the site.

Make a "test run" the evening before the test. Find the parking areas. If your hotel is within four to six blocks of the test site, walk to the site; this is a terrific way to help reduce anxiety and get the blood circulating to your brain! Whether you drive or walk to the site, go the day before to make sure you know where you are going.

Go to bed early; do not study, cram, or party! Plan to eat a light dinner, something that will not upset your stomach—you do not need to be up half of the night with heartburn and/or diarrhea!

The BIG DAY Is Here

Eat a well-balanced breakfast, not sweet rolls and coffee. Protein and complex carbohydrates will help sustain you during the examination. Eat light, something that is nourishing, but not heavy. Do not drink a lot of coffee; you do not need to have the caffeine jitters or be distracted by frequent bathroom trips.

Dress comfortably, but look nice. Anticipate that the temperature at the testing sites will be a little cool rather than too warm. Do not wear tight clothes that restrict your breathing when you sit down! Dress casually and comfortably, and be prepared with a sweater or light jacket just in case you need it. Arrive at the test site a little early. This will allow you time to get checked in and prevent anxiety about being late.

HOW DO I SELECT AN NCLEX REVIEW COURSE?

There are many review courses available to assist the graduate nurse in preparing for the NCLEX. Before you sign up, evaluate which course will be most beneficial to you. In considering a review course, remember that the objective is review, not primary learning (Box 5-2).

What Types of Review Courses Are Available? Evaluate your geographic location. Which review courses are easily accessible? Are you considering traveling to another city to attend a review course? Collect data on all of the courses, then compare them to see which one best meets your needs and budget. Check with your prospective employer regarding time off and scheduling. Plan ahead, and make an intelligent decision regarding review courses. Do not feel that you must sign up with the first review company that contacts you!

Carefully evaluate your need for a review course. Are you the type of student who can plan study time, establish a study review schedule, and stick to it? Were you in the top 25% of your graduating class? Have you had experience working in a hospital with adult medical-surgical patients, other than while you were in school? As a new graduate, do you feel prepared for this examination? If you can answer yes to all of these questions, you may not want to consider a review course in your preparation for the NCLEX-RN. Most graduates can say yes to one or two of these questions, but not to all of them.

What Are the Qualifications of the Review Course Instructors? To teach a review course effectively, the instructor needs to be familiar with the NCLEX. That ability is most often found in instructors who have teaching experience in a school of nursing. Some hospitals provide in-house review courses taught by excellent educators and clinical specialists. Determine if these instructors are familiar with the

BOX 5-2 Selecting an NCLEX Review Course

Here are some questions to consider:

WHERE AM I GOING TO WORK?
Will the institution pay for the review? ______________________
Will the institution pay the initial fee or do I need to plan for reimbursement? ______________________

DOES THE INSTITUTION PROVIDE AN ON-SITE REVIEW?
Who teaches it? ______________________
Is it an independent company or hospital employees? ______________________

REVIEW COURSE INSTRUCTORS
Who will teach the class? Your faculty from school? Or review course faculty trained by the review company? ______________________

WHAT TYPE OF INSTRUCTIONAL MATERIAL IS USED?
Does it cost extra outside the registration fee? ______________________
If it is additional to registration fee, where do I get it? ______________________
Can I keep all of the instructional materials (e.g., books, testing booklets, audiotapes, DVDs, CDs)? ______________________
Does the instructional material include practice test questions in the NCLEX format? ______________________
Can I get any of the course materials ahead of time to begin studying?
____

HOW ARE THE CLASSES CONDUCTED?
How many days? ______________________
Are days consecutive or spread over several weeks? ______________________
What are the hours each day? ______________________
What type of audio-visual aids are used? ______________________
What is the teaching style (e.g., group work, lecture, home study, group participation, testing practice)? ______________________
What is the average size class for the area? ______________________

HOW MUCH DOES IT COST?
What is the total price? ______________________
Does this include all of the class materials? ______________________
What is the per-hour or per-day cost? *(This will help to evaluate cost-effectiveness of various types of programs.)* ______________________
Are there group rates, and what are they? ______________________
Are there early registration discounts? ______________________
When does the money have to be in? ______________________
Are there any "extra incentives"? ______________________

BOX 5-2 Selecting an NCLEX Review Course—cont'd

HOW DO I PAY FOR IT?
Is there a payment plan? ______
Can I make an early deposit to hold my space? ______
When is the deposit due? When is the final amount due? ______
If I change my mind after I make the deposit, can I get the deposit back?
______

IS THERE A GUARANTEE?
What is the guarantee? ______
Can I take the review over again? ______
Does it have to be in the same location as the first time? ______
What do I have to do to qualify for the guarantee? ______
Do I get further assistance in identifying areas of need and studying for next time? ______

WHAT IS THE PASS RATE AND HOW IS IT DETERMINED?
Is it based on all new graduates who took the review? ______
Is it a company survey of participants after NCLEX? ______
Is it based on all participants or only the first-time takers? ______
Is it based on the company projected success rate? ______
Did the review company answer all of my questions in a courteous manner and seem interested in my business? ______
Do you know anyone who has taken a review? ______
What are their recommendations? ______

NCLEX test plan. Information that is not a focus of the NCLEX plan does not need to be included in a review course. It is also important to find out if the review course faculty is from a school of nursing in your immediate area. It is possible that you will be paying for a review course to be taught by someone from your nursing school faculty. A review course may be more effective and help you to more effectively confirm knowledge if it is taught by someone other than your school faculty. You need to hear information from a different perspective. This helps to anchor information and reinforce previous learning. Look for a course that brings faculty in from areas outside your school.

What Type of Instructional Materials Are Used in the Course? Are the materials an additional course expense? Do you get to keep the materials after the course is over? Are handouts, workbooks, CDs, audiotapes, books, and other materials used to enhance learning? Be concerned if there are no course outlines, workbooks, handouts, or books; you might spend all of your time writing and miss listening to the necessary information. Do the course materials include practice test questions that are similar in format to the NCLEX? Ask about the format used to organize the material (e.g., integrated, blocked, systems). How does the format compare with the NCLEX plan of patient needs and nursing process that is described in your *Candidate Bulletin* from the National Council?

How Is the Course Taught? Are visuals used to enhance learning? Is the presentation given by a "live person?" Some courses may be conducted on line, or may be presented through videos and audiotapes rather than through a person who will speak to you and answer your questions.

Does the Course Include Instruction in Test-Taking Skills and Practice? Test-taking skills and practice are a very important aspect of a review course. The graduate needs to practice testing strategies and use them in answering questions written by someone other than their nursing school faculty.

How Much Does the Course Cost? Most review courses cost between $200 and $350. Frequently, there is a discount for early registration, and there may also be a discount for group registration. Make sure you understand the review company policy regarding deposit and registration fees. Make sure you understand the cancellation policy. Some companies will let you pay a deposit, with the total amount due by a certain date. Check out the possibility of organizing a group; some courses give a free review or a discount to the group organizer.

How Long Does It Last? Is the course 3, 4, or 5 consecutive days? Is it given only in the evenings? Is it taught only on the weekend for 6 weeks? This is very important to determine early in your evaluation of review courses. Compare the price with the length of the course—are you getting your money's worth? Notify your employer as soon as possible if you need to fit the review into your work schedule. Most hospitals will arrange the new graduate's schedule to allow attendance at a review course. Some hospitals even provide a review course as a benefit to the new graduate nurse employee! Once you have determined which review course you wish to take, discuss it with your prospective employers or notify your current employer as soon as possible. It is important to provide adequate advance notice to your employer so that staffing schedules may be planned.

Where Is the Course Held? Are you going to have to drive for an hour every day? Will you need to obtain a hotel room? Ask about parking. What is the availability of inexpensive restaurants in the area? Is food going to be a major expense?

What Are the Statistics Regarding the Pass Rate for the Company? It is very appropriate to inquire about how the pass rate statistics are determined by the review company. Check the webpage for the NCSBN (*www.ncsbn.org*) to determine the most current statistics for passing the NCLEX. Appendix A has a listing of the Web addresses for the State Boards of Nursing. The review company must obtain the results directly from course participants or from schools of nursing. The National Council does not make this information available to the review companies. Find out whether the advertised pass rate is based on actual responses from participants or on projected figures from the company.

Does the Review Company Offer any Type of Guarantee? Some review companies will offer you a guaranteed "refund" or a free review course, or further assistance if you are not successful on the examination. Find out what the guarantee means and who is eligible for it. Sometimes the "guaranteed refund" is not easily accessible. Make sure you get in writing what you must do to be eligible and to file for the benefit.

What Is the Size of the Class? Some review course classes will have several hundred participants. One problem resulting from a large class is that if you do not get there an hour early, you do not get a seat where you can see or hear. There are some review companies that limit the enrollment depending on the classroom environment. Ask about the size of the class and the classroom environment.

When Is the Course Offered? Some graduates prefer to take a review course just before the examination so that the information is still fresh in their minds. Most graduates prefer to take the review within 1 to 2 weeks before the examination. This time frame generally works very well; the review course is scheduled during the time you are waiting for your Authorization to Test. When you receive your authorization, you have completed your review course, and you are ready to schedule the examination. This schedule allows time to organize and study those areas that are your weakest. If you have only one review course available, how does it fit with your plans for scheduling the examination? Another aspect to consider is your employment schedule. Can you get time off from work? If your employer will not give you the time off, you may need to take a review course as early in the day as possible so that you can go to work. Try to arrange your review course time, so that you can focus on reviewing the information. If you have to work nights or evenings during the course, you will not benefit as much from the review.

Call the review company to get your questions answered. Do they spend time on the telephone with you, or are they in a rush to get you off the telephone? Ask what makes their course better than another course. Is the company representative friendly and knowledgeable, and does that person demonstrate concern for answering all of your questions?

Ultimately, each graduate must decide whether to take a review course and which review course is right. The more informed you are regarding a review course, the more intelligent a decision you can make.

NCLEX-RN REVIEW BOOKS: WHICH ONE IS RIGHT FOR YOU?

It is important to select a review book that meets your study needs. The first step is to check out your choices. Nursing faculty, friends with review books, the school library, and the local nursing textbook stores are all sources of information regarding review books. There are two main kinds of nursing review books: those with content review and those that consist totally of review test questions. Evaluate how the book will be used: Is it for study during school, or is it specifically for review for the NCLEX? For example, if you bought the review book to study pediatric nursing, you may be disappointed. The focus of the NCLEX is not on pediatrics; therefore, it is not often a strong component in review books. If you wish to use a review book to identify priority aspects of care in the medical–surgical patient, a review book can be of great benefit. The following discussion of review-book selection is directed primarily toward review books that contain content review. Take notes as you read the different selections; it is hard to remember all the positive and negative points of each book (Box 5-3). Frequently, students find the review books to be of great benefit during school in assisting them to organize and consolidate a large amount of information. Plan to purchase a review book while you are still in nursing school. Review books are revised about every 3 years.

BOX 5-3 Selecting a Review Book: Where Do I Start?

Here are some questions to consider:
Does the review course I am considering provide a review book? __________
What does the review book look like? __________
- Type style: is it easy to read? __________
- Outline or narrative format? __________
- Quality of the paper: does it bleed through when highlighted? __________

Is the table of contents helpful? __________
What is the organization pattern of the book? __________
Is the information blocked or integrated? __________
Is the primary focus on nursing care? __________
Are the high-priority areas easily identified and adequately covered? __________
Is there a comprehensive index? __________
How easy is the information to find and to understand? __________
Does it cover the priorities of nursing care? __________
Where are the medications, treatments, and diagnostics for each of these topics? __________
Are there test questions included in the content review book? __________
Are there questions at the end of each chapter? __________
Are there sample tests to practice test-taking skills? __________
Are the sample tests integrated, blocked (pediatrics, obstetrics, medical), or reflective of previous chapter material? __________
Does the book include the correct answers and rationale for all of the test questions? __________
Is information repeated in different areas? __________
What is the focus of the content? __________
Are test-taking strategies included in the book and easy to understand? __________

Do an Overview. Is the type style and size comfortable to read? Does the page layout enhance reading and finding information? Are there graphics, charts, or diagrams? Is the information outlined, or is it narrative in style? Is it difficult to read a constant narrative text?

Scan the Table of Contents. Is the information presented in a logical sequence? How is the information organized? It is important that the information be organized in a manner that is logical to you. The NCLEX is based on an integrated format, with a focus on the nursing process and client needs. Read the introduction to see how these areas were considered in the organization of the text. Quickly scan the table of contents, and check the number of pages in various areas of subject material. What is the focus of the material?

Evaluate Chapter Layout. How well is the material organized within the chapter? Are there major headings and subheadings to assist you in finding information quickly? Some texts use two-toned shading, boxes, or a second color to highlight divisions of content or priority information. These may not be points you have identified in previous textbooks; however, these devices help to decrease the monotony of constant reading and to increase interest in the material presented.

Evaluate Content. Select a topic or topics you would like to read about in each of the review books you are considering. Select the priority nursing concepts and interventions you want to identify (e.g., nursing care of a patient with diabetes). Evaluate the information regarding the adult, pediatric, and obstetric patient. How does the information compare in the review books you are considering? Is the material logically organized? Does it contain the major concepts of care for that particular example? The focus of the book should be toward nursing care, not medical diagnosis, pharmacology, or pathophysiology. In evaluating the currency of content, keep in mind that you cannot expect information that came out last month to be reflected in any textbook. The focus of NCLEX is to evaluate entry-level nursing care that is common practice across the country. Remember, the NCLEX is more heavily weighted toward the medical–surgical patient.

Evaluate the Index. Take several common topics, and look them up in the index. A good index is critical to finding information in a timely manner.

Test Questions. Are test questions included in the text? Questions may be found after each of the main chapters or grouped together at the end of the book. Check to see if a rationale for the correct answer is included for each question. Does a computer disk of questions come with the book? How many questions are on the disk? Are the computer questions different from the questions in the book? You may be expecting the disk to have new practice questions, and it only has the questions that are in the book. If a computer disk of questions comes with the book, can the disk be used indefinitely, or does it disintegrate after so many uses?

Test-Taking Strategies. Does the book include information on test-taking strategies for multiple-choice questions? Test-taking strategies help you to be more "test-wise." These strategies can be of great benefit while you are still in school, in addition to practicing them as a method to prepare for the NCLEX.

TEST ANXIETY: WHAT IS THE DISEASE? HOW DO YOU GET RID OF IT?

Frequently, students and graduates focus on their "test anxiety" as the reason for not doing well on examinations. Test anxiety is something that only you can change. You are the one allowing the anxiety to affect you in a negative way. The only person responsible for your test anxiety is you, and the only one who can do anything about it is you. Look at some simple steps to decrease your anxiety regarding testing.

- **Plan ahead.** Do not wait until the last minute to read the 150 pages in your textbook, review all your classroom notes, and read the 10 articles assigned for the test. Plan study time, and stick to it!
- **Set aside study time for when you are at your best.** Frequently, study time is scheduled at a time when everything else (laundry, meals, housecleaning, yard work, and so on) is completed. You are defeating your purpose and increasing your anxiety when you try to study at a time when you are tired and not receptive to learning.
- **Study smart.** Plan for 45 minutes to an hour of review on the day after a 90-minute class lecture. This will greatly enhance your retention of the classroom information. Plan for an hour to review/scan assigned reading or information

prior to class, so that you will know where information is located and what you will need to take as notes in class.

- **Give yourself a break!** Plan your study time to include a break about every hour. Your retention of information begins to decrease after about 30 minutes and is significantly decreased after an hour.
- **Think positively!** If your friends are "negative thinkers," do not plan to study with them. Go to the movies or play sports with them, but do not study with them. Anxiety and negative thinking are contagious—do not expose yourself to the disease!
- **Do not cram.** The NCLEX is not written to evaluate memory-based information. Test questions focus on the higher levels of cognitive ability. Application of principles and the analysis of information will be required to determine an appropriate nursing response or action (Wendt, 2003). Do not jeopardize your critical-thinking skills by staying up late and cramming.

Just thinking about an examination can cause some students an increase in anxiety. It seems as though during the last year of school, particularly the last semester, tests become a major source of anxiety. Everyone knows fellow students who become obsessed with the idea that they are going to fail an important examination. View an examination as a positive step—an opportunity to demonstrate your knowledge, get rid of those negative thought "tapes"! Put yourself in charge of your feelings. Replace those negative thoughts and ideas with positive ones: "I will pass this test; I will be so glad when this test is behind me; it is going to feel good to get this one done!" Write down positive affirmations, and put them on your bathroom mirror, on your refrigerator, anywhere you will see them often. Potential employers, state boards of nursing, your spiritual advisers, and your neighbors are not going to think less of you if you are not at the top of the class. Keep in mind that your employers and the state boards do not care what your grades were in school or on the NCLEX—they just want to know that you can pass the NCLEX and practice nursing safely. Give yourself permission to be in the middle—an average student on grades, but one who is concerned about professional, safe nursing practice.

WHAT KIND OF QUESTIONS CAN I EXPECT ON THE NCLEX?

On the NCLEX, most of the questions are in the multiple-choice format; they have a stem in which the question is presented and four options from which to choose an answer. Of these four options, three are meant to distract you from the correct answer. With the four-item, multiple-choice questions, there is only one correct answer. The multiple-choice NCLEX questions give you the choice of four answers, not a combination of the four options (e.g., 1. A, B, C) (Figure 5-2).

The focus of NCLEX is on nursing care. The questions will ask you to use nursing concepts in the situation presented.

What Are "Alternate Format Questions," and Why The Big Fuss About Them? In the mid-1990s, the National Council began an investigation to determine if different types of questions, other than the four-item, multiple-choice question, could more effectively assess the entry-level nursing competence. In April of 2003, these different types of questions were included on the NCLEX. These questions are included in the test bank of questions that will be used to select the test items for a candidate's examination. There is no preset number of alternate format questions that will be presented to a candidate; the question or items will be randomly selected as the adaptive testing process selects questions that meet the parameters of the test plan. The National Council anticipates that candidates who take a minimum number (75) of questions may be presented with one operational or scored alternate format item (NCSBN, *Fast facts about alternate item formats and the NCLEX examination*, 2005).

Candidates should keep in mind that there are 15 pretest questions for which the National Council is gathering data to measure the validity of the question. These 15 items may or may not contain several alternate format items. There is no special or additional nursing knowledge needed to answer the alternate format questions. There is no attempt to hide or camouflage the questions; they are randomly selected. The same nursing concepts are being tested, and the questions are based on the same test plan. The question is just asked in a different format. There is not anything you need to do differently with regard to the alternate format questions; just be aware of types of format, and pay attention to how the question is asking for the information.

What Are the Different Types of Alternate Format Questions?

Fill in the blank. These are questions in which a short answer is required. Frequently, this is a question that requires a calculation, maybe a drug calculation, or an intake and output calculation, or assessment scoring. Only the numbers should be entered in the space provided. No units of measurement should be included with the answer (Figure 5-3).

Multiple-response item. These are a different type of multiple-choice question. There will be more than four options presented, and the question will very clearly ask you to select all of the options that apply to this question. With the mouse, you will select each option you want to include in the answer, and click the button at the bottom to continue, then confirm your answer. There is only one correct combination of answers (Figure 5-4).

Hot spot. These items will present a diagram, and you will be asked to select an area on the diagram to answer the question. For example, the diagram might be that of the anterior thorax, and the question is to click on the area where you would place the stethoscope to listen for the apical heart rate, or click on the area where you would listen for the characteristic sounds of the mitral valve (Figure 5-5).

Drag and drop. You will be presented with a list of activities, clients, or, perhaps, steps in a procedure. The question will ask you to click on each item and "drag" it to the right side of the screen, then place the items in the order in which they would be performed, or order of priority of care. Determine what is the first or priority action, then the next one. Determine how all of the options will be ranked. After you have determined your answer, click on the option you want to place first, "drag" that option over, and place it in the box. You will then select the next option you want to place second, "drag" that option over, and place it in the box. You will continue this process until you have used all of the options present. This is called an "ordered response" (Figure 5-6).

Chart or exhibit item. This item will present a problem, then give a chart or exhibit information. You can click on areas of the exhibit/chart to find information that will assist you in solving the problem that is presented. There will still be four options from which to select the correct answer, but you will need to evaluate the data in the exhibit/chart to determine the correct answer. Do not attempt to select the correct answer without evaluating the exhibit/chart information (Figure 5-7).

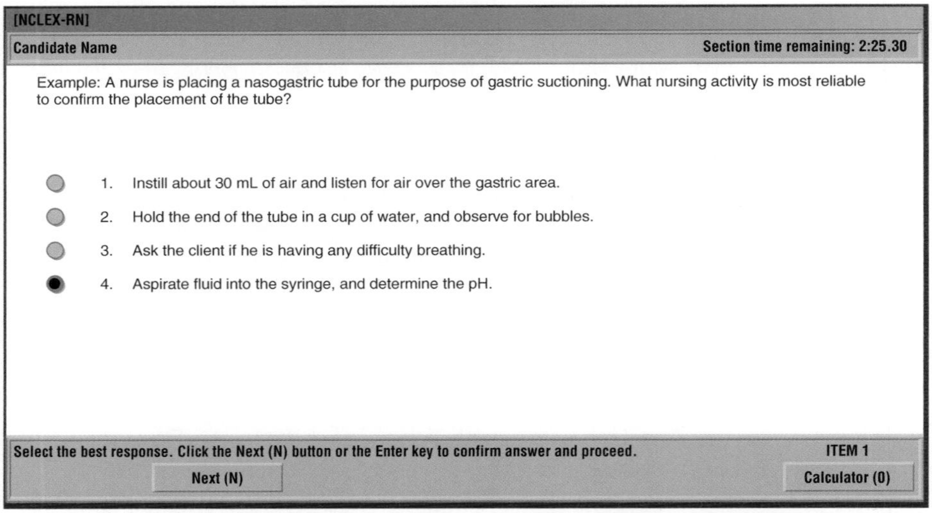
[NCLEX-RN]
Candidate Name
Section time remaining: 2:25.30
Example: A nurse is placing a nasogastric tube for the purpose of gastric suctioning. What nursing activity is most reliable to confirm the placement of the tube?
1. Instill about 30 mL of air and listen for air over the gastric area.
2. Hold the end of the tube in a cup of water, and observe for bubbles.
3. Ask the client if he is having any difficulty breathing.
4. Aspirate fluid into the syringe, and determine the pH.
Select the best response. Click the Next (N) button or the Enter key to confirm answer and proceed.
ITEM 1
Next (N)
Calculator (0)

Answer - 4: The most reliable method of checking placement is to determine the pH of the aspirated fluid. The most common method used is to insert air and listen for the air movement into the stomach. The second and third options are not reliable.

FIGURE 5-2
Sample of multiple-choice test question.

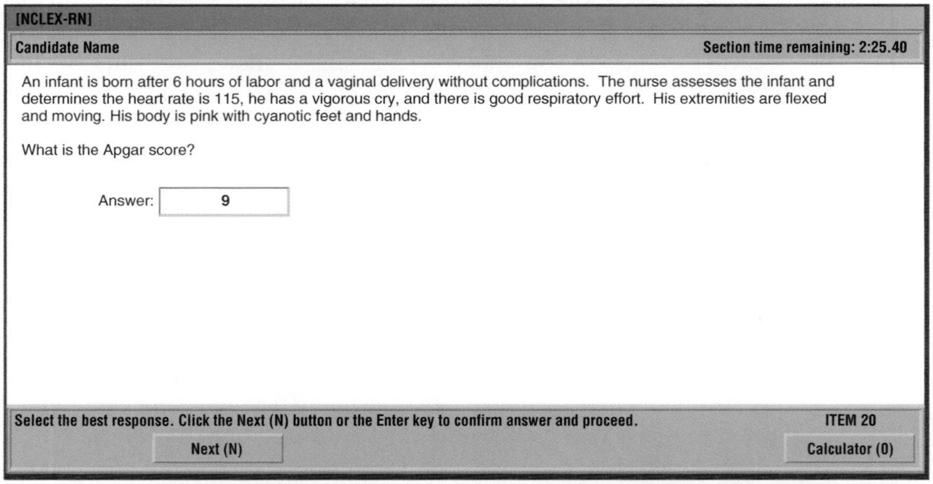
[NCLEX-RN]
Candidate Name
Section time remaining: 2:25.40
An infant is born after 6 hours of labor and a vaginal delivery without complications. The nurse assesses the infant and determines the heart rate is 115, he has a vigorous cry, and there is good respiratory effort. His extremities are flexed and moving. His body is pink with cyanotic feet and hands.
What is the Apgar score?
Answer: 9
Select the best response. Click the Next (N) button or the Enter key to confirm answer and proceed.
ITEM 20
Next (N)
Calculator (0)

Answer - 9: The Apgar is scored on the infant assessment. Two points are assigned to the folllowing areas: heart rate over 100, respiratory rate - good cry, muscle tone - well flexed, reflex irritability - cry, and color is completely pink. There is a possible total of 10 points. In the infant described, all of the areas received 2 points with the exception of color, the infant described has cyanotic feet and hands. There would only be 1 point for that area with a total of 9 points.

FIGURE 5-3
Fill in the blank.

[NCLEX-RN]

Candidate Name **Section time remaining: 3:15.20**

The nurse is caring for an 85-year old client who has a diagnosis of *Mycoplasma* pneumonia. What precautions will the nurse implement in assisting the client with morning care?

Select all that apply:

- [x] 1. Wear clean gloves.
- [ ] 2. Remove all extra suctioning supplies from the room.
- [ ] 3. Dispose of the gown and mask in container outside client's door.
- [x] 4. Wear face mask when working within 3 feet of the client.
- [x] 5. Put on a gown prior to entering the room.
- [ ] 6. Remove the stethoscope from the room if it did not come in contact with the client.

Select the best response. Click the Next (N) button or the Enter key to confirm answer and proceed. **ITEM 21**

Next (N) **Calculator (0)**

Answer: The answer is based on standard precautions, plus respiratory precautions for the pneumonia. Nothing should be removed from the room and the gown should be removed prior to leaving the room, not outside the room.

FIGURE 5-4
Multiple response.

[NCLEX-RN]

Candidate Name **Section time remaining: 3:15.40**

The nurse is caring for a client who is receiving .25 mg Digoxin each morning. On the graphic, identify the correct location where the nurse should place the stethoscope to determine the client's pulse.

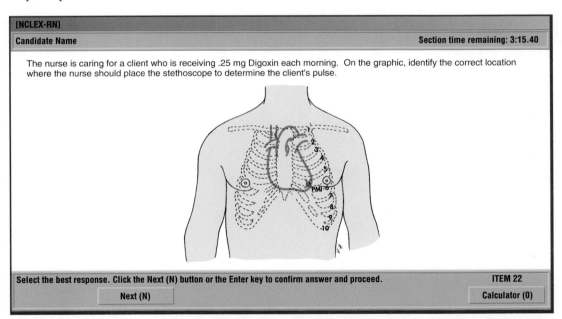

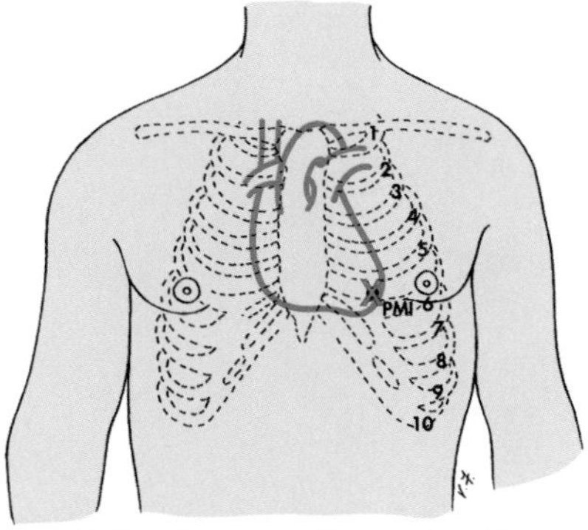

Select the best response. Click the Next (N) button or the Enter key to confirm answer and proceed. **ITEM 22**

Next (N) **Calculator (0)**

Answer: To evaluate the apical pulse the stethoscope should be placed on the area of the PMI - left midclavicular line, 5th intercostal space. To answer this question, you would simply click the area on the graphic. The correct location is noted in the figure.

FIGURE 5-5
Hot spot.

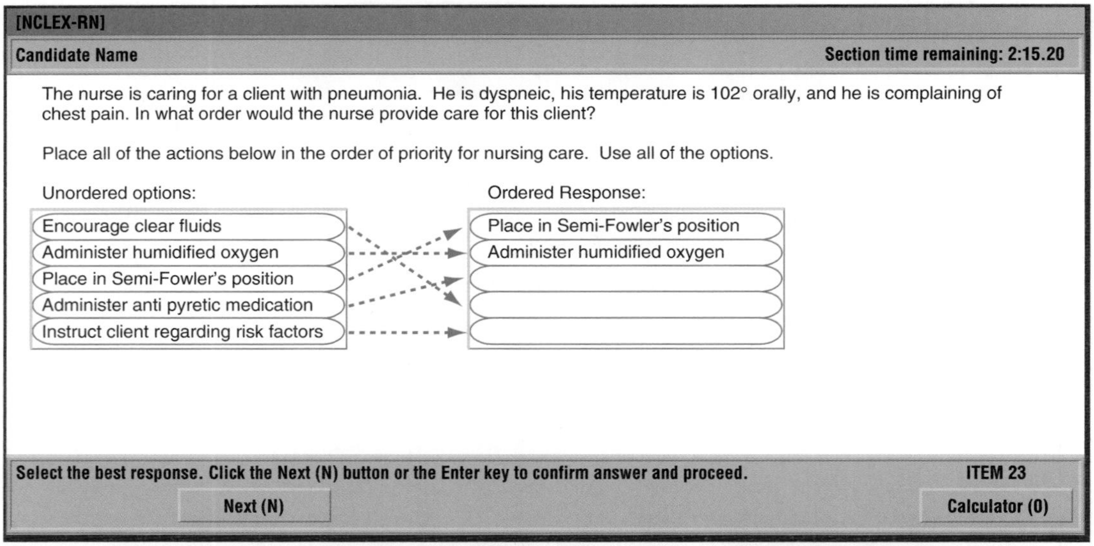

Need to know: Review each of the items in the list. Determine what is the most important action to take first, then second, etc. This question is asking you to provide care for a client who is experiencing difficulty breathing and has chest pain. The dyspnea and chest pain are most likely a result of the client's pneumonia. Position is the first thing that you can do that will benefit the client the most, then begin the oxygen, administer the antipyretic medication, encourage clear liquids, and teaching is last. Remember Maslow when setting priorities.

FIGURE 5-6
Drag and drop (ordered response).

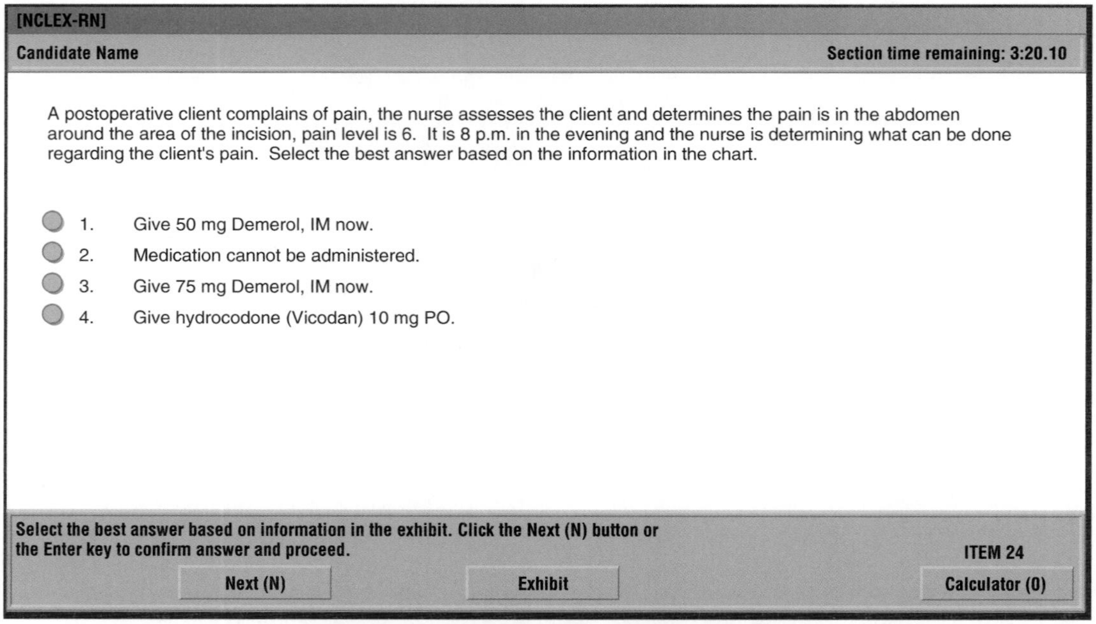

Need to know: Click on the first exhibit and evaluate the information.

FIGURE 5-7
Exhibit/chart.

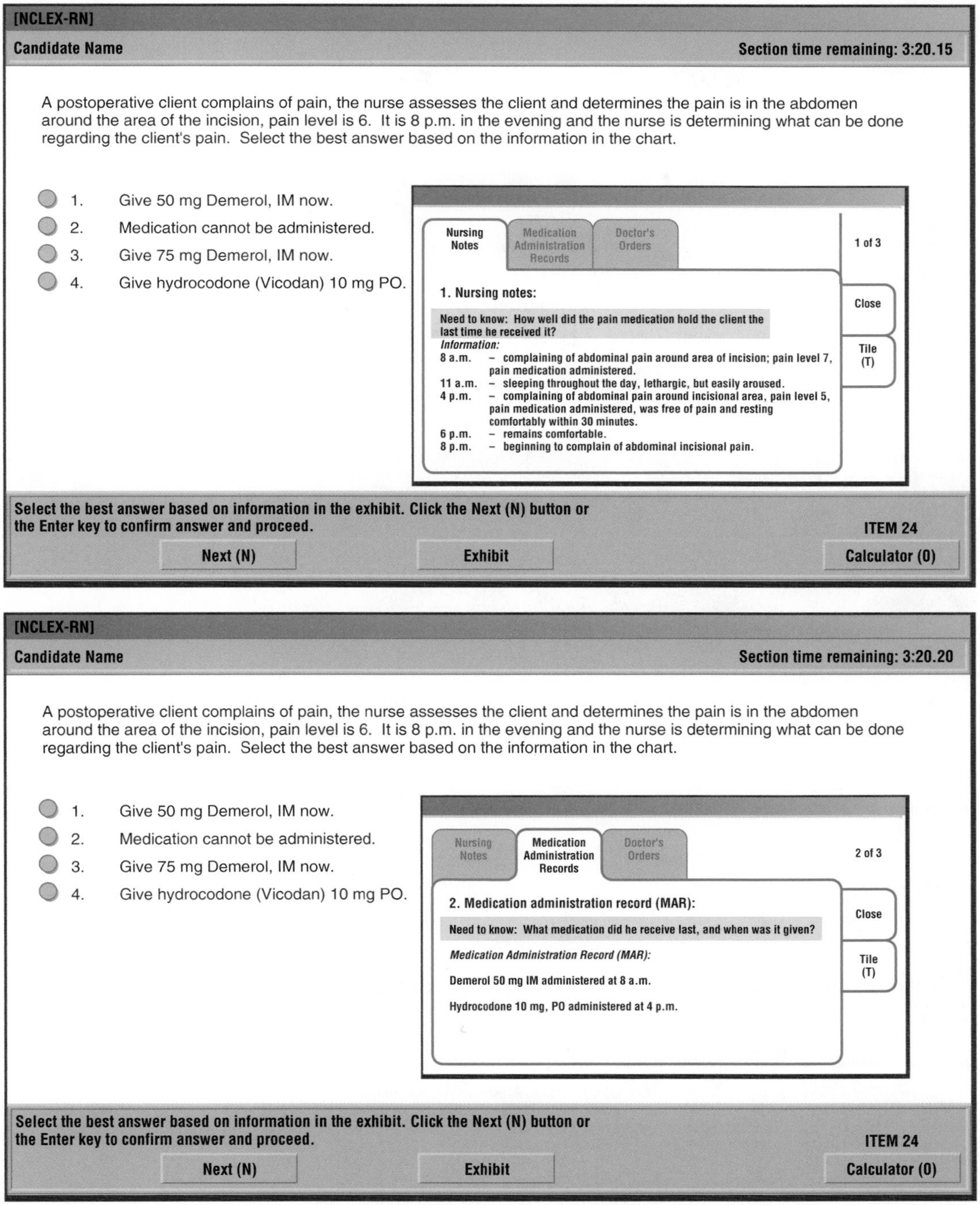
[NCLEX-RN]
Candidate Name
Section time remaining: 3:20.15
A postoperative client complains of pain, the nurse assesses the client and determines the pain is in the abdomen around the area of the incision, pain level is 6. It is 8 p.m. in the evening and the nurse is determining what can be done regarding the client's pain. Select the best answer based on the information in the chart.
1. Give 50 mg Demerol, IM now.
2. Medication cannot be administered.
3. Give 75 mg Demerol, IM now.
4. Give hydrocodone (Vicodan) 10 mg PO.
Nursing Notes
Medication Administration Records
Doctor's Orders
1 of 3
1. Nursing notes:
Need to know: How well did the pain medication hold the client the last time he received it?
Information:
8 a.m. – complaining of abdominal pain around area of incision; pain level 7, pain medication administered.
11 a.m. – sleeping throughout the day, lethargic, but easily aroused.
4 p.m. – complaining of abdominal pain around incisional area, pain level 5, pain medication administered, was free of pain and resting comfortably within 30 minutes.
6 p.m. – remains comfortable.
8 p.m. – beginning to complain of abdominal incisional pain.
Close
Tile (T)
Select the best answer based on information in the exhibit. Click the Next (N) button or the Enter key to confirm answer and proceed.
ITEM 24
Next (N)
Exhibit
Calculator (0)
[NCLEX-RN]
Candidate Name
Section time remaining: 3:20.20
A postoperative client complains of pain, the nurse assesses the client and determines the pain is in the abdomen around the area of the incision, pain level is 6. It is 8 p.m. in the evening and the nurse is determining what can be done regarding the client's pain. Select the best answer based on the information in the chart.
1. Give 50 mg Demerol, IM now.
2. Medication cannot be administered.
3. Give 75 mg Demerol, IM now.
4. Give hydrocodone (Vicodan) 10 mg PO.
Nursing Notes
Medication Administration Records
Doctor's Orders
2 of 3
2. Medication administration record (MAR):
Need to know: What medication did he receive last, and when was it given?
Medication Administration Record (MAR):
Demerol 50 mg IM administered at 8 a.m.
Hydrocodone 10 mg, PO administered at 4 p.m.
Close
Tile (T)
Select the best answer based on information in the exhibit. Click the Next (N) button or the Enter key to confirm answer and proceed.
ITEM 24
Next (N)
Exhibit
Calculator (0)

FIGURE 5-7
Exhibit/chart—cont'd.

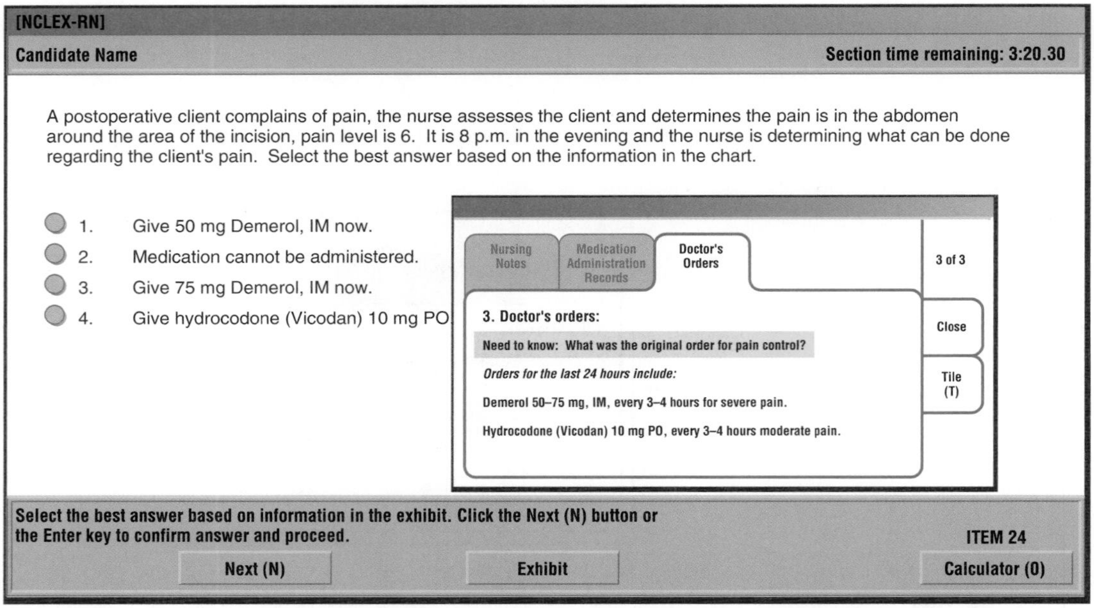

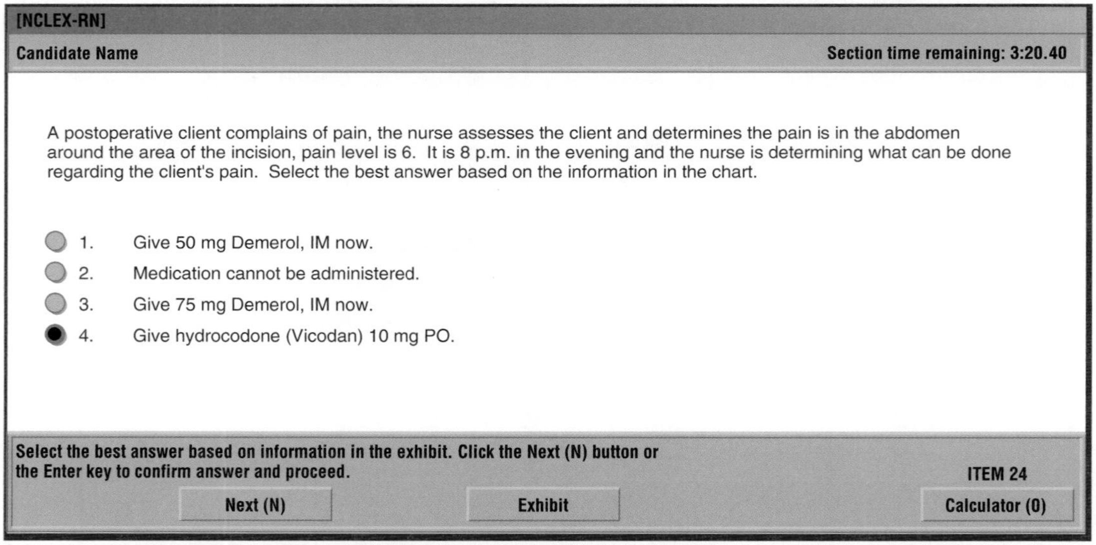

Need to know: Analysis of information.
Client received Demerol 50 mg IM at 11 a.m. and he was lethargic and sleeping for the next 5 hours. He received hydrocodone PO at 4 p.m. and he was comfortable for the next 4 hours. The doctor's orders are current for both the IM and the PO medication for pain. Give the hydrocodone, PO for pain at this time. It held him for 4 hours the last time, and the doctor's order is current.

FIGURE 5-7
Exhibit/chart—cont'd.

WHAT DIFFERENCE DO TEST-TAKING STRATEGIES MAKE?

Knowing how to take an examination is a skill that is developed through practice. Look back at the beginning of nursing school and your first nursing examination; you have come a long way from there! How many times during school have you reviewed a test and discovered you knew the right answer, but marked the wrong one? Nursing faculty and those responsible for the NCLEX are not sympathetic to your claim that you "really meant this answer and not the one I marked." How many times did you go back and change an answer from the correct response to the wrong one? If these are common errors you experienced during nursing school, you need to incorporate testing strategies into your testing skills. Some of the testing practices you have developed over the years may be positive, some may be negative. Information on test-taking strategies can be of benefit to you now and later. Start using testing strategies now. This will help you with your current examinations, and they will be second-nature when you take the NCLEX. Take the time to implement good testing practices—get the question right the first time! Analyze where you are with testing skills, get rid of the negative, and retain the positive.

WHAT ARE STRATEGIES FOR ANSWERING MULTIPLE-CHOICE QUESTIONS?

Read the Question (Stem) Carefully. Do not read extra meaning into the question. Make sure you read the "stem" correctly and understand exactly what information is being requested. (Do you tend to make the patient sicker than he really is by the time you finish the question?)

Create a Pool of Information. What are the concepts of care regarding a patient with the condition or problem presented? Get a general idea of the condition and type of care required before you read the options.

Evaluate All the Options in a Systematic Manner. Focus on what information is being requested, then carefully go through each option. Do not stop with the first correct answer; the last option may be more correct or more inclusive of information.

Eliminate Options You Know Are Not Correct. And leave them alone! Once you have eliminated an option, do not go back to it unless you have gained more insight into the question. Frequently, your initial response in evaluating an option is correct. Go through all of the options and eliminate incorrect ones. What is left is frequently the correct answer, even if it is not what you were looking for.

Identify Similarities in the Options. Find the one that is different. The option that is different may be the correct answer. For example, in a question dealing with a low-residue diet, three of the options might contain a vegetable with a peeling, but one might not—that one is probably the correct answer. Evaluate options that contain several suggested patient activities. Are the activities similar, with one that is different?

Evaluate Priority Questions Very Carefully. Keep in mind the nursing process and Maslow's hierarchy of needs. You must obtain adequate assessment information before proceeding with the nursing process. According to Maslow, physical needs must be met before psychosocial needs—the physical needs of your mental health patient must be met before you can focus on the mental health needs. When considering the physical needs, respiratory needs are a priority. (You've got to breathe first!)

Select Answers That Focus on the Client. Choices that focus on hospital rules and policies are most often not correct. Analyze your testing skills so that you will know where to start to improve them. Once you have identified your testing weaknesses, organize a plan to correct the problem areas. One of the most difficult things to do is to change the way you are used to doing something, even when it makes life easier. Get an early start on evaluating testing skills; it can make a significant difference in the remaining examinations in nursing school.

NCLEX TESTING TIPS

NCLEX Hospital. For the NCLEX examination to be appropriate to all candidates nationwide, it is important that there be a base for the vast knowledge that is to be tested. Therefore, when you are taking the NCLEX, consider yourself working in the NCLEX Hospital. It is a great place to work—everything works like it is supposed to, great equipment, plenty of staff, and the best nursing care possible. The clients (the patients are most frequently referred to as clients on the NCLEX) all have conditions that respond just like the book says they are supposed to respond. Study according to your textbooks. Your clinical experience is complementary with your academic study. Do not focus on the unusual, unexpected, or strange things that happened to you during clinical rotations.

NCLEX Clients. Focus on the client in the question you are working on. As far as the NCLEX Hospital is concerned, that is the only client you are to be concerned about. Do not worry about the five or six other clients you may have assigned to your care. In the NCLEX Hospital, you are taking care of one client/patient at a time, unless it is designated otherwise. Your priority concern is the client in the current question you are trying to answer.

Medication Administration. Know the five rights and the common nursing implications of medications. Usually, both the trade name and generic name are provided in the question. A good strategy is to study the medications according to the classification. For example, study the nursing implications regarding administration of corticosteroid medications and be able to identify common corticosteroid medications.

Calling for Assistance. Be careful with questions for which the right answer appears to be to call someone else to take care of the problem. This is a nursing examination; therefore, identify the best nursing management. This includes questions that include calling the doctor, respiratory therapist, housekeeping, chaplain, or social worker. Be sure there is not something you need to do for the client before notifying someone else regarding the problem. If the client is experiencing difficulty, his condition is changing, and there is nothing you can do, call the doctor. This is particularly true in situations in which the patient is experiencing a problem with impaired circulation. However, if the client is having difficulty breathing, the priority focus is to maintain an open airway, and/or to begin oxygen as well as assess the status of the client prior to calling the doctor.

Positioning. Watch questions that have particular positions in the stem of the question, or include positions in the options. Is the client's position necessary to prevent complications or treat a current problem, or is it primarily for comfort? As you are reviewing, be aware of questions that include conditions that require a specific position in the care of that client.

Delegation and Supervision. The NCLEX frequently includes questions in these areas. Some common considerations to make when evaluating these questions:

- Delegate to someone else the most stable patient with the most predictable response to care.

- Delegate tasks to most qualified person to perform the task.
- Do not delegate teaching or evaluating responsibilities.
- Delegate tasks to nursing assistants that have the most specific guidelines (e.g., collecting a urine sample, feeding, providing hygiene, ambulating).

Setting Priorities. Determine the most unstable client who requires nursing care to prevent immediate problems—take care of this client first. Keep in mind the steps of the nursing process (assessment is first), and Maslow's hierarchy of needs (breathing is first).

Doctor's Orders. Most often when an option is presented that requires a doctor's order, you can consider there is already a doctor's order for the action. If the question states "a dependent nursing action…" or "the nurse would initiate what action… ," consider the possibility of whether or not you need an order for the activity.

Be aware that the expected answer frequently will not be included in the options! This is not uncommon on NCLEX questions. Consider the principles and concepts of care for a patient with the problem presented.

CONCLUSION

Wow! NCLEX deadlines, review courses, testing skills, review books, money, license—and all you thought you needed to do was graduate from nursing school! There are a lot of steps in between graduating from nursing school and being successful on the NCLEX. The key to surviving it all with a smile is careful planning and implementing those plans during your role transition. (That sounds a lot like the nursing process, doesn't it?) The NCLEX-RN is one of the most incredible opportunities of your life. This examination will open the doors for you as you begin one of the most fantastic experiences of a lifetime: a career in nursing.

Just say to yourself, "I can do it. I can pass NCLEX!"

REFERENCES

National Council of State Boards of Nursing: *Fast facts about alternate item formats and the NCLEX examination*, Chicago, National Council of State Boards of Nursing. Accessed April, 2005 at *www.ncsbn.org*.

National Council of State Boards of Nursing: *NCLEX candidate bulletin*, Chicago, 2005, National Council of State Boards of Nursing.

National Council of State Boards of Nursing: *Nurse licensure compact*, Chicago, National Council of State Boards of Nursing. Accessed April, 2005 at *www.ncsbn.org*.

Smith J, Crawford L: *RN practice analysis linking the NCLEX-RN examination to practice*, Chicago, 2003, National Council of State Boards of Nursing.

Wendt A, Harris L: *NCLEX RN examination: detailed test plan for the national council licensure examination for registered nurses*, Chicago, 2003, National Council of State Boards of Nursing.

UNIT III

Nursing: A Developing Profession

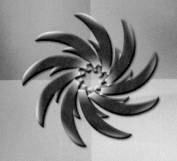

CHAPTER 6

HISTORICAL PERSPECTIVES: INFLUENCES OF THE PAST

JOANN ZERWEKH, EdD, RN, FNP, APRN, BC

History repeats itself because each generation refuses to read the minutes of the last meeting.

—*Anonymous*

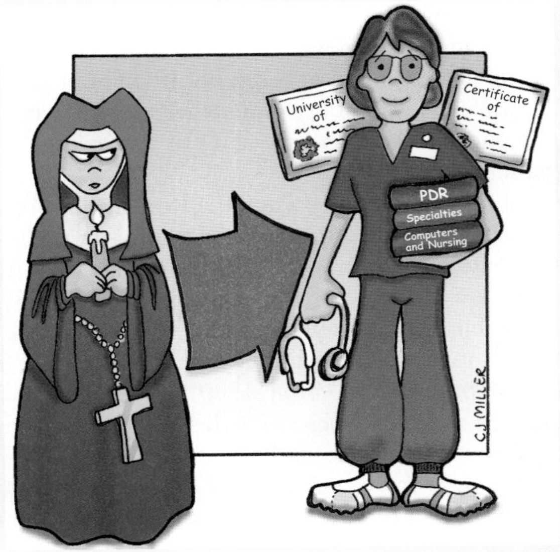

Nursing has come a long way; it is not what it used to be.

After completing this chapter, you should be able to:

- Explain the early European contributions to nursing.
- Explain the forces that affected the roles of American nurses.
- Discuss what nurses do.

So, you have to study the history of nursing. Generally, the topic is considered boring. Well, be prepared for a different approach to the topic. Knowing the history of our profession guides our understanding of why we do what we do today. This understanding can be useful to us as we set our professional goals. Threads of nursing history can be found throughout the book. Chapters 7 and 9 on the image of nursing and nursing education contain brief historical reviews of these areas. Understanding the history can often help in deciding what changes are needed, what changes are helpful, and what changes may be unnecessary. Let us begin with a look at where nursing began.

NURSING HISTORY: PEOPLE AND PLACES

WHERE DID IT ALL BEGIN?

Most nursing historians agree that nursing, or the care of the ill and injured, has been done since the beginning of human life and has generally been a woman's role. A mother caring for a child in a cave and someone caring for another ill adult by boiling willow bark to relieve fever are both examples of nursing. The word nurse actually is derived from the Latin word *nutricius*, meaning *nourishing*.

Roman mythologic figures included the goddess Fortuna, who was usually recognized as being responsible for one's fate and who also served as Jupiter's nurse (Dolan, 1969).

Even before Greek and Roman times, ancient Egyptian physicians and nurses assembled voluminous pharmacopoeia with more than 700 remedies for numerous health problems. Great emphasis was placed on the use of animal parts in concoctions that were generally drunk or applied to the body. The physician prescribed and provided the treatments and usually had an assistant who provided the nursing care (Kalisch & Kalisch, 1986). Some ancient medicine was based on driving out the evil spirit rather than curing or treating the malady. The treatments were often very foul and often included fecal material. By now you may be thinking of the saying, "The treatment was successful, but the patient died."

Advancement of medical knowledge halted abruptly when the Roman Empire was conquered. Any medical and health care knowledge that survived these dark times did so only through the efforts of Jewish physicians who were able to translate the Greek and Roman works (Kalisch & Kalisch, 1986). One bright spot was in Salerno, when a school of medicine and health was established for physicians and women to assist in childbirth. In fact, a midwife named Trotula wrote what may be considered the first nursing textbook on the cure of diseases of women (Dalton, 1900). Generally, nursing was performed by designated priestesses and was associated with some type of temple worship. Little information has survived about this early period. Historians have assumed that Hippocrates was assisted by women, but there is little information to support that. From these roots, nursing began to develop as a recognized and valued service to society (Jamieson & Sewall, 1949).

WHY DEACONS, WIDOWS, AND VIRGINS?

Paralleling the fall of the Roman Empire was the rise of Christianity. The early organization of the young Christian church, which was directly affected by the vision of

Paul, included a governing bishop and seven appointed deacons. These individuals assisted the apostles in the work of the Church (the word *deacon* means *servant*). The deacon was directly responsible for distributing all the goods and property that apostles relinquished to the Church before they "took up the cross and followed." The apostles were required to give up all material resources to achieve full status in the Church.

Women sympathetic to the Christian cause of aiding the poor were encouraged in this work by the bishops and deacons. Eventually, the deacons relinquished aiding the poor to women and established the position of deaconess for that purpose. To maintain a pure heart, these women were required by the Church to be either virgins or widows. The stipulation for widows, however, was that they had to have been married only once (Jamieson and Sewall, 1949). The deaconesses carried nursing forward as they ministered to the sick and injured in their homes. Phoebe, a friend of Paul's and the very first deaconess in the young Christian church, has been called the first visiting nurse (Dana, 1936).

Treatments continued to be a mixture of scientific fact, home remedies, and magic. Eventually, an order of widows evolved that was composed of women who were free from home responsibilities and thus were able to give a total commitment to work among the poor. The widows, although not ordained, continued to do the same work as the deaconesses. This was soon followed by the creation of the Order of Virgins as the Church began placing greater value on purity of body. Although deaconess orders were abolished in the Mediterranean countries, they thrived in other European countries. The traditional commitment to care for the poor and sick became invaluable in a society that generally had neither the time nor the inclination to aid them. Eventually, these women became known as *nuns* (*non nuptae*, not married).

During this time, tremendous upheavals were constantly occurring in the world. Wars, invasions, and battles were constant, and as a result of these encounters, the number of widows was significant. Society during this time did not have the sophistication or the means to deal with the dependents of the soldiers killed in battle. As a means of survival, women joined the nuns as a form of protection from starvation and poverty. This was a dark and dreary time in which superstition, witchcraft, and folklore were predominant influences. Because of the need for physical protection, convents were built to shelter these women (Jamieson and Sewall, 1949). The convents became havens to which women could withdraw from ignorance and evil and be nurtured in traditional Christian beliefs (Donahue, 1985). The deaconesses, widows, and virgins continued to minister to and nurse the ill within the safety of the convent.

HOW DID KNIGHTHOOD CONTRIBUTE TO NURSING?

The Holy Wars furthered the development of nursing in a rather interesting way. Because many Christian crusaders became ill while in Jerusalem, a hospital known as the Hospital of St. John was built to accommodate them. Those who fought in these Holy Wars were known as knights—men who had taken oaths of chivalry, justice, and piety. They often had men trained in the healing arts accompany them into battle to care for them, should they be stricken. These male nurses usually wore a red cross emblazoned on their tunics so that in the heat of battle they could be easily identified and avoid injury or death (Bullough & Bullough, 1978).

The Hospital of St. John gave excellent nursing care. Many of the nurses who survived stayed to work with the hospital organizers. As the battles in the Holy Land continued, the nurses and knights organized a fighting force with a code of rules and a uniform consisting of a black robe with a white Maltese cross, the symbol of poverty, humility, and chastity. They ventured out to rescue the sick and wounded and transported them to the hospital for care, and thus they became known as the Hospitalers (Kalisch and Kalisch, 1986). Male nurses dominated these orders. Other orders that emulated the Hospitalers developed in Europe, and more hospitals were opened that used the Hospital of St. John as a model (Donahue, 1985).

The altruistic spirit of nursing was also seen in the craftsmen's guilds. Although their primary purpose was to provide training and jobs through the practice of apprenticeship, the guilds provided care and aid for their members when they became old and could no longer work at their trade. The guilds also assisted members and their families in times of illness and injury. The apprenticeship system—in which experience is gained on the job but no formal education is given—once served as a model for the training of nurses (Donahue, 1985). It is no longer used, however, and is now considered to have been detrimental to the evolution of nursing.

What nursing gained during this period of history was status. The altruistic ideal of providing care as a service performed out of humility and love became the foundation for nursing. The recognition of the value of hospitals grew; all across Europe, cities were building their own hospitals. A general resurgence in the demand for trained doctors and nurses contributed to the building of medical schools and the development of university programs in the art and science of healing.

WHAT ABOUT REVOLTS AND NURSING?

Revolts—not the kind that incurred battles, but revolts of a social nature—were common. There were battles, too; however, the social revolts had a more direct impact on nursing. The revolution of the spirit, more commonly known as the Renaissance, ushered in new concepts of the world: the discovery of the laws of nature by Newton, the exploration of unknown lands, and the growth of secular interests (humanism) over spiritual ones. In this era emerged several outstanding humanists who were to become saints (Donahue, 1985). Interestingly, in depictions of these saints, they are shown as needing nursing care or as giving care to a wounded or injured person.

In Europe, the Protestant Reformation began primarily as a religious reform movement, but ended with revolt within the Church. Many hospitals in Protestant countries were forced to close, and those loyal to the Church that operated them were driven out of the country, which resulted in a significant shortage of nurses (mostly nuns) to care for the ill and injured. The poor and ill were considered a burden to society, and those hospitals that remained operational in the Protestant countries became known as "pest houses." To fill the need for nurses, women, many of whom were alcoholics and former prostitutes, were recruited. Generally, a nurse was a woman serving time in a hospital rather than a prison (Jamieson & Sewall, 1949; Donahue, 1985).

The industrial and intellectual revolutions that followed the Reformation all had a significant impact on nursing. During the Industrial Revolution, as production of much-needed goods was streamlined through industrial innovation, craftsmen left the rural life to work in factories. The intellectual contributions of scientists, many of whom were physicians, combined with the inventions of the microscope, thermometer, and pendulum clock, advanced our knowledge and understanding of the world. The invention of the printing press allowed for easier sharing of information, which further contributed to experimentation. Finally, a disease that was feared worldwide was conquered when Edward Jenner (1749-1823) proved the effectiveness of the smallpox vaccination.

Throughout these revolutions, however, the maternal and infant death rates continued to be high. In fact, before his pioneering work in antisepsis in obstetrics, Ignaz Phillipp Semmelweis (1818-1865) observed that patients giving birth in hospitals under the care of educated physicians had significantly higher death rates than women giving birth at home or at clinics with the assistance of midwives.

Despite all of the knowledge gained during this time of revolution, society was generally callous to the plight of children. Children were abandoned without apparent remorse, and infanticide was practiced by poor families desperate to reduce the number of mouths to feed. They had no reliable form of birth control except abstinence. Because it was common practice for the woman hired as a wet nurse to sleep with the infant, many infants were inadvertently suffocated. Donahue (1985) reported that, during this period, 75% of all children baptized were dead before they reached the age of 5 years. Because of the persistence of these sad conditions, children and foundlings' hospitals were established. Eventually, laws were enacted to aid these unfortunate victims (Donahue, 1985).

Existing health care conditions for the ill and injured continued to contribute to high mortality rates. Some sources reported hospital mortality rates as high as 90%. Conditions in the armies were no better. In any military action, mortality rates were high. Reports from the battlefront during the Crimean War suggested that battles were postponed because there were too few able-bodied soldiers to fight. Dysentery and typhoid were the military's nemeses. If a soldier was wounded, infection invariably resulted. Hospitals generally offered no guarantee of survival. In any event, these occurrences had a serious effect on military strategies. If men are ill or injured, battles cannot be won.

Upon this scene entered Florence Nightingale.

FLORENCE NIGHTINGALE: THE LEGEND AND THE LADY

First, let us discuss the legend. Published works about Florence Nightingale before the 1960s generally presented the legend. Most authors agreed that she was beautiful, intelligent, wealthy, socially successful, and educated. She certainly had an ability to influence people and used every Victorian secret to accomplish her desires. Although Nightingale believed it improper for her to accept payment for her services, she did demand financial support for materials, goods, and staff to accomplish her programs and goals. Some historians believe that it was through Nightingale's influence that Jean Henri Dunant, a Swiss gentleman, provided the aid to the wounded that lay the foundation for the organization of the International Red Cross (Dodge, 1989; Bullough, Bullough, & Stanton, 1990; Dossey, 2000).

Regardless of what actually happened between Dunant and her, Nightingale's interest and ambition lay in becoming a nurse. Her family was in an uproar over this decision.

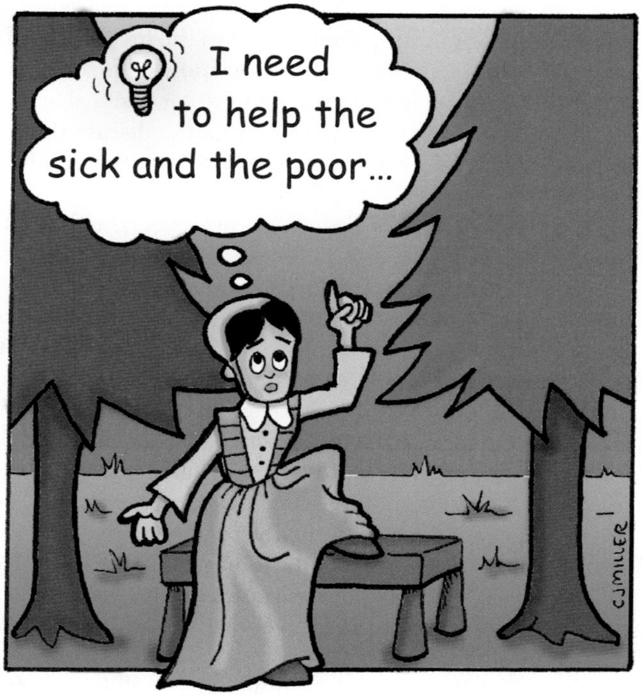

FIGURE 6-1
Florence Nightingale: The Legend (Mystic, Visionary, Healer) and the Lady.

As described by Dossey (2000), Florence (or Flo as her family and friends called her) began her journey as a *mystic* when she was 16 years old. Her experience of a sudden, inner "knowing" took place under two majestic cedars at Lebanon in Embley, one of her sacred spots for contemplation. She received the following in her awakening moment. "That a quest there is, and an end, is the single secret spoken." Energized by her contact with the Divine Reality or Consciousness, Florence "worked very hard among the poor people" with "a strong feeling of religion" for the next 3 months (Dossey, 2000, p. 33) (Figure 6-1, Critical Thinking Box 6-1, and Box 6-1).

Nightingale's parents felt that hospitals were terrible places to go, and nurses were, in most cases, the dregs of society. Hospitals were certainly not places for women of proper social upbringing. Although she was forbidden to, Nightingale studied

CRITICAL THINKING BOX 6-1

Consider all that you have heard about Florence Nightingale. Now, think about the idea that she was a mystic. What does that mean?

BOX 6-1 Nightingale and Mysticism

What is mysticism? Considered to be a universal experience of enlightenment obtained via meditation or prayer that focuses on the direct experience of union with divinity, God, or Ultimate Reality, and the belief that such experience is a genuine and important source of knowledge. It is characterized by a call to personal action, because the person is uncomfortable with the world as it is. Underhill (1961) describes five (nonlinear or nonsequential) phases in the spiritual development of a mystic.

Awakening: A profound experience that changes life forever, where the person hears the voice of God. At age 16, Nightingale experienced her first Call from God, and again on three other occasions later in life when she heard the voice of God again.

Purgation: A time where the person realizes that they are not worthy, as they become more aware of the Divine Reality. Nightingale spent her later teen years and young adulthood (approximately 17 years) separating herself from the affluent lifestyle and worldly possessions that characterized her early life.

Illumination: Person is completely consumed with passion for and a sense of God or Divine Absolute. For Nightingale, this period began when she accepts her first superintendent position at Harley Hospital in London that propelled her to battle for better conditions during the Crimean War invasion and reform of the army medical department, when she returned to England.

Surrender: Typically referred to as the "dark night of the soul," as the person searches for inner significance in every aspect of life. This period for Nightingale is thought to have been approximately 6 years after the Crimean War from the time she was in her late 30s to her late 60s and associated with her chronic ill health and episodes of stress, overexertion, and depression.

Union: The realization that the person has reached a level of deep inner connectedness with the Divine Reality. The last 20 years of Nightingale's life (age 70 through 90) are engendered with an appreciation of the blessings in her life and feelings of peace, joy, and power. The driving force in her life was no longer spurred by social action and issues.

From Dossey B: *Nursing as a spiritual practice: the mystical legacy of Florence Nightingale.* Retrieved April 5, 2005 from *http://www.altjn.com/perspectives/spiritual_practice.htm.*

nursing (in secret). After a fortuitous meeting, a relationship developed between Nightingale and Sidney and Elizabeth Herbert, an influential couple who were interested in hospital reform. Impressed with Nightingale's analytical mind and her ability to apply nursing knowledge to the critical situation in the hospitals (Bullough & Bullough, 1978; Bullough, Bullough, & Stanton, 1990), they encouraged her to study nursing at Kaiserswerth School, run by Lutheran deaconesses (Dolan, 1969). Her family, of course, was very unhappy. In fact, Dodge (1989) reported that the event precipitated a family crisis because they threatened to withdraw financial support.

Nightingale accepted a position as administrator of a nursing home for women, the Institution for the Care of Sick Gentlewomen in Distressed Circumstances. She hired her own chaperone and went to work at reforming the way things were done. Nightingale's interest in hospital reform was insatiable. She visited hospitals and took copious notes on nursing care, treatments, and procedures. She sent reports on hospital conditions to Sidney Herbert, the British secretary of war. Secretary Herbert then assigned her other hospitals to review. The reviews always included recommendations for improving nursing care. From this early background of experiences, Nightingale was now ready for her greatest mission—the Crimean War. The legend was on the way (Bullough, Bullough, & Stanton, 1990).

In 1854, soldiers were dying, more from common diseases than from bullets. Bullough, Bullough, and Stanton (1990) reported that the Crimean War was a series of mistakes. No plan was made for supplying the troops, no plan was in place to maintain the environment in camps, and no provisions were available to care for the injured after the battle. When Herbert appointed Nightingale as head of a group of nurses to go to Crimea, she had already developed a plan of action. In fact, some historians believe that she was already planning to go in an unofficial capacity. The announcement caused a sensation, and when Nightingale began a rigorous selection process for accepting nurses, many volunteered, but few were chosen. She cleaned up the kitchens, the wards, the patients, and the mess. From there, the legend grew.

She was clever; after demonstrating the effectiveness of her methods, she withdrew her services. Naturally, all that she had accomplished was done under the scrutiny, skepticism, suspicion, and anger of the physicians. Without the services of the nurses, the abominable conditions quickly returned, and finally the physicians begged her to do whatever she wished—just help! Nightingale responded to the pleading. The actual number of soldiers who benefited from the care of her nurses was immeasurable.

The nurses made rounds day and night, and the legend of the lady with the lamp was born.

Nightingale's great success prompted her to begin developing schools of nursing based on her knowledge of what was effective nursing. Eventually, many schools in Europe and America used the Nightingale model for nursing education. The program was generally 1 year in length, and classes were small. Many women wanted to become nurses; however, only 15 to 20 applicants were accepted for each class. The goals of her programs included training hospital nurses, training nurses to train others, and training nurses to work in the district with the sick poor (Dolan, 1969). In any event, Nightingale had changed society's view of the nurse to one of dignity and value and worthy of respect.

In any legend, the truth is often mixed with myth. The stories surrounding Florence Nightingale are many. What is interesting is that, before the 1970s, authors tended to deify Nightingale or establish her as a saintly person. These myths make for interesting reading. Early nurse historians also contributed to these myths by their interpretations of Nightingale's work. But myths have a purpose. They can be used to explain world views of groups of people or professions at a given time, and they provide explanations for practice beliefs or natural phenomena. Myths tend to maintain a degree of accuracy when the truth is lost. The trick is to separate myth from fact and story from legend and to draw conclusions regarding the occurrences. This is no easy task when one studies Florence Nightingale. Therefore, it is important to read a variety of studies across several time periods before drawing conclusions about the legend and the lady, Florence Nightingale.

In summary, Florence Nightingale had certain characteristics that assisted her in becoming successful during the strict Victorian times in which she lived. She was extremely well educated for her time. She had traveled throughout the world and had the advantage of personal wealth and a gift for establishing relationships with persons of influence and philanthropic spirit. Most portraits depict her as an attractive woman with pleasant features. Contemporary historians agree she had tremendous compassion for all who suffered. She was very strong-willed, a characteristic that carried her through the period of the Crimean War. She had the ability to analyze data and draw relevant conclusions, on which she based her recommendations. Her students of nursing received better preparation than most physicians. She was 36 at the end of the war, and when she returned home, she became a virtual recluse until she died at age 90. She did have some physical ailments: Crimean fever, sciatica, rheumatism, and dilation of the heart, each of which could have crippling side effects and contributed to her becoming bedridden (Bullough, Bullough, & Stanton, 1990). "In 1995, D.A.B. Young, a former scientist at the Wellcome Foundation in London, proposed that the Crimean fever was actually Mediterrean fever, otherwise known as Malta fever; this disease is included under the generic name brucellosis" (Dossey, 2000, p. 426). Because of the widespread Crimean fever that the soldiers encountered, it is thought that Nightingale was exposed to this disease most likely from ingesting contaminated food, such as meat or raw milk, cheese, or butter. It seems a logical assumption that Nightingale's 32-year history of debilitating, chronic symptoms are compatible with a diagnosis of chronic brucellosis. In any event, the legend and the lady had a significant effect on American nursing as we know it today (Dolan, 1969; Bullough & Bullough, 1978; Dodge, 1989; Bullough, Bullough, & Stanton, 1990; Dossey, 2000).

AMERICAN NURSING: CRITICAL FACTORS

WHAT WAS IT LIKE IN COLONIAL TIMES?

In colonial times, nursing responsibilities were shared by all able-bodied persons; however, if there was a choice, women were preferred to do the nursing. Early colonial historians described care for the ill and house chores as the responsibilities of nurses. Although most women of this era were considered dainty (Bradford, 1898), nurses were usually depicted as willing to do hard work. Some colonies organized nursing services that sought out the sick and provided comfort to those who were ill with smallpox and other diseases (Bullough & Bullough, 1978). There were few trained nurses, however, and most of the individuals who delivered nursing care in the five largest hospitals were men (Dolan, 1969). Eventually, women were hired at the command of George Washington to serve meals and care for the wounded and ill. The era ended with the enactment of the first legislation to improve health and medical treatment and to provide for formal education for society as a whole (Dolan, 1969).

WHAT HAPPENED TO NURSING DURING THE U.S. CIVIL WAR?

The period of the U.S. Civil War witnessed an improvement in patient care through control of the environment in which the patient recovered. The greatest problems for the Army stemmed from the poor sanitary conditions in the camps, which bred diseases such as smallpox and dysentery. The results were many deaths from inadequate nutrition, impure water, and a general lack of cleanliness.

Nurses who had some formal training were recognized as being major contributors to the relative success of hospital treatments. It was in this era that the value of primary prevention, or the prevention of the occurrence of disease by measures such as immunization and the provision of a pure water supply, became understood. Volunteer nurses, mostly women, served in hospitals caring for those wounded soldiers fortunate enough to have survived the trip from the battlefield. Their patients were nursed in a clean environment and were provided with adequate nutrition. The likelihood of their recovering was significantly improved. Astute physicians observed that patients cared for by nurses generally recovered well enough to return to the battlefield. Families, too, saw that when nurses had control over the environment, their ill or injured loved one was more likely to recover—and return home.

As the United States moved into the industrial age of the early 1900s, Victorian values began to permeate the middle and upper-middle classes. Social concerns focused on protecting families from the diseases of the crowded urban areas, and the demand for improved health care increased.

HOW DID THE ROLES OF NURSES AND WIVES COMPARE DURING THE VICTORIAN ERA?

The Victorian era had a significant effect on nurses, primarily because they were women. The parallelism between the idealized Victorian woman and the traditional nurse is stunning. The effect of many of the values and beliefs of this era, some historians report, is still felt by women today.

The typical upper-class Victorian household consisted of a husband, who earned a living outside of the home and maintained total control of the family finances, and his wife, who maintained harmony within the home and raised their children. Women's work was generally restricted to philanthropic and voluntary work; they attended teas and other social functions to raise money for organizations and people in need.

Most women were considered fragile and dainty. They were often ill. It has been suggested that their illnesses and frailty were used as a form of birth control to prevent the numerous pregnancies that most women experienced. Some historians concluded that it was through their weaknesses that women gained control and attention. If the wife was ill or frail, maids or servants were hired, but if the wife were healthy, the husband would expect more from her. The Victorian wife was expected to "be good." She was esteemed by her husband, but had limited power within the confines of the home and society. She was expected to be hard-working and able to maintain harmony while at the same time being submissive to the demands of her husband. Generally, this fostered dependence on the dominant male figure—the Victorian husband (Rybczynski, 1986).

Let us examine nursing during this same time, especially within the hospital organization. Nurses generally were women who wanted to avoid the drudgery of a Victorian marriage. They were required to be single to make a complete commitment to their vocation. Schooled in submission, women were expected to be equally accommodating within the hospital organization. A good nurse worked for harmony within the hospital. She was expected to be hard-working and submissive. The doctor and the hospital administrator were frequently the same person, usually a man, who expected position and power to go hand in hand. Patients were admitted only if they had income and could afford to pay for the services. It was the physician who generated income, and good nurses were expected to help them continue to maintain power. Because the system rewarded people for being ill, there was little incentive to be healthy. Social values contributed to dependence on the health care system. From this milieu came the reformers (Stewart, 1950; Davis, 1961; Bullough & Bullough, 1978; Kalisch & Kalisch, 1986).

WHO WERE THE REFORMERS OF THE VICTORIAN ERA?

The Victorian era, although a time of repression for women, was also a time of reform. A list of important names in nursing reform includes M. Adelaide Nutting, Minnie Goodnow, Lavinia L. Dock, Annie W. Goodrich, Isabel Hampton Robb, Lilian D. Wald, Isabel M. Stewart, and Sophia Palmer, among others (Jamieson & Sewall, 1949; Kalisch & Kalisch, 1986). These women, who had in common a comfortable upper-middle–class background, intelligence, and education, also had in common a desire to reach beyond the constraints that society imposed on them. As society began to realize the important role that nurses played in treating the ill and injured, it also began to understand the need for training programs that would educate better nurses. Reformers focused on establishing standards for nursing education and practice. Among their accomplishments were the organization of the American Nurses Association and the creation of its journal, the *American Journal of Nursing*, and the enactment of legislation to require the licensure of prepared nurses. This protected the public from inadequate care given by people who were not trained to nurse (Christy, 1971; Dock, 1900).

THE NURSE'S ROLE: THE STRUGGLE FOR DEFINITIONS

WHAT DO NURSES DO?

As a student, you study nursing texts that explain theories, skills, principles, and the care of patients. Every text has at least one introductory chapter that describes nursing and its significance. By examining many of these introductory chapters of nursing texts, you can generate a rather extensive list of roles (Anglin, 1991). From this list of roles, six major categories can be determined (Table 6-1). The most traditional role for

TABLE 6-1

What Nurses Do

Caregiver	Teacher	Advocate	Manager	Colleague	Expert
Care provider	Patient educator	Interpreter	Administrator	Collaborator	Academician
Comforter	Counselor	Learner	Coordinator	Communicator	Historian
Handmaiden	Patient teacher	Protector	Decision maker	Facilitator	Nursing instructor
Healer		Risk-taker	Evaluator	Peer reviewer	Professional educator
Helper		Change agent	Initiator	Professional	Researcher
Nurturer			Leader	Specialist	Research consumer
Practitioner			Planner		Teacher
Rehabilitator					Theorist
Support agent					Practitioner
					Leader

nurses is that of *caregiver.* The nurse as *teacher* is often referred to when discussing patient care or nursing education. The role of *advocate* has been very controversial since 1900. Nurses were also expected to be *managers* ever since the first formal education or training program was instituted. Another interesting role for the nurse is that of *colleague.* The final role is that of *expert.*

WHAT IS THE TRADITIONAL ROLE OF A NURSE?

The role of the nurse as caregiver has engendered the least amount of controversy. This role has been thoroughly documented, not only in writing but also through art, since early times. Nurses and nursing leaders agree that this is their primary role. As students, your caregiving skills will be measured constantly through skill laboratories, clinical evaluation proficiency, and, eventually, through licensure testing and staff evaluations. All of these mechanisms are used to evaluate your ability to be a caregiver. When we think of the role of caregiver, we think of someone who is moved to take action so that suffering can be relieved. What is difficult to measure is the level of feeling related to caring. There is a great debate in nursing as to whether nurses can be taught to care. However, despite this controversy, most nurses agree that they are caregivers. Because our current education is based on Nightingale's principles of caring, it is no surprise that all of you believe that you will provide care to those in need. You may choose to provide this care in various settings, but basically all of you desire to be caregivers and are expected to be so.

Caregiving is probably the only role about which there is agreement as to what it means and how we do it.

Imagine a nurse giving care. Generally, the picture that most often comes to mind is someone, usually female, in a white uniform caring for a patient who is ill. This picture is the romanticized version of caregiving continually portrayed in movies, television, and novels. We know that caregiving takes place in many settings: clinics, homes, hospitals, offices, businesses, and schools, among others. We can probably agree that caregiving is an important role for nurses and is probably why most of us chose nursing. Studies examining the role of caregiver continue, and our understanding of the role is expanding (Benner, 1984; Leininger, 1984; Watson, 1985). Without a doubt, this is an important role, one that is essential to nursing.

DID YOU KNOW YOU WOULD BE A TEACHER?

When you take care of patients, it soon becomes apparent that certain information must be shared with them so that they can participate in their care. Teaching patients about their therapy, condition, or choices is critical to the successful outcome of some prescribed treatments. For example, nurses have learned through research that knowledge can reduce anxiety before and after surgery. We teach patients about almost everything related to their care. Knowledge can enhance compliance with medications and can encourage healthy lifestyles and behaviors. Teaching becomes

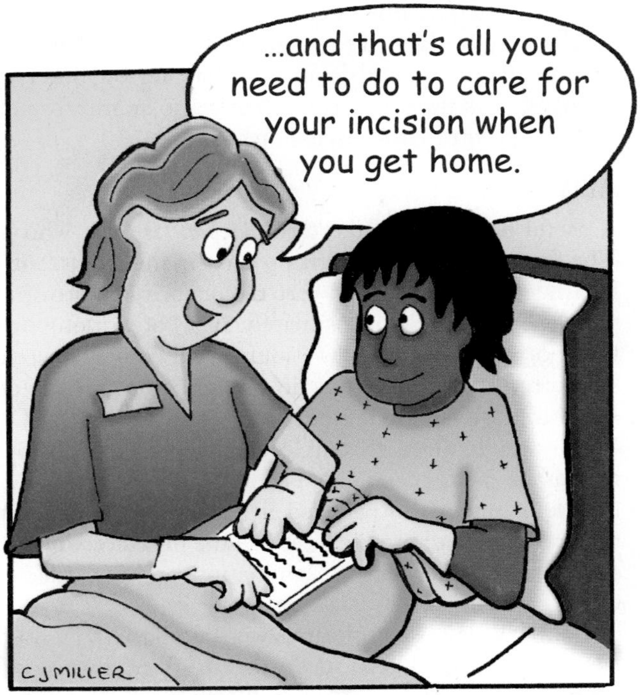
...and that's all you need to do to care for your incision when you get home.
CJMILLER

FIGURE 6-2
Did you know you would be a teacher?

especially important when patients have to make treatment choices and decisions about their care. With the volumes of information available regarding health care, it is even more important that nurses help patients understand what they need to know to make wise decisions. Without exception, standardized care plans have included, as a nursing action, *patient education*. Discharge plans also provide for patient education. Home care includes teaching as a reimbursable activity. Agency charting procedures all require documentation of patient education. All nursing textbooks include sections on what the nurse needs to emphasize regarding patient education. With all this evidence, there is little doubt that the teacher role is an important one for the nurse.

The role of the nurse as teacher of other nurses is rooted in the evolution of nursing education; however, as schools of nursing developed, nurses were taught by physicians. Gradually, nurses began supervising students of nursing and taught them on the job. Eventually, the influence of Nightingale resulted in qualified nurses teaching students about nursing. This method has prevailed in nursing schools.

In America, the greatest impetus to nurses as teachers occurred in 1948 when recommendations from the Brown report included the separation of the nursing schools from hospital administrative budgets. This was a major step in nurses' gaining control over the budget and the educational processes of students (Brown, 1948). Numerous nursing curricula since 1900 have included sections on what the nurse needs to teach the patient about the illness. This continues to be a very important role for the nurse at a time when treatment choices and lifestyle choices are numerous.

Teaching is planned to strengthen a patient's knowledge of making decisions about treatment options and is an essential nursing intervention (Alfaro-LeFevre, 1998). In many ways the nurse as teacher is also an interpreter of information, and this leads us to the next role for discussion.

WHO WILL ADVOCATE?

A useful definition of the term *advocate* is "one who pleads a cause before another." The first advocacy issue, arising early in the 1900s, concerned nursing practice. Public health and visiting nurses were the majority (approximately 70%), and hospital nurses were the minority (approximately 30%) of working nurses. Working as a private duty nurse or visiting nurse was a source of income for women who had no other means of support. Because there was no way to determine the credentials of the visiting nurse, many impostors worked in that capacity. Lavinia L. Dock, Sophia Palmer, and Annie W. Goodrich, three nursing leaders, deplored this situation and endeavored to protect the public from unscrupulous "nurses" (Goodnow, 1936; Dolan, 1969). Dock was an excellent nurse who believed in fairness to qualified nurses and to the public. She advocated that all practicing nurses be measured by a "fair-general-average standard," as determined by written examination, and rewarded with licensure upon attainment of the standard (Christy, 1971).

Palmer's proposed solutions were similar. Many hospitals were sending out inexperienced undergraduates to do private-duty nursing while keeping the income. She advocated a training school in which students of nursing would learn to give care under a qualified nurse and supported the implementation of a registration process for all qualified nurses to protect the public from incompetent, unqualified nurses.

Goodrich advocated compulsory legislation that would ensure that graduates or trained nurses would be the only ones who could work as nurses. She pleaded for the registration of qualified nurses, not only for the protection of the nurse but for the protection of the community. Goodrich also fought against correspondence or home-study programs for nurses, which were a greater menace to the public's safety than people realized. Such legislation, she believed, would encourage talented young women who were intellectually prepared for scientific education to select nursing as a career. The role of the advocate, as understood by these three early nursing leaders, was to protect the public from unqualified nurses (Christy, 1969; Dock, 1900; Palmer, 1900).

From this beginning, the role of advocate grew. Public-health nurses served as advocates in factories and communities during the Industrial Revolution. Many municipal boards of health hired visiting nurses to work as inspectors in the factories to protect the workers from health hazards and to help prevent accidents. Communities were finding that the nurse as advocate for the factory worker had inestimable value. Visiting nurses were also proving very effective in preventing the spread of communicable diseases.

Hospital nurses also worked as advocates for the patients while giving care. Nurses were crucial in protecting patients from harm when they were too ill to protect themselves. Nurses were also responsible for providing measures to relieve pain, and they strove to make their patients happy and comfortable, even if it meant breaking the rules sometimes (Hill, 1900). During the 1970s and 1980s, the responsibility of the nurse as advocate was expanded to include speaking for their clients when they could not speak for themselves (Sovie, 1978). Nurses returned to work in churches in the primary role of advocate under the Granger Westberg model for parish nursing. The members of the congregation where a parish nurse practiced found affirmation and support as they reached to improve their physical, emotional, and spiritual health (Striepe, 1987).

However, consumers, administrators, and courts do not share the perception of the nurse as advocate. The findings of a study done in 1983 indicated that consumers did not recognize the nurse as an initiator of health care (Miller, Mansen, & Lee, 1983). Consumers also believed that physicians would protect the rights of the patient. Miller, Mansen, and Lee (1983) concluded that although nurses were serving as mediators between patients and institutions, changes rarely occurred within the institutions as a result of this role. Patient advocacy was directly related to the power and authority allowed the nurse by the particular system. Nurses generally became advocates whenever the issue was care; however, they had little power to be truly effective as an advocate when the concerns involved the medical regimen or health care services (Miller, Mansen, & Lee, 1983). Examples of advocacy included questioning doctors' orders, promoting client comfort, and supporting patient decisions regarding health care choices.

Advocacy is a critical role for nurses today. Nurses are in a vital position to be effective in this role.

With the need for informed consent, advance directives, and treatment choices, patients more than ever need an advocate to interpret information, identify the risks and benefits of the various treatment options, and support the decision they make. Being an advocate does involve taking personal and professional risks. When the issue is care, nurses are willing advocates, but when the issue is the profession, nurses seem reluctant (Anglin, 1991).

WHY ARE NURSES MANAGERS?

Even Florence Nightingale recognized the need for nurses to be managers. She insisted that nurses needed to organize the care of the patient so that other nurses could carry on when they were not present. There were four major eras in the development of the nurse as manager. During the first period, lasting until about 1920, the nurse was known as the *charge nurse*. Charge nurses were responsible for teaching the nursing students what they needed to know and for directing the care that the students gave. The charge nurse was autocratic. This nurse had absolute authority over the student.

During the second era, lasting until 1949, the term *supervisor* was used to describe the role. The supervisor continued to be responsible for the students; however, the role had expanded to include enforcing agency policies, developing improvements in the care of the ill, and being responsible for the effective use of the ward's resources. The supervisor served on hospital committees but had no vote. Supervisors continued their autocratic management styles and established high standards of nursing practice. At the end of this period, management techniques were beginning to focus on a more humanistic approach, which was a more effective use of human resources. Nurses were more involved in the patient-care process. Hospital administrators were relying on nursing expertise to establish policies for patient care and hospital administration. This era ended with the publication of Esther Lucille Brown's report (1948) recommending that nursing education be separated from hospital administration.

During the third period, lasting until 1970, the nurse was referred to as a *coordinator*. The nurse coordinator no longer had responsibility for the nursing education of the students but was expected to motivate staff, be innovative, and solve problems. Coordinators were active in improving patient care and were expected to maintain harmony within the institution. Many nurse coordinators had few skills in and little knowledge of middle management. They basically learned by trial and error how to be effective.

The last period, from 1970 to the present, is a series of waves. Nurses gained recognition as managers and were able to function in that role. Hospital nurses gained middle-management positions and proved their abilities. The period before diagnostic-related groups (DRGs) saw escalating hospital costs and growth in the numbers of employees and services. From this growth came significant efforts to control the costs of health care. The term *manager* is used most often now in the nursing literature, but you may find it used to describe any of the four periods.

No matter what era in history you study, the expectation is that the nurse manager will coordinate patient care and supervise nurses in the delivery of quality care.

One cannot leave the discussion of this important role without some comments about the pressure of economics on the delivery of health care. Because nurse-managers are responsible for budgets and monitor reimbursement, the movement toward a case-management system is much like a tidal wave in nursing as a whole—unexpected and unprepared for. However, the reality is that nurses have always been case managers—not as contemporary critics might define it, but as working nurses, especially in community health. Zander's classic interpretation of case management—that is, a nurse manages nursing care while containing costs and maintaining quality (Zander, 1987; 1988)—has guided the practice of community-health nurses for as long as this area of practice has existed, even before the definition was developed. However, the model is relatively innovative in hospital settings. The knowledge and skills required for the nurse as manager have become increasingly complex. Nurse-managers are expected to solve problems, evaluate care and personnel, develop budgets, delegate responsibility, negotiate, and be critical-thinkers in an effort to maintain harmony within the institution. Without a doubt, the role of the nurse as manager has evolved into a complex one that includes organizing patient care, directing personnel to achieve agency goals, and allocating resources (Anglin, 1991).

CAN NURSES BE COLLEAGUES?

The role of colleague is a vital one for any profession. The status of colleague within health care generates pictures of nurses, doctors, and pharmacists discussing, on an equal basis, problems and concerns related to health care. In nursing, however, a review of our history reveals that we have not quite achieved the status of colleague. Interdisciplinary collegial relationships currently are tenuous. More surprising is that, even among nurses, intradisciplinary collegial relationships are strained. Three periods in the evolution of this role can be identified.

The first period, that of the *assistant role*, ended in 1940. This early category of colleague was clearly defined by nursing leaders as one who was cooperative, loyal, and obedient to the physician and the hospital (Anglin, 1991). These characteristics were considered critical to being a competent nurse. In 1905, Jan Hodson actually set the standard by insisting that loyalty to the doctors was the most important factor for a faithful nurse to be successful. Hodson supported blind faith in carrying out doctors' orders, no matter how different or unusual. She also recommended a strong sense of responsibility when working with subordinates and superiors (Hodson, 1905; Anglin, 1991). However, she encouraged collegial exchange of information and emphasized asking for advice in serious or delicate matters (Hodson, 1905). Obviously, physicians encouraged and rewarded this type of subordinate role (Lawman, 1907; Aikens, 1935; Hamilton, 1949).

From 1941 to 1959, the role of colleague fell under the title of *coordinator*. A major effort to evaluate nursing service delivered during World War II revealed this more authoritarian principle of management (Brown, 1948). Nurses were caught between their hospital's administration, the physicians, and, unfortunately, the highly authoritarian managers within their own profession. Few contributions from nurses were incorporated into the planning of the organizations. In public-health nursing, however, the role of colleague was fully realized (Brown, 1948). Public-health nurses served on boards of health and were major contributors in public-health planning and programs within local health departments. One important recommendation that came from the Brown report (1948) was that nurses should work to improve their actions and words based on their understanding of human behavior, and learn to deal effectively with people. Brown continued by recommending an even more important goal for nurses. Once nurses learned to deal effectively with people, they could make major contributions to the total effort of health care delivery and other disciplines (Brown, 1948). Great emphasis was placed on developing collegial relationships for the good of the health care system. From these significant recommendations came team-nursing approaches to care and the coordination of activities for improved patient care. However, the theme of cooperation remained (Anglin, 1991).

Between 1960 and the present, the term *collaborator* has been adopted for this role. The root of this word means "to exchange information with the enemy." This may be the most fitting description of the role. Nurses were interested in developing collaborative relationships with doctors, pharmacists, and other health professionals. The literature is abundant with discussions of these relationships and consistently describes these relationships as collaborative (Hahm & Miller, 1961; Quint, 1967; Seward, 1969; Kelly, 1975; Wisener, 1978; Tourtillott, 1986).

WHERE DOES THIS LEAVE THE ROLE OF COLLEAGUE?

Nursing education has promoted the term collaborator over colleague. The dilemma is that employers neither recognize nor reward the role. Students in their educational experiences are seldom offered the opportunity to practice the role of colleague and, therefore, have only a vague understanding of the role. However, public-health nurses throughout American history have not only understood the role, but probably have attained a greater degree of collegiality than any other practice area of nursing. Public-health nurses are not the majority within the profession. Nevertheless, they continue to enjoy and maintain the essence of the role (Anglin, 1991). As a colleague, one recognizes nurses with expertise and relies on those nurses for their expertise in the interest of improving patient care and advancing the profession. The essence of the role is mutual respect and equality among professionals, both intradisciplinary and interdisciplinary (Anglin, 1991). Until nurses can respond to each other with respect, it will be difficult to move from collaborator to true colleague.

WHAT ABOUT EXPERTS?

There is one other role in which nurses are often found. For lack of a better name, this role is called *expert*. It is a conglomerate of advanced formal or informal education and acquired or recognized expertise. The role includes academicians, historians, nursing educators, clinicians, professional educators, researchers, research consumers, theorists, nurse technologists, and the leaders within the profession. The American Academy of Nursing recognizes some of these individuals and votes to bestow on them the honor of Fellow. There are many nurses who are experts in an area of practice, whether it be in clinics, at the bedside, in nursing homes, or in other settings. As nurses with special expertise, they are called on to provide testimony in courts and at government hearings or to share information and knowledge with other nurses, which is their obligation to the profession. This sharing can be done through mentoring, guest-speaking, performing in-services, offering continuing-education programs, contributing to publications, and writing technical articles. These experts are usually the nurses who create the momentum that moves the profession forward. This is a role that should be recognized, encouraged, and rewarded.

CONCLUSION

What do nurses do? There is no simple answer. We agree that nurses care for patients—and, hence, are caregivers. We agree that nurses teach patients what they need to know to make informed choices—and therefore are teachers. We also agree that the role of manager exists in some form, and so we manage our practice and patients' care. We can even define the role of advocate, although, based on the history of the role, nurses are reluctant to take risks to fully carry the role into the future. The role of colleague is less clear. We are consistent in using the term collaborator; however, the term colleague is deemed more fitting for professionals, and that is the role to which we should aspire.

Finally, we have experts, who we may or may not recognize and upon whom the profession depends to provide the leadership for the whole. These roles merely provide a beginning for you to understand the profession you have chosen—nursing. May you become proficient in these roles and develop into an expert, and then provide the leadership for nursing in the future.

The future is not the result of choices among
Alternative paths offered;
It is a place that is created,
Created first in the mind and will,
Created next in activity.
The future is not some place we are going to,
But one we are creating.
The paths to it are not found, but made.
And the activity of making them
Changes both the maker and the destiny.

—*Anonymous, 1987*

REFERENCES

Aikens CA: *Studies in nursing ethics*, Philadelphia, 1935, Saunders.

Alfaro-LeFevre R: *Applying nursing process: a step-by-step guide*, New York, 1998, Lippincott Williams & Wilkins.

Anglin LT: *The roles of nurses: a history, 1900 to 1988*, Ann Arbor, Mich, 1991, University of Michigan.

Benner P: *From novice to expert: excellence and power in clinical nursing practice*, Menlo Park, CA, 1984, Addison-Wesley.

Bradford W: *History of Plymouth plantation: book II (1620)*, Plymouth, Mass, 1898, Wright & Potter.

Brown EL: *Nursing for the future*, New York, 1948, Russell Sage Foundation.

Bullough V, Bullough B: *The care of the sick: the emergence of modern nursing*, New York, 1978, Prodist.

Bullough V, Bullough B, Stanton MP: *Florence Nightingale and her era: a collection of new scholarship*, New York, 1990, Garland.

Christy TE: Portrait of a leader: Isabel Hampton Robb, *Nurs Outlook* 17(3):26-29, 1969.

Christy TE: First fifty years, *Am J Nurs* 71(9): 1778-1784, 1971.

Cohen EL, Cesta, TG: *Nursing case management: from essentials to advanced practice applications*, St. Louis, 2005, Mosby.

Dalton R: Hospitals: their origins and history, *Dublin J Med Sci* 109(3), 17-19, 1900.

Dana CL: *The peaks of medical history*, New York, 1936, Paul B. Hoeber.

Davis MD: I was a student over 50 years ago, *Nurs Outlook* 61:62, 1961.

Dock L: What may we expect from the law?, *Am J Nurs* 1:9, 1900.

Dodge BS: *The story of nursing*, ed 2, Boston, 1989, Little, Brown.

Dolan JA: *History of nursing*, Philadelphia, 1969, Saunders.

Donahue MP: *Nursing: the finest art*, St Louis, 1985, Mosby.

Dossey B: *Florence Nightingale: mystic, visionary, healer*, Springhouse, Penn, 2000, Springhouse.

Goodnow M: *Outlines in the history of nursing*, Philadelphia, 1936, Saunders.

Hahm H, Miller D: Relationships between medical and nursing education, *J Nurs Educ* 39:849-851, 1961.

Hamilton JA: Success or failure in nursing administration, *Am J Nurs* 49:496, 1949.

Hill J: Private duty nursing from a nurse's point of view, *Am J Nurs* 1(2):129, 1900.

Hodson J: *How to become a trained nurse*, New York, 1905, William Abbott.

Jamieson EM, Sewall MF: *Trends in nursing history*, Philadelphia, 1949, Saunders.

Kalisch PA, Kalisch BJ: *The advance of American nursing*, Boston, 1986, Little, Brown.

Kelly LY: *Dimensions of professional nursing*, ed 3, New York, 1975, Macmillan.

Lawman JH: The evolution and development of the nurse, *Am J Nurs* 8:8, 1907.

Leininger M: *Care: the essence of nursing and health*, Thorofare, NJ, 1984, Charles B. Slack.

Miller BK, Mansen TJ, Lee H: Patient advocacy: do nurses have the power and authority to act as patient advocate?, *Nurs Leadersh* 6(2):56-60, 1983.

Palmer S: The editor, *Am J Nurs* 1(4):166-169, 1900.

Quint GC: Role models and the professional nurse identity, *J Nurs Educ* 6:11, 1967.

Rybczynski W: *Home: a short history of an idea*, Middlesex, England, 1986, Penguin.

Seward JM: Role of the nurse: perceptions of nursing students and auxiliary nursing personnel, *Nurs Res* 18(2):164-169, 1969.

Sovie L: Nursing. In Chaska N, editor: *The nursing profession*, New York, 1978, GP Putnam's Sons.

Stewart IM: A half-century of nursing education, *Am J Nurs* 50:617, 1950.

Striepe J: *Nurses in churches: a manual for developing parish nurse services and networks*, Spencer, IA, 1987, Iowa Lake Area Agency on Aging.

Tourtillott EA: *Commitment—a lost characteristic*, New York, 1986, JB Lippincott.

Watson J: *Nursing: human science and human care—a theory of nursing*, East Norwalk, Conn, 1985, Appleton-Century-Crofts.

Wisener S: *The reality of primary nursing care: risks, roles and research. Role changes in primary nursing*, New York, 1978, National League of Nursing.

Zander K: Nursing case management: a classic. *Definition* 2(2):1-3, 1987.

Zander K: Managed care within acute care settings: design and implementation via nursing case management, *Health Care Supervisor* 6(2):24-43, 1988.

CHAPTER 7

Nursing Education

GAYLE VARNELL, PhD, RN, CPNP

Education should not be a destination—but a path we travel all the days of our lives.

—*Anonymous*

Education is the ability to listen to almost anything without losing your temper or your self-confidence.

—*Robert Frost*

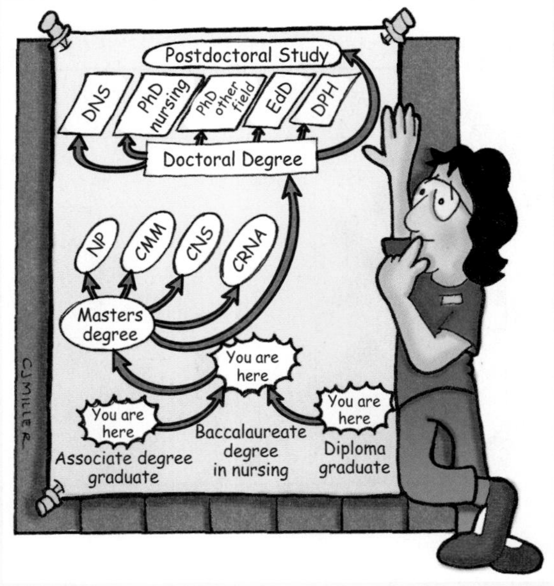

Pathway to career goals.

After completing this chapter, you should be able to:

- Compare the various types of educational preparation for nursing.
- Describe the educational preparation for a graduate degree.
- Compare the alternative options provided by career-ladder or bridge programs, external degree, Bachelor of Science in Nursing–completion, and online universities.
- Describe the purpose of nursing program accreditation.
- Discuss the future of nursing education.

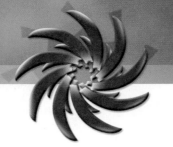

After struggling to complete your basic educational preparation for nursing, you are probably looking forward to that first paycheck as a registered nurse.

The last thing on your mind is returning to school for more education! The purpose of this chapter is not to discuss the issue of entry into practice or to debate which educational program is best. Instead, the purpose of this chapter is to help you look at where you are educationally and to offer direction regarding educational opportunities to enhance your career goals. Before looking down the path at the variety of educational offerings available to help you meet those goals, let us look at the variety of pathways that lead to the basic educational preparation for an RN.

Which path did you travel? There are three primary paths (diploma, associate's degree, and baccalaureate degree) that lead to one licensing examination: the National Council Licensure Examination for Registered Nurses (NCLEX-RN). These programs usually require a high school diploma or the equivalent for admission. Some of the other, less common, paths include master's and doctoral degree programs, both of which accept college graduates with liberal arts majors. Other paths that are becoming increasingly more popular include career ladder programs (from practical nurse to associate-degree nurse), two-plus-two programs (from associate's degree to baccalaureate nurse), and the increasingly popular accelerated baccalaureate program for non-nursing college graduates.

The distribution of the RN population according to basic nursing education is illustrated in Figure 7-1. In 1980, the diploma education tract was the highest level of education for most nursing graduates. In the year 2000, the associate degree was the highest level of education for most nursing graduates, with diploma and baccalaureate graduates approximately equal in number.

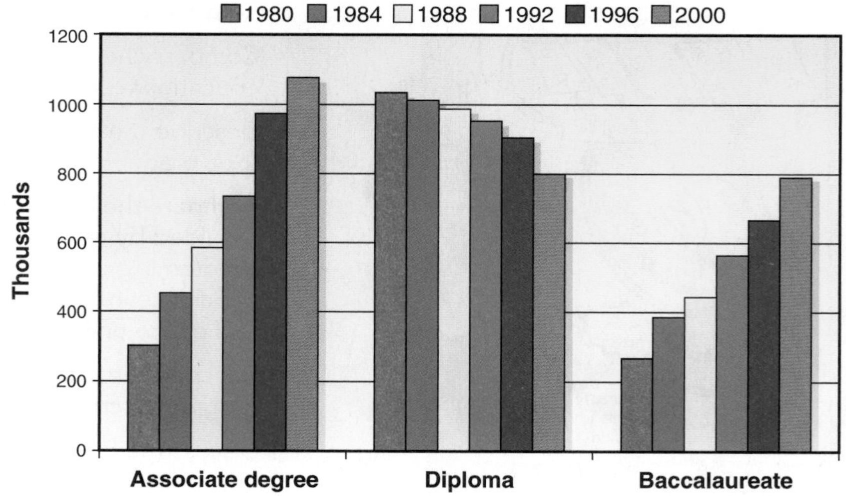

FIGURE 7-1

Distribution of RNs according to basic nursing education, 1980-2000. *(From Health Resources and Services Administration:* HRSA Bureau of Health Professions Division of Nursing sample survey, *2000, Health Resources and Services Administration.)*

PATH OF DIPLOMA EDUCATION

WHAT IS THE HISTORY OF DIPLOMA NURSING?

The oldest form of educational preparation leading to licensure as a RN in the United States is the diploma program. Many nurses practicing in the United States today received their basic educational preparation in a diploma program.

Education in diploma schools emphasized the skills needed to care for the acutely ill patient. Graduates received a diploma in nursing, not an academic degree. From 1872 until the mid-1960s, the hospital diploma program was the dominant nursing program. Diploma programs currently represent less than 10% of all basic RN programs (AACN, 2004 Media relations nursing fact sheet, 2004). Perhaps one of the reasons for this decline was that the courses offered by hospitals frequently did not confer college credit. Although most diploma programs are associated with institutions of higher learning, where the graduates receive some college credit, they still may not receive college credit for the nursing courses. Other diploma programs have evolved into what is called a *single purpose institution*, having baccalaureate-degree-granting privileges for nursing only.

WHAT IS THE EDUCATIONAL PREPARATION OF THE DIPLOMA GRADUATE?

The current preparation of a diploma nurse varies in length from 2 to 3 years and takes place in a hospital school of nursing. This type of program may be under the direction of the hospital or incorporated independently. The diploma program may include general education subjects such as biology and physical and social sciences, in addition to nursing theory and practice. Graduates of diploma programs are prepared to function as beginning practitioners in acute, intermediate, long-term, and ambulatory health care facilities. Because there is a close relationship between the nursing school and the hospital, graduates are well prepared to function in that institution; on graduation, many graduates are employed by that hospital and therefore experience an easier roll transition.

Standards and competencies for diploma programs are developed and maintained by the National League for Nursing (NLN) Council of Diploma Programs. Graduates of diploma programs are awarded a certificate and are eligible to take the NCLEX-RN state board examination for licensure.

PATH OF ASSOCIATE-DEGREE EDUCATION

WHAT IS THE HISTORY OF ASSOCIATE-DEGREE NURSING?

The associate-degree nursing program has the distinction of being the first and, to date, only educational program for nursing that was developed from planned research and controlled experimentation. Since its beginning in 1951, the associate-degree nursing program has grown to more than 880 programs, producing more graduates annually than either diploma or baccalaureate programs. According to the Seventh National Sample Survey of Registered Nurses, conducted in 2000, 55.4% of the RNs who graduated in the past 5 years received their initial nursing education from an associate-degree program. Graduates are employed in hospitals, outpatient departments, nursing homes, physicians' offices, and home-care agencies.

In 1951, Mildred Montag published her doctoral dissertation, *The Education of Nursing Technicians*, which proposed education for the RN in the community college. Dr. Montag suggested that the associate-degree program be a terminal degree to prepare nurses for immediate employment. According to Dr. Montag, there was a need for a new type of nurse, the "nurse technician," whose role would be broader than that of a practical nurse but narrower than that of the professional nurse. The technical nurse was to function at the "bedside." The duties of the technical nurse, according to Dr. Montag, would include (1) giving general nursing care with supervision, (2) assisting in the planning of nursing care for clients, and (3) assisting in the evaluation of the nursing care given (Montag, 1951).

In 1952, an advisory committee was established by the American Association of Junior Colleges. Along with the NLN, this committee was to conduct cooperative research on nursing education in the community college. The goals of this Cooperative Research Project were threefold: (1) to describe the development of the associate-degree nursing program, (2) to evaluate the associate-degree graduates, and (3) to determine the future implications of the associate degree on nursing. The original project was directed by Dr. Montag at Teachers College of Columbia University and included seven junior colleges and one hospital from each of the six regions of the United States.

In the proposed technical nursing curriculum, there was to be a balance between general education and nursing courses. Unlike the diploma programs, the emphasis was to be on education, not service. At the end of 2 years, the student was to be awarded an associate's degree in nursing and was to be eligible to take the state board examinations for RN licensure. This degree was seen as terminal and not a step toward obtaining a baccalaureate degree (Montag, 1959).

WHAT IS THE EDUCATIONAL PREPARATION OF THE ASSOCIATE-DEGREE GRADUATE?

The current preparation of an associate-degree nurse usually begins within a community college, although some programs are based within a senior college or university. The program is 18 to 21 school calendar months in length. The NLN recommends that the program of learning be within 60 to 72 semester credits (90 to 108 quarter credits) and that there be a balanced distribution of no more than 60% of the total number of credits allocated to nursing courses (NLN, 2001). In some programs, the student must complete the general education and science course requirements before beginning the nursing courses. At the end of the program, the student receives an associate's degree in nursing.

Associate-degree nursing education has helped to bring about a change in the type of student who enrolls in nursing programs. Prior to the emergence of associate-degree nursing programs, nursing students were traditionally single, white females younger than 19 years of age from middle-class families (Kaiser, 1975). Associate-degree programs attract a more diverse student population of older individuals, minorities, men, and married women from a variety of educational backgrounds. Many of these individuals have baccalaureate and higher degrees in other fields of study and are seeking a second career. Along with their maturity, these students bring life experiences that are applicable to nursing. The students tend to be more goal-oriented and have a more realistic perspective of the work setting. The community college curriculum is conducive to students who want to attend school on a part-time basis.

Standards and competencies for associate-degree programs are developed and maintained by the NLN Council of Associate Degree Programs. At the NLN 1998 Education Summit, the associate degree in nursing (ADN) competencies were revised to include multiculturalism, long-term care, systems management, and interdisciplinary collaboration. Graduates of associate-degree programs are eligible to take the NCLEX-RN state board examination for licensure.

Dr. Montag's original proposal for the associate-degree program to be a terminal degree is no longer applicable. In 1978, the American Nurses Association proposed a resolution regarding associate-degree programs that stated that they be viewed as part of the career upward-mobility plan rather than as terminal programs. The associate-degree program has provided students with the motivation to further their education and the opportunity for career mobility. Although many nursing students end their education with an associate's degree, many enter the associate-degree program with every intention of continuing their nursing education to the baccalaureate level and even further.

PATH OF BACCALAUREATE EDUCATION

In this discussion, only the "generic" baccalaureate programs are addressed. A generic student is defined as a student who enters a baccalaureate nursing program with no training or education in nursing. A traditional generic baccalaureate program includes lower-division (freshman and sophomore) liberal arts and science courses with upper-division (junior and senior) nursing courses. RNs entering baccalaureate programs are discussed later in this chapter.

WHAT IS THE HISTORY OF BACCALAUREATE NURSING?

A few early training schools were affiliated with universities to provide some of the science courses. In 1889, Mercy Hospital in Chicago affiliated with Northwestern University. The science courses offered to nursing students were outside the academic curriculum and did not lead to a degree. Teacher's College of Columbia University also played a critical role in the establishment of baccalaureate nursing education by establishing a 1-year course in hospital economics in 1899. The course was extended to 2 years in 1905 (Anderson, 1981).

The early baccalaureate nursing programs were usually 5 years in length and consisted of the basic 3-year diploma program with an additional 2 years of liberal arts. In 1919, there were eight baccalaureate programs. Currently, there are 673 baccalaureate programs in the United States (Peterson, 2004).

WHAT IS THE EDUCATIONAL PREPARATION OF THE BACCALAUREATE GRADUATE?

The current preparation of a baccalaureate nurse is 4 to 5 years in length (120 to 140 credits) and emphasizes courses in the liberal arts, sciences, and humanities. Approximately half to two thirds of the curriculum consists of nonnursing courses. To qualify for a baccalaureate program, the student must first meet all of the college's or the university's entrance requirements. Usual entrance requirements include college preparation courses in high school (e.g., foreign language, advanced science, and math courses) and a specified cumulative grade-point average. Most colleges also require a college entrance examination such as the Scholastic Aptitude Test (SAT) or the American College Test (ACT).

During the first 2 years of a traditional baccalaureate nursing program, the student is usually enrolled in liberal arts and science courses with other nonnursing students. It is not until late in the sophomore or early junior year that nursing courses are introduced. There are some baccalaureate programs that incorporate nursing courses throughout the 4-year nursing curriculum. The emphasis in the baccalaureate nursing program is on developing critical decision-making skills, exercising independent nursing judgment, and acquiring research skills.

The graduate of a baccalaureate program must fulfill both the degree requirements of the nursing program and those of the college. On completion of the program, the usual degree awarded is a Bachelor of Science in Nursing (BSN).

The graduate of a baccalaureate program is prepared to provide health promotion and health restoration care for individuals, families, and groups in a variety of institutional and community settings. Graduates of baccalaureate nursing programs are eligible to take the NCLEX-RN state board examination for licensure. BSN graduates are also prepared to continue their education by moving directly into graduate education. An increasing number of BSN graduates are continuing their nursing education by going directly into graduate programs.

NONTRADITIONAL PATHS FOR NURSING EDUCATION

WHAT ABOUT A MASTER'S DEGREE AS A PATH TO BECOMING AN RN?

Master's degree (MSN) programs are particularly attractive to the growing number of college graduates who later in their lives decide to enter nursing (Berlin, Stennett, & Bednash, 2003). There are a few colleges and universities that offer master's degree programs leading to the initial professional degree in nursing. Yale University, the University of Texas at Austin, and the University of Tennessee are among the institutions that have such programs. Generally, the program is 2 years long. On graduation these students are expected to demonstrate the same entry-level competencies in nursing as baccalaureate graduates. MSN graduates are then eligible to take the NCLEX-RN.

WHAT ABOUT A DOCTORAL PATH TO BECOMING AN RN?

The last path, and the least common, leading to the RN licensure examination is the doctoral degree. This program was begun in 1979 at Case Western Reserve University. Rush University in Chicago initiated a similar program in 1988, and the University of Colorado began one in 1990 (Forni, 1989). These programs provide basic nursing courses, along with advanced nursing courses. On completion, the graduate is eligible to take the NCLEX-RN.

GRADUATE EDUCATION

WHAT ABOUT GRADUATE SCHOOL?

Whatever path you chose to become an RN, there is one thing for certain: It was not easy. After putting life, liberty, and the pursuit of happiness on hold while you worked toward becoming an RN, it may seem like pure insanity to subject yourself to more education!

Graduate nursing education, like other graduate programs, is responding to changes in social values, priorities in the public sector, and student demographics, in addition to technologic advances, knowledge development, and maturity of the profession (McCloskey & Grace, 2001).

Graduate education programs are available on either a part-time or a full-time basis. Graduate programs require a good grade-point average at the undergraduate level. Prerequisites for most graduate programs are satisfactory scores on the Graduate Record Examination (GRE) or the Miller Analogies Test (MAT). Although an increasing number of graduate programs are waiving the entrance examination requirements, it is strongly recommended that all students, whether they plan to pursue graduate studies or not, take the GRE after completing their undergraduate studies. Taking another test may be the last thing you want to do, but it is much easier to do it now, while the information is current in your mind, than later, when you decide that you want to continue your education.

WHAT IS THE HISTORY OF GRADUATE NURSING EDUCATION?

Graduate nursing programs in the United States originated during the late 1800s. As more nursing schools sought to strengthen their own programs, there was increased pressure on nursing instructors to obtain advanced preparation in education and clinical nursing specialties.

The Catholic University of America, in Washington, DC, offered one of the early graduate programs for nurses. It began offering courses in nursing education in 1932 and conferring a master's degree in nursing education in 1935.

The NLN's Subcommittee on Graduate Education first published guidelines for organization, administration, curriculum, and testing in 1957. These guidelines have been revised throughout the years and reflect the focus in master's education on research and clinical specialization.

Until the 1960s, the master's degree in nursing was viewed as a terminal degree. The goal of graduate education was to prepare nurses for teaching, administration, and supervisory positions. In the early 1970s, the emphasis shifted to developing clinical skills, and the roles of clinical specialists and nurse practitioners emerged. By the late 1970s, the focus again shifted back to teaching, administration, and supervisory positions (McCloskey & Grace, 2001).

In response to health care reform, the number of master's programs has increased. The total number of master's programs is now 398, with an enrollment of 34,181 students. A large number of these students (63%) are attending graduate school part-time (Berlin, Stennett, & Bednash, 2003).

WHY WOULD I WANT A MASTER'S DEGREE?

You've got to be kidding! More school?

Sure, an advanced degree may not be in your career plans right now, but later on, after you have been practicing nursing, you may change your mind. Policy statements from the nursing profession reflect the need for more education in preparation for nursing's changing role, a result of health care reform. As care delivery moves increasingly from the acute-care center to the community setting, there will be an increased need for advanced clinical practice nurses. Nursing programs are already responding to this changing need.

Master's nursing programs vary from institution to institution, as do the admission and course requirements and costs. The master of science (MS) and the master of science in nursing (MSN) are the most common degrees. The usual requirements for admission include the following: a baccalaureate degree from an NLN accredited program in nursing, licensure as a registered nurse, completion of the GRE or MAT, and a minimum undergraduate grade point average (GPA) of 3.0.

The majority of programs are at least 18 to 24 months of full time study. Unlike undergraduate school, master's students usually choose an area of role preparation, such as education or administration as well as an area of clinical specialization such as pediatrics or adult health. Some of the more common areas of role preparation include education, administration, case management, health policy/health care systems, informatics, as well as the increasingly popular advanced clinical practice roles.

Areas of specialty within the master's nurse practitioner programs include family, acute care, pediatric, psychiatric, geriatric, school health, and adult nursing practice. There are more family nurse practitioner programs than any other program. According to the national sample survey of registered nurses March 2000, information on RNs prepared for advanced practice, there are 88,186 nurse practitioners, 54,374 clinical nurse specialists, 9232 nurse-midwives, 29,844 nurse anesthetists, and 14,643 nurse practitioner/clinical nurse specialists (Figure 7-2). To take advantage of these trends and better position yourself in the job market, you might find that the benefits of returning to school far outweigh the sacrifices.

In the more traditional programs, the student takes the courses required for the degree, and then, depending on institutional requirements, may also be required to take a written or oral comprehensive examination or write a thesis, or both. There are

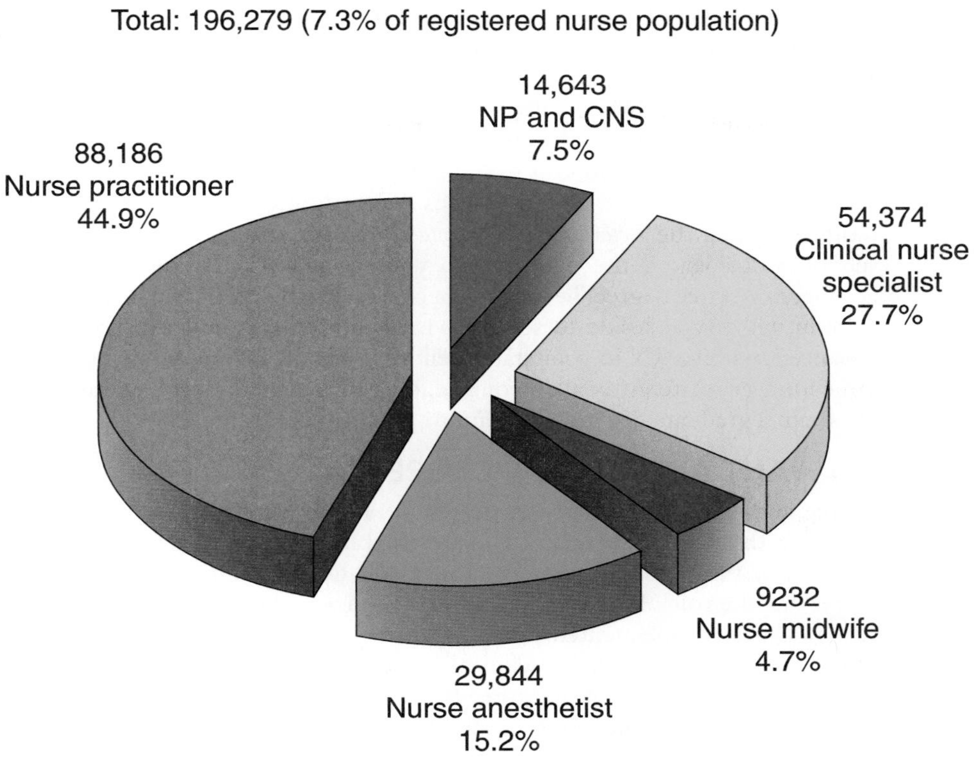

FIGURE 7-2
Registered nurses prepared for advanced practice, March 2000. Total: 196,279 (7.3% of registered nurse population). CNS, clinical nurse specialist; NP, nurse practitioner. *(From Health Resources and Services Administration:* HRSA Bureau of Health Professions Division of Nursing sample survey, *2000, Health Resources and Services Administration.)*

also nontraditional models that include outreach programs, summers-only programs, and RN-to-MSN tracks for RNs who do not have undergraduate degrees and RNs who have bachelor's degrees in other fields.

Advances in technology have also made it possible for graduate programs to become more creative in the way courses are being offered. It is now possible for students to obtain all or part of their course offerings by means of the Internet, distance-learning, computer-based programs, and teleconferencing. This flexibility is making it easier for students in rural communities and part-time students to obtain advanced degrees.

HOW DO I KNOW WHICH MASTER'S DEGREE PROGRAM IS RIGHT FOR ME?

Your career goals and interests will help you to determine which choice is best for you. Do some reading on your area of special interest, and find out what advanced education would help you to obtain your career goals. As an example, a nurse with a nonnursing master's degree would need to complete master's in nursing to become an advanced practice nurse. If you think that you might want to become a nurse practitioner at some point in your life, be sure that you obtain your master's in nursing. You can always go back and obtain a post-master's certificate as a nurse practitioner. If your master's is in another field, this would not be possible.

Once you have decided on a master's degree, there are several resources available online, such as the *Peterson's Guide (www.petersons.com)*, to help you find the right school. Consider all the options. Do your homework. If you are considering an advanced-practice degree, be sure to check with the Board of Nurse Examiners for the state in which you reside to see what the requirements are to be recognized as an advanced practice RN in your state. Believe it or not, the requirements are NOT the same for every state. After all, if you are going to expend the time, energy, and finances to obtain a graduate degree, you want to get the most from it.

WHY WOULD I WANT A DOCTORAL DEGREE?

Power, authority, and professional status are usually associated with a doctoral degree. Nurses with doctoral degrees provide leadership in the improvement of nursing practice and in the development of research and nursing education programs. It is no secret that the role of the nurse is changing and will continue to change as health care reform is being implemented. There is a growing need for administrators, policy analysts, clinical researchers, and clinical practitioners within both the community and governmental agencies. Nurses need to position themselves to take on these new leadership roles, and the way to do this is through advanced education, particularly at the doctoral level.

There are two basic models of doctoral education in nursing: the academic degree, or Doctor of Philosophy (PhD), and the professional degree, or Doctor of Nursing Science (DNS, DSN, or DNSc). For either of these degrees, you must have a master's in nursing. The total number of doctoral programs in nursing in the United States is now 83 (Berlin, Stennett, & Bednash, 2003). The PhD continues to be the most highly esteemed degree in higher education. Nurses also have other doctoral-degree options available to them, such as the Doctor of Education (EdD), the Doctor of Public Health (DPH), the Doctor of Philosophy (PhD) in a discipline besides nursing, the nontraditional external-degree doctorate, and the Nurse Doctorate (ND).

In August of 2004, the American Association of Colleges of Nursing (AACN) drafted a position statement on the practice doctorate in nursing (DNP). The term *practice doctorate* would be used instead of *clinical doctorate*, and the ND degree would be phased out. The DNP would become the educational preparation for all advanced-practice nurses. This move toward a DNP is to take place over a 15-year period (AACN, Draft position statement on the practice doctorate, 2004). Again, this is only a draft, but it is very important for you to be aware of this when you are making a major decision such as graduate education.

The doctorate in nursing is basically a new concept. Before 1965, the most common doctoral degree earned by nurses was the EdD. It was not until the establishment of the federally supported Nurse Scientist Training Program in 1962 that a shift toward obtaining a PhD began. The DNS has been awarded since the early 1960s (Rowland & Rowland, 1984).

HOW DO I KNOW WHICH DOCTORAL PROGRAM IS RIGHT FOR ME?

As with the master's degree, it is important to look at your career goals before deciding which doctoral program is best for you. To help you with that task, look at the NLN publications specific to doctoral education. Ask yourself how much time you can devote to obtaining a doctorate degree. The average time needed to complete a doctoral program is 4.5 years (Rowland & Rowland, 1984). Can you be a full-time student, or must you continue to work? What do you plan to do with the degree once you get it?

"Today, a doctorate in nursing should be the first choice for nurses seeking doctoral education" (Allen, 1990). Is this a realistic goal? Is there an institution available to you that offers a doctorate in nursing or would you have to consider moving? What are your career and professional goals? Do you want to teach? The PhD is considered the research degree. It prepares an individual for a lifetime of intellectual inquiry and has an increased emphasis on postdoctoral study. In contrast, the DNS is viewed as the practical degree. The goal of this program is to prepare an advanced practitioner for the application of knowledge with an emphasis on research. The original intent of the DNS was to prepare nurses to do clinical research.

OTHER TYPES OF NURSING EDUCATION

WHAT ARE THE OTHER AVAILABLE EDUCATIONAL OPTIONS?

In the 1960s, baccalaureate programs made it very difficult for the RN to return to school to earn a baccalaureate in nursing. Most of the time, these nurses found themselves receiving no credit for their past education or experience. A resolution passed in 1978 by the American Nurses Association (ANA) that urged the creation of quality career-mobility programs with flexibility to assist individuals desiring academic degrees in nursing helped to change this philosophy. There are several basic patterns for achieving upward mobility in nursing, and within these basic patterns there are many variations. Career-ladder programs or bridge programs, BSN-completion programs, external-degree programs, and online universities are the basic patterns that will be addressed in this section. In assessing the educational options that are available, one source of information is All Nursing Schools' website at *www.allnursingschools.com/find/*. The potential student should also contact individual schools for information regarding their particular programs. The career-ladder or bridge concept focuses on the articulation of educational programs to permit advanced placement without loss of credit or repetition. There are many variations on this type of program. Multiple-exit programs provide opportunities for students to exit and reenter the educational system at various designated times having gained specific education and skills. An example is a program that ranges from practical nurse to RN at the associate's, baccalaureate, master's, and doctoral levels. A student in such a program may decide to leave the educational system at the completion of a specific level and be eligible to take the licensure examination applicable to that educational level. On termination, the student may choose to work for a while and later return for more education at the next level without having to repeat courses on previously acquired knowledge or skills.

One such program is Project LINC (Ladders in Nursing Careers), which was developed in the city of New York for the purpose of providing educational advancement opportunities for individuals who are in entry-level or midlevel jobs in nursing. It is a collaborative effort involving more than 40 hospitals and long-term care facilities in the New York metropolitan area and serves as a state and national model of educational mobility.

A growing number of basic nursing education programs within the community-college setting are beginning to offer career-ladder–type programs, affiliating themselves with upper-division colleges in the area. A student can enter the community college to spend 1 year studying to become a practical or vocational nurse. After a year, the student can decide to stop and take the practical nurse licensure examination or continue and complete the associate's degree in nursing. At the end of the second year, the student is eligible to take the RN licensure examination and may choose either to exit as an associate-degree nurse or to attend an affiliated upper-division college to obtain a baccalaureate degree (Figure 7-3).

WHAT IS A BSN-COMPLETION PROGRAM?

A BSN-completion program is a baccalaureate program designed for students who already possess either a diploma or an associate's degree in nursing and hold a current

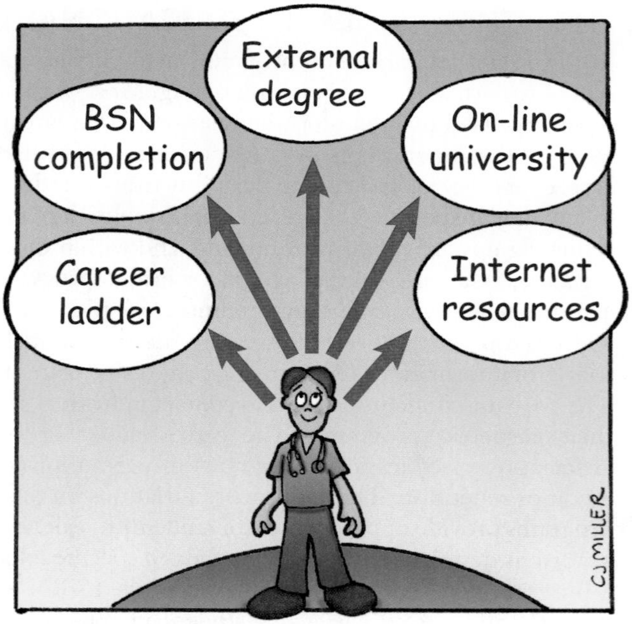

FIGURE 7-3
What are other available educational options?

license to practice as an RN. Depending on the part of the country, these programs may also be known as RN baccalaureate (RNB) programs, RN/BSN programs, baccalaureate RN (BRN) programs, two-plus-two programs, or capstone programs. In most of these programs, nurses receive transfer credit in basic education courses taken at other institutions plus either some transfer credit for their previous nursing courses or the opportunity to receive nursing credit by passing a nursing challenge examination. The usual length of such programs is 2 years, depending on the number of course requirements completed at the time of admission to the program. In an effort to meet the needs of the returning student, many BSN-completion programs offer flexible class scheduling, which allows the student to continue working while going to school. Another innovation being implemented to address the needs of individuals seeking baccalaureate degrees in outlying geographic areas is telecommunication-assisted studies and Internet courses. There are a growing number of programs available completely online.

What Is an External-Degree Program? The external-degree program gives credit for an individual's knowledge, regardless of how that knowledge was acquired. The external-degree program is a nontraditional program that allows a student to gain credit, meet external-degree requirements, and obtain a degree from a degree-granting institution without attending classes. Two examples of external-degree programs for RN education are the New York Board of Regents external degree programs (REX) for associate (ADN) and BSN education. Both of these programs are designed to allow individuals to obtain a degree in nursing without leaving their jobs or their communities. These programs are NLN-accredited. In these programs, all students are required to pass specific college-level tests and performance examinations in two components: general education and nursing. Tests are administered in several cities throughout the United States. On completion of the external-degree program, students are eligible in most states to take the RN licensure exam. There are also external-degree programs in which a person can earn a doctoral degree.

In summary, there are many paths that all lead to the same destination: the opportunity to take the licensure examination to become an RN.

Internet Resources. Besides the traditional method of education, more and more colleges and universities are offering courses and even entire programs by means of the World Wide Web. One of the largest NLNAC (National League for Nursing Accrediting Commission)–approved programs for BSN completion and graduate education is the University of Phoenix Online campus. Nursing education online is a rapidly expanding part of the Internet. At times, it can be confusing and overwhelming trying to find these courses. There are several sites that are available to help locate the courses (and course descriptions) that are being taught on the Internet, in addition to the colleges and universities that are offering the courses. See the Internet resources listed on this book's Evolve site.

ACCREDITATION

Why should you be concerned whether the nursing program you are attending, or thinking about attending, is accredited? Accreditation assures you, the student, and the public that educational standards over and above the legal requirements of the state have been achieved. It guarantees the student the opportunity to obtain a quality education. Accreditation is strictly a voluntary process. The U.S. Department of Education approves the professional association that is allowed to accredit nursing schools. Until 1997, the NLN was the only accrediting body for nursing programs. In 1997 the NLNAC was established, and responsibility for all accrediting activities was transferred to this new independent subsidiary. Around the same time, the AACN sought recognition from the U.S. Department of Education to accredit baccalaureate and graduate degree nursing programs, because membership in AACN is restricted to deans and directors of baccalaureate and graduate programs. The Task Force on Accreditation of Health Professions Education of the Pew Commission issued a report in June 1999. The accreditation report may be accessed on the UCSF Center for the Health Professions Web site at *http://futurehealth.ucsf.edu.*

Some graduate nursing programs require completion of an NLN-approved undergraduate program as a prerequisite for admission to their master's or doctoral program. The NLN publishes an official complete list of NLN-accredited programs annually. Accreditation becomes a major concern as more and more courses and programs are offered by means of distance-learning.

With two organizations offering accreditation to schools of nursing, it was difficult for schools of nursing to develop competency statements that were consistent. Rather than listing competency statements for three levels of nursing, the competency statement accepted by the 1996 annual meeting of the National Council of State Boards of Nursing (NCSBN) is presented. According to the NCSBN, "Competence is defined as the application of knowledge and the interpersonal, decision-making and psychomotor skills expected for the practice role, within the context of public health, safety and welfare" (NCSBN, 1996, p. 47).

The promotion of competency requires a collaborative approach; it involves the individual nurse, employers of nurses, nursing educators, and the regulating board of nursing. The roles of each of these in competence accountability are described in Figure 7-4.

NURSING EDUCATION: FUTURE TRENDS

Education is a lifelong process and an empowering force that enables an individual to achieve higher goals. Student access to educational opportunities is paramount to nursing education. A chapter on nursing education would not be complete without taking a look at the future.

THE CHANGING STUDENT PROFILE

Future nursing programs will need to be flexible to meet the learning needs of a changing student population. It has previously been stated that there is a growing population of nontraditional students—individuals who are making midlife career changes in part because of job displacement or job dissatisfaction. The student population tends to be older, married, and with families. More poor, minority, and foreign students are looking toward nursing education for career opportunities. There are a growing number of students choosing to attend school part time.

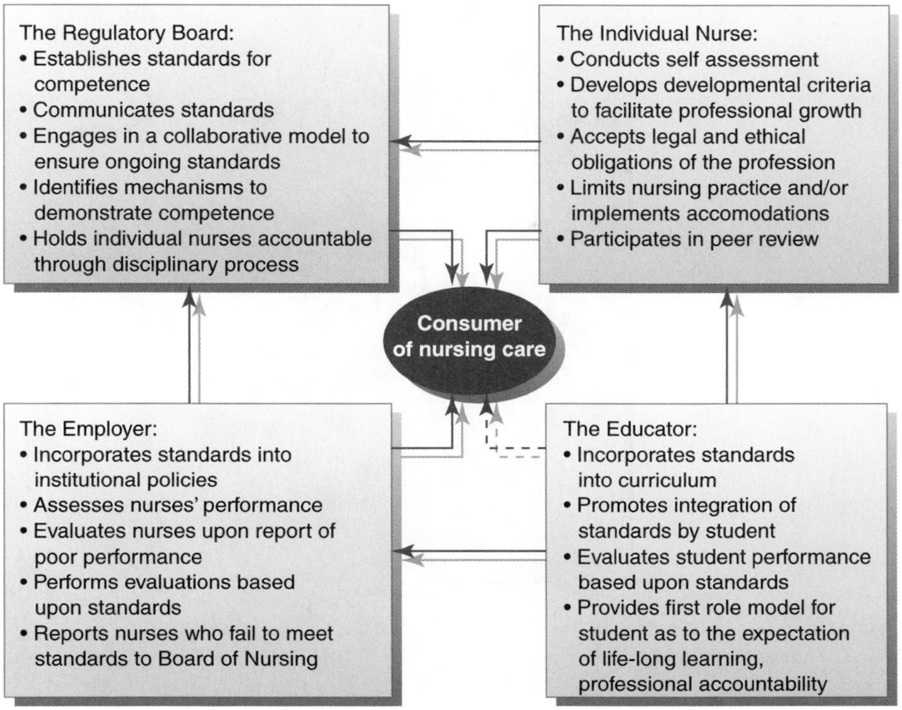

The Regulatory Board:
• Establishes standards for competence
• Communicates standards
• Engages in a collaborative model to ensure ongoing standards
• Identifies mechanisms to demonstrate competence
• Holds individual nurses accountable through disciplinary process
The Individual Nurse:
• Conducts self assessment
• Develops developmental criteria to facilitate professional growth
• Accepts legal and ethical obligations of the profession
• Limits nursing practice and/or implements accomodations
• Participates in peer review
Consumer of nursing care
The Employer:
• Incorporates standards into institutional policies
• Assesses nurses' performance
• Evaluates nurses upon report of poor performance
• Performs evaluations based upon standards
• Reports nurses who fail to meet standards to Board of Nursing
The Educator:
• Incorporates standards into curriculum
• Promotes integration of standards by student
• Evaluates student performance based upon standards
• Provides first role model for student as to the expectation of life-long learning, professional accountability

Actions of boards of nursing that ensure competence to the public:

1. Establish competence requirements for safe and effective practice.
2. Communicate standards to the consumers, nurses, nursing educators, employers, and other regulators.
3. Hold individual nurses accountable for continued competence.
4. Engage in collaborative activities with nurses, educators, employers, and consumers to ensure nurses practice safely and effectively.
5. Identify a variety of techniques nurses may use to demonstrate competence.
6. Discipline nurses who fail to meet standards for safe and effective practice.
7. Inform the public of disciplinary actions taken against nurses.
8. Establish nondisciplinary model to monitor and/or limit the practice of nurses who demonstrate an inability to carry out essential nursing role functions.

FIGURE 7-4
Competence accountability. *(From National Council of State Boards of Nursing: Annual meeting. In* Book of reports, *Chicago, 1996, National Council of State Boards of Nursing, p 51).*

These changes mean that nurse educators will have to further address the needs of the adult learner. More programs will be needed that permit part-time study and allow students to work while attending school. One option may be for more night or weekend course offerings. There will continue to be a need for emphasis on remedial education such as developmental courses in math, English, and English as a second language. The diversity in the student population means diversity in learning rates, which might be addressed with more self-paced learning modules (Figure 7-5).

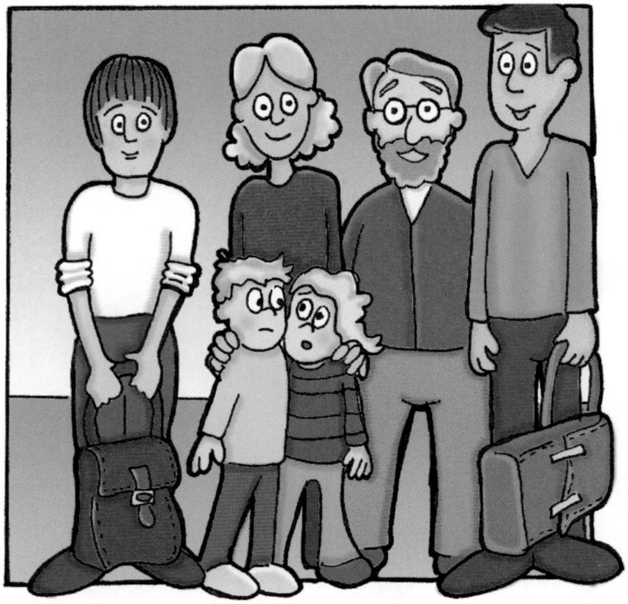

FIGURE 7-5
The changing student profile.

EDUCATIONAL MOBILITY

Educational mobility will also need to be addressed further. A growing number of individuals in health care are seeking more education. The issue is not one of entry into practice, but rather of how to best facilitate the return of these individuals to nursing school for educational advancement.

A SHORTAGE OF QUALIFIED NURSING FACULTY

Data on faculty reported by the AACN for 1999 and 2000 indicate that the average age of faculty has increased to a mean of 50.2 years for all faculty (AACN, 2004). Because of the decrease in the number of students entering the nursing profession and then choosing to teach, the number of qualified faculty will continue to decline. Predictions have one third of the nursing faculty retiring or resigning from 1992 through 2006 (Buerhaus, 2000).

TECHNOLOGY AND EDUCATION

Educational learning will continue to change with technologic advances in telecommunication and computer-assisted instruction. Nurses and nurse educators will need education to implement these advances into the curriculum and into nursing practice. As with cable television, which has extended the boundaries of the classroom, these new technologies will facilitate the offering of outreach programs.

CHANGING HEALTH CARE SETTINGS

There has been a major shift from inpatient to outpatient nursing services as health care and nursing focuses on maintaining health rather then dealing with illness. However, with an increase in the age of the population, there are more patients in the hospital with multiple chronic problems. Society is now developing a variety of new health care settings. Are nurses educated for these new roles? What will be the role of the advanced nurse practitioner? Will there be enough nurses educationally prepared to meet these new challenges?

THE AGING POPULATION

There is a growing aging population. According to the Administration on Aging, by 2030 there will be approximately 70 million people over the age of 65 years, representing 20% of the population (2004). Naisbitt and Aburdene stated in their book *Megatrends 2000*, published in 1990, "If business and society can master the challenge of daycare, we will be one step closer to confronting the next great care giving task of the 1990s—eldercare." This is still a critical issue in the 21st century. Already, the United States has well over 2000 adult daycare centers. Nursing educators need to address the provision of health care to the elderly and include it in the curricula.

What great opportunities in nursing!

CONCLUSION

The future of nursing looks bright and exciting. With technologic advances, changes in health care settings, increased demand for the services of the RN, and the shift back to the acute-care setting, nurses now have increased opportunities to chart their own destinies.

Nurses who have career plans and career goals will see the future trends in health care as a challenge and an opportunity for career growth in areas such as case manager, independent consultant, nurse practitioner, policy maker, or entrepreneur. In contrast, nurses without career goals may find themselves displaced or obsolete. There has never been a more exciting time to be entering the profession of nursing than right now. Opportunities in nursing are wide open to those with the sensitivity and the creativity to embrace the future.

REFERENCES

Administration on Aging website. Retrieved November 24, 2004, from *http://www.aoa.gov.*

Allen J, editor: *Consumers guide to doctoral degree programs in nursing*, National League for Nursing Publication No. 15-2293, New York, 1990, National League for Nursing.

American Association of Colleges of Nursing: *Draft position statement on the practice doctorate*, approved by the AACN Board July 2004.

American Association of Colleges of Nursing: *2004 Media relations nursing fact sheet, http://www.aacn.nche.edu/Media/FactSheets/nursfact.htm.*

Anderson NE: The historical development of American nursing education, *J Nurs Educ* 20(1):18-36, 1981.

Berlin L, Stennett J, Bednash G: *Enrollment and graduations in baccalaureate and graduate programs in nursing*, Washington, DC, 2003, American Association of Colleges of Nursing.

Buerhaus PI: A nursing shortage with a fundamental difference, *Syllabus Am Assoc Coll Nurs* 26(5):3-4, 7, 2000.

Bullough B, Bullough V: *Nursing issues for the nineties and beyond*, New York, 1994, Springer.

Forni PR: Models for doctoral programs: first professional degree or terminal degree?, *Nurs Health Care* 10(8):429-434, 1989.

Kaiser JE: *A comparison of students in practical nursing programs and in associate degree nursing programs*, National League for Nursing Publication No. 23-1592, New York, 1975, National League for Nursing.

McCloskey J, Grace HK: *Current issues in nursing*, ed 6, St. Louis, 2001, Mosby.

Montag ML: *The education of nursing technicians*, New York, 1951, GP Putnam's Sons.

Montag ML: *Community college education for nursing*, New York, 1959, McGraw-Hill.

Naisbitt J, Aburdene P: *Megatrends 2000: new directions for tomorrow*, New York, 1991, William Morrow.

National Council of State Boards of Nursing: *Definition of competence and standards for competence*, National Council of State Boards of Nursing annual meeting. In *Book of reports*, Chicago, 1996, National Council of State Boards of Nursing.

National League for Nursing, Council of Associate Degree Nursing Competencies Task Force: *Educational competencies for graduates of associate degree nursing programs*, bookcode 1404-6, New York, 2001, National League for Nursing.

Peterson T: *Peterson's nursing programs 2005*, ed 10, Lawrenceville, NJ, 2004, Thomason-Peterson.

Rowland HS, Rowland B: *The nurse's almanac*, ed 2, Rockville, MD, 1984, Aspen.

U.S. Department of Health and Human Services, Health Resources and Services Administration: *The registered nurse population, March 2000: findings from the national sample survey of registered nurses*, Washington, DC, 2001, Government Printing Office.

CHAPTER 8

NURSING THEORY

ANNE SULLIVAN, RN, MSN

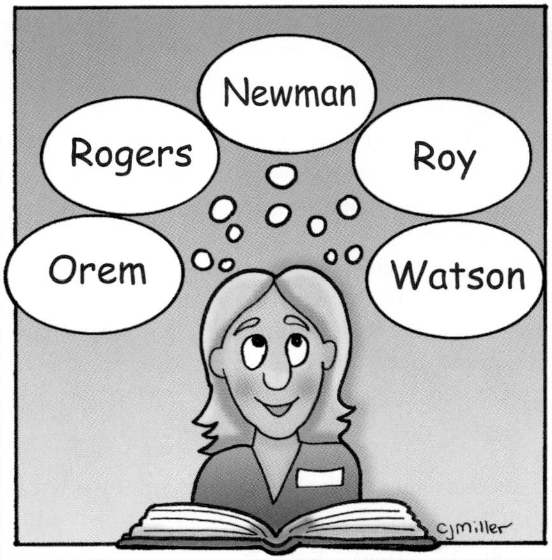

There are many nursing theories available to help guide my practice.

After completing this chapter, you should be able to:

- Identify the purposes for nursing theory.
- Describe the origins of nursing theory.
- Describe some of the key words associated with nursing theory.
- Identify some of the more well-known and well-developed nursing theories.
- Discuss some of the main points of each of these theories.

Just mentioning the word *theory*, let alone *nursing theory*, can make many nurses' yawn reflexes start to work overtime. What is theory? Who are nursing theorists? Most nurses are not aware of theory, nor can they name a nursing theorist. Nursing theories are a way to organize and think about nursing, and the people who wrote theories are part of our nursing history. Theory provides an overall "theme" to what nurses do. In this chapter, the key words related to theory are defined, and the theories of eight nursing theories are summarized.

Buckle your seatbelts, we might be in for a bumpy ride—and no yawning!

NURSING THEORY

WHAT IS THEORY?

Quite simply, theories are words or phrases (concepts) joined together in sentences, with an overall theme, to explain, describe, or predict something. A more complex definition might be a theory is "a set of interrelated concepts, definitions, and propositions that present a systematic way of viewing facts/events by specifying relations among the variables, with the purpose of explaining and predicting the fact event" (Kerlinger, as cited in Hickman, 2002).

Theories help us understand and find meaning in our nursing experience and also provide a foundation to direct questions that provide insights into new ways of knowing. Ellis (1997) stated in 1968, "A theory is a coherent set of hypothetical, conceptual and pragmatic principles forming a general frame or reference for a field of study." You might see theory referred to as a conceptual model or a conceptual framework.

Nursing theory is, according to Meleis (Hickman, 2002) "…an articulated and communicated conceptualization of invented or discovered reality in or pertaining to nursing for the purpose of describing, explaining, predicting or prescribing nursing care."

The bottom line is that words and phrases (concepts) are put together into sentences (propositions that show the relationships among the words/concepts), with an overall theme to create theories. Theories also have some basic assumptions (jumping-off points; what is assumed to be true), such as patients need nurses. Nursing theories also define four metaparadigms (big, comprehensive concepts) and address the nursing process.

WHAT NURSING THEORY IS NOT

Nursing theory is *not* managed care, primary nursing, team nursing, or any other more business-related method of delivering care. Nursing theory is *not* obstetric nursing, surgical nursing, home health nursing, nor any other nursing specialty, but nursing theory can be applied to all of the areas of nursing, including administration, education, patient care, and research. Nursing theory is by nurses and for nurses, providing care to their patients or clients, either directly or indirectly.

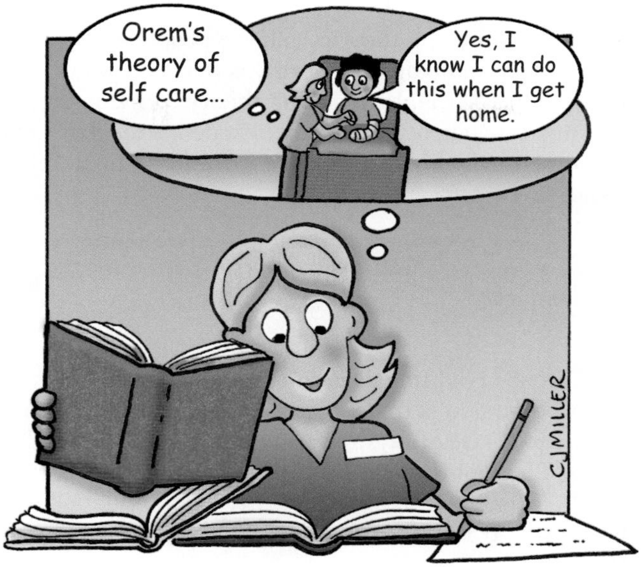
Orem's theory of self care...
Yes, I know I can do this when I get home.
CJMILLER

FIGURE 8-1
Theory guides both research and nursing practice.

WHY THEORY?

Consider all that you do as a nurse. What you do is based on principles from many different professions, such as biology, sociology, medicine, ethics, business, theology, psychology, and philosophy. What is specifically based on nursing? Also, if nursing is a science (and it is), there must be some scientific basis for it. Finally, theory ties in with the professionalism that we see as part of nursing (Figure 8-1).

According to Klein and White (Hanson et al., 1998), theory is a means to gather information, to more clearly and specifically identify ideas, to guide research, to show how ideas are connected to each other, to make sense of what we observe or experience, to predict what might happen, and to provide answers. A nurse is not a "junior physician," although for years nursing care has been based on the medical model. Because nursing is a science (as well as an art) and a unique profession in its own right, nurses need nursing theory upon which to base their principles of care (Critical Thinking Box 8-1).

CRITICAL THINKING BOX 8-1

What are some advantages and disadvantages that you can see to using nursing theory?

WHAT IS THE HISTORY OF NURSING THEORY?

In studying nursing theories and the people who created them, it is important to look at the background of the theorist, as well as how life experiences, beliefs, and education influenced what is the resulting theory. What is the overall theme and main ideas of the theory, and how does the theorist define the four nursing metaparadigms (or another way to say really BIG concepts, or words, with many different meanings or ways in which to use the word)? (Box 8-1)

The four metaparadigms for nursing are nursing, person, health, and environment.

Florence Nightingale is considered to be the first nursing theorist. She saw nursing as "A profession, a trade, a necessary occupation, something to fill and employ all my faculties, I have always felt essential to me, I have always longed for; consciously or not... The first thought I can remember, and the last was nursing work... " (Dunphy, 2002). Now, you might not feel that dedicated, but Nightingale also stated, "Nursing is an art... It is one of the Fine Arts; I had almost said, the finest of the Fine Arts." (Dunphy, 2002).

BOX 8-1 Definition of Metaparadigms

PERSON
Individuals, families, communities, and other groups who are participants in nursing.

ENVIRONMENT
A person's significant others and physical surroundings, as well as to the setting in which nursing occurs, which ranges from the person's home to clinical agencies to society as a whole.
All local, regional, national, and worldwide cultural, social, political, and economic conditions that are associated with the person's health.

HEALTH
A person's state of well-being at the time that nursing occurs, which can range from high-level wellness to terminal illness.

NURSE
The actions taken by nurses on behalf of or in conjunction with the person, and the goals or outcomes of nursing actions. Nursing actions typically are viewed as a systematic process of assessment, labeling, planning, intervention, and evaluation.

From Fawcett J: *Analysis and evaluation of contemporary nursing knowledge: nursing models and theories,* Philadelphia, 2000, FA Davis.

Nightingale had various influences, including her education, which was fairly comprehensive for a 19th century English woman, her religion (Unitarianism), the history of the time (the Crimean War and invention of the telegraph), and her social status. The Unitarian belief involved salvation through health and wholeness, or our modern day "wholism." Nightingale believed that there was no conflict between science and spirituality. Science was necessary for the development of a mature concept of God. Nightingale also studied many other religions throughout her lifetime and considered starting a Protestant religious order of nuns (Dunphy, 2002).

Nightingale came from a very wealthy family and enjoyed traveling throughout Europe, one of the destinations being Kaiserwerth in Germany, where she observed and was moved by nuns caring for the ill. Nightingale felt a "calling" to care for others and began training with various groups, usually nuns who cared for the sick. When the Crimean War broke out, Nightingale was asked and volunteered to go to care for the wounded English soldiers. The Crimean War was the first war since the invention of the telegraph, so the news of the War was more immediate than had been previously experienced (Dunphy, 2002).

The overall theme of Nightingale's theory was that the person is influenced by the environment. When she went to help soldiers during the Crimean War, her initial intent was to feed the soldiers healthy food and to clean up. When soldier mortality rates fell, a legend was born! (Dunphy, 2002). (Figure 8-2).

Nightingale felt that nursing was separate from medicine and that nurses should be trained (although I like the word educated better, signifying your professionalism

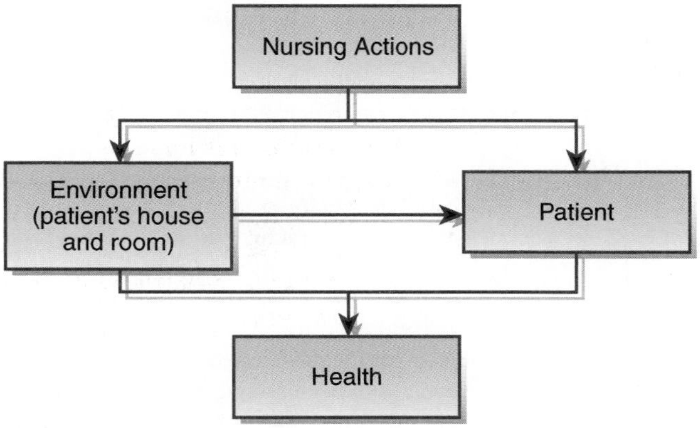

FIGURE 8-2

Nightingale's Conceptual Model of Nursing. *(From Fitzpatrick J, Whall A:* Conceptual models of nursing: analysis and application, *ed 3. Stamford, Conn, 1996, Appleton & Lange, p 38, Figure 3-1.)*

versus being potty trained or trained to rollover and heel). She also believed that the environment was important to the health of the person and that the nurse should support the environment to assist the patient in healing (Dunphy, 2002).

To define the metaparadigms (or big, comprehensive words), Nightingale noted that the person is the center of the model, and incorporated a holistic view of the person, someone with psychologic, intellectual, and spiritual components. The nurse was a woman (because only women were nurses in Nightingale's day) who had charge of the health of a person, whether in providing wellness care, such as with a newborn, or in providing care to the sick. Health was the result of environmental, physical, and psychological factors, not just the absence of disease (Dunphy, 2002).

No other theories were identified or published until the 1950s when Peplau published her theory based on the interpersonal process. Various other nurses were working on theories throughout that time and into the 1960s. In the 1970s, nursing was beginning to see itself as a scientific profession based on theoretic ideas (Table 8-1). In 1972, the National League for Nursing (NLN) required that nursing curricula be based on conceptual frameworks (McEwen, 2002).

TABLE 8-1

Nursing Theories

Year	Theorist	Theory Description
1860	Florence Nightingale	Although her model did not have a specific name, the basic underpinnings revolve around how a person is influenced by the environment. Nursing was a "calling" to help the patient in a reparative process by directly working with the patient or indirectly by affecting the environment to facilitate health and recovery from illness.
1952	Hildegard Peplau	Interpersonal Relations Model—described the four phases of the dynamic relationship between nurse and patient; orientation, identification, exploitation, and resolution.
1960	Faye Abdellah	Patient Centered Approach—developed a list of 21 unique nursing problems related to human needs; promoted the use of a problem-solving approach to practice rather than merely following physician orders. Responsible for changing the focus of nursing theory from a disease-centered to a patient-centered approach and moved nursing practice beyond the patient to include care of families and the elderly.
1961	Ida Jean Orlando	Theory of Deliberative Nursing Process—focuses on the interpersonal process between nurse and patient through a deliberative nursing process; most concerned with what was uniquely nursing.
1966	Virginia Henderson	Her "unique functions of nurses" was one of the many topics that she wrote about; however, all of her materials provided a focus for patient care via 14 basic needs.

Continued

TABLE 8-1

Nursing Theories—cont'd

Year	Theorist	Theory Description
1969	Myra Estrin Levine	Conservation Model—focuses attention on the wholeness of the person, adaptation, and conservation, which is guided by four principles (conservation of energy, structure, personal integrity, and social integrity).
1970	Martha Rogers	Science of Unitary Human Beings—an abstract model addressing the complexity of the "unitary human being," which allows for the examination of phenomena (energy fields, paranormal) that other theories do not describe, as the nurse promotes synchronicity between human beings and their environment/universe.
1971	Dorothea Orem	Self-Care Nursing Theory—three interwoven theories of self-care, self-care deficit, and nursing system help the nurse to identify strategies to meet the patient's self-care needs.
1971	Imogene King	Theory of Goal Attainment—client goals are met through the transaction between nurse and client involving three systems (personal, interpersonal, and social).
1972	Betty Neuman	Neuman Systems Model—focus on wellness and mitigating stress within three levels of prevention—primary, secondary, and tertiary.
1974	Sister Callista Roy	Roy's Adaptation Model—individual seeking equilibrium through the process of adaptation; identified six physiological needs (exercise and rest, nutrition, elimination, fluid and electrolytes, oxygenation and circulation, regulation of temperature, senses and the endocrine system).
1976	Josephine Paterson and Loretta Zderad	Humanistic Nursing Theory—focus on the nurse and the patient where dignity, interests, and values are of greatest importance; felt there was more to nursing that was not explainable by scientific principles.
1978; 1991	Madeline Leininger	Theory of Culture Care Diversity and Universality—a grand theory that considers the impact of culture on the person's health and caring practices.
1979	Margaret Newman	Theory of Health as Expanding Consciousness—every person in every situation is ever changing in a unidirectional, unpredictable, all-at-once pattern involving movement, time, space, and consciousness; emphasized the importance of viewing patients in the context of their holistic patterns.
1979	Jean Watson	Theory of Human Caring—identifies 10 carative factors focusing on the interactions between the one who is caring and the one who is being cared for that foster caring.
1980	Dorothy Johnson	Behavioral Systems Model—focus on human behavior rather than the person's state of health, which helped clarify the differences between medicine and nursing.
1981	Rosemarie Rizzo Parse	Theory of Human Becoming—focus on the human-health-universe; views nursing as a participation effort with the patient that focuses on health.
1983	H. Erickson, E. Tomlin, and M. Swain	Modeling and Role Modeling Theory—uses the understanding of the client's world to plan interventions that meet the client's perceived needs that will assist the client to achieve holistic health; focus is on the person receiving the care, not the nurse, not the care, and not the disease.

Continued

TABLE 8-1

Nursing Theories—cont'd

Year	Theorist	Theory Description
1984	Pat Benner	Professional-Advancement-Model—applied the Dreyfus model of skill acquisition to nursing; area of concern was not how to do nursing but, rather, "how do nurses learn to do nursing"; identified seven domains of practice-helping, teaching/coaching, diagnosing and monitoring, managing changes, administering and monitoring therapeutic interventions, monitoring quality care, and organizing to enact the work role.

From Fawcett J: *Analysis and evaluation of contemporary nursing knowledge: nursing models and theories*. Philadelphia, 2000, FA Davis; and George JB: *Nursing theories: the base for professional nursing practice*, ed 4, Norwalk, Conn, 1995, Appleton & Lange.

Among the most well known and well formulated theories or models include those by Dorothea Orem, Martha Rogers, Sr. Callista Roy, Dorothy Johnson, Betty Neuman, Imogene King, Jean Watson, and Madeleine Leininger (Box 8-2). Each theory has been around for at least 20 years, and each theorist has practiced nursing at the bedside, in the community, and in administration or education. They are not women writing theories in an "ivory tower" with no idea about what nurses do.

BOX 8-2 Definitions of Metaparadigms by Each Theorist

THEORIST: NIGHTINGALE
Person: center of model; holistic view, incorporating psychological, intellectual, and spiritual components
Nurse: a woman who is in charge of the health and illness of people
Health: result of environmental, physical, and psychological factors
Environment: all that surrounds a person affects the state of health; sanitary conditions

THEORIST: OREM
Person: physical, psychological, interpersonal, and social aspects
Nursing: the actions to overcome or prevent self-care limitations or provide self-care
Health: conditions that permit self-care

THEORIST: ROGERS
Person: energy field that exhibits patterns
Environment: energy field interacting with the person
Health: indication of the pattern of the energy field
Nursing: purpose is to repattern the person and environment

Continued

BOX 8-2 Definitions of Metaparadigms by Each Theorist—cont'd

THEORIST: ROY
Person: biopsychosocial being seeking equilibrium
Nursing: manipulates the stimuli to promote coping
Health: successful coping with stressors

THEORIST: JOHNSON
Person: behavior and biological systems
Nursing: restore or maintain the balance
Health: balance or stability

THEORIST: NEUMAN
Person: physiologic, psychological, sociocultural, developmental, and spiritual variables
Health: continuum from wellness to illness
Nursing: helps reduce the stressors through prevention
Environment: internal, external, created

THEORIST: KING
Person: interacts with environment
Health: dynamic state of being
Nursing: interacts with patient to set and achieve goals

THEORIST: WATSON
Person: mind-body-soul connection
Health: unity and harmony with mind, body, and soul
Nursing: promotes sense of inner harmony with "caring moments"
Environment: social environment

THEORIST: LEININGER
Person: caring and capable
Nursing: transcultural caring
Health: culturally defined

WHO ARE THE NURSING THEORISTS?

SELECTED NURSING THEORISTS

Dorothea Orem—Self-Care Nursing Theory. Orem's theory includes the overall theme of self-care. She sees the person as one who is composed of physical, psychological, interpersonal, and social aspects. Nursing consisted of those actions to overcome or prevent self-care limitations (self-care deficits) or to provide self-care for someone who is unable to do so. A nurse may need to do everything for the patient (wholly compensatory, such as for a patient who is under general anesthesia or is critically ill), to do some things for the patient (partly compensatory, such as with a patient who is two days post-op and may be able to do some, but not everything for himself or herself), or to educate the patient (supportive educative, such as with postpartum parents). Health, to Orem, is internal and external conditions that permit self-care needs to be met. The environment is anything outside of or external to the person. So, in assessing a patient, a nurse using Orem would ask, "What can the patient do for himself or herself? And what do I, as the nurse, need to do for the patient? What are the patient's self-care deficits (or things that he/she cannot do)?" (Leddy & Pepper, 1998).

Orem's nursing process includes assessing the client and deciding if nursing care is needed and if so, which self-care deficits are present? Does the client need wholly or partly compensatory or supportive-educative nursing care? The nurse needs to identify interventions and decide which interventions the client can do (if any) and which interventions the nurse will do. The nurse describes which helping methods are used for the interventions (acting for or doing for another, guiding and directing, providing physical or psychologic support, providing a therapeutic environment, or teaching) (Foster & Bennett, 2003). And all interventions fall under one of these five helping methods (Figures 8-3 and 8-4).

Martha Rogers—Science of Unitary Human Beings. Martha Rogers is one of the most original thinkers of the nursing theorists. Her overall theme is that the person and environment are one thing and cannot be separated. Rogers takes wholism to a new level. The person, for Rogers, is an energy field that exhibits patterns (think of electrocardiogram [ECG] patterns, fetal heart rate patterns, biorhythms, auras). Health is an "indication of the complexity and innovativeness of patterning of the energy field that is the person" (Leddy & Pepper, 1998, p. 188). Rogers, however, did not like to define the word "health," as she felt that it was a value judgment (e.g., what your patient thinks is healthy about himself may not be what you think is healthy about the patient). The environment for Rogers was also an energy field that was interacting constantly with the energy field of the person (kind of like what Nightingale thought too). The role of nursing was to repattern the person and environment to achieve

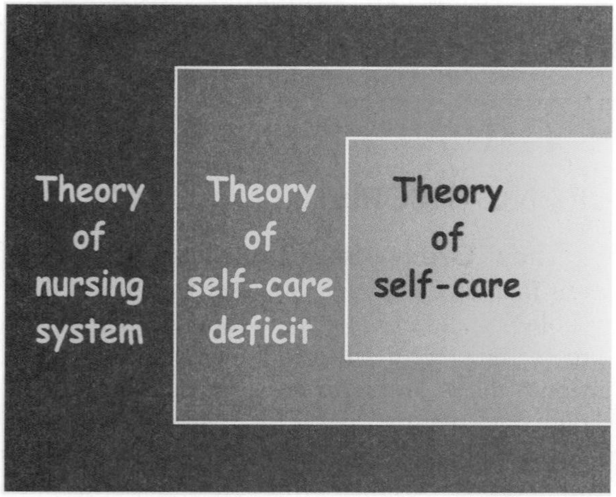

FIGURE 8-3

Orem's Self-Care Deficit Model. *(From Orem DE:* Nursing concepts of practice, *ed 6, St Louis, 2001, Mosby, p 141.)*

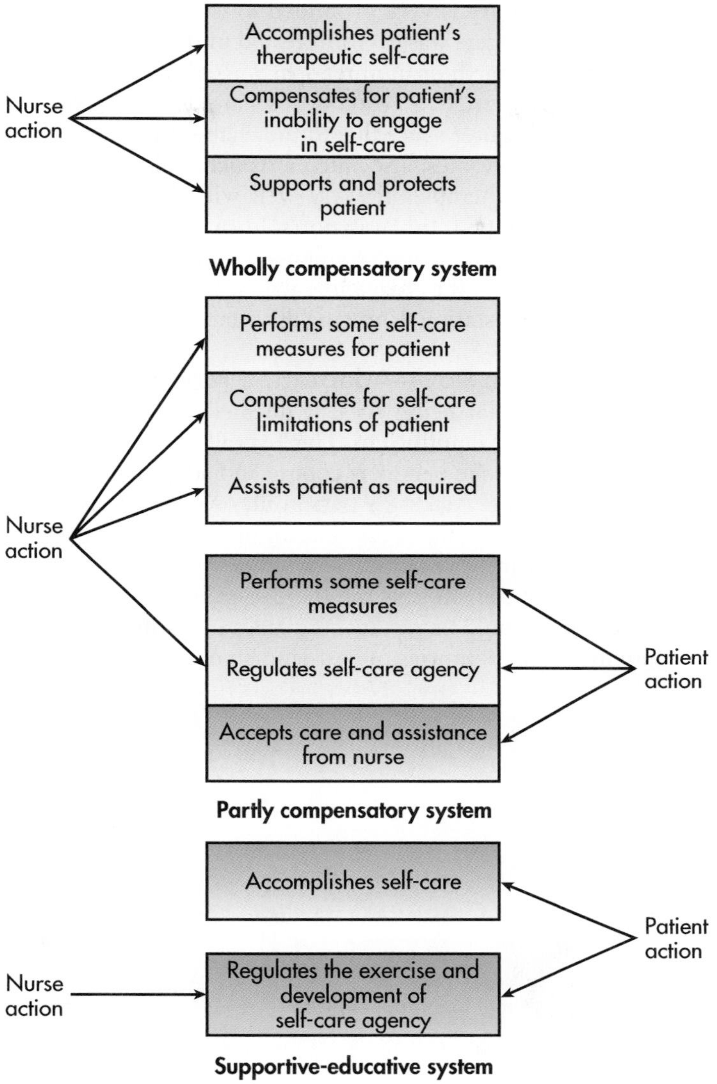

FIGURE 8-4
Orem's Basic Nursing Systems. *(From Orem DE:* Nursing concepts of practice, *ed 6, St Louis, 2001, Mosby, p 351.)*

maximum health potential for the person. While this may all sound a little far-fetched, many nurses, when first entering a patient's room in a hospital, will assess the patient and rearrange/clean up the room to make it more convenient and/or therapeutic for caring for the patient. That is, the patient and environment were "repatterned" to achieve maximum health for the patient (Leddy & Pepper, 1998).

Rogers' theory is very grounded in the science of physics and the ideas of matter and energy. Rogers was very interested in space travel and saw nurses as providing care for people on earth or in outer space. Rogers felt that some pathology was due to our being earthbound, (e.g., osteoporosis and arthritis), but that these diseases would not be an issue in outer space due to the changes in gravity. Rogers felt that nursing could use creative therapies, also, such as touch, color, sound, motion, and humor. The use of alternative therapies fit very well with Rogers' ideas. Rogers' nursing care plan that she developed, but was not sold on, included Pattern Manifestation Knowing-Assessment (our idea of assessment), Voluntary Mutual Patterning (whereby the nurse and client pattern the environmental energy to promote health—or interventions), and Pattern Manifestation Knowing-Evaluation (our idea of evaluation) (Muth Quillen, 2003) (Figure 8-5).

Sister Callista Roy—Adaptation Model. Sister Callista Roy saw the person as a biopsychosocial being (yes, it does seem like these theorists make up their own words), seeking equilibrium. Her overall theme was adaptation. As nurses, we are to assess how well the person is coping and adapting to stimuli. The stimuli could be any stressors that are making a person ill, or causing him/her to not adapt. The stimulus could be a focal stimulus (or the stimulus that is the greatest concern at the moment—e.g., labor pain); the stimulus could be contextual (all other stimuli in the area that contribute to the effect of the focal stimulus, such as noise in the background); and/or the stimulus could be residual (an unknown stimulus to the nurse that is bothering the patient—e.g., memories of past labors and births).

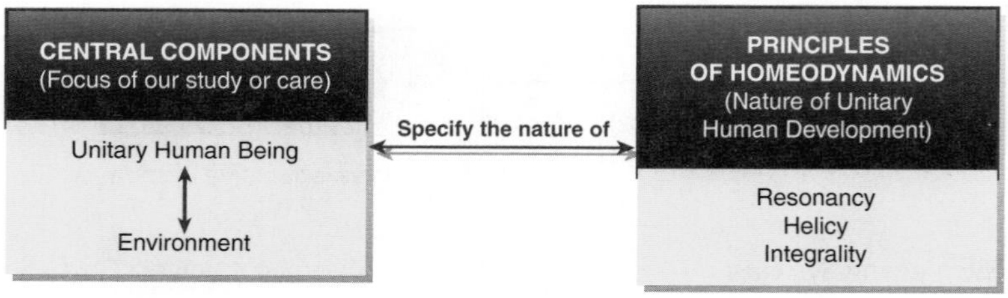

FIGURE 8-5

Roger's Science of Unitary Human Beings. *(From Fitzpatrick J, Whall A:* Conceptual models of nursing: analysis and application, *ed 3, Stamford, Conn, 1996, Appleton & Lange.)*

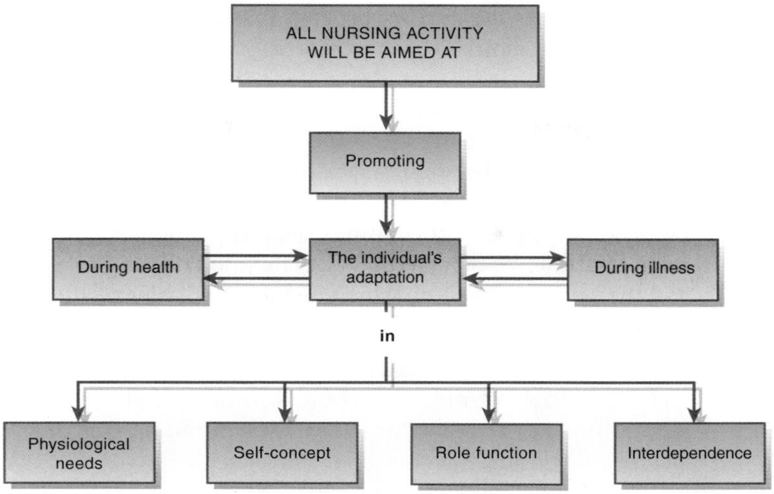

FIGURE 8-6
Roy's Adaptation Model *(From Pearson A, Vaughan B, Fitzgerald M:* Nursing models for practice, *ed 3, Edinburgh, 2005, Butterworth & Heineman, p. 129.)*

Health is defined as successful coping with stressors, and the environment is defined as influences that affect the development of a person. Illness is unsuccessful coping. The nursing process is a problem-solving approch that encompasses steps to gather data, identify capacities and needs of the human adaptive system, select and implement approaches for nursing care, and evaluate the outcome of the care provided. In Roy's nursing process, she adds two assessment parts: What is the stimulus? and What is the person's response to the stimulus? The nurse's role would be to manipulate stimuli to improve successful coping (Leddy & Pepper, 1998) (Figure 8-6).

Dorothy Johnson—Behavioral Systems Model. Dorothy Johnson was one of Roy's teachers at UCLA. Johnson's theme was balance within a behavior system. The person is a behavior system that is orderly and seeks balance. The person is seen as a behavior system and a biological system. The person is made up of seven subsystems. The environment is anything outside of the person or behavior system. Health is balance or stability. The nurse's role is to restore or maintain the balance in the person or behavior system. A visual example could be learning to crutch walk after a leg fracture. The person needs to literally learn to balance on crutches, but also needs to learn to "balance" other aspects of his life that are affected by the broken leg (Leddy & Pepper, 1998).

Johnson sees the nursing process as assessment, diagnosis, intervention, and evaluation. The person's seven subsystems are assessed. These subsystems include the achievement subsystem, which includes mastery or control of the self or environment; the aggressive/protective subsystem, which includes protecting oneself or others; the dependency subsystem, which includes obtaining attention or assistance from others; the eliminative subsystem, which includes elimination as we think of it; but also being able to express one's feelings or ideas, the ingestive subsystem, which includes eating, but also "taking in" other things such as pain medication or information; the attachment or affiliative subsystem, which includes relating to another or achieving intimacy; and the sexual subsystem, which includes activities related to sexuality, such as procreating and sexual identity (Holaday, 2001) (Figure 8-7).

Consider how patients for whom you care could fall into each of these seven subsystems, or which subsystems would most apply to the patients for whom you provide care.

Betty Neuman—Systems Model Betty Neuman's conceptual model focuses on prevention, or prevention as intervention as a response to stressors. Primary prevention is what a person does to prevent illness—e.g., exercise, sleep 8 hours, eat a balanced diet. Secondary prevention is what is done when an illness strikes. For example, when a person with a myocardial infarction comes into the ER, what is done by the staff to prevent this person from dying or from having further heart damage? Tertiary prevention can be thought of as what is done to rehabilitate a person after an illness or accident, such as with cardiac rehabilitation or stroke rehabilitation. Tertiary prevention can move the person back to primary prevention again. The nurse's role is helping to reduce the stressors through the three levels of prevention.

Neuman also talks about the flexible lines of defense, the normal lines of defense, and lines of resistance. The flexible lines of defense are the outermost boundary and is the initial response to stressors. Neuman describes it as accordion-like, in that it can expand and contract depending on our health practices—e.g., lack of sleep, lack of eating well. Our normal lines of defense are what usually protect us from stressors—e.g., our age, physical health, genetic make-up, spiritual beliefs, and gender. When the flexible lines of defense can no longer protect us from stressors, the person's equilibrium is affected, and a reaction occurs. The lines of resistance come into play to help restore balance, such as the immune system (Leddy & Pepper, 1998; George, 2003a). The person, for Neuman, has physiological, psychological, sociocultural, developmental, and spiritual variables (George, 2003a).

Think of how Neuman's ideas accurately portray the life of a student, as he or she struggles to keep up with coursework, work, and family life, but maybe finding himself or herself sleeping less, eating less or eating poorly, and then getting sick or having less energy. Neuman's nursing process has just three steps: diagnosis, nursing goals (interventions are included with this step), and nursing outcomes (George, 2003a). Neuman also has a unique way of looking at the environment, which she identifies as internal, external, and the created environment. The created environment is developed by the client and serves as a protective device for the client (George, 2003a). The created

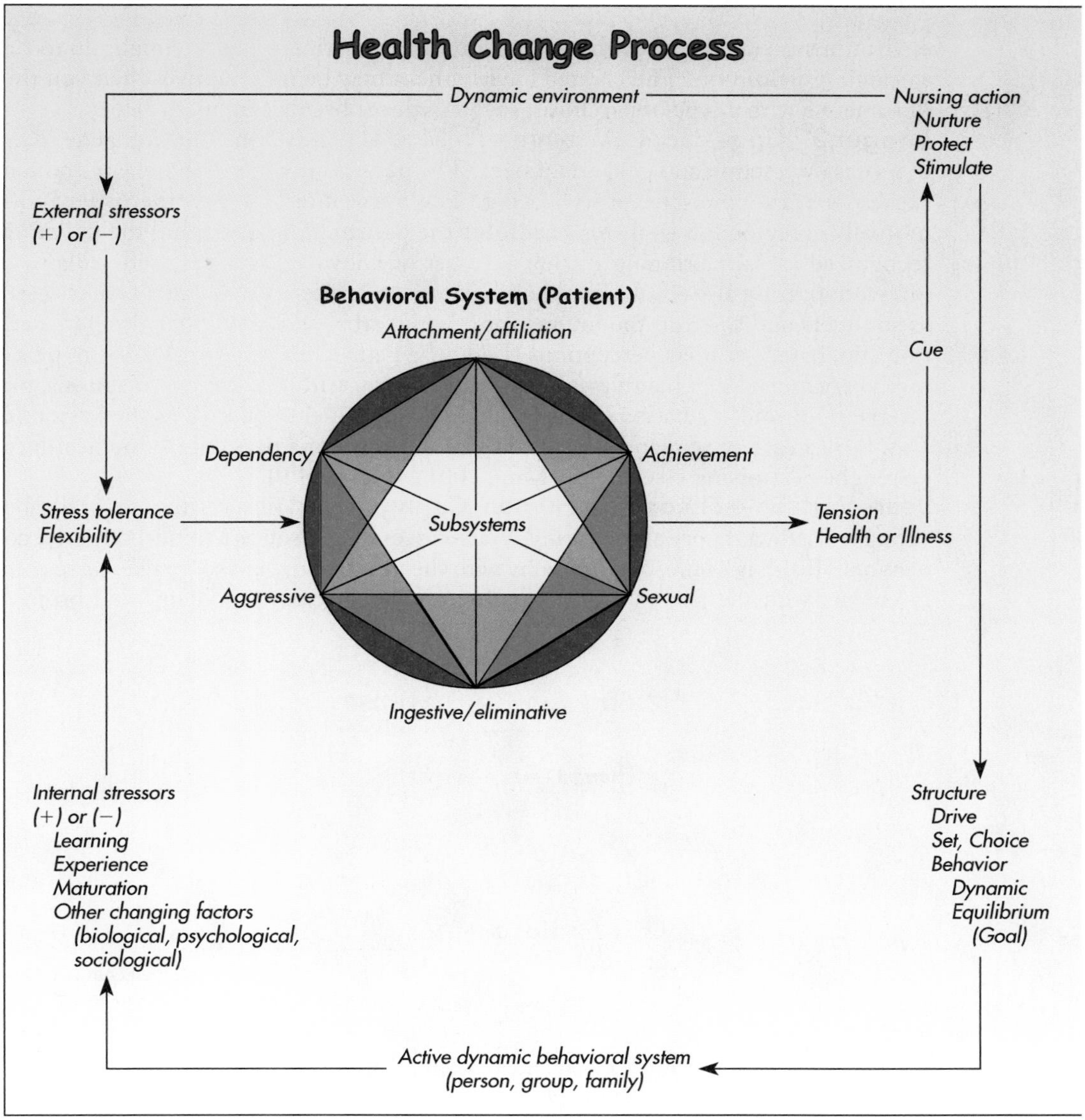

FIGURE 8-7

Johnson's Behavioral Systems Model. *(From Marriner Tomey A:* Nursing theorists and their work, *ed 5, St Louis, 2002, Mosby, p 256.)*

environment could be a healthy adaptation in considering what one might do to relax through visualization. The created environment may be maladaptive when you think of someone with a type of psychosis, such as schizophrenia (Figure 8-8).

Imogene King—Goal Attainment Model The theme of Imogene King's theory is interaction and goal attainment. The person interacts with the environment. Health is a dynamic state of well being. The nurse interacts with the patient to set mutually agreed upon goals for health for the patient. The nurse and the patient are recognized as each bringing his/her own set of knowledge, values, and skills to the interaction. King also emphasizes that the nurse and patient usually first come together as strangers and through the interactions, both verbal and nonverbal, develop a relationship, based on their perceptions (Leddy & Pepper, 1998). King's nursing process looks very much like what nurses are already familiar with: assessment, diagnosis, plan, intervention, and evaluation. King would like her model to be used as the basis of the U.S. health care system and also would like the entry of a person into the health care system be via nursing assessment (King, 2001)! (Figure 8-9).

Jean Watson—Theory of Human Caring. Jean Watson's theory is all about caring—finally, a theory about caring. Watson sees the person as a mind-body-soul connection. Health is a unity and harmony with the mind, body, and soul. The nurse comes in contact with the person in a "caring occasion" or "caring moment" and promotes

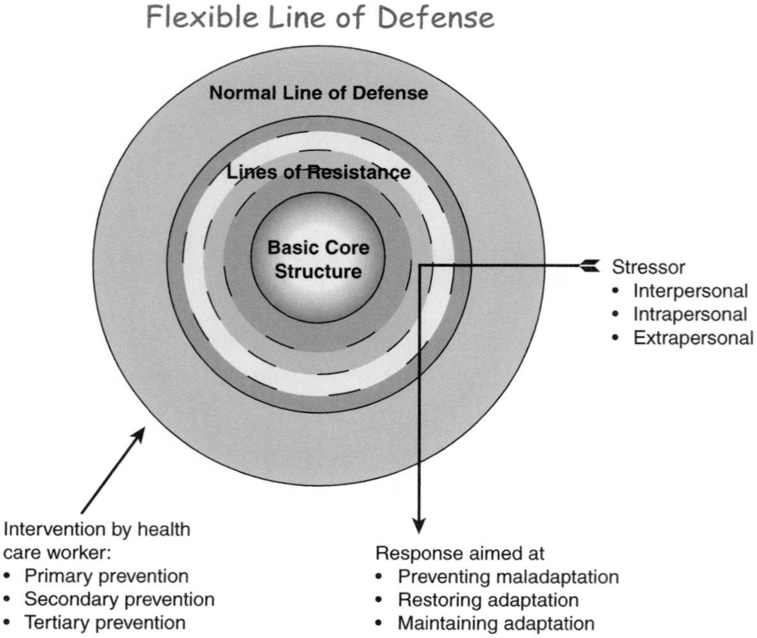

FIGURE 8-8

Neuman Systems Model. *(From Pearson A, Vaughan B, Fitzgerald M:* Nursing models for practice, *ed 3, Edinburgh, 2005, Butterworth & Heineman, p 145.)*

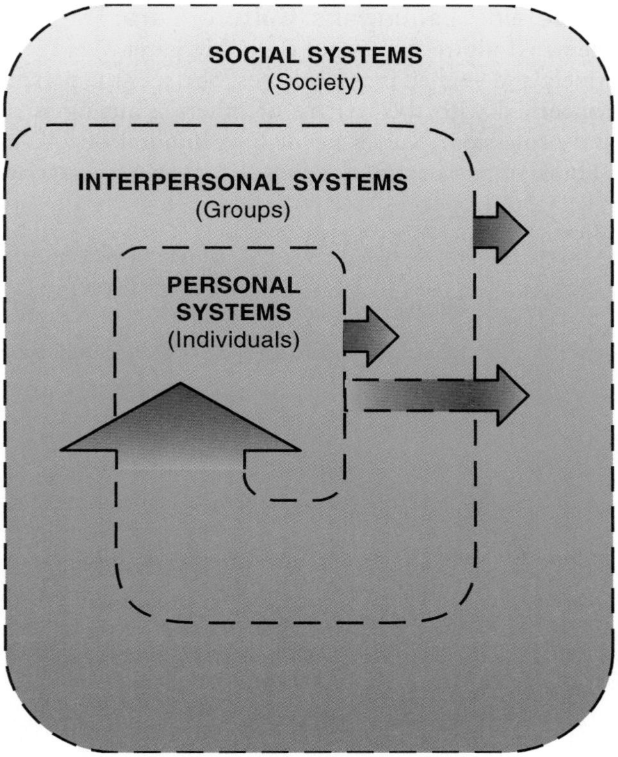

FIGURE 8-9
King's Goal Attainment Model for Nursing. *(From Pearson A, Vaughan B, Fitzgerald M:* Nursing models for practice, *ed 3, Edinburgh, 2005, Butterworth & Heineman, p. 162.)*

restoration of a sense of inner harmony through Watson's 10 carative factors. Caring to Watson is a moral idea, rather than an interpersonal technique (Leddy & Pepper, 1998).

Watson's 10 carative factors include (see what nursing interventions you can identify with each one):

1. The formation of a humanistic-altruistic system of values
2. The instillation of faith-hope
3. The cultivation of sensitivity to one's self and to others
4. The development of a helping-trust relationship
5. The promotion and acceptance of the expression of positive and negative feelings
6. The systematic use of the scientific problem solving methods for decision making
7. The promotion of interpersonal teaching-learning
8. The provision for a supportive, protective, and corrective mental, physical, socio-cultural, and spiritual environment
9. Assistance with the gratification of human needs
10. The allowance for existential-phenomenologic forces (Alligood, 2002; Wills, 2002)

Madeleine Leininger's Culture Care Theory. Madeleine Leininger's overall theme is culture. Leininger is the Margaret Mead of the health field and has traveled widely and studied many cultures. She sees the person as caring and capable of being concerned with the welfare of others. Nursing is a transcultural caring discipline and profession. Nurses need to be mindful of folk or generic health care practices. (Think of any health care practices that were practiced when you were a child that

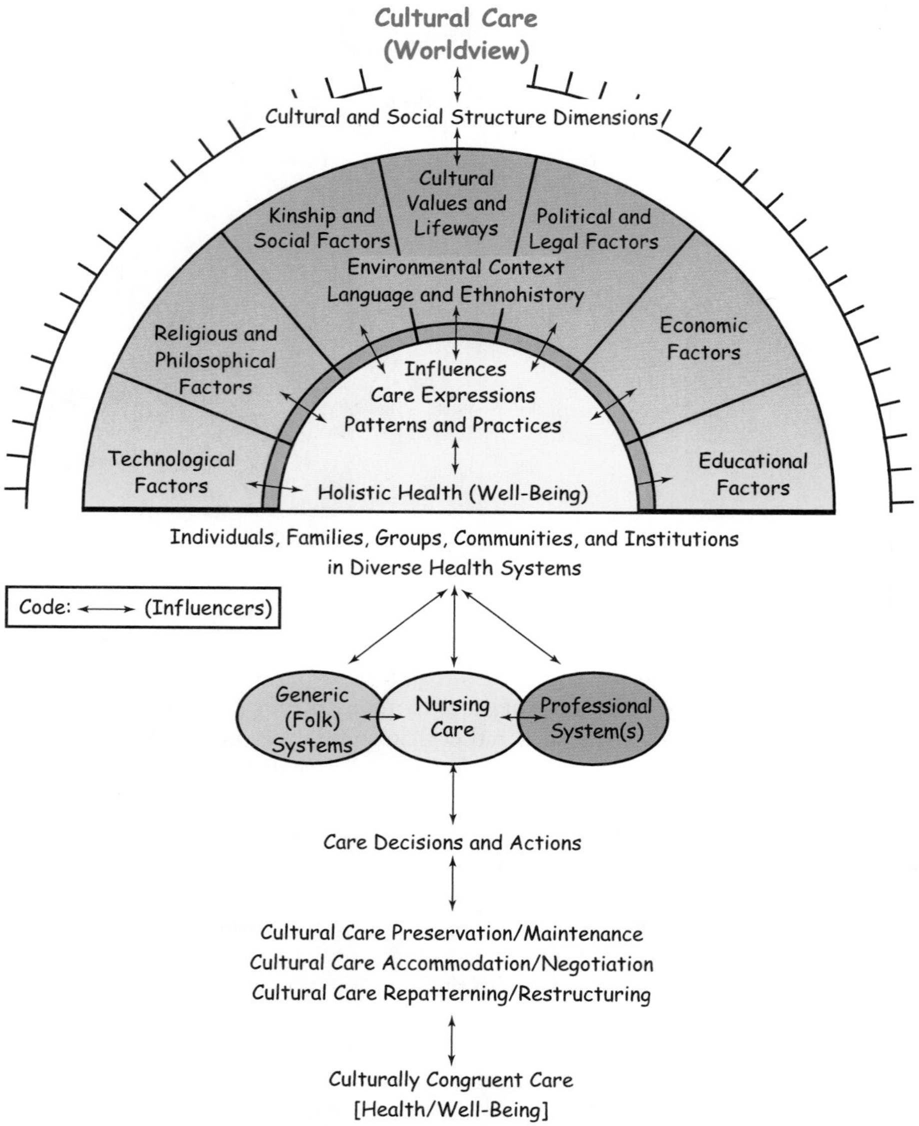

FIGURE 8-10
Leininger's Sunrise Model. *(From Alligood MR:* Nursing theory: utilization and application, *ed 2, St Louis, 2002, Mosby, p. 389.)*

would be considered folk or generic health care—e.g., Vick's Vapo-Rub applied to your chest during a cold, not drinking hot or cold beverages depending on the illness, not sitting too closely to the TV set to watch TV because it was "bad" for your eyes.) The nurse needs to be aware of and use culture care data that is influenced by religion, kinship, language, technology, economics, education (both formal and informal), cultural values and beliefs, and the physical (or ecological) environment. Leininger believes that there can be no curing without caring. Health is culturally defined (George, 2003b).

The health care professional needs to examine the prescribed health care requirements and decide if there can be culture care preservation or maintenance (where the relevant care values can be retained), or if there needs to be culture care accommodation or negotiation (where the cultural practices need to be adapted or negotiated to return the patient to health), or if culture care repatterning or restructuring is required (where the patient needs to change or significantly alter culturally based health practices to promote good health). Leininger's theory can be summarized in her Sunrise Model. The upper half of the model is for collecting data and the lower half is for decision making (George, 2003b) (Figure 8-10).

CONCLUSION

In reviewing the nursing theories, you may find that some especially appeal to you and others do not. That is okay. What nurses need to learn from the theories is that they are a rich part of our nursing history, and that the theories are a way to organize, delivery, and evaluate the care that we provide (Critical Thinking Box 8-2).

CRITICAL THINKING BOX 8-2

In reviewing the theories, which one would best fit in your clinical practice?
Which theory most appeals to you and why?
Which theory/theories would fit best with the following client settings and why?

- Pre-op patient
- Labor patient
- Psychiatric patient
- Nursing curriculum
- Managing a nursing unit
- Organizing an internal medicine clinic
- Organizing a computer generated acuity form
- Pediatric patients
- Home health
- Hospice care
- Long-term care facility

REFERENCES

Alligood MR, Marriner Tomey A: *Nursing theory: utilization and application*, ed 2, St Louis, 2002, Mosby.

Dunphy LH: Florence Nightingale caring actualized: A legacy for nursing. In ME Parker (Ed.): *Nursing theories and nursing practice*, Philadelphia, 2002, FA Davis, pp 31-53.

Ellis R: Characteristics of significant theories. In LH Nicoll (Ed.): *Perspectives on nursing theory*. Philadelphia, 1997, Lippincott, pp 373-381.

Fawcett J: *Analysis and evaluation of contemporary nursing knowledge: nursing models and theories*, Philadelphia, 2000, FA Davis.

Fitzpatrick J, Whall A: *Conceptual models of nursing: analysis and application*, ed 3, Stamford, Conn, 1996, Appleton & Lange

Foster PC, Bennett AM: Dorothea E. Orem. In University of Phoenix College of Health Sciences and Nursing (Eds.): *Theoretical foundations of nursing practice*, Boston, 2003, Pearson Custom Publishing, pp 137-168.

George JB: *Nursing theories: the base for professional nursing practice*, ed 4, Norwalk, Conn, 1995, Appleton & Lange.

George J: Betty Neuman. In University of Phoenix College of Health Sciences and Nursing (Eds.): *Theoretical foundations of nursing practice*, Boston, 2003a, Pearson Custom Publishing, pp 243-267.

George J: Madeleine M. Leininger. In University of Phoenix College of Health Sciences and Nursing (Eds.): *Theoretical foundations of nursing practice*, Boston, 2003b, Pearson Custom Publishing, pp 289-303.

Hanson SM, Kaakinen JR, Friedman MM: Theoretical approaches to family nursing. In MM Friedman (Ed.): *Family nursing*, Stamford, Conn, 1998, Appleton & Lange, pp 75-98.

Hickman JS: An introduction to nursing theory. In University of Phoenix College of Health Sciences and Nursing (Eds.): *Theoretical foundations of nursing practice*, custom text, Boston, 2002, Pearson Custom Publishing, pp 15-28.

Holaday B: Dorothy Johnson: Behavioral system models of nursing. In M. Parker (Ed.): *Nursing theories and nursing practice*, Philadelphia, 2001, FA Davis, pp 83-101.

King I: Imogene M. King: Theory of goal attainment. In M Parker (Ed.): *Nursing theories and nursing practice*, Philadelphia, 2001, FA Davis, pp 273-286.

Leddy S, Pepper J: *Conceptual bases of professional nursing*, ed 4, Philadelphia, 1998, Lippincott.

McEwen M: Overview of theory in nursing. In M McEwen & EM Wills (Eds.): *Theoretical basis for nursing*, Philadelphia, 2002, Lippincott, pp 23-47.

Muth Quillen S: Rogers' model: science of unitary persons. In University of Phoenix College of Health Sciences and Nursing (Eds.): *Theoretical foundations of nursing practice*, custom text, Boston, 2003, Pearson Custom Publishing, pp 309-323.

Pearson A, Vaughan B, Fitzgerald M: *Nursing models for practice*, ed 3, Edinburgh, 2005, Butterworth & Heineman.

Wills E: Grand nursing theories based on interactive process. In M McEwen & EM Wills. (Eds.): *Theoretical basis for nursing*, Philadelphia, 2002, Lippincott, pp 152-181.

CHAPTER 9

Image of Nursing: Influences of the Present

LINDA STEVENSON, PhD, RN

Oh, the power the gift He gives us, to see ourselves as others see us.

—*Robert Burns, 1786*

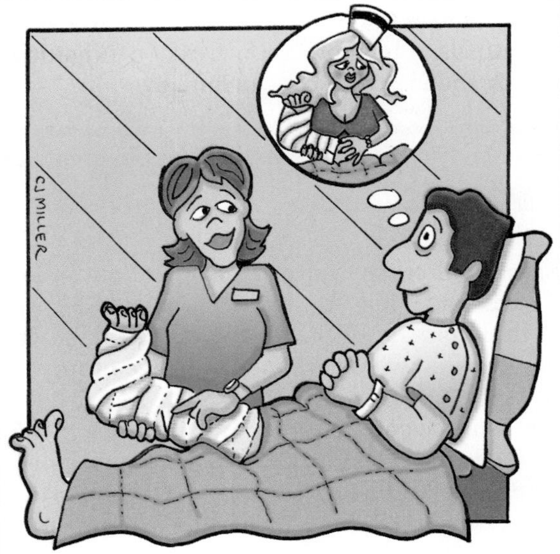

Nursing image—how is nursing perceived?

After completing this chapter, you should be able to:

- Identify selected literature that has influenced the image of professional nursing.
- Describe different sociologic models that characterize "professionalism."
- Apply Pavalko's characteristics as a framework to describe modern-day nursing practice.
- Identify the role that nursing organizations have in professional practice.
- Describe the role of credentialing and certification in professional practice.

Nursing image—how is it perceived? What does it mean to be a professional nurse? How does the public view nursing? How does nursing define and view itself?

Within the profession of nursing there is no single definition of nursing on which all nurses agree. To describe the current image of the professional nurse would be analogous to the old Indian folk tale in which three blind men attempt to define an elephant by touching three separate parts of the animal.

Modern-day nursing has many exciting professional dimensions, one of which includes the debate surrounding its identification as a profession. A current movement in nursing is to change the public image of the nurse. In this chapter, the development of nursing into a profession is discussed, and the present and future dimensions of nursing's "image" are explored. Historical knowledge about our "rites of passage" gives us an appreciation of where nursing is today as a profession, and what the future of nursing may hold for you, the recent graduate, in our complex and evolving health care world.

IMAGE OF NURSING

WHAT DO WE MEAN BY THE "IMAGE" OF NURSING?

Nursing has been identified as an "emerging profession" for at least 150 years. The historical context of nursing's image is usually traced back to Florence Nightingale, the "founder of nursing." But, in Great Britain, nurses believe that the association with Nightingale has held nursing into the subservient shadows of health care owing to her beliefs that nurses should be subordinate to doctors, and should not speak in public; she also was not in favor of registration (licensing in today's verbiage) and the formal training of nurses (The In/Visibility of Nurses in Cyberculture, 2005). Little is noted of this in the American nursing journals, and more is focused on Nightingale's successes in terms of statistical research and infection-control initiatives.

Is it time for nursing to look at Florence Nightingale in a different perspective? Will this change the current image of nursing?

The image of professional nursing continues to evolve and is significantly affected by the media, women's issues and roles, and a high-technology health care environment. How nursing views itself in the evolution of the profession and how actively nurses are involved in the definition process will determine the image of nursing in the future.

The idea that "a nurse is a nurse" is inaccurate. Nurses are professionals who are science driven, technically skilled, and caring (Dukes, 2003). In 1997, the Woodhull study on Nursing and the Media found that less than 10% of newspaper and magazine articles are related to health care, and when nurses are discussed, they are portrayed as incidental to health care (Kirschling & Ryan, 1997). Currently, a survey shows that 80% of the nurses on the Internet were female, white, middle class, blonde, and between 20 and 35 years of age (The In/Visibility of Nurses in Cyberculture, 2005).

Dombeck (2003) noted that "the portrayal of nurses generally parallels the portrayal of women in the media" (p. 351), and that image of nursing has continued to demonstrate a general lack of knowledge regarding the role of professional nurses (Ward et al., 2003). As more men are entering the profession, and there is a push to increase minorities in nursing, will the image of nursing change?

Most nurses would like to be thought of as autonomous and competent decision-makers within their nursing-practice areas. Throughout the 1990s, a nationwide advertising campaign supported by the National Commission on Nursing Implementation Project produced radio and television ads that said, "If caring were enough, anyone could be a nurse." Nurses of America, an advocate organization sponsored by the National League for Nursing (NLN), implemented a very successful program directed toward improving the image of nursing as depicted on television, on radio, in print, and on lecture circuits. Consultants were contracted to work with executives, politicians, and celebrities on presenting nursing in a positive manner. This approach reinforced the image of the modern-day professional nurse as having decision-making and problem-solving skills.

The Center for Nursing Advocacy was founded in April 2001 by a group of seven graduate students at Johns Hopkins University School of Nursing. The focus of the Center is to improve the portrayal of nursing in the media. The Center lists as its mission to increase understanding of the role nurses play in modern health care, with the end result fostering growth and diversity in the nursing profession. The Center for Nursing Advocacy has successfully worked with companies to remedy several advertising campaigns that portrayed nurses in an unflattering and inaccurate manner. The Center also lists the best and worst media portrayals of nursing annually (Center for Nursing Advocacy, 2005).

Nursing associations are working together to promote a positive image and deal with nursing shortage issues. Nurses for a Healthier Tomorrow, an alliance of 37 nursing organizations, has launched a national media campaign that demonstrates, through print and broadcast media, the many opportunities for the career of nursing. One tangible example of this effort is the website *www.nursesource.org*. Sigma Theta Tau International, the national honor society for nursing, is the coordinator of Nurses for a Healthier Tomorrow. Check out their website at *www.nursingsociety.org*. The American Nurses Association published a flyer titled, *Every Patient Deserves a Nurse*, along with other promotional materials for the lay public. The promotional message of these materials reinforces the positive image of nurses as patient advocates and critical resources both to patients and families, and emphasizes the right of people to a safe health care environment.

In 2002, the Johnson and Johnson Company developed a nationwide campaign to support the nursing profession. This program, entitled "The Campaign for Nursing's Future," was developed along with health care leaders and nursing organizations such as the National Student Nurse's Association (NSNA), the American Nurse's Association (ANA), the National League for Nursing (NLN), the American Organization for Nurse Executives (AONE), and Sigma Theta Tau. The goal was and continues to be to increase the numbers of young adults entering nursing through increasing the visibility of nurses of varied races, gender, and roles. The website for the campaign can be found at www.discovernursing.com.

Sigma Theta Tau International also produced the television program Nursing Approach, from January 1993 to April 1994. This series aired weekly in 350 cities in the United States and Canada. In its 15 months of programming, Nursing Approach disseminated the latest nursing knowledge for patient care, presented by nurses in all areas of nursing research and clinical practice. This very positive television profile of nursing enhanced the professional image and the presence of men in nursing and used the media as an innovative tool to show the diverse role of nursing in caring for patients and families.

The image of nursing continues to evolve as media shows the many roles of nurses in the restructuring of health care environments and in a variety of settings, such as emergency rooms and in wartime (e.g., in Desert Storm). Studies continue to verify that competent nursing care affects mortality rates in critical-care patients, and the future for many nursing jobs lies in the expanding role of nursing into community-based practice settings. The role and image of the nurse will continue to change as the many facets of health care delivery evolve into this century. The current nursing shortage will play a significant role in the creation of the future image and role of the nurse. How will nurses respond to these changes? The journey toward attaining a professional image has been and will continue to be challenging.

WHAT CONSTITUTES A PROFESSION?

There are many ways to describe a "professional." What meaning does the word have for you as a graduate professional nurse? Controversy over the definition of the term professional as it relates to nursing is not a new issue. Strauss (1966), a noted sociologist, found the word professional used in reference to nursing in a magazine article published in 1892 titled "Nursing, a New Profession for Women." The nurses of the twentieth and twenty-first centuries owe a lot to Isabel Adams Hampton (later Isabel Hampton Robb) for her visionary focus in the late 1800s. She was an outstanding advocate for the professionalization of nursing. In the textbook *Nursing Ethics* (1901), she wrote that:

> The trained nurse, then, is no longer to be regarded as a better trained, more useful, higher class servant, but as one who has knowledge and is worthy of respect, consideration, and due recompense.... She is also essentially an instructor; part of her duties have to do with the prevention of disease and sickness, as well as the relief of suffering humanity.... These are some of the essentials in nursing by which it has become to be regarded as a profession, but there still remains much to be desired, much to work for, in order to add to its dignity and usefulness

In Caplow's classic work from the early 1950s, *The Sociology of Work*, several steps in the process of "becoming professional" were defined further, and the value of forming an association that defined a special membership was addressed. Caplow suggested that making a name change to clarify an area of work or practice would subsequently produce a new role. With the creation of this new role, the group would then establish a code of ethics and legal components for licensure to practice and educational control of the profession (Caplow, 1954). This process of becoming professional was taking place in nursing in 1897 with the establishment of the ANA. Other aspects of professionalization were also beginning to develop. For example, the Code for Nurses was suggested as early as 1926, although it was not written or published by the ANA until the early 1950s. Revisions were made in 1956, 1960, and 1976, with changes made in

1985 that included interpretative statements. In the summer of 2001 at the ANA convention, delegates again updated and changed the name to the *Code of Ethics for Nurses with Interpretive Statements (www.ana.org/ethics/ecode.htm)*.

Almost 20 years after Caplow's work, Pavalko (1971) described eight dimensions of a profession. Pavalko's dimensions of a profession and their specific application to nursing are examined in more detail later in this chapter. Nursing continues to apply these dimensions to support nursing's move away from the occupational focus on "professionalism." Is nursing a profession or semiprofession?

By responding to the questions in Critical Thinking Box 9-1, which presents a fourth model of professionalism, Levenstein's model, you will be able to identify common themes in describing a profession. What are your thoughts about the nursing profession in light of these criteria?

Others have written about professions and their development, but these sociologic models present some logical characteristics for you to use to examine professionalism.

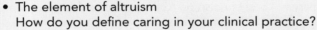

CRITICAL THINKING BOX 9-1

LEVENSTEIN'S CHARACTERISTICS OF A PROFESSION

What do you think about . . .

- The element of altruism
  How do you define caring in your clinical practice?
- Code of ethics
  Are you familiar with the ANA Code of Ethics?
- Collaboration with groups and individuals for the benefit of the patient
  What other groups do you work with in your clinical setting that affect the health needs of the patient and family?
- Colleagueship demonstrated by:
  An Organization for licensing—
  What is the role of the State Board of Nursing in your state?
  A group that helps ensure quality—
  Are you aware of the role of national nursing organizations that accredit nursing programs?
  There are two national nursing organizations that accredit nursing programs; do you know what they are?
  Peer evaluations of practitioners—
  What is the role of job evaluations in terms of professional growth?
- Accountability for conduct and responsibility for practice decisions
  Who monitors professional conduct issues from a legal and ethical point of view?
  Does shared governance reflect more control of one's nursing practice?
- Strong research program
  Are you aware that a national center for nursing research is now operating in Washington, DC?

According to Henshaw, a noted nursing leader and researcher, a profession includes "self-regulation and autonomy with ultimate loyalty and accountability to the professional group" (Talotta, 1990). Nursing is a dynamic profession and continues to strive to enhance a professional image—which leads us to the next question.

IS NURSING A PROFESSION?

Eunice Cole, past president of the ANA, described nursing as a dynamic profession that has established a code of ethics and standards of practice, education, service, and research components. The standards for both the professional and practical dimensions of nursing are continually reviewed and updated. Nurses, strong in numbers but splintered professionally in many ways, represent the largest group of health care providers in the United States. There are nearly 2.7 million registered nurses in the workforce with an average age of 45 years, and an estimated 71% of this population is working full time in nursing, with another 28% working part time (HRSA, 2002). By using Pavalko's eight dimensions to describe a profession, let us examine nursing and issues that challenge the collective whole.

1. A Profession Has Relevance to Social Values. Does nursing exist to serve self or others? Nursing historically had its roots in true altruism with lifelong service to others. Nursing defined itself in the ANA's Social Policy Statement (1988) as the "diagnosis and treatment of human responses to actual or potential health problems," and this definition remains today. As nurses, we focus not only on the treatment component of patient care, but also on wellness and health promotion issues, as a part of our nursing practice. The goal is to shift the focus of health care so that primary prevention becomes more valued. As this shift occurs, nurses will become increasingly important because of their ability to be teachers of health promotion activities and managers of wellness, activities that have an impact on social values.

2. A Profession Has a Training or Educational Period. According to Florence Nightingale, a nurse's education should involve not only a theory component, but also a practice component. An educational process for any professional is critical because it transmits the knowledge base of the profession and, through research and other scholarly endeavors, advances the practice of the profession. Luther Christman, noted nursing leader, has suggested that without a uniform educational base, it is difficult for nurses to communicate what they do as professionals, have clear standards of nursing care, stabilize colleagueship with other professionals, and ensure adequate funding of the profession. The diversity of educational programs for nurses has stimulated debate regarding the entry practice level for registered nurses. Some questions surrounding the issues include the following:

- Can associate-degree programs continue to provide an adequate educational base for the profession?
- Is the nurse prepared for current and future nursing functions, if educated at the diploma level?
- How critical is it to complete a 4-year Bachelor of Science in Nursing (BSN) program to handle the challenges of the health care environment, complex patient-family needs, and the expanding community-based settings for clinical work?
- Will the Doctor of Nursing degree that was pioneered at Case Western University become the minimum background for entry into the profession?

These questions have been debated since the publication in 1965 of an ANA position paper that charged the profession with the goal of establishing nursing education at the baccalaureate level within 25 years. Almost 40 years have passed since then, and the issue continues to challenge the profession. The inability of nursing organizations and educational systems at all levels to come to agreement on this issue has affected the solidarity of the profession.

Other states (such as Maine and Idaho) had serious debate in the mid-1990s on regulatory issues concerning the BSN as the entry credential. Beyond this generic-degree controversy are the issues associated with specialization: What should the entry-level degree be to enter into specialty nursing practice: the Master of Science (MSN) degree or a doctorate (PhD)? This issue was not resolved in the twentieth century. Will the twenty-first century bring a resolution to the issue?

3. Elements of Self-Motivation Address the Way in Which the Profession Serves the Patient or Family and Larger Social System. In 1990, the Tri-Council of Nursing, along with the American Association of Colleges of Nursing, designed a "Nursing Agenda for Health Care Reform" to collectively express the views of nurses concerning health care. Endorsed by 39 major specialty nursing organizations, along with the ANA and the NLN, the Tri-Council emphasized a restructured health care system that would provide universal access to health care, direct health care expenditures toward primary care, and reduce costs.

Political activity is a way of translating social values into action. Nursing faces special challenges when, for example, nurses must "strike" for pay and benefits or demonstrate a united front to gain federal funding rather than continuing a passive role in such issues.

> "It is time for the nursing profession to define a new narrative that reflects how much the profession has changed, how critical nursing skills are to today's patient care, how the profession has stayed abreast of medical and technological innovation, and what nursing is going to look like in the future" (Kaplan, 2005).

4. A Profession Has a Code of Ethics. Nursing, like other professions, has ethical dimensions. As noted earlier in the chapter, the nursing *Code of Ethics* published by the ANA dates to the 1950s. Key points of the *Code* are given in Box 9-1. The *Code of Ethics* is discussed in more detail in Chapter 19.

BOX 9-1 Code of Ethics for Nurses

The ANA House of Delegates approved these nine provisions of the new Code of Ethics for Nurses at its June 30, 2001, meeting in Washington, DC. In July 2001 the Congress of Nursing Practice and Economics voted to accept the new language of the interpretive statements, resulting in a fully approved revised Code of Ethics for Nurses with Interpretive Statements, as follows.

1. The nurse, in all professional relationships, practices with compassion and respect for the inherent dignity, worth, and uniqueness of every individual, unrestricted by considerations of social or economic status, personal attributes, or the nature of health problems.

Continued

BOX 9-1 Code of Ethics for Nurses—cont'd

2. The nurse's primary commitment is to the patient, whether an individual, family, group, or community.
3. The nurse promotes, advocates for, and strives to protect the health, safety, and rights of the patient.
4. The nurse is responsible and accountable for individual nursing practice and determines the appropriate delegation of tasks consistent with the nurse's obligation to provide optimum patient care.
5. The nurse owes the same duties to self as to others, including the responsibility to preserve integrity and safety, to maintain competence, and to continue personal and professional growth.
6. The nurse participates in establishing, maintaining, and improving health care environments and conditions of employment conducive to the provision of quality health care and consistent with the values of the profession through individual and collective action.
7. The nurse participates in the advancement of the profession through contributions to practice, education, administration, and knowledge development.
8. The nurse collaborates with other health professionals and the public in promoting community, national, and international efforts to meet health needs.
9. The profession of nursing, as represented by associations and their members, is responsible for articulating nursing values, for maintaining the integrity of the profession and its practice, and for shaping social policy.

5. A Professional Has a Commitment to Lifelong Work. By this statement, Pavalko means that a professional sees his or her career as more than just a steppingstone to another area of work or as an intermittent job. Nursing continues to be a female-dominated profession, and prevailing definitions of masculinity have acted as a barrier to men entering the profession. This needs to change if we are to increase the numbers of men in nursing and alter the patriarchal nature of the profession. Government data show that 81% of the nearly 2.7 million registered nurses work in health care (HRSA, 2002). Nursing constitutes the largest health care occupation, and more jobs are expected for registered nurses than for any other occupation. This faster than average growth is being driven by technologic advances. Thus, nursing as a career has great potential for financial rewards, involvement in a variety of professional endeavors, and commitment to lifelong work.

6. Members Control Their Profession. Nurses are not entirely autonomous. Although nurses work under professional control, they are under legislative control as well. Among these controls are the 50 state boards of nursing, which control the scope of nursing practice within each state and professional practice standards that are supported both at local and national levels. In 1973, the ANA wrote the first Standards of Nursing Practice and since then has had a leadership role in the development of general and many specialty nursing practice standards.

Another publication by the ANA, the *Standards of Clinical Nursing Practice* (1991), discusses the use of nursing process and professional practice standards. The development of professional practice standards indicates to the larger social system that nursing can define and control its quality of practice. These national standards are incorporated into institutional standards to help guide nursing practice. Most recent publications by the ANA can be found on their website at *www. nursingworld.org.* The issue at hand, however, is that these professional practice standards authorize nurses to practice nursing. Nurses are expected to take responsibility for their own actions and not just follow the physician without thinking critically.

Nurses practice in varied settings, and the advanced-practice nurse is in more of an autonomous professional practice role, such as the nurse midwife, psychiatric clinical specialist, or nurse practitioner. In 1992, there were 100,000 advanced-practice nurses in the United States. In March 2000, the number of RNs with at least one advanced-practice credential was 196,000, with the largest percentage of that group working as nurse practitioners (HRSA, 2002). These changes represent the largest-growing segment of specialty nursing practice. Advancing one's education level is often paired with increased autonomy.

Most nurses in this country work within a structured setting; three out of five jobs are in hospital, inpatient, or outpatient settings. Trends in those settings are slowly changing to give nurses a stronger voice. For example, nursing care delivery systems that have case management and shared governance reflect more progressive and autonomous environments (see Chapter 15). Nursing can control its scope of practice through professional organizations and publishing documents, along with an active voice in regulatory bodies, such as state boards of nursing.

7. A Profession Has a Theoretical Framework on Which Professional Practice is Based. Nursing continues to be based in the sciences and humanities, but nursing theory is evolving. It was not until the 1950s that nursing theory was "born." In 1952, Dr. Hildegard Peplau published a nursing model that described the importance of the "therapeutic relationship" in health and wellness. Since then, other nursing theorists such as Martha Rogers, Sister Callista Roy, Dorothea Orem, and Betty Neuman have contributed to our evolving theory-based nursing science.

8. Members of a Profession Have a Common Identity and a Distinctive Subculture. The outward image of nursing has changed remarkably within the past 50 years. Nurses were once identified by how they looked rather than by what they did. The nursing cap and pin reflected the nurse's school and educational background. The modern-day trend emphasizes that it is not what is worn but what is done that reflects one's role in the nursing profession. The struggle to shift out of rigid dress codes was a major issue in the 1960s. Clothing and other symbols identify a subculture, and changes in that identification process occur slowly. What kind of an image do you want to project as a professional nurse? (Critical Thinking Box 9-2).

Nursing colleagues reflect attitudes and values about the profession. Many schools of nursing have alumni associations, student nurse associations, and nursing honor societies or clubs on campus. These groups provide social interaction during the nursing

CRITICAL THINKING BOX 9-2

WHAT DO YOU THINK?

WHAT KIND OF IMAGE DO YOU WANT TO PROJECT AS A "PROFESSIONAL"?

- Should nurses wear visible body jewelry or tattoos? Is it acceptable to wear a nose ring because it is a part of your culture? What if it is not? How many earrings should a nurse be allowed to wear?
- What do professionals call each other in the clinical setting? Do you wear your name badge with proper credentials? Are the doctors on your unit called by their first name or last name? How do they address you?
- Do you wear your school pin? What other credentials and symbols indicate additional competence?
- What should nurses wear? Do scrubs look professional? Can a nurse wearing cartoon character scrubs be taken seriously? Why? Why not? Should nurses leave the hospital in their scrubs and go to the grocery store?

DOES THE PUBLIC EXPECT TO SEE NURSES WEARING A WHITE DRESS, HOSE, AND WHITE SHOES? WHAT IMPACT DOES THIS HAVE ON IMAGE?

- How should a professional look and behave? What other professions are associated with a "uniform"?

education years and are great ways to network later in one's career. Sigma Theta Tau has the Chiron Mentoring program to assist individual nurses to achieve their professional goals related to leadership, scholarship, and evidenced-based nursing. Their website is *www.nursingsociety.org/programs/chiron.html.* Belonging to a professional organization such as the ANA, the NLN, or a specialty organization helps professional nurses continue to network and maintain collegiality in our practice areas.

> "Nurses should choose optimism, making positive strides each day to celebrate who they are and the differences they make. Just a nurse—no, never."
> —Melissa Fitzpatrick, 2001

When will the conflicts in educational preparation be resolved? How will we use further refinement and application of nursing theories in our clinical practice? What can nurses do to have more control of nursing practice regardless of the clinical setting? Will there be an increase in the percentage of people who are choosing nursing as a career? What are the forces that will help nursing "come together" and become not only a true profession, but the largest and most powerful of all the health care professional groups (there is always strength in numbers)?

NURSING ORGANIZATIONS

WHAT SHOULD I KNOW ABOUT PROFESSIONAL ORGANIZATIONS?

Nursing organizations have significant roles in empowering nurses in their emerging professionalism. Yet, many nurses do not belong to a national organization such as the American Nurses Association (ANA) or their state affiliate organization, or even to specialty-focused groups like the American Association of Critical Care Nurses (AACN) or the National Black Nurses Association (NBNA). During the past few years, researchers have examined the issue of belonging to a professional organization, with no conclusive findings regarding why or how nurses choose nursing organizations. Some have suggested that organizations that represent nursing as a whole, such as the ANA and the National League for Nursing (NLN), do not meet the needs of the individual nurse practicing in today's changing health care environment.

In the early 1950s, belonging to a professional nursing group was popular. By the 1980s, membership in both the ANA and the NLN had declined by 10% to 15%, whereas the nursing population had increased by 150%. During this same period, specialty organizations such as the Association of Operating Room Nurses (AORN) and the Oncology Nursing Society (ONS) increased their membership. Does this shift in affiliation reflect a shift in practice settings from the generalist area to specialist areas and suggest that nurses are selecting a specialty organization that represents their current practice? Affiliation with a nursing organization to facilitate networking with colleagues is valuable and meaningful. As a recent graduate, you will need to examine your options for joining a professional group and then demonstrate your professional commitment by active involvement.

The question should be "Which ones should I join?" rather than "Should I even join an organization?" Some organizations give discount memberships to recent graduates the first 6 to 12 months after graduation and provide payment options (Figure 9-1). In the next section, various organizations are reviewed, with some historical notes to assist you in making the best choice as you begin your nursing career. A more complete directory of nursing organizations can be found in Appendix B (also see Critical Thinking Box 9-3).

WHAT ORGANIZATIONS ARE AVAILABLE TO THE RECENT GRADUATE?

A few of these key professional organizations for individual and organizational membership are described in the next section in alphabetical order. Many of these organizations

CRITICAL THINKING BOX 9-3

WHAT DO YOU THINK?

- How are nurses in your organization socialized?
- Is there an informal initiation process? (can be looked on as hazing)
- Ask new nurses if this has happened to them.
- How can this be changed? How can new nurses be nurtured?

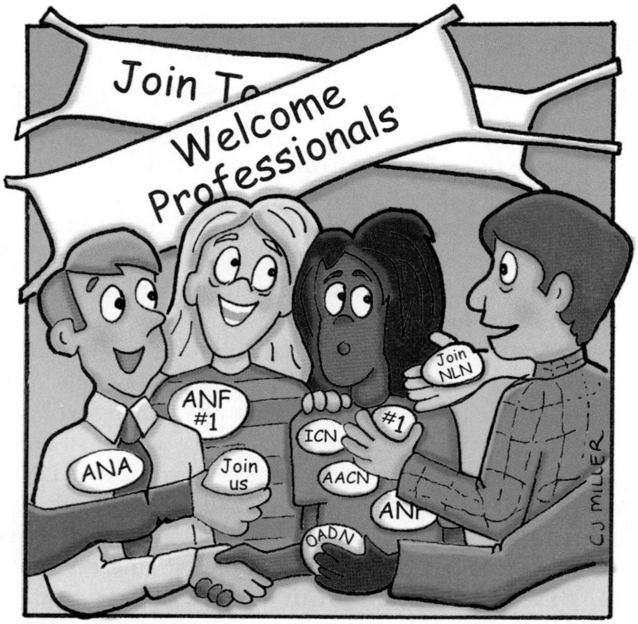

FIGURE 9-1
There is a nursing organization to fit your needs.

publish a newsletter or professional journal, and most have websites. Individual membership in one or more organizations is a great way to maintain current knowledge about changes in your career field.

American Nurses Association. The ANA is identified as the professional association for registered nurses. It was through the early efforts of Isabel Hampton Robb and others that the Nurses Associated Alumnae of the United States and Canada was formed. At the World's Fair in 1890, a group of 15 nursing leaders began discussions about forming a professional association. Six years later, alumnae from the training schools organized the professional association now called the ANA. Canadian members split from the original group in 1911 and formed their own professional association. The organizational structure of the ANA has undergone many changes over the years.

Currently, when an individual joins the ANA, he or she joins the national organization along with the constituent associations at the state and local level. This method geographically groups smaller clusters of members together according to their practice interests. The current membership of the ANA represents totals more than 180,000.

In 1974, an amendment to the Taft-Hartley Act allowed professional nursing organizations to be considered to be labor unions. United American Nurses is the collective bargaining organization representing the ANA. After this significant event, some nursing administrators and managers withdrew their memberships in ANA because of the potential conflict of interest between professional affiliation and the workplace. However, this change generated the development of other major nursing organizations: the Center for the American Nurse (CAN) and the American Association of Nurse Executives (AONE).

The ANA has been at the forefront of policy issues and represents nursing in legislative activities. The cabinets and councils of the ANA have provided standards of practice for both the generalist and the specialist. The 1988 Social Policy Statement document defines nursing practice at both the generalist and specialist levels. The certifying organization of the ANA is the American Nurses Credentialing Center (ANCC), which has certified more than 150,000 RNs in different practice areas at both the generalist and the specialist level. The ANCC, a subsidiary of the ANA since 1991, identifies its mission as improving nursing practice and promoting quality health care service through several types of credentialing programs. The ANCC has created a modular approach to certification that enables the nurse to be recognized for multiple areas of expertise, not simply for competency in a core clinical specialty. There are 30 generalist care clinical specialties or advanced-practice care areas. As a result of their "open door 2000" program, all qualified registered nurses, regardless of their educational preparation, can become certified as a generalist in any of the following specialty areas: gerontology, medical-surgical, pediatrics, perinatal, and psychiatric–mental health nursing.

In addition to certifying individual nurses, the organization also accredits educational providers (i.e., organizations that issue continuing-education credits for professional programs), recognizes excellence in Magnet nursing services, and educates the public about credentialing and professional nursing. This organization is electronically linked on the home page of the ANA *(www.nursingworld.org)*.

American Nurses Foundation and the American Academy of Nursing. Two other organizations associated with the ANA are the American Nurses Foundation, founded in 1955, and the American Academy of Nursing (AAN), founded in 1973. Briefly described, these organizations serve special purposes in support of research and recognition of nursing colleagues. The American Nurses Foundation was established as a tax-exempt corporation to receive money for nursing research. With the establishment of the National Nursing Research Institute, the focus has changed to one of support in the areas of policy-making and research or educational activities. The AAN has a membership of more than 1500 nursing leaders and was established as an honorary association for nurses who have made significant contributions to the nursing profession. When a nurse is elected to the AAN, she or he is called a Fellow, and the credential following the individual's name is FAAN. The official publication of this organization is *Nursing Outlook*.

International Council of Nurses. The International Council of Nurses, established in 1899, is the international organization representing professional nurses. The focus of this nursing organization is on worldwide health care issues and nursing issues; it meets every 4 years and is headquartered in Geneva, Switzerland.

National League for Nursing. The NLN, established in 1952, can be traced to the 1893 organization of the American Society of Superintendents of Training Schools for Nurses of the United States and Canada. Between the late 1800s and the early 1900s, seven nursing organizations formed and joined under the collective name and function of the NLN. One of the unique features of the NLN is that both individuals and agencies are members. The NLN adopted a strategic plan in 1995 to place community-based health care education and health care delivery at the center of its focus and activities (NLN, 1995). The NLN continues to foster improvement in nursing services and nursing education and offers annual educational summits for nursing faculty and leaders in all types of nursing-education programs to come together to discuss nursing education. A nonnurse can join the NLN to fulfill its purpose of promoting the consumer's voice in some nursing policies. The NLN has a biennial convention and publishes *N&HC: Perspectives on Community* (called *Nursing & Health Care* before 1995) bimonthly, NLN Update, and numerous other publications that can be obtained by calling 800-669-1656 or by visiting their website at *www.nln.org*.

Before 1997, the NLN functioned as an accrediting body in all levels of nursing education. In 1997, the NLN created an independent organization called the National League for Nursing Accrediting Commission, Inc. (NLNAC) to accredit educational and professional nursing programs. This organizational change was in response to the new standards established by the US Department of Education. This step was taken to separate accrediting activities from membership activities and to respond to the Higher Education Act Amendment of 1992. Is your school an NLNAC-accredited institution? Visit their website at *www.nlnac.org*.

National Student Nurses' Association. The National Student Nurses' Association (NSNA) is a fully independent organization and publishes its own quarterly journal, *Imprint*. It was formed in 1952 for students enrolled in nursing programs. Becoming a member of the NSNA may be viewed as a way to begin the "professional" socialization process. Often, members of the NSNA serve on selected committees of the ANA and speak to the ANA House of Delegates regarding student-related issues. There are state and national chapters.

National Organization for Associate Degree Nursing (NOADN). This group was organized in 1986 as an outgrowth of several state organizations. Texas was the first state to have a chapter, which was started in 1984. Membership is open to associate-degree nursing graduates, educators, and students. Individuals, states, agencies, and other organizations may also join. There are state and national chapters. The mission of this organization is to be the leading advocate for associate degree nursing education and practice. NOADN strives to maintain eligibility for RN licensure for graduates of associate-degree (AD) programs; to promote AD nursing programs in the community, to provide a forum for discussion of issues impacting AD nursing, to develop partnerships and increase communication with other health care professionals, to increase public understanding of the AD nurse, to participate in state and national levels in the formation of health care policies, and to facilitate legislative action supporting the activities of NOADN. Visit their website at *www.noadn.org*.

American Association of Colleges of Nursing. This organization is the national voice for university and 4-year college educational programs in nursing and has a membership of more than 500 colleges. The mission of the organization is to serve the public interest by assisting deans and directors in improving and advancing nursing education, research, and practice. This organization publishes a newsletter and a bimonthly nursing journal called the *Journal of Professional Nursing*.

In the past few years, it has formed a subsidiary for credentialing purposes. That organization is the Commission on Collegiate Nursing Education. This autonomous accreditation agency serves only baccalaureate and higher degree programs in the accreditation process. Additional information on either organization can be found at *www.aacn.nche.edu*.

American Board of Nursing Specialties. The past 15 years have demonstrated significant growth in specialty practice in nursing. Throughout the 1980s and 1990s, these organizations met annually as the National Federation of Specialty Nursing Certifying Organization to discuss issues in certification and nursing practice. This organization dissolved, and many of the specialty organizations joined the American Board of Nursing Specialties in 1991. The ABNS was established to create uniformity in nursing certification, and, as such, now represents more than 25 specialty nursing organizations that promote specialty practice, in addition to the certification issues associated with specialty practice. The ABNS functions as a consumer advocate in promoting nursing certification.

As a recent graduate, are you interested in a particular specialty nursing practice area? How and when do you anticipate obtaining specialty certification? How will you include membership in a professional organization in your 5-year career-educational plan?

The American Red Cross. This is an international organization of approximately 120 Red Cross organizations around the world. Nurses of the American Red Cross pioneered public health nursing in the early 1900s. The American Red Cross is a voluntary agency that is supported by contributions and plays an important role in providing disaster relief and education in first aid and home health and in organizing volunteers to assist in hospitals and nursing homes.

In summary, the roles that professional organizations have in enhancing the image of nursing are significant. Their impact is seen in both educational and practice issues for generalist and specialist nurse roles. Organizations provide a voice for nursing in policy issues and serve to unite nurses as a group of professionals. Ultimately, it may be nursing organizations that will serve as the catalyst for change in the health care system, and their impact will be felt in the next century.

CREDENTIALING: LICENSURE AND CERTIFICATION

WHAT IS CREDENTIALING?

In the early days of nursing before the Nightingale era, anyone could say they were a nurse and practice their "trade" as they wished. It was only during the past century that nursing became a credentialed profession. A credential can be as simple as a written document of an individual's qualifications. A high school diploma is a credential that indicates a certain level of education has been attained. A credential can also signify a person's performance. The attainment of a title (e.g., FAAN) signifies excellence in performance; a postgraduate degree from an institution of higher learning (PhD or EdD) indicates success in terms of academic achievement and advanced nursing knowledge.

In nursing, the educational credentials that an individual holds indicate not only academic achievement, but also that a minimum level of competency in nursing skills has been attained. Academic achievement is represented by an associate degree in nursing (ADN), a diploma in nursing, or a baccalaureate degree in nursing (BSN or BS). After academic preparation and successful completion of NCLEX, you will have a legal credential—your nursing license—that permits you to practice as an RN. Additional nursing credentials may reflect areas of practice in special areas, such as Critical Care Registered Nurse (CCRN) and Certified Addictions Registered Nurse (CARN) Figure 9-2 summarizes how professional and legal regulations affect the individual, the institution, and the public.

WHAT ARE REGISTRATION AND LICENSURE?

Licensure affords protection to the public by requiring the individual to demonstrate minimum competency by examination. By 1923, all 48 states had some form of nursing licensure in place. Nursing licensure is a process by which a governmental agency grants "legal" permission to an individual to practice nursing. This accountability is maintained through a governmental agency responsible for the licensing and registration process. The state boards of nursing are the governmental agencies responsible for this process. Boards of nursing vary in structure and design on the basis of the nurse practice act within each state. The state boards of nursing also exercise legal control over schools of nursing within their respective states. In 1978, all boards of nursing formed a national council, the National Council of State Boards of Nursing (NCSBN), to present a more collective front on nursing education and licensure.

Foreign nurse graduates who want to practice nursing in the United States must contact the board of nursing in the state in which they want to practice to obtain licensure, because each state controls the requirements for licensure. The state's board of nursing will review the candidate's nursing education and determine requirements needed to obtain a license in that respective state. Most states require that foreign nurses take the Committee on Graduates of Foreign Nursing Schools (CGFNS) examination before the NCLEX-RN. This examination determines proficiency both in nursing and the English language, thus assisting in the prediction of success on the NCLEX-RN. All foreign graduates, regardless of licensure in their home countries, must successfully complete the NCLEX-RN.

WHAT IS CERTIFICATION?

In the classic article on credentialing published by the ANA in the late 1970s, certification is defined as a "voluntary process by which a nongovernmental agency or association certifies that an individual licensed to practice a profession has certain predetermined standards specified by that profession for specialty practice" (ANA, 1978-1979). Certification is a different credential than licensure and has a variety of interpretations—both for the nursing profession and the public.

The movement toward certification in nursing practice areas has grown significantly within the past 40 years. It was in 1946 that credentialing was first required for entry into practice as a nurse anesthetist (i.e., Certified Registered Nurse Anesthetist [CRNA]). Twenty-five years later, nurse midwives followed suit by requiring certification through the American College of Nurse Midwives as an entry-level credential.

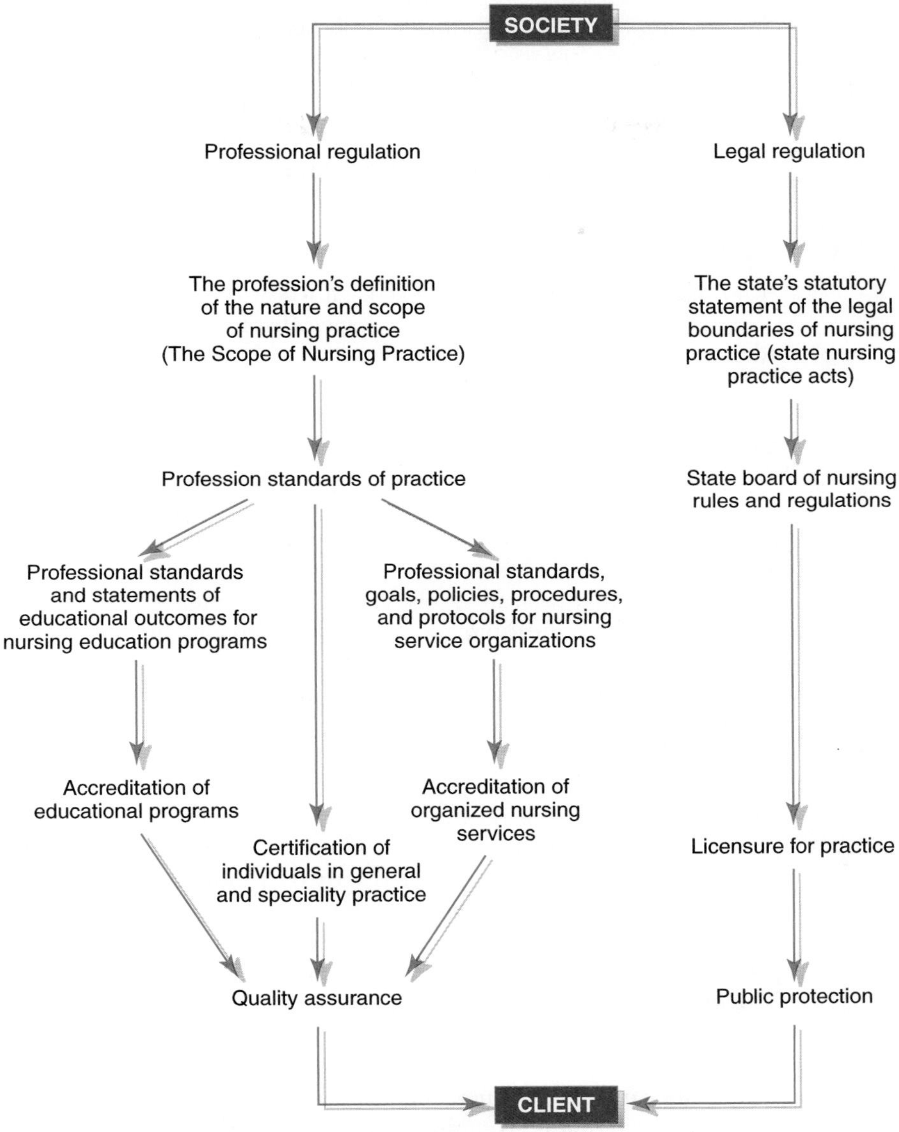

FIGURE 9-2
Flow chart on professional and legal regulation of practice. *(From American Nurses Association:* The scope of nursing. *Kansas City, Mo, 1987, ANA.)*

> The nursing license is recognized as indicating minimum competency, whereas the certification credential indicates preparation beyond the minimum level.

An August 2000 press release by the ANCC of the largest study ever conducted in the United States and Canada with credentialed nurses indicated that nurses who have professional certification made fewer health care errors (ANCC, 2003).

CERTIFICATION: GENERALIST OR SPECIALIST?

According to the ANA, a generalist is an RN who may practice in a general or special area of nursing. To be identified as a specialist nurse, the individual needs to have an advanced degree beyond the baccalaureate and to practice in a special area of nursing (ANA, 1990). Since the establishment of the first certification program by the ANA in 1973, certification is the credential that provides recognition of professional achievement in a defined functional or clinical area of nursing practice.

Specialty and generalist nursing organizations represent the largest number of nurses in the nation. More than 350,000 of the nearly 2.7 million RNs in this country hold certification in a specialty area of nursing (Miller, 2000). Research data from the ANCC indicate that there are 67 organizations that certify nurses, 95 different credentials, and more than 134 different specialty areas. Credentials, such as professional certification, are the stamps of quality and achievement to communicate professional competence. The process of becoming certified engages a full circle of accountability to patients and families, along with professional colleagues (Nardini, 2000).

WHAT IS ACCREDITATION?

The term accreditation is often confused with certification. The term is defined as a process by which a voluntary, nongovernmental agency or organization approves and grants status to institutions or programs (not individuals) that meet predetermined standards or outcomes. The accreditation of nursing programs by either the NLNAC or the Commission on Collegiate Nursing Education (CCNE) is an activity that you, the recent graduate, may have been involved with during your nursing education. The organizations that accredit programs were enumerated in an earlier part of this chapter.

Accreditation is a peer review and voluntary process. The use of standards and criteria are supported by member schools for the evaluation peer review process. The process of accreditation is similar for both accrediting organizations—the Commission on Collegiate Nursing Education and the NLNAC. The NLNAC is the only organization that accredits all levels of nursing program education from the practical nurse to the graduate-level nurse.

WHAT NURSING JOURNALS OR LITERATURE ARE AVAILABLE?

Nursing journals were first published as a way of maintaining communication with other nurses. At the turn of the century, two nursing journals existed in the United States: *The Nightingale*, a monthly publication started by Sarah Post, and *The Trained*

Nurse (later called *Nursing World*), started by Mary Francis. The *American Journal of Nursing* was first published in 1900 by the ANA and is still in publication today. *Nursing "Year"* and *RN* are two other widely read nursing journals, but they are not affiliated with any professional organization. Numerous nursing journals are published by specialty organizations, such as *Emergency Room Nursing*, *Oncology Nursing*, *Addictions Nursing*, and the *Journal of Pediatric Nursing*.

Because of the changing health care environment and the proliferation of knowledge in health care and nursing, much of the knowledge acquired in your nursing education program may be out of date 5 years after you graduate. Naisbitt and Aburdene (1990) talked about this issue in *Megatrends*, and concluded that we have moved from the Industrial Age to the Information Processing Age, with nursing in an information-provider role. Nursing journals continue to be a major link between nursing organizations and professionals in this age of information explosion. Connectivity is the buzzword of this millennium and with this there has been a proliferation of online journals and web-based information resources. As a new graduate, the ease of accessibility of online journals will facilitate staying abreast of the current trends.

How will you stay current after graduation? How do you plan to maintain practice skills and a current knowledge base? Will you be a lifelong learner?

CONTEMPORARY ISSUES

Florence Nightingale once described nursing as a "progressive art in which to stand still is to step backward." Those thoughts from more than 100 years ago still hold true today with regard to changes that are occurring in nursing professional practice areas. Major shifts in the health care setting mandate that modern-day nurses embrace flexibility and adaptability in their professional behaviors. The greater need for advanced-practice nurses represents a role shift that can move nursing forward to influence and effect a more powerful position as a profession. Flexibility in work behaviors, additional educational credentials, and certification can be viewed as positive responses to the changes taking place in health care. Opportunities have never been better for the recent graduate, as your career launches you into the future. Let us look at two of the issues that will likely affect your professional practice.

WHAT IS GOING ON IN THE JOB MARKET?

Nurses are health care's front-line professionals and number as the nation's largest health care profession, but there is a growing disparity between the supply of and the demand for nurses that is leading to a potentially overwhelming nursing shortage. In the early 1990s, a major downsizing of RN staff occurred through attrition and layoffs, and an increased use of nonlicensed personnel was added to the nursing-care delivery system. Currently, the demand for health care and the demand for registered nurses will increase at the same time as the supply of RNs in the workforce will be declining (Buerhaus, 2001) (Figure 9-3).

The acute-care setting remains the major job placement area for recent graduates. Although there has been an increase in nurses working in community settings overall, NCSBN research reveals that very few recent graduates are working in

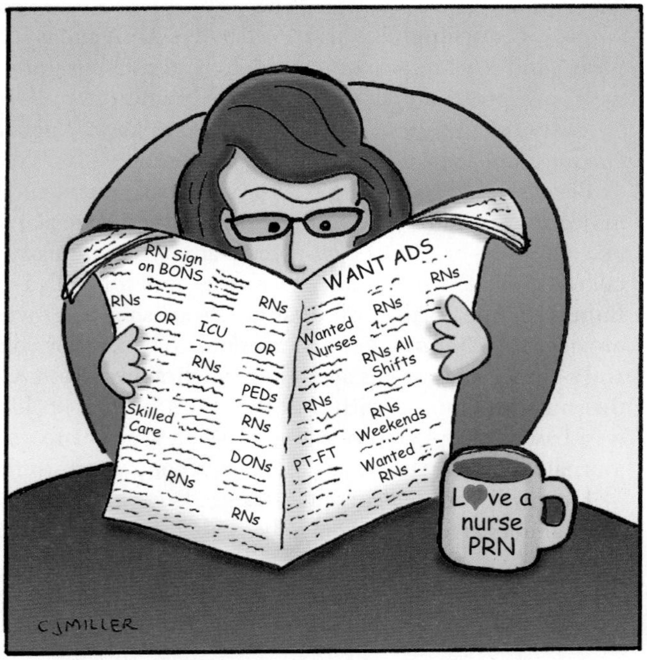

FIGURE 9-3
What is going on in the job market?

community-based settings. Most (84%) of recent graduates are working in hospitals providing direct patient care.

With today's job market changes, a major health care problem has developed in acute care. With the aging of RNs across the country and the increased level of patient acuity in the hospital, a staffing crisis has again developed in acute-care hospitals. According to the Joint Commission for Accreditation of Hospitals in 2002, inadequate nurse staffing has been a factor in 24% of the 1609 cases of patient deaths, injury, or loss of function reported since 1997.

Nursing shortages are a cyclical phenomenon that has occurred throughout the history of nursing. At the core of past shortages have been the increased availability of alternate career choices for women, poor working conditions, and cost-containment strategies (McCabe, 2002). Today's shortage is due to a confluence of factors, including: an aging population, fewer workers coming into nursing, an aging workforce, more options for women, the generation gap, the work environment with increased workloads, and inadequate support systems (Kimball, 2004). These issues call for all those who have a stake in the issue to "break out of their professional silos and work together" to realize an effective long-term change (Kimball, 2004). As nurses, we need to examine our responsibility for and contribution to building professional cohesion to increase effectiveness in implementing positive roles for the future of nursing and health care (McCabe, 2002)

In spite of the dire forecasts, there have been some positives. Vanderbilt School of Nursing reported that between 2001 and 2002 there was an increase in the numbers of registered nurses younger than age 35, and for the first time the number of men in the nursing workforce has increased to 9%. In West Virginia, a consortium of health care organizations and colleges within 11 counties created a teaching mechanism to promote nursing as a career. The 11 counties now have a surplus of nurses and expect that this will continue for the next few years.

In today's market-driven reform of all health care jobs, the recent graduate must use a variety of strategies to maintain employability. A well-known consultant with expertise in corporate transitions and job markets has identified three characteristics that an individual needs for future job security in any area: employability, vendor-mindedness, and resiliency (Bridges, 1994). Employability is the skills and knowledge that the nurse brings to the health care agency. The nurse's knowledge and abilities that enhance quality patient outcomes can translate into dollar savings for the institution. Vendor-mindedness means that the nurse needs to ask, "What can I offer as a professional that would make the employer want my specific qualities and flexibility as an individual?"

Resiliency describes the professional's ability to blend into system needs in a chaotic time of health care change. The nurse who is shifted from the charge nurse position to staff level needs to keep a positive attitude within the job arena. Nurses need to promote job security within the system by adding new skills and abilities that help them maintain viability as professionals—perhaps cross-training to the emergency room or perinatal areas of the hospital or strengthening clinical skills through an added certification credential of management. The clinical role is demanding more delegation skills and fewer clinical skills with the influx of health care workers and the advent of working for several institutions rather than just one system (contract work).

Although there is a definite shortage, health care institutions continue to expect new graduates to have a current knowledge base with critical-thinking abilities. As Leah Curtin (1995) so succinctly stated, "Job security is not found in the job but rather in the person who holds the job..." Nursing is a career, and nurses must take charge of their professional futures.

WHAT ABOUT ADVANCED-PRACTICE NURSING?

A University of Colorado nursing professor, Dr. Loretta Ford, founded the first nurse practitioner (NP) program in 1965. As early as the mid-1960s, Dr. Ford believed that the NP would evolve from the graduate setting. There are more than 150 programs that educate NPs in a variety of clinical tracks, and more than 1000 publications address the role of the nurse practitioner (Watson, 1995). Advanced practice has since greatly diversified, with a variety of clinical roles, methods of educational preparation, and scopes of clinical practice, with more than 7.3% of today's registered nurses having advanced-practice credentials (HRSA, 2002). As master's degree programs proliferated in the 1970s with government funding, the clinical nurse specialist (CNS) emerged from university settings. The CNS had a focus area that was equated with graduate education. Ford, in 1965, had envisioned that the NP would evolve from graduate settings.

Historically, NPs were able to enter the practice field in a variety of ways, as defined by the scope of their practice rather than their educational credentials. The scope of practice was defined by the board of nursing of the state in which the person was licensed as an RN. Thus, historically, a nurse could become an NP through a certificate program or other non–master's degree program. In 1987 the ANA, in its *Scope of Nursing* document, addressed the differences between the generalist and the specialist, making the distinction that the specialist has a graduate degree (ANA, 1987). Nurse practitioner programs have become integral parts of master's and even post-master's programs.

All types of advanced-practice nurse (APN) roles are responding to the changes in the health care arena. The need to redefine and clarify the terms and roles of professional nursing has never been more pressing, not only for the profession, but for the public. The movement toward a consensus on the definitions and the roles in advanced-practice nursing is occurring. Table 9-1 summarizes the terms and information regarding advanced-practice roles. As nursing struggles to develop this consensus, the issues of educational preparation and certification continue to challenge the profession. State boards of nursing reflect great variability in credentialing and advanced-practice roles in the legal language of scope of practice. For example, one of the oldest credentialed professional groups, nurse anesthetists, used certification—not education—to enter their professional specialty in 1952. Today, nurse anesthetists obtain certification at the graduate or the postgraduate level for entry into practice.

As a recent graduate you may want to explore the option of advanced-practice nursing as part of your long-term career goals. Both the NLN and the ANA have publications and videos about advanced-practice nursing. Check their websites for up-to-date information that may help you include specialty practice in the design of your 5-year career plan. In addition, reading about career roles for advanced practice and talking with APNs in your work sites can help you expand your career vision and plan for the future.

CONCLUSION

Nursing over the past century has portrayed many images—from the "angel of mercy" to Sairy Gamp, who was all things unprofessional. The nurse then moved from the heroine of the war years to the sex object. How will we reshape the image of nursing for the future? What are the ways in which nursing will be ready to meet the challenges of the changing health care environment?

The questions can go on and on, but the answers to these questions will have to come from nurses in practice, education, and research in a collective fashion. The issues, which have a significant impact on nursing's professional image, must be resolved so that nursing can move forward. As a recent graduate, you will be a part of this exciting transition as nursing takes control and directs the course of its future.

Why, then the world's mine oyster, which I with sword will open.
Merry Wives of Windsor—Shakespeare

TABLE 9-1

Advanced-Practice Nursing

	Education	What They Do
Nurse practitioner (NP)	Most of the approximately 150 NP education programs in the United States today confer a master's degree. At least 36 states require NPs to be nationally certified by the ANA or a specialty nursing organization. In March 2000, almost 45% of advanced-practice nurses were NPs.	Working in clinics, nursing homes, hospitals, or their own offices, NPs are qualified to handle a wide range of basic health problems. Most have a specialty—for example, adult, family, or pediatric health care. NPs conduct physical examinations, take medical histories, diagnose and treat common acute minor illnesses or injuries, order and interpret laboratory tests and radiographs, and counsel and educate patients. In all states they may prescribe medication according to state law. Some work as independent practitioners and can be reimbursed by Medicare or Medicaid for services rendered. Others work for hospitals, HMOs, or private industry.
Certified Nurse-Midwife (CNM)	An average 1.5 years of specialized education beyond nursing school, either in an accredited certificate program or, like NPs, increasingly at the master's level.	CNMs provide well-woman gynecologic and low-risk obstetric care including prenatal, labor and delivery, and postpartum care. In 1998, the most current year data are available from the National Center for Health Statistics, there were 277,811 CNM-attended births in the United States. This accounted for 9% of all vaginal births that year. The number of CNM-attended births has increased every year since 1975. An ANA meta-analysis of CNM care found that nurse-midwives performed fewer fetal monitors, episiotomies, and forceps deliveries; administered fewer intravenous solutions; delivered fewer low–birth-weight and premature infants; and had shorter patient hospital stays. CNMs have prescriptive authority in all 50 states.

Continued

TABLE 9-1

Advanced-Practice Nursing—cont'd

	Education	What They Do
Clinical Nurse Specialist (CNS)	CNSs are the second-largest advanced-practice group. They are registered nurses with advanced nursing degrees—master's or doctoral—who are experts in a specialized area of clinical practice such as mental health, gerontology, cardiac or cancer care, or community or neonatal health. In 1998, it is estimated that there were 61,601 RNs prepared to practice as CNSs, including 7802 who were also licensed as NPs. Almost 91% of the 53,799 who were licensed solely as CNSs were employed in a nursing position; however, only 23% were practicing in a position with the title of CNS. Twenty-five percent were employed in nursing-education positions. Only 31% maintained national certification or state recognition, or both, as an advanced-practice nurse or CNS. In March 2000, almost 30% of advanced-practice nurses were CNSs.	CNSs work in hospitals, clinics, nursing homes, their own offices, and other community-based settings, such as industry, home care, and HMOs. Qualified to handle a wide range of physical and mental health problems, CNSs provide primary care and psychotherapy. They conduct health assessments, make diagnoses, deliver treatment, and develop quality-control methods. In addition to delivering direct patient care, CNSs work in consultation, research, education, and administration. Some work independently or in private practice and can be reimbursed by Medicare, Medicaid, Champus, and private insurers.
Certified Registered Nurse Anesthetist (CRNA)	CRNAs are registered nurses who complete a graduate program and meet national certification and recertification requirements.	In this oldest of the advanced nursing specialties, CRNAs administer approximately 65% of the 26 million anesthetics given to patients each year in the United States. As of October 2001, CRNAs were the sole anesthesia providers in nearly 50% of all hospitals and more than 65% of rural hospitals in the United States, enabling these health care facilities to provide obstetric, surgical, and trauma stabilization services. CRNAs provide anesthetics to patients in collaboration with surgeons, anesthesiologists, dentists, podiatrists, and other qualified health care professionals.

REFERENCES

American Nurses Association: *The study of credentialing in nursing: a new approach*, vol 1-2: Report of the committee, Kansas City, MO, 1978-1979, ANA.

American Nurses Association: *The scope of nursing*, Kansas City, Mo, 1987, ANA.

American Nurses Association: *Social policy statement*, Kansas City, Mo, 1988, ANA.

American Nurses Association: *The career credentials: professional certification: the 1990 certification catalog*, Kansas City, Mo, 1990, Center for Credentialing Services.

American Nurses Association: *Standards of clinical nursing practice*, Kansas City, Mo, 1991, ANA.

American Nurses Credentialing Center: *2003 Certification catalog*, Washington, DC, 2003, ANCC.

Bridges W: *Job shifts: how to prosper in a workplace without jobs*, New York, 1994, Addison-Wesley.

Buerhaus P: It starts with you, *Nurseweek*, November 28, 2001, *www.nurseweek.com/news/features/01-11/genrn_2.html.*

Center for Nursing Advocacy. *Fictional portrayals of nurses: original research*, February 2005, *www.nursingadvocacy.org/research/fict_original.html.*

Caplow T: *The sociology of work*, Minneapolis, 1954, University of Minnesota.

Curtin L: Job Security: Is nothing sacred anymore?, *Nurs Manage* 26(7):7-9, 1995.

Dombeck M: Work narratives: Gender and race in professional personhood. *Res Nurs Health* 26:351-365, 2003.

Dukes ME: Writer hopes to change nurses image, *Stripe*, May 9, 2003, *www.dcmilitary.com/army/stripe/8_18/local_news/23071-1.html.*

Health Resources and Services Administration: *National sample survey of registered nurses*, Washington, DC, 2002, HRSA, Bureau of Health Professions, Division of Nursing, *http://bhpr.hrsa.gov/healthworkforce/reports/rnsurvey/default.htm.*

Kaplan M: Speech: why isn't nursing more newsworthy?, *Medscape Nursing*, January 2005, *www.medscape.com.*

Kimball B: Health care's human crisis. *Online J Issues in Nurs* 9(2), 2004, *www.medscape.com/viewarticle/490771.*

Kirschling J, Ryan S: *The Woodhull Study on Nursing and the Media: healthcare's invisible partner. Summary findings*, Indianapolis, 1997, Sigma Theta Tau.

McCabe S: Recruiting the 21st century nurse: getting to the heart of the matter, *Tennessee Nurse* 65(3): 10-18, 2002.

Miller N: Leadership roundtable. *Nurs Econ* 18(2): 91-94, 2000.

Naisbitt J, Adurdene P: *Megatrends 2000*, New York, 1990, William Morrow.

Nardini J: Certification and credentialing—what does it mean to the patient?, *Nephrol Nurs J* 27(5), 457-459, 2000.

National League for Nursing: *NLN updates*, New York, 1995, NLN.

Pavalko R: *Sociology of occupations and professions*, Itasca, Il, 1971, Peacock.

Peplau H: *Interpersonal relationships in nursing*, New York, 1952, Putnam Press.

Smith J, Crawford L: *2002 RN practice analysis*, Chicago, 2003, National Council of State Boards of Nursing.

Strauss A: *The Structure and Ideology of American Nursing: An Interpretation in the Nursing Profession.* New York, 1966, Wiley.

Talotta D: Role conceptions and professional role discrepancy among baccalaureate nursing students, *Image J Nurs Sch* 22(2):111-115, 1990.

The in/visibility of nurses in cyberculture, March 2005, *www.nursing-informatics.com/visiblenurse7.html.*

Ward C, Styles I, Bosco A: Perceived states of nurses compared to other health care professionals, *Contemporary Nurse* 15(1/2):20-24, August 2003, *www.contemporarynurse.com/15-1p20.htm.*

Watson J: Advanced nursing practice and what might be, *J Nurs Health Care* 16(2):78-83, 1995.

UNIT IV

NURSING MANAGEMENT

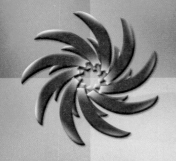

CHAPTER 10

Challenges of Nursing Management

JOANN WILCOX, MSN, RN

Leaders don't force people to follow—they invite them on a journey.

—*Charles S. Lauer*

Outstanding leaders go out of their way to boost the self-esteem of their personnel. If people believe in themselves, it's amazing what they can accomplish.

—*Sam Walton*

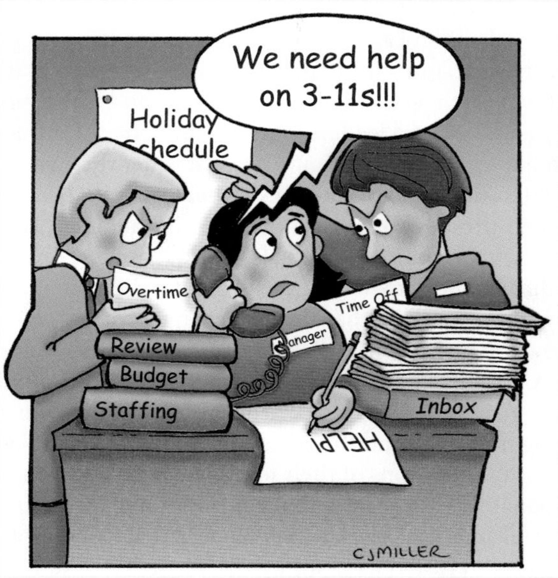

Nursing management can be challenging.

After completing this chapter, you should be able to:

- Differentiate between management and leadership.
- Describe various types of management.
- List characteristics of a good leader.
- Compare various leadership styles.
- Identify characteristics of today's workforce.
- Distinguish between power and authority.
- Apply problem-solving strategies to clinical management situations.
- Identify work characteristics of future generations.
- Identify the characteristics of effective work groups.
- Discuss the change process.

As you get closer to meeting your goal of becoming a graduate nurse, consideration should be given to understanding the role of the nurse as a leader and manager. You might be thinking:

I don't want to be a manager, I'm a recent graduate!
OR
I want to take care of patients, not be a paper pusher!

Consider this: Nursing, in any role, is a *people business*. *Management* is the process of effectively working with people. When you accept your first position as a graduate nurse, you must realize that you are entering a work group where members spend at least one third of the day interacting with each other. Nurses must use interpersonal, leadership, and management skills to be effective in their roles.

Management requires different levels of functioning depending on the role of the individual nurse. For instance, as a recent graduate, you will have primary management responsibility for the patients to whom you are assigned to provide care. This may include planning and coordinating the care with other nursing personnel, such as nursing assistants. It may also require working with other members of the health team to meet patient needs. With more experience, you may become a team leader or charge nurse with responsibility for managing a group of staff members who provide care for a larger number of patients, perhaps even an entire unit.

MANAGEMENT VERSUS LEADERSHIP

WHAT IS THE DIFFERENCE BETWEEN MANAGEMENT AND LEADERSHIP?

Although the terms *management* and *leadership* are frequently interchanged, they do not have the same meaning. A leader selects and assumes the role; a manager is assigned or appointed to the role. Managers have responsibility for organizational goals and the performance of organizational tasks such as budget preparation and scheduling. Although it is desirable for managers to be good leaders and to be effective at influencing others, there are leaders who are not managers and, more frequently, managers who are not leaders! So, let us discuss the actual differences in more detail.

Management is a problem-oriented process with similarities to the nursing process. Management is needed whenever two or more individuals work together toward a common goal. The manager coordinates the activities of the group to maintain balance and direction. There are generally four functions that the manager performs: *planning* (what is to be done), *organizing* (how it is to be done), *directing* (who is to do it), and *controlling* (when and how it is done). All of these activities go on continuously and simultaneously, with the percentage of time spent on each varying with the level of the manager, the characteristics of the group being managed, and the nature of the problem and goal.

Managers must be attentive to both dimensions of their job: the mission and goals of the organization and the interpersonal relationships among the staff and between the staff and the manager. The successful manager is one who respects the people of the organization as individuals and who is interested in ensuring the work is well done.

Leadership, in contrast, is a way of behaving; it is the ability to cause others to respond, not because they have to, but because they want to. Leadership is needed as much as management for effective group functioning, but each differs. The manager determines the agenda, sets time limits, and facilitates group functioning. The leader focuses a group's efforts on identifying goals and carrying out the activities needed to reach those goals.

Florence Nightingale was an early nursing leader. What characteristics of a manager did she also demonstrate?

WHAT IS MEANT BY MANAGEMENT STYLE?

There are a variety of different management styles that you will experience in your nursing practice. These styles are a continuum between *autocratic* and *laissez-faire* styles (Figure 10-1).

The *autocratic manager* uses an authoritarian approach to direct the activities of others. This individual makes most of the decisions alone without input from other staff members. Under this style of management, the emphasis is on the tasks to be done, with less focus on the individual staff members who perform the tasks. The autocratic manager may be most effective in crisis situations when structure and control are critical to success, as, for instance, during a cardiac arrest or code situation.

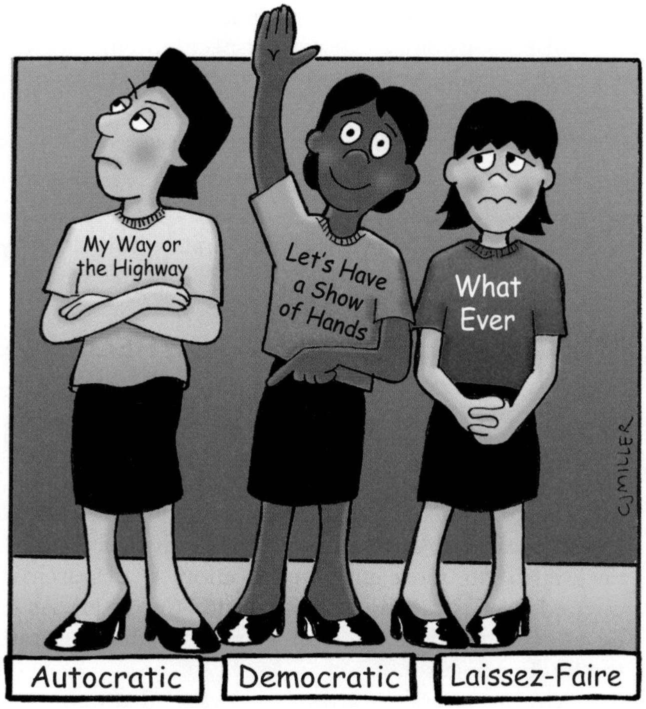
My Way or the Highway
Let's Have a Show of Hands
What Ever
CJMILLER
Autocratic
Democratic
Laissez-Faire

FIGURE 10-1
Management styles.

On the other end of the continuum is the *laissez-faire manager* who maintains a permissive climate with little direction or control exerted. This manager allows staff members to make and implement decisions independently and relinquishes most of his/her power and responsibility to them. Although this style of management may function effectively in highly motivated groups, it may not be effective in a bureaucratic health care setting that requires many different individuals and groups to interact.

In the middle of the continuum is the *democratic manager*. This individual is people-oriented and emphasizes effective group functioning. The goals of the group are identified, and the manager is perceived as a group member who is its organizer and who keeps it moving in the defined direction. The environment is open, and communication flows both ways. The democratic manager encourages participation in decision making; he or she recognizes, however, that there are situations in which such participation may not be appropriate and is willing to assume responsibility for a decision when it is necessary.

As you can see, the continuum of management styles includes approaches ranging from almost total control to almost complete freedom for subordinates. Behaviors vary from telling others what to do to delegating authority for meeting objectives to the work group. In choosing a management style, the manager must decide between control and freedom and determine which trade-offs are acceptable in a particular situation.

An example of an action a democratic manager might take is to create a Nurse Practice Committee on his/her unit. This committee would have some defined authority and responsibility to address specific items in the practice environment such as schedules, practices on the unit, and the purchase of supplies under a specific dollar limit. This type of committee supports the fact that staff and management are interdependent in governing the successful practice environment (Tonges, Baloga-Altieri, & Atzori, 2004)

Look at managers on your clinical units—how do they fit into these categories?

WHAT ARE THE CHARACTERISTICS AND THEORIES OF LEADERSHIP?

The many attempts to define what makes a good leader have resulted in a variety of concepts and proposals. Researchers have tried to identify the characteristics or traits necessary to be a good leader. Several of these studies defined the concept of a *born leader*, implying that the desired traits are inherited. With later research, it became clear that desired leadership traits could be learned through education and experience. It also became clear that the most effective leadership style for one situation was not necessarily the most effective for another. Research indicated that the effectiveness of the leader is influenced by the situation itself. As leadership theories continue to develop, emphasis is more on what the leader does rather than focusing on the traits the leader possesses.

There are several theories of leadership that we should discuss. The first is *contingency leadership*, which says leadership should be flexible enough to address varying situations. Although this may sound complicated, it can be compared with your approach to patient care. As a nurse, you individualize a patient care plan on the basis of the needs of a particular patient. Then you implement the plan using available resources. The effective leader, using contingency leadership, brings the same flexible approach to each situation where leadership is required.

Interactional leadership is the next type of leadership to consider. With interactional leadership, the focus is on the development of trust in the relationship (Marquis & Huston, 2003). This leader is high in both *job-centered behavior* and *employee-centered behavior* and is equally concerned for the needs and feelings of the employee and the effective and efficient completion of the job. This individual uses democratic concepts in management and views the tasks to be accomplished from the standpoint of a team member.

Other leaders may be high in either job-centered behavior or employee-centered behavior and low in the other aspect of the leadership role. A leader who uses the autocratic style of management, for example, would probably be high in job-centered behavior and lower in employee-centered behavior. At the other extreme would be the individual who has little concern for either the employee or the task to be accomplished. This individual could be expected to approach management with a laissez-faire attitude and may not be considered to be an effective leader.

Finally, leadership can also be described as *transactional* or *transformational*. The transactional/transformational leader is one who has a greater focus on vision, defined as the ability to envision some future state and describe it to others so they can begin to share that vision.

Let us look at the following few examples:

Tom is a high employee-centered and high job-centered democratic manager who could be considered an interactional leader. He is a person who is equally concerned about the employee as a person as well as getting the job done efficiently and effectively and is flexible enough to vary the emphasis on the employee or the job based on the situation to be addressed.

Another type of leader is Jean, who is high job-centered and low employee-centered. She is a person who focuses on the job to be done with less focus on the needs or feelings of her employees. A great deal of work is accomplished with her autocratic style of management.

Randy, in contrast, demonstrates a high interest in his employees and in their needs more than getting the job done. He is a high employee-centered and low job-centered leader.

Laura, the individual with laissez-faire behaviors, is the kind of person who just does not seem to demonstrate interest in either her employee's needs and feelings or the need to get the job done. She would be considered a low employee-centered and low job-centered, neither of which is indicative of an effective leader.

One would anticipate the Chief Executive Officer and the Chief Nurse Executive in the hospital where you work would both be transformational leaders. It is their responsibility to see the bigger picture and to be able to describe that vision or picture to others. Porter-O'Grady (2003b) describes this as the leader who can "stand on the balcony." From this position, the leader can monitor the ebb and flow of the organization and determine which direction the organization is moving. Seeing the big picture and communicating this vision are needed for a leader to be effective, because it helps to have a vision that can be put into words for others to understand.

Although most agree that every individual leans toward one of these styles, it has been found that fluctuations from one to another can occur depending on the

CRITICAL THINKING BOX 10-1

Consider your educational and clinical experiences. What leadership qualities have you observed? What management characteristics have you observed? Are there specific personality traits that enhance a person's performance of these two roles?

particular situation. In the health care setting, good leaders carefully balance job-centered and employee-centered behaviors to meet both staff and patient needs effectively (Critical Thinking Box 10-1).

A good leader works toward established goals and has a sense of purpose and direction. A good leader must also be aware of how her/his behavior impacts the workplace. Emotions, moods, and patterns of behavior displayed by the leader will create a lasting impression on the behavior of the team involved. It is critical for the leader to be aware of this impact if she/he is going to be effective in managing and leading a team (Porter-O'Grady, 2003a). Rather than push staff members off in many directions, this leader uses personal attributes to organize the activities and pull the staff toward the goals.

Remember, it is easier to pull than to push!

Let us take a moment now to summarize the main concepts of leadership that we have discussed.

- Leadership can be learned.
- Leaders are developers of people.
- A person's style of leadership is dependent on that individual's basic personality and the particular situation in which he or she is functioning.
- The demands of the situation in which a leader is to function influence the qualities, characteristics, knowledge, and skills necessary for successful leadership.
- The degree to which the leader is knowledgeable and competent directly influences the subordinates' feelings of security and their ability to cooperate to meet goals.

THE TWENTY FIRST CENTURY: A DIFFERENT AGE FOR MANAGEMENT AND FOR LEADERSHIP

The face of leadership is changing, and that is very evident in nursing and health care. A major problem in nursing is the continuation of doing the same activities when the demand is changing. The change in health care is altering some of the foundations of nursing practice. The short stay and emerging therapeutics require less clinical time and challenge the need for specific nursing interventions. Nurses are becoming increasingly frustrated with the reality that the nursing care they were taught to provide and they feel they need to do is not possible due to the decreased time spent with the patients (Porter-O'Grady, 2003b). This dissatisfaction may be compounded even more by the characteristics of the upcoming generations, especially if we do not learn how to bridge the gaps in working and managing others from different generations.

"For the first time in decades, there are four separate and distinct generations potentially working together in a stressful and competitive nursing workplace." (Boychuk-Duchscher & Cowin, 2004, p. 493)

The leadership of health care in the twenty-first century is impacted by the diverse generations in today's workplace: the Silent or Veteran Generation (born between 1925 and 1942—account for 10% of the current workforce); the Baby Boomers (born between 1943 and 1960—account for 45% of the current workforce); Generation X (born between 1961 and 1977—account for 30% of the current workforce); and the newest group to the job market, Generation Y (born between 1978 and 1995—account for 10% of the workforce). There are major differences in these groups —in communication styles, what motivates them, what turns them off, and their workplace ideals (Martin, 2004, p. 62; Boychuk-Duchscher & Cowin, 2004).

WHO ARE THE SILENT OR VETERANS?

This retiring group of nurses, as well as the oldest generation were taught to rely on tried, true, and tested ways of doing things. This group's early experience with economic hardship and their witness to the Great Depression of the 1920s and 1930s, World War II destruction and genocide, the eradication of polio, and the control of other diseases (e.g., tuberculosis, whooping cough) via the development of antibiotics and immunizations, place value on loyalty, discipline, teamwork, and respect for authority (Boychuk-Duchscher & Cowin, 2004, p. 494).

WHO ARE THE BABY BOOMERS?

The Baby Boomers make up the largest group of nurse employees working today, with the majority of management positions filled by the Baby Boomers. This group has a multitude of family responsibilities, frequently spanning three generations—they have their own children and they are caring for aging parents. This group is frequently referred to as the "sandwich generation"—they are caught between caring for their own children as well as caring for their aging parents. This group is very ambitious. They put in long hours and have a strong sense of idealism, both in family and in work. The Baby Boomers value what others think, and it is important that their achievements be recognized. The Baby Boomers have set and maintained a grueling pace between their family and employment responsibilities. This group has embraced technology as a method for being more productive and to have more free time (Cordeniz, 2003).

WHO IS GENERATION X?

The Generation X group grew up in the information age. They are an energetic and innovative generation. They are hard workers, but unlike the Baby Boomers, the Generation X employees have little loyalty or confidence in leaders and institutions. They change jobs frequently and will stay in a position as long as it is good for them. Their independence and reliance grew out of their childhood experiences of being alone, as both Baby Boomer parents worked. "Latch-key" generation is another term used to describe this group. They have no aspirations for retirement. The use of technology has initiated an expectation of instant response and satisfaction. Their learning style has been shaped by technology—they want immediate answers from a variety of sources. They want different employment standards—they want opportunities for self-building and responsibility for work outcomes. They want extensive learning and precepting, and they want their questions answered immediately. They value their free time; therefore, flexible scheduling and benefits (daycare centers, liberal vacations, working from home) are important. They claim to be motivated by work that agrees with their values and demands (Cordeniz, 2003).

WHO IS GENERATION Y?

Generation Y, also known as Generation "Net," Nexter, or the Millennium Generation was born between 1978 and 1995. They are the largest group, perhaps three times the size of Generation X. They are going to have a formidable impact on the employment market. Many of them are still children, but there are a large number of them that are adolescent. Those in their early 20s are entering the job market now. This generation represents a large number of the children of the Baby Boomers. While the Baby Boomers were and are still trying to master Windows, these kids are playing with computers in day care centers!

The impact of this generation remains to be seen, but the research has several predictions. This generation is smart and believe education is the key to success, diversity is a given, technology is as transparent as air, and social responsibility is a business imperative (Martin, 2004). They are optimistic, and they are interactive. Traits in this group include individuality and uniqueness. They can multitask, think fast, as well as being extremely creative. Managing this group will require a totally different set of skills than what is in the market today. They are not team players. They are in the driver's seat, and work for them is there if they want it. Focusing on understanding their capabilities, treating them as colleagues, and putting them in roles to push their limits will help the manager to recognize the potential of this group to become the highest-producing workforce in history (Martin, 2004).

The challenge to nursing will be to develop a workplace as well as a profession that will be attractive to all three generations who represent the mainstream of the workforce. Initially, there must be a focus on recruiting the younger generations into the health care fields, and specifically into nursing. There must also be an emphasis on retention of experienced nurses. They are necessary to mentor the younger generations, and their experience is invaluable. Eric Chester works with young people and has outlined strategies for managing and motivating the younger generation (Box 10-1). Review these strategies; they are not new. These strategies work well for every generation as well as every organization at any time (Critical Thinking Box 10-2) (Verret, 2000).

CRITICAL THINKING BOX 10-2

What generation do you belong to? How do your work values and personal characteristics fit that generation?

BOX 10-1 Motivational Strategies for Generation X and Y

1. **Let them know that what they do matters.**
   When was the last time a letter from a patient that was very pleased with the care on a unit was shared with the staff? When was the last time management sat down with all of the unit personnel to tell them what a good job they are doing? When was the last time the Chief Executive Office complimented the staff on a job well done?
2. **Tell them the truth.**
   When did the managers on a unit acknowledge to the staff exactly what was going on? For example, the surgery schedule is going to be heavy this next week, there are going to be a lot of new admissions as well as a lot of patients that will be going home. Acknowledge that the work level is going to increase, and see if any of the staff have suggestions for improving the coordination and workload assignments.
3. **Explain why you are asking them to do it.**
   When a difficult time is anticipated, explain to the staff what is happening and why. Maybe a particular area of the hospital is overloaded and additional staff are being pulled from their regular units to help out. These patients must be accommodated and cared for—this is why the hospital is there, and maintaining patient census is what pays the bills.
4. **Learn their language.**
   When was the last time the unit manager, head nurse, or other manager actually sat down with the staff (all levels) to find out who they are and what they like to do? What are their priorities, family situations, what do they do on their days off?
5. **Be on the look out for rewarding opportunities.**
   When did a staff member handle a particular difficult patient situation very well and the staff member was acknowledged at that time? Give positive feedback when opportunities arise, do not wait for a performance evaluation to do so.
6. **Praise them in front of their peers and other staff.**
   Acknowledge a job well done at a staff meeting, or in the presence of people who are important to that person.
7. **Make the workplace fun.**
   Making the hospital work environment fun can sometimes be a little difficult, but there are opportunities for humor if we just look for them. Clients share a lot of humor with the staff, is the staff encouraged to share that with the rest of the unit personnel? When something funny happens to staff, are they encouraged to laugh and share with others?
8. **Model behavior.**
   Does the behavior of the unit manager or head nurse model the behavior they are expecting others to exhibit? What about confidentiality—it is expected of the personnel, does the manager practice it as well?
9. **Give them the tools to do the job.**
   What about effective communication skills, or perhaps good customer service skills—the health care industry is in the job of providing a service for the customer—the client. Training is offered for the technical skills—new equipment, procedures, policies, but what about training for the skills necessary in dealing with people? How about skills to deal effectively with the angry patient, the difficult doctor, the outraged family? (Verret, 2000)

These strategies are from Eric Chester, as presented by Carol Verret in her article, "Generation Y: Motivating and Training a New Generation of Employees."

Data taken from Verret C: Generation Y: motivating and training a new generation of employees. *In Ideas and trends: hotel online*, November 2000, *www.hotel-online.com/Trends/CarolVerret/GenerationY_Nov2000.html*.

POWER AND AUTHORITY IN NURSING MANAGEMENT

DO YOU KNOW THE DIFFERENCE BETWEEN POWER AND AUTHORITY?

Power is having the ability to effect change and influence others to meet identified goals. Authority relates to a specific position and the responsibility associated with that position. The individual with authority has the right to act in situations for which one is held responsible within the institutional hierarchy.

Today there is much discussion in nursing about the importance of power and the concept of *empowerment.* To *empower* nurses is to provide them with greater influence and decision making in their roles. The realization of greater power in the profession depends on the willingness of administrators to allocate this power and of nurses to accept it, along with the accompanying responsibility.

Remember, power and responsibility always go hand in hand!

WHAT ARE THE DIFFERENT TYPES OF POWER?

There are many different types of power, so let us discuss those that are most common. *Legitimate power* is power connected to a position of authority. The individual has power as a result of the position. The head nurse has legitimate power and authority as a result of the position.

Reward power is closely linked with legitimate power in that it comes about because the individual has the power to provide or withhold rewards. If supervisors have the power to authorize salary increases or scheduling changes, then they have reward power. Coercive power is power derived from fear of consequences. It is easy to see how parents would have coercive power over children on the basis of the threat of punishment. This type of power can also be used against staff members when, for example, there is the threat of receiving unfavorable assignments. However, in considering the characteristics of the upcoming generations, this may not be effective with them.

Expert power is based on specialized knowledge, skills, or abilities that are recognized and respected by others. The individual is perceived as an expert in an area and has power in that area because of this expertise. For instance, the enterostomal therapist has expertise in the care of individuals who have had ostomies. Therefore, staff nurses seek out the therapist as a resource and use the expert's knowledge to guide the care of these patients.

Referent power is power a person has because others closely identify with that person's personal characteristics; they are liked and admired by others. Individuals who have knowledge that is needed by others to function effectively in their roles possess information power. This type of power is, perhaps, the most abused! An individual may, for example, withhold information from subordinates to maintain control. The leader who gives directions without providing needed information on rationale or constraints is abusing information power.

Leaders and managers need to understand the concept of power and how it can be used and abused in working with others. Nurses, on the whole, need to identify ways to increase their power within the health team. Graduate nurses need to be aware of and willing to implement methods and resources to increase their personal power. As they gain experience in the staff nurse role, they can develop expert power by increasing competency in their roles and clinical skills.

Refining interpersonal skills that enhance the ability to work with others can expand many types of power, such as information and referent power. These skills include communicating clearly and completely what people need to know and delegating tasks to those who know how to accomplish them. Demonstrating a willingness to give and receive feedback and being positive in communicating are also important. All of these are ways that can help individuals develop and enhance power in working with others.

It is also important to recognize what detracts from power. Impressing others as disorganized, either in personal appearance or in work habits, engaging in petty criticism or gossip, and being unable to say *no* without qualification are some of the behaviors that can detract from power.

MANAGEMENT PROBLEM SOLVING

HOW ARE PROBLEM-SOLVING STRATEGIES USED IN MANAGEMENT?

Management is a *problem-oriented* process. The effective manager analyzes problems and makes decisions throughout all the planning, organizing, directing, and controlling functions of management. Problem solving can be readily compared with the nursing process (Table 10-1). This is because the nursing process is based on the scientific method of problem solving. The two are essentially the same, as can be seen by comparing the steps of one to the other.

As with the nursing process, problem solving does not always flow in an orderly manner from one step to the next. Throughout the process, feedback is sought, which may indicate a need for altering the plan to reach the desired objective. The most critical step in either process is identifying the problem (identified as the *nursing diagnosis* in the nursing process). Frequently what was originally identified as *the problem*

TABLE 10-1

Nursing Process vs. Problem Solving

Nursing Process	Problem Solving
Assessment	Data gathering
Analysis/nursing diagnosis	Definition of the problem
Development of plan	Identification of alternative solutions
Implementation of plan	Implementation of plan
Evaluation/assessment	Evaluation of solution

may be too broad or unclear. Only the symptoms of the problem may be seen initially, or there may be several problems overlapping. If an approach is used to relieve only the symptoms, the problem will still exist. The good manager will guide the process of identifying the problem by asking questions such as "What is happening?" "What is being done about it?" "Who is doing what?" and "Why?" It is important to differentiate among facts and opinions and to attempt to break down the information to its simplest terms. Think of it as being a detective looking for every clue!

Once the problem is clearly identified, the group should *brainstorm* all possible solutions. Often the first few alternatives are not the best or most practical. Identifying a number of viable alternatives usually provides more flexibility and creativity. All possible solutions must fall within existing constraints, such as staff abilities, available resources, and institutional policies. The more complex the problem, the more judgment is required. In some cases the problem may extend beyond the manager's scope of responsibility and authority, and, therefore, it may be necessary to seek outside help.

After identifying all the alternatives, each must be evaluated in relation to changes that would be required in existing policies, procedures, staffing, and so forth, and what effect these changes would have. Ask "What would happen if . . ." questions to clarify the short- and long-term implications of each alternative. Always keep in mind that the perfect solution is not possible in most situations.

Problem solving represents a choice made between possible alternatives that are thought to be the best solution for a particular situation. At its best, problem solving should involve ample discussion of the possible solutions by those who are affected by the situation and who possess the knowledge and power to support the possible solution. Once an alternative has been selected, it should be implemented unless new data or perspectives warrant a change. Feedback should be sought continuously to provide ongoing evaluation of the effectiveness of the solution. Remember that simply choosing the best alternative does not automatically ensure its acceptance by those who work with it!

Frequently, implementing the solution to a problem causes several other problems to arise. This can be avoided if the selected solutions are tested before implementation to identify any areas that may be negatively impacted by the new solution. Many of you will be given the opportunity to work with others to complete an analysis of new procedures, for example, before that new procedure is fully implemented. If problems arise after the analysis, testing, and implementation, the new problems should not be allowed to impede the implementation process. Instead, pause and consider each problem individually, solve it, and then return to the plan that was tested. After a period of trial, an evaluation should be completed to determine the progress made. A complete solution may not have been reached, but some progress should have been made. If not, a slight modification in the approach or a completely new alternative may be needed. The old adage—*if at first you don't succeed, try, try again*—is most appropriate when applying the problem-solving process! Remain positive, confident, and flexible! Eventually, a possible solution will work! Let us apply the process to an actual problem.

John is the head nurse on a busy medical-surgical unit with 32 patients. Staff members have complained to him that too much time is being spent during morning change-of-shift report. After asking questions and seeking out additional information, John determines that a more clear definition of the problem is that the night charge nurse does not give a clear, concise report. Involving the night charge nurse in the problem-solving process helps to define the problem, because the nurse does not have adequate knowledge of how to give a change-of-shift report.

Can you see how, once the problem has been clarified, it becomes more amenable to an acceptable, and perhaps even easy, solution?

HOW DO WE RELATE PROBLEM SOLVING AND DECISION MAKING?

By definition, problem solving and decision making are almost the same process, with one very notable difference. Decision making requires the definition of a clear objective to guide the process. A comparison of the steps of each illustrates this difference (Table 10-2). Although both problem solving and decision making are usually initiated in the presence of a problem, the objective in decision making may not be to solve the problem, but only to deal with its results. It is also important to distinguish between a good decision and a good outcome. A *good outcome* is the objective that is desired, and a *good decision* is one made systematically to reach this objective. A good decision may or may not result in a good outcome. Although it is desirable to have both good decisions and good outcomes, the good decision-maker is willing to act, even at the risk of a negative outcome.

Susan is the evening charge nurse on a medical unit that has a total of 24 patients. One of the patients is terminally ill and seems to be having a particularly difficult evening. The patient requires basic comfort measures but little complex care. Susan has a choice of assigning the patient to another RN or delegating care to a nursing assistant. If she assigns the RN, the workload for the other staff will be heavier and she, herself, will be assigned to the terminally ill patients to provide the care that cannot be delegated to the nursing assistant. She decides to assign the RN, because this patient requires the emotional and physical support best provided by an RN. During the shift, the RN spends time sitting with the patient. Close to the end of the shift, the patient dies. Was this a good decision with a bad outcome or a good decision with a good outcome?

Decision making is values-based, and problem solving is a more scientific process. Nurses make decisions on the basis of personal values, life experiences, perceptions of the situation, knowledge of risks associated with possible decisions, and their individual ways of thinking. Because of these variables, it is possible, even probable, that two individuals given the same information and using the same decision-making process would arrive at different decisions.

In today's ever-changing health care environment, it is important for nurses and nurse managers to be effective in both problem solving and decision making. The good manager will evaluate the problem-solving or decision-making process on the basis of criteria that provide a view of the big picture. These criteria include the likely effects on the objective to be met, on the policies and resources of the organization, on the individuals involved, and on the product or service delivered.

TABLE 10-2

Problem Solving vs. Decision Making

Problem Solving	Decision Making
Define problem	Set objective
Identify alternative solutions	Identify and evaluate alternative decisions
Select solution and implement	Make decision and implement
Evaluate outcome	Evaluate outcome

The quality of patient care is dependent on the ability of the nurse to effectively combine problem solving with decision making. To do so, nurses must be attuned to their individual value systems and understand their effect on thinking and perceiving. The values associated with a particular situation will limit the alternatives generated and the final decision. For this reason, the fact that nurses typically work in groups is beneficial to the decision-making process. Although the process is the same, groups generally offer the benefits of a broader knowledge base for defining objectives and more creativity in identifying alternatives. The effectiveness of the group decision-making process is dependent on the dynamics of the group. It is, therefore, important for nurses to understand the roles of individuals within the group and the dynamics involved in working in groups to take full advantage of the group process. Chapter 11 focuses on communication, group process, and working with teams.

WHAT EFFECT DOES THE LEADER HAVE ON THE GROUP?

The leader's philosophy, personality, self-concept, and interpersonal skills all influence the functioning of the group. A leader is most effective if members are respected as individuals who have unique contributions to make to the group process. Can you remember our earlier discussion of the characteristics of a good leader? The ability to influence and motivate others is particularly important in the group process.

Whenever the combination of people in a group is altered, the dynamics are changed. If the group is in the working phase, it will revert to the initiating phase when a new person or persons are added and will remain there until they have been assimilated into the group and a new dynamic has been formulated. The most effective groups are those that have had consistent membership and are highly developed. These groups demonstrate friendly and trusting relationships; the ability to work toward goals of varying difficulty; flexible, stable, and reliable participation of members; and productivity, with high-quality output. Leadership within these groups is democratic, and the members feel positive about their participation and the outcomes of the group process. Now let us apply these principles to a real situation!

When you graduate and accept a nursing position, you will become a new nurse in the work group, causing it to regress to the initiating phase. You must demonstrate to the members of the group that you are worthy of being included in the group. If this is your first nursing position, you must also demonstrate to the group that you are worthy of entering the nursing profession. During this time, you should anticipate experiencing feelings of loneliness, isolation, and distance that accompany the initiating phase. Expect to feel as though you are being excluded, and understand that it is part of the process. Instead of focusing on these feelings, put your energy into forming supportive professional relationships, including the social aspects of these relationships. Seek and use feedback, and ask for help in areas that are not as familiar to you, such as priority setting. As you contribute your individual talents to the group, you will move from being a dependent new person to full group membership. It is important that you do not underestimate the length of time that may be needed to accomplish this task! Group processes proceed very slowly in most cases, and it may be 6 months or more before you are accepted as a full member of the work group. Do not be discouraged!

Remember that management skills come with experience in nursing, so do not be too hard on yourself during the transition phase. Identify nurse managers who have the skills you would like to incorporate into your management style. Look at the positive side of working for various nursing managers as a means to assist you in the development of your personal management style. Develop the ability to think like a nurse manager as you carry out your assignments—always look at the big picture.

THE CHALLENGE OF CHANGE

How many times have you heard staff nurses complain about how powerless they feel about the lack of control they have over their work environment? They state that they are frustrated that they cannot give the amount and quality of patient care that they desire and that staffing patterns are placing undue stress on them. Do they talk about leaving the acute-care environment and trying some other aspect of nursing (perhaps home health) as a less stressful option? Why do they run away from a situation, rather than thinking about how they can act to change it? Do they feel powerless to do so? Is it easier to withdraw and escape?

One thing we all know is that change is inevitable, particularly in today's health care delivery system. Economic factors have taken center stage, and cutbacks in all aspects of health care services are occurring. But change can be like a truck with no driver at the wheel: It moves slowly and steadily toward you (Figure 10-2). You have three options: You can move out of the situation and perhaps miss some opportunities; you

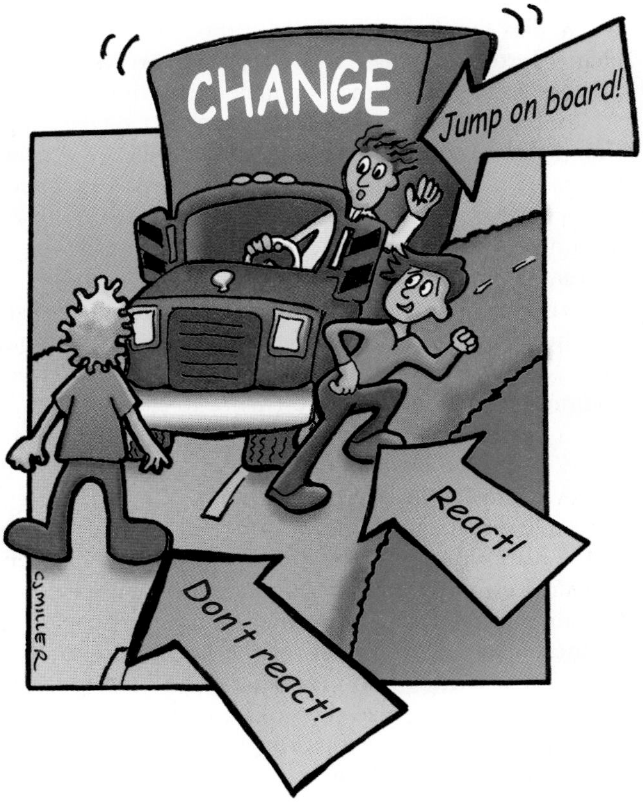

FIGURE 10-2
Change: react, do not react, or jump on board.

TABLE 10-3

Nursing Process vs. Problem Solving vs. Change Process

Nursing Process	Problem Solving	Change Process
Assessment	Data gathering	Recognition that a change is needed; collect data
Identification of possible nursing diagnoses	Definition of problem	Identification of problem to be solved
Selection of nursing diagnosis	Selection of one of possible alternatives	Selection of one of possible alternatives
Development of plan	Development of plan	Implementation of plan
Implementation of plan	Implementation of plan	Implementation of plan
Evaluation	Evaluation of solution	Evaluation of effects of change
Reassessment	Evaluation of solution	Stabilization of change in place

can just stand there and withdraw, doing what you are told to just to avoid conflict; or you can start to run with it, jump on, and try to steer it in a positive direction.

So, how do you begin to direct the *change truck*? The first thing to know about the change process is that it, too, has similarities to problem solving and the nursing process. Let us lay them out and compare the three processes (Table 10-3).

Look familiar? Maybe it is not that hard to take control and be a change agent! The first thing that you need to know about the change process is that resisting change is a natural response for most people. All of us are most comfortable in our state of equilibrium, where we feel in control of what we are doing. To deal effectively with change, it is important to understand that every change involves adaptation. It requires a period of transition in which the change can be understood, evaluated in light of its impact on the individual, and, one hopes, eventually be embraced.

There are various reasons why people resist change, and understanding them will help you to implement the change process more effectively. Following are the most common factors that cause resistance to change:

- A perceived threat to self in how the change will affect the individual personally
- A lack of understanding regarding the nature of the change
- A limited ability to emotionally cope with change
- A disagreement about the potential benefits of the change
- A fear of the impact of the change on self-confidence and self-esteem

Kurt Lewin sought to incorporate these concepts in his Change Theory. He identified three phases in an effective change process: *unfreezing*, *moving*, and *refreezing*. In the unfreezing phase, all of the factors that may cause resistance to change are considered. Others who may be affected by the change are sought out to determine whether they recognize that a change is needed and to determine their interest in participating in the process. You will need to determine whether the environment of the institution is receptive to change and then convince others to work with you.

The *moving* phase occurs once a group of individuals has been recruited to take on responsibilities for implementing the change. The group begins to sort out what must be done and the sequence of actions that would be most effective. They identify individuals who have the *power* to assist in making the plan succeed. *(What types of power would be most effective?)* They also attempt to identify strategies to overcome the natural resistance to change—how to effect a cooperative approach to implement the change. Once developed, the plan is then put into place.

The *refreezing* phase occurs when the plan is in place and everyone involved knows what is happening and what to expect. Publicizing the ongoing assessment of the pros and cons of the plan is an important part of its ultimate success. Be certain someone is responsible for continuing to work on the plan so it does not lose momentum. Finally, make the changes stick—or *refreeze*. This will make the change a part of everyday life and will no longer be perceived as something new. Now let us apply this process to a real situation!

> **Patti is working in a medical-surgical unit at a 200-bed acute-care hospital. She constantly hears her peers complaining about the lack of adequate nursing staff, and over the past 3 months, two full-time staff nurses have resigned. To cover the unit, part-time staff from temporary agencies and from the hospital staffing pool are being used to supplement the remaining regular staff. Because this staff has little orientation to the unit and is frequently assigned where they are needed the most, the continuity of care and a potential for increased errors in patient care became a major concern.**

Rather than continuing to complain about the situation or considering leaving it, Patti decided to act and try to steer the change truck. She approached a few of the nurses and initiated a discussion about the changes in staffing and how scheduling had become a nightmare for the charge nurse. She enlisted the support of several of the staff to begin problem solving possible solutions. They agreed that increased staffing was probably not a possible immediate solution and determined to work within the constraints that they had.

Several of the pool nurses were receptive to requesting that their assignment be limited to this one unit and agreed to schedule their hours to complement each other. This, in essence, would add a shared full-time position, at no additional cost, and would also provide consistency of patient care. When the proposal was presented to administration, they agreed to support the idea on the basis of its economic and patient-centered benefits.

The Change Truck—how will you respond?

React—move out of the way. Let the truck (change) pass you by. However, opportunities may be missed.

Do not act—just stand there and let the truck run over you. It will leave you behind and more than likely in worse shape than when you started.

Act—start running when you see it coming. Pace with it until you can decide when to jump on and steer it in the direction you want to move.

WHO INITIATES CHANGE AND WHY?

Another aspect to consider when evaluating change is who wants the change and why. Is it the system? Is it management? Is it you, the nurse? Or is it the patient? Change should be carefully planned and implemented for specific reasons. By identifying who is initiating the change, the implementation can be better understood.

System. The most common reason for change is that what you did before is no longer effective. For example, the handwritten medical record system is largely being replaced by the electronic medical record because the old system does not allow for the integration of the information in the record, generates volumes of paper, and is not adequate to keep pace with the number of patients and the need to access key information quickly from various individuals both inside and outside of the traditional hospital (home health nurse or hospice nurse at the patient's home).

Management. Change frequently occurs when new management enters the scene. This provides a new perspective and view regarding how the system operates. For example, a new vice president of nursing decides to implement critical pathways. The overall organization may benefit from the change; however, the employee may be wondering "How will the implementation of critical pathways change my job? Do I know how to implement a critical pathway?" (Critical Thinking Box 10-3).

Patient. When customers are not happy, something within the system needs to change. What are the specific patient problems, and how can they be resolved? For example, patients are complaining about lengthy admission procedures. Faxing physician orders or allowing direct admission to units may streamline the admission process.

Yourself. Sometimes we impose change on ourselves—we may or may not like it, but we see a need for it. Who ever wanted to go on a diet and enjoyed doing it? Stop to consider how you are going to implement the change. How will your work environment be affected? Can you delegate any part of it? If change involves other employees, make them a part of that change. They will own the results—that is, you will use the WIIFM principle (Wilson, 1996, p. 21).

WIIFM Principle: What's In It For Me?

Again, change depends on your own perspective. You will be either actively involved in changes or choose to take a passive role. The choice is always yours. There are typical

CRITICAL THINKING BOX 10-3

What changes have you made in your life?
How long did one situation last before it changed again?
You have just learned to deal successfully with the changes associated with being a student. Now you are facing the challenge of change again as you prepare for your role as a practicing registered nurse.

emotional phases encountered in the change process. It is important for nurse managers to recognize and plan interventions to effectively deal with these emotions. Table 10-4 summarizes the characteristics and helpful interventions associated with the change process. Only when you feel threatened by a change will you go through the steps (i.e., resistance, uncertainty, assimilation, transference, integration) to conquer it (Wilson, 1996) (Figure 10-3). All change will elicit some type of resistance. It is up to you to increase the impetus for change while decreasing resistance. The decision to be involved with change will help steer you in a direction that will be most beneficial.

TABLE 10-4

Emotional Phases of the Change Process

Phase	Characteristics	Interventions
Equilibrium	High energy; feelings of balance, peace, and harmony	Explain how changes will impact the status quo.
Denial	Denies reality that change will occur; experiences negative changes in physical health, emotional and cognitive behavior.	Actively listen, be empathetic and use reflective communication. Offer stress-management programs.
Anger	Blames others; may demonstrate envy, rage, or resentment.	Be assertive and assist with problem solving. Encourage employee to determine the source of his/her anger.
Bargaining	Efforts made to try and eliminate the change; frequently talks in such terms as "If only."	Search for real needs and problems and explore ways to achieve outcomes through conflict management and win-win negotiation skills.
Chaos	Diffused energy; feelings of powerlessness and insecurity and a sense of disorientation.	Encourage quiet time for reflection as inner search for identity and meaning occur.
Depression	No energy left; nothing seems to work; sorrow, self-pity and feelings of emptiness.	Encourage expression of sorrow and pain. Have lots of patience as employees learn to let go.
Resignation	Lack of enthusiasm as change is accepted passively.	Allow employees to move at own pace.
Openness	Some renewal of energy and willingness to take on new roles or assignments resulting from change.	Patiently explain again, in detail, the desired change.
Readiness	Willingly expends energy to explore new events that are occurring, reunification of emotions and cognition.	Assume a directive management style; assign tasks, provide direction.
Reemergence	Feelings of empowerment as new projects ideas are initiated.	Mutually explore questions and develop an understanding of role and identity. Employees take actions based on own decisions.

Adapted from Perlman D, Takacs GJ: The ten stages of change, *Nurs Manage* 21(4):34, 1990.

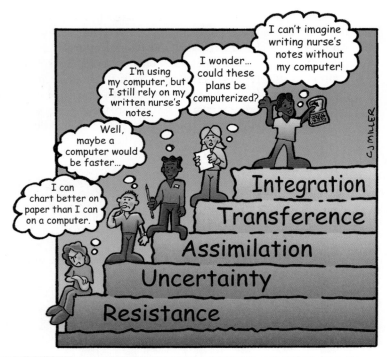

FIGURE 10-3
Five steps toward conquering change.

CONCLUSION

As a new graduate, you will be facing many transitions, including the transition from staff nurse to a leadership position of nursing manager. Having a good understanding of management styles and your own early adoption of a leadership and management style that fits both your personality and needs of your particular place of employment's nursing staff will be important to your success. Decision-making skills and understanding change theory will provide you with the tools to build effective nursing management practices.

REFERENCES

Boychuk-Duchscher J, Cowin L: Multigenerational nurses in the workplace, *J Nurs Admin* 34(11):493-501, 2004.

Cordeniz J: Recruitment, retention and management of generation X: a focus on nursing professionals, *J Healthcare Manage* 47(4):237-249, 2003.

Marquis BL, Huston CJ: *Leadership roles and management functions in nursing*, ed 4, Philadelphia, 2003, Lippincott Williams and Wilkins.

Martin C: Transcend generational lines, *Nursing Manage* 34(4):24-28, 2003.

Martin C: Bridging the generation gap, *Nursing* 34(12): 62-63, 2004.

Perlman D, Takacs GJ: The ten stages of change, *Nurs Manage 21*(4):34, 1990.

Porter-O'Grady T: A different age for leadership. Part 1: new context, new content. *J Nurs Admin* 33(2):105-110, 2003a.

Porter-O'Grady T: A different age for leadership. Part 2: new rules, new roles, *J Nurs Admin* 33(3):173-178, 2003b.

Sherman R: Growing our future nursing leaders, *Nurs Admin Q 29(2):125-132, 2005.*

Tonges M, Baloga-Altieri B, Atzori M: Amplifying nursing's voice through a staff-management partnership, *J Nurs Admin* 34(3):134-139, 2004.

Verret C: Generation Y: Motivating and training a new generation of employees. In *Ideas and trends: hotel online*, November 2000, *www.hotel-online.com/Trends/CarolVerret/GenerationY_Nov2000.html.*

Wilson P: Change: coping with tomorrow today, Shawnee Mission, Kan, 1996, National Press.

CHAPTER 11

EFFECTIVE COMMUNICATION AND TEAM BUILDING

TOM GAGLIONE, RN, MSN

To effectively communicate, we must realize that we are all different in the way we perceive the world and use this understanding as a guide to our communication with others.

—*Anthony Robbins*

If you can laugh together, you can work together.

—*Robert Orben*

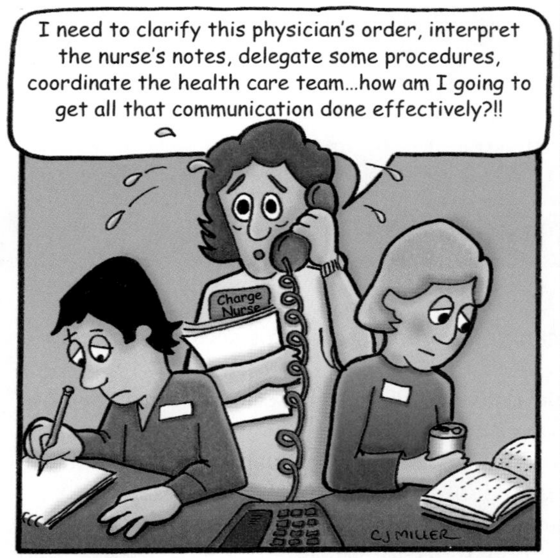

Communication should be clearly stated and directed to the appropriate, responsible individual.

After completing this chapter, you should be able to:

- Describe the basic components of communication.
- Identify effective ways of communicating with other health care workers.
- Describe an assertive communication style.
- Apply effective communication skills in common nursing activities.
- Identify different types of groups and group process.
- Analyze group member roles.
- Discuss team building and group problem solving.

Communication is like breathing—we do it all the time, and the better we do it the better we feel. At times communication can be so subtle; others are not able to comprehend the sender. Communication between people in everyday life is an exercise in subtleties and interpretations. The more personal the information, the more indirect and obscure the message becomes. In nursing, indirect communications and obscure terminology can be the difference between life and death. When you say, "I want to be clear when I communicate to others," it is no different from washing windows. The clearer the window, the better we see. Communicating what we see, what needs to be done, and teaching a client what they need to know is part of the foundation of nursing care.

THE COMMUNICATION PROCESS

WHAT ARE THE PARTS OF THE COMMUNICATION PROCESS?

Communication begins with a person who creates a *message* on the basis of his or her own perception of a situation. This person is the sender, who transmits the message using words, actions, body language, tone of voice, and facial expression. The message goes to a *receiver*, who has to interpret and evaluate the message, including all the words and the signals. When the receiver sends a message back to the sender to let the sender know what he or she heard or saw, that is called *feedback*. So, communication is basically the giving and receiving of information that involves responding with meaning.

Much of the skill involved in effective communication involves how clear the message is. The actual words that are used are known as the message's *content*. Sometimes the words are very clear and the message is easily understood. But at other times, the words might mean different things to different people. The way in which the words are said may also change how they are interpreted. Check Critical Thinking Box 11-1 for an example of how many different ways information can be interpreted. The reciprocal process of communication is illustrated in Figure 11-1.

CRITICAL THINKING BOX 11-1

TRY THIS...

1. How many different ways can you communicate this sentence to change its meaning?
   "I do not care how you've done that procedure before; do it my way now."
2. When the instructor says to you:
   "Come to my office at 2:00. There's something I want to talk to you about." What are some possible interpretations of the message?
3. When a patient's spouse says to you:
   "I do not need your help when we go home."
   How many possible explanations can you come up with regarding the meaning of the communication?

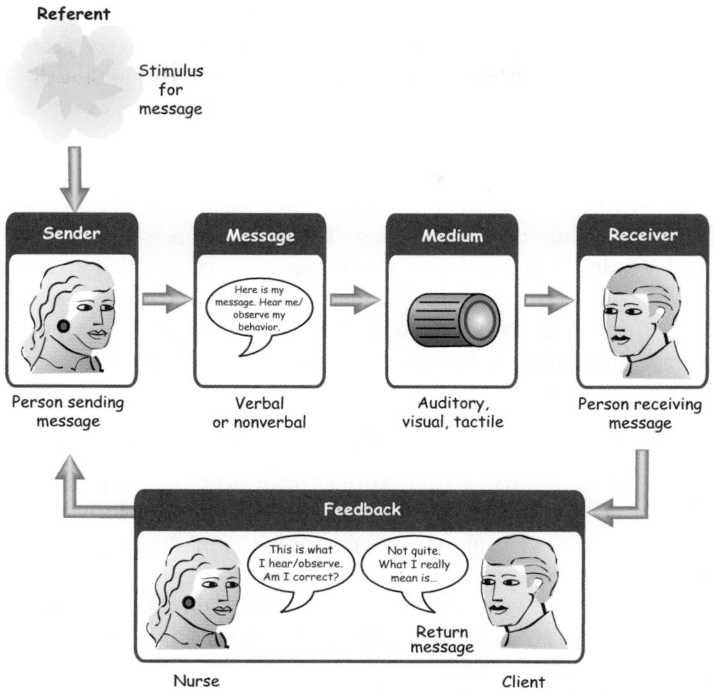

FIGURE 11-1
Communication Model. (*From* *Varcarolis EM:* Foundations of psychiatric mental health nursing: a clinical approach, *ed 4, Philadelphia, 2002, Saunders, p. 248.*)

We all know that spoken words make up what we call *verbal communication.* When we include body movements, facial expressions, and tone of voice, we are adding the nonverbal communication components that make up nearly 90% of the message. An angry voice and crossed arms can change a friendly, supportive message to a hostile and critical one. The way we choose to communicate is known as *process*. The process may clarify the message or confuse the receiver. Consider the following one-act play as an example:

SCENE ONE

Susan has been working on a very busy surgical unit for 6 weeks since she graduated from nursing school. She is approached by the dietitian, who says to her, "I was so relieved when I got to the unit and saw that you had already requested a dietary modification for Mr. Smith following his surgery. Imagine that; I didn't even have to tell you to do it."

SCENE TWO

Susan: "Can you believe the arrogance of that dietitian? Just because she's been here forever and I'm new, does that give her the right to treat me like I'm a stupid third-grader?"

Nancy (another recent graduate): "How do you know that's what she meant?"

Susan: "I could just tell by the frustration in her voice and how she moved away from me so quickly. It was as if she couldn't stand to talk to me anymore."

SCENE THREE (THE NEXT DAY ON THE UNIT)

Dietitian: "Susan, I wanted to thank you again for your initiative yesterday with Mr. Smith. I was having a particularly stressful day, and the thought of having to do one more task just seemed to overwhelm me. You really helped me out."

Susan: "I'm glad you said something about it. I wasn't sure what you meant then, and I feel much better."

Huber (2000) suggests several reasons why communication fails to be effective that can be applied to our one-act play. Nonverbal signals may mean different things to different people and can easily be misinterpreted; so can the words we use. In addition, if we are short of time, it is hard to hear clearly and remember pieces of important information. Finally, the personalities of the sender and the receiver may create a bias or distortion of the message.

WHAT ARE THE BASIC PRINCIPLES OF EFFECTIVE COMMUNICATION?

Here are some suggestions for improving our communication with others.

1. Communication is a process involving interaction between at least two people. Merely giving information is not communication unless the opportunity for a response is given.
2. The sender has a responsibility to make the message as clear as possible. You can verify what has been received by asking "Would you share with me how you interpreted what I just said?"
3. Whenever possible, use the simplest, most precise words you can. Your words must be understood by the listener.
4. Encourage the receiver of your message to provide feedback so you can verify that the message has been interpreted in the way it was intended. The receiver might say "So, what you're saying is ... " or "Let me make sure I understand you ...."
5. Remember that nonverbal behavior communicates a message even when words are not used. Try to match your nonverbal behaviors to the feeling or tone of the message you want to send to others.
6. Your reputation and credibility will make it easier for you to communicate during difficult situations. When you are trustworthy, reliable, and competent, people will listen more carefully and be more likely to interpret your messages in a positive way.
7. Because communication is an interactive process, it is much more successful within the context of a sound relationship. To create and maintain that positive relationship with others, you need to acknowledge the needs, feelings, and contributions of others. This helps create a climate more open to communication.
8. Whenever possible, communicate directly with the person you want to receive your message. This allows for immediate feedback and verification and can reduce the chances of misunderstanding.
9. Concentrate on the communication happening in the present. Avoid the temptation to daydream or plan ahead what you might say or do next.
10. Be aware of your personal values and biases, and try to keep them from interfering with your ability to communicate.
11. When you are caring for a patient in his or her home, be especially respectful of the personal nature of the surroundings.

WHAT ARE FACILITATIVE MESSAGES?

Strayhorn (1977) divides messages into two types: facilitative and obstructive. Table 11-1 details some types of facilitative messages. These messages create a positive outcome in which the people communicating with each other feel good about their interaction. It takes self-awareness and practice to send facilitative messages, but it is worth it. Your relationships with other health care workers will be satisfying and, ultimately, the patients you care for will benefit.

TABLE 11-1

Facilitative Messages

Type	Definition	Example	Effect
1. I want statement	Asks for a specific behavior	"I want you to let me practice this skill by myself and then check me in 3 days."	Simplest way to communicate what you want within a relationship
2. I feel statement	Shares your feeling in response to the other person's specific behavior	"I felt irritated just then when you told me to clean the nurses' station."	Allows you to get in touch with and share you feelings in a way undistorted by assumptions
3. I like and I do not like statements	Indicates your pleasure or displeasure with a specific behavior	"I liked it when you told me I did a good job with that patient."	Helps define what would make you happier; positive reinforcement most effective in changing another's behavior
4. Reflection	Tells the other person what you think you heard so he or she can verify or deny your interpretation.	"Sounds like that really upset you."	Helps increase listening skills, reduces distorted messages, acknowledges feelings.
5. Open-ended statement	Indicates general area of interest, but leaves specifics to other person	"Tell me your reactions to the new medication cart."	Offers attention and encourages communication to begin
6. Agreeing with part of a criticism or argument	Refuses to argue by agreeing or sympathizing with some part of the other's statement	The head nurse has just said to you, "You do not have any sense." You say, "It's true that I could be smarter than I am."	Avoids wasting time arguing; allows you to remember that you do not have to be perfect; focuses energy on negotiation of wants
7. Asking for more specific criticism	Allows you to ask what behaviors the critic didn't like, what behavior he or she would like in the future	The patient's family says, "You're doing that all wrong." You reply, "What would you like me to be doing instead?"	Turns an argument into an opportunity for productive negotiation; keeps anger at a minimum

Continued

TABLE 11-1

Facilitative Messages—cont'd

Type	Definition	Example	Effect
8. Bargaining	Sender offers to sacrifice for the other if the other will sacrifice in return	"OK, I'm hearing that you do not want me to criticize you publicly. If I work on quitting doing that, will you work on asking me for help when you do not know how to do something?"	Offers positive incentives for meeting others' needs
9. Citing specific behaviors and observations	Names specific behaviors and events and describes them without drawing conclusions about meaning	"I noticed during the meeting that you weren't saying much, weren't smiling. I'm wondering what was going on."	Allows the other person to hear about his or her behavior and clarify what specific behaviors mean; reduces misperception
10. Asking for feedback	Asks the other person's reaction to what you have just said	"I'm interested in how you react to that idea."	Allows the sender to be sure the message was received as it was intended; allows further clarification
11. You are good, you did something good, your something is good statement	Conveys something was worthwhile	"You've really grown in your ability to handle complex situations." "That was good."	Draws attention to positive aspects of the other person and makes the other person feel good, appreciated
12. I intend statement	Conveys independent action the person plans to take	"I intend to be more careful about my charting."	Indicates the person accepts responsibility for his or her behavior
13. Communication postponement	Asks for postponement of a discussion until a more favorable time	"I'm feeling hurt and angry right now and would like some time to think before we talk more."	Allows you to be in emotional control

Modified from Strayhorn JM Jr: *Talking it out: a guide to effective communication and problem solving,* Champaign, Ill, 1977, Research Press, pp 53-76.

Strayhorn (1977, p. 7) summarizes the benefits of learning to use facilitative messages: "If I can avoid antagonizing the other person, make my wishes known, find out the other person's wishes, explore various options, and make decisions accordingly, then I am much better equipped to bring happiness to others and to allow them to bring happiness to me."

WHAT ARE OBSTRUCTIVE MESSAGES?

Strayhorn (1977) says that obstructive messages generally make it much more difficult for people to communicate effectively within a positive relationship. Table 11-2 has some examples of obstructive messages. Noting the distinction between facilitative and obstructive messages will make you more attentive to the process of communication and more effective at getting your needs met. Try to identify facilitative and obstructive responses in Critical Thinking Box 11-2.

TABLE 11-2

Obstructive Messages

Type	Definition	Example	Effect
1. Communication cutoff	Statement or action that cuts off communication in order to avoid unpleasant feelings or to express hostility	"Just forget it—I won't ever bring it up again." "You do not care about me, just like everybody else."	Makes it impossible to negotiate a mutually acceptable solution to needs
2. Put-down question	Rhetorical question used to communicate a dissatisfied feeling in an indirect way	"What's the use in my doing anything for you when you always screw it up later anyway?"	Creates a need to attack or defend
3. You are bad, you did something bad statement	Conveys a negative value judgment about the other person	"You do not care about anybody but yourself."	Makes the other person feel threatened and less worthy; leads to further attack
4. You should statement	Statements that begin "you should have . . . ," "you shouldn't have . . . ," or "you ought to . . . "		
5. Defending oneself	Response to criticism in which person tries to prove that what he or she did was right	"It wasn't my fault that patient started screaming; I was trying to be nice. That doctor sure was rough and uncaring, though."	Creates focus on placing blame, rather than looking for a solution
6. Sarcasm	Making a humorous statement, opposite of what is meant, to express hostility	"Oh sure, you're never late. We all really believe that."	Promotes attack and defense; allows the sender to avoid responsibility for expressing anger honestly and directly
7. Commanding	Directing another person to do something in an authoritarian voice that implies no choice	"You can't do that sort of thing around here."	Creates a power struggle and resentment

Continued

TABLE 11-2
Obstructive Messages—cont'd

Type	Definition	Example	Effect
8. Expressing dissatisfaction through a third party	Communication not directed at the person to whom it is intended	Susan says to the head nurse, "You really ought to speak to Mary. She refuses to help any of the rest of us when we are really busy."	Allows attack and avoidance, may also lead to distorted messages
9. Assuming rather than checking it out	Assume your perception of an ambiguous or nonverbal message was correct without checking it out verbally	Susan sees the head nurse and a doctor in conversation at the door of one of her patient's rooms. The head nurse looks angry and is shaking her head. Susan concluded that they think she gave terrible care to that patient. In reality, they are talking about a hospital policy committee meeting.	Misunderstandings persist without being cleared up, and actions are based on mistaken assumptions
10. Premature advice	Offer advice without first having encouraged the person to explore his or her feelings freely	Susan: "My head nurse really bothers me. She keeps giving me too much work." Mary: "If I were you, I'd tell her off. She has no right to treat you that way. Do not let her push you around."	Often the advice is not appropriate and closes off exploration of the real issue

Adapted from Strayhorn JM Jr: *Talking it out: a guide to effective communication and problem solving*, Champaign, Ill, 1977, Research Press, pp 53-76.

CRITICAL THINKING BOX 11-2

TRY THIS…

See if you can come up with some facilitative responses and some obstructive responses to these situations.

1. You are trying to finish your assignment, and your patient's family keeps asking you questions. This is interfering with your work.
2. One of your co-workers repeatedly asks you for money and never pays you back.
3. You need to be off this weekend to take care of a family emergency. Your head nurse tells you that her staffing needs must come first and you will have to work.

COMMUNICATION IN THE WORKPLACE

Sharing information with the members of the health care team requires different approaches. This communication on a daily basis may involve delegation of a nursing procedure to an LVN (LPN) or aide, clarification of a physician's orders, reevaluation of a patient care assignment of another health care team member, or coordination of various hospital departments (e.g., radiology, dietary, pharmacy) to provide nursing care. Create role-playing situations with your peers by taking turns being in the supervisor and subordinate roles (Critical Thinking Box 11-3).

HOW CAN I COMMUNICATE EFFECTIVELY WITH MY SUPERVISOR?

Upward communication with supervisors takes on a formal nature. It is important to learn and then use the channels of communication. If you are a team member, this means you share information with your team leader. The team leader shares information with the supervisor, who shares information with the assistant vice president of nursing, who shares information with the vice president of nursing, and so on. You can see that there are many levels of nursing between the bedside nurse and the people with major decision-making responsibility.

Do you remember the game you played as a child in which someone whispers a secret to the next person, and each person repeats the secret down the line until the last person speaks the secret aloud? The secret may have started out as "Jenny was out picking berries today so she can bake a pie." By the end of the line, it may have become "Jenny is so allergic to cherries that she breaks out into hives." The point is that messages can get very distorted when they travel through many people in the upward flow of communication. Arredondo (2000) says it is important in communicating with superiors to state needs clearly, explain the rationales for requests, and suggest the benefits to the larger unit. It is also important to listen objectively to the response of the supervisor because there may be good reasons for granting or not granting the request.

CRITICAL THINKING BOX 11-3

TRY THIS...

Role play these situations with your classmates. Try taking turns being in the boss and subordinate roles.

1. The head nurse has asked the team leader and the nurse providing care to Mr. Smith to explain his progress.
2. You are the team leader giving reports to two nursing assistants and one LPN who will be working on your team today.
3. You are discussing the care of a newly diagnosed insulin-dependent diabetic patient with the dietitian, the social worker, and the patient's wife.

Arredondo (2000) gives the following tips for talking to your supervisor:

1. Keep your supervisor informed.
2. If a problem is developing, make an appointment to talk it over. Have specific information available, especially written documentation of facts. Focus on problem solving, not just the problems.
3. Show that you have important information to share and a sense of responsibility.
4. Be careful which words you use. Avoid blaming others, exaggeration, and overly dramatic expressions.
5. Do not talk to your supervisor when angry, and do not respond with anger. Use "I" statements, and explain what you think.
6. If you want to present a new idea, give your supervisor a written proposal, then meet to discuss it after the supervisor has read it.
7. Accept feedback, and learn from it.
8. Never go above or around your supervisor. Always communicate directly with your supervisor first before going further up the chain of command.

HOW CAN I COMMUNICATE EFFECTIVELY WITH OTHER NURSING PERSONNEL?

When you speak with other professional nurses, you are communicating in a lateral, or horizontal, flow of information. This flow is based on a concept of equality, in which no person holds more power than the other. This type of communication is best done in a work climate that promotes a sense of trust and respect among colleagues. When nurses work well together, their cohesiveness makes success more likely. This takes work and the deliberate use of facilitative messages (Northouse, 2001).

Ideally, professional nurses should view themselves as equals in their interactions with members of other health care disciplines, and their approach to communication should be a lateral one, even with physicians. At the basis of this communication is the ability of the nurse to see himself or herself as competent and worthy of being an equal to physicians, social workers, dietitians, and others. To gain this self-confidence is a major goal of every recent graduate. The use of effective communication practices, as described in this chapter, will help you achieve that goal.

HOW CAN I COMMUNICATE EFFECTIVELY WITH PATIENT CARE ASSISTANTS?

Even a recent graduate will soon be providing direction to licensed nursing personnel and unlicensed assistive nursing personnel. (See Chapter 14 for further information on delegation.) It is important to remember that these people have needs for satisfaction and self-esteem, too. Directions do not need to be given in the form of authoritative commands unless an emergency demands immediate action in a prescribed way. Marquis and Huston (2000) suggest that when you provide direction, you need to think through exactly what you want to be done, by whom, and when. You need to get the full attention of the other person so that you know he or she is hearing you accurately. You should then give clear, simple instructions in step-by-step order, using a supportive tone of voice. Before the other person goes to do the task, ask for feedback to verify that he or she has accurately heard your instructions. Finally, follow-up is necessary to be sure your directions were carried out and to find out what happened, in case something more needs to be done. Involving personnel who are at other levels of nursing care in the planning and evaluation of the care will increase their sense of responsibility for the outcomes and will help you to seem less authoritarian. Use the checklist in Critical Thinking Box 11-4: Facilitation Skills Checklist to identify areas needed for growth.

CRITICAL THINKING BOX 11-4

FACILITATION SKILLS CHECKLIST

Directions: Periodically during the clinical experience, use this checklist to identify areas needed for growth and progress made. Think of your clinical patient experiences. Indicate the extent of your agreement with each of the following statements by marking the scale: ***SA, strongly agree; A, agree; NS, not sure; D, disagree; SD, strongly disagree.***

1. I maintain good eye contact.	SA	A	NS	D	SD
2. Most of my verbal comments follow the lead of the other person.	SA	A	NS	D	SD
3. I encourage others to talk about feelings.	SA	A	NS	D	SD
4. I am able to ask open-ended questions.	SA	A	NS	D	SD
5. I can restate and clarify a person's ideas.	SA	A	NS	D	SD
6. I can summarize in a few words the basic ideas of a long statement made by a person.	SA	A	NS	D	SD
7. I can make statements that reflect the person's feelings.	SA	A	NS	D	SD
8. I can share my feelings relevant to the discussion when appropriate to do so.	SA	A	NS	D	SD
9. I am able to give feedback.	SA	A	NS	D	SD
10. At least 75% or more of my responses help enhance and facilitate communication.	SA	A	NS	D	SD
11. I can assist the person to list some alternatives available.	SA	A	NS	D	SD
12. I can assist the person to identify some goals that are specific and observable.	SA	A	NS	D	SD
13. I can assist the person to specify at least one next step that might be taken toward the goal.	SA	A	NS	D	SD

Adapted from Myrick D, Erney, T: *Caring and sharing*, Minneapolis, 1984, Educational Media Corporation, p 154.

WHAT DOES MY IMAGE COMMUNICATE TO OTHERS?

Remember that old saying "Do not judge a book by its cover"?

Unfortunately, we know that most people do not follow that suggestion. People get impressions about us from the way we look, sound, talk, and act. Often we are less careful about the messages we send with our appearance and behavior than we are when we choose our words. But our image may speak louder than our words. Think about it. Would you feel comfortable accepting nutrition advice from a 300-pound nurse? How would you like it if your instructor criticized your professionalism while wearing dirty shoes, a wrinkled uniform, bright red nail polish, and four earrings in each earlobe? What would you think about a physician whose progress notes contain many misspelled words and poor grammar? (Figure 11-2)

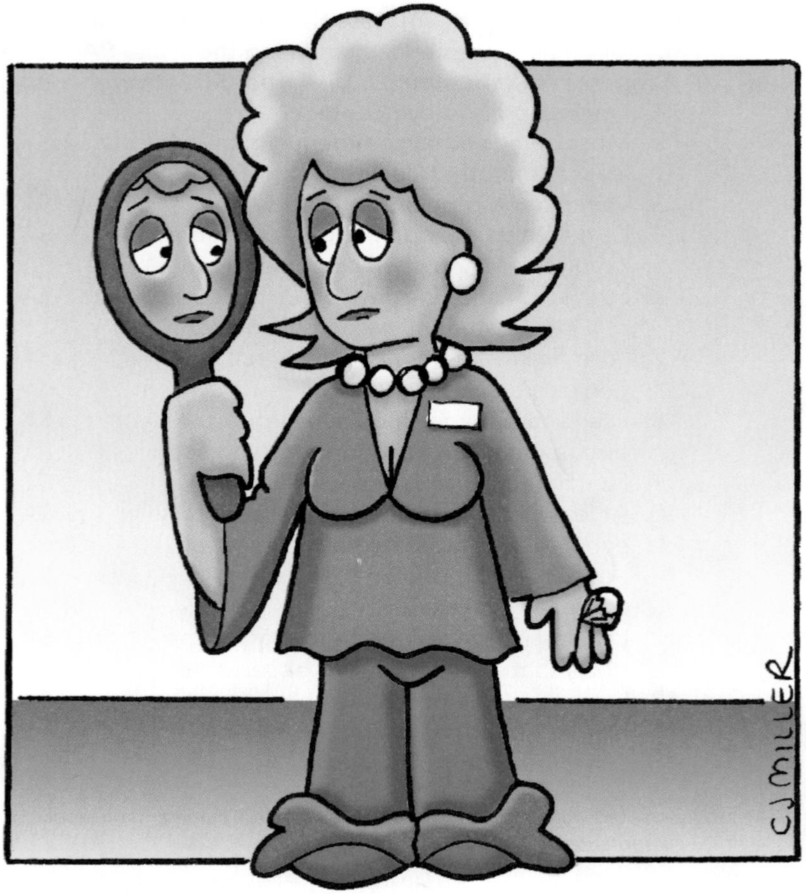

FIGURE 11-2
What does my image communicate to others?

Communication is enhanced by your credibility. And people listen more to people they respect. Your image will help you communicate your professional credibility. The place to start projecting a positive image is with the first impression your appearance creates (Vengel, 2000). Good personal hygiene is a must. Each day you have to pay attention to your grooming. This means a flattering, neat haircut; clean, well-fitting clothes; reasonable makeup and perfume; minimal jewelry; and clean, sensible shoes. Your image is improved greatly if your weight is appropriate for your height and bone structure. Your appearance at work should conform to the norms for professionals in your work setting; save your individuality for your personal time away from work.

Another aspect of your image is your depth and breadth of knowledge. You need to know your particular area of nursing thoroughly if you want the respect of others. However, you also need to know something about a wide variety of subjects so that you can have conversations with people beyond nursing. This means keeping up with current events, learning things about art or sports, and reading books. When people discover common interests, they are more willing to communicate with you.

Flexibility is necessary for effective communication with different kinds of people. This means that you are willing and able to adapt your behavior to relate more comfortably or effectively with others. Flexibility is part of a positive image because it says to people that you are willing to accept responsibility for changing your behavior to meet the professional needs or requirements of others.

People who achieve success in their professional careers are enthusiastic. They let others know they are happy to be at work. They work harder, longer, and more accurately. They are pleasant to be around. They are sincere in their efforts to create a professional image that can be trusted.

Take an inventory of your appearance, knowledge, and attitude. If you are not sure what kind of image you are communicating, ask several trusted friends.

HOW DO SEX DIFFERENCES INFLUENCE COMMUNICATION STYLES?

Men and women view their work environments from different perspectives (Vengel, 2000; Mindell, 2001). Men often see the world from a logical, sequential, focused perspective. Women often tend to see the big picture and to seek solutions based on what makes people feel comfortable rather than on logic. Subtle communication differences can create barriers to open, healthy communication between men and women in the workplace. Men may ask fewer questions in a public situation, especially if they feel that their questions might suggest ignorance. Women seem to be more comfortable asking questions (Mindell, 2001). In fact, there are times when a person can benefit from remaining silent and looking up information later in private so that others do not conclude that the asker lacks sufficient knowledge. At other times, a person must be assertive and ask questions so that he or she does not threaten the health of patients.

Within the workplace, the dominant communication style is direct, confident, and assertive. This style may be more familiar to men because they are often raised hearing more aggressive, direct language from their parents, whereas many women may be more used to a soft, supportive tone of voice and choice of words. Cultural values learned in childhood also play a role in the communication style a person chooses. This style may have to be modified to make interactions more successful. A woman who is communicating with a man may need to be more direct and assertive than usual, whereas a man may need to learn to be less aggressive in many situations.

Another sex difference in communication is related to childhood experiences with sports. Men often grow up with participation in team sports. They have worked toward a goal and have learned to strategize together for the good of the team, building a network of allies. Women have tended to be less involved with team sports than men. Women are more likely to have spent more time interacting with a few people they really like who share similar values and behaviors. Women are generally taught to be polite and to say nice things about and to others, whereas men are encouraged to do whatever it takes to help the team win. In the workplace, men and women need to understand their different points of view so that they can be team players and value cooperation and respectful relationships with each other.

To summarize, men and women have innately different communication styles, often developed from childhood experiences. To be successful in the workplace, we all have to learn as much as we can about communication differences, identify our own styles, and have the flexibility to use other communication techniques in situations that call for it.

WHAT SHOULD I KNOW ABOUT THE "GRAPEVINE"?

The grapevine is like the tabloid papers. Would you bet your job on its accuracy? So, when in doubt, check the facts out!

In addition to formal messages, informal communication flows upward, downward, and horizontally and is known as the *grapevine*. Whereas some people think of this kind of communication as gossip, others say it is the way things really get done. No matter how we describe the grapevine, we know it flourishes in all settings. People enjoy the satisfaction of the social interaction and recognition associated with the grapevine. It also provides information to employees that may not be easily obtained in any other way. It may be the quickest way to find out what the supervisor really values or what the new job openings are (Marquis & Huston, 2000) (Figure 11-3).

Mindell (2001) provides the following tips for controlling the grapevine, which can provide much distorted information:

1. Provide factual information to answer questions before they are asked. Few employees get all the information they feel they need.
2. Communicate face-to-face whenever possible. Do not trust the accuracy of messages through a third party.
3. Whenever rumors are running through the grapevine, hold a meeting to provide information and answer questions.
4. Do not spread rumors. Make sure you have all the facts from their source.
5. Enlist the support of respected leaders to spread the truth.
6. Address significant issues as soon as possible with your manager so that negative feelings can be defused.
7. Make sure what is put in writing is clear and accurately understood.

HOW CAN I DEAL WITH CULTURAL DIVERSITY AT WORK?

Dochterman and Grace (2001) tell us that culture is a pattern of values and beliefs that is reflected in the behaviors we demonstrate. Whenever a group of people spend an

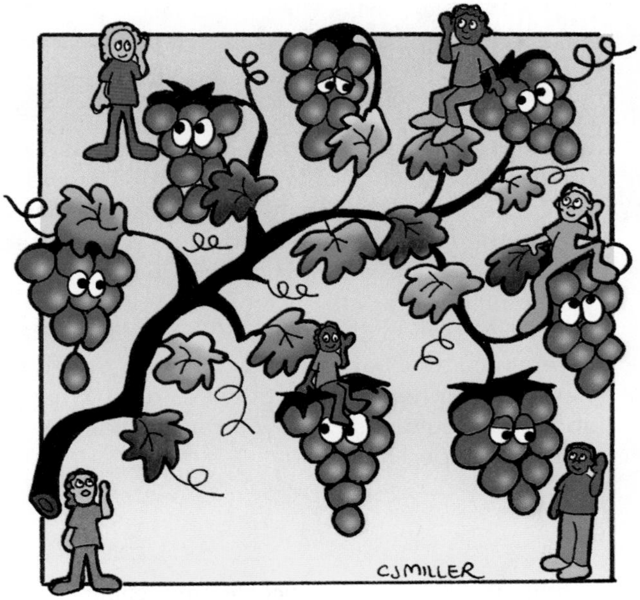

FIGURE 11-3
What should you know about the grapevine?

extended period of time together, they develop a culture. Each of us comes from a cultural background, and we have beliefs, values, and behaviors that result from that background. In our workplaces, we will encounter many different types of people coming from diverse cultural backgrounds. To communicate effectively, we need to understand our own culture as well as the other person's culture. In addition, we must acknowledge and adhere to the cultural norms or rules that have developed in our workplace.

We must be aware of stereotypes that may interfere with our ability to see people as individuals. If we view people according to stereotypes, we might limit the way we perceive their communication. Even positive stereotypes make assumptions about people that may be inaccurate and thus may limit the nurse's ability to use all of his or her work skills effectively (Critical Thinking Box 11-5).

According to Arredondo (2000), communication goes through many filters when a person interacts with someone whom he or she perceives as different. Some of those filters are related to culture, sex, education level, age, and experience. When messages go through these filters, they may change because the actual communication symbols are interpreted according to a person's own cultural values and beliefs. This change may lead to misperceptions and misinterpretations. Communication is improved when we become more aware of the filters we use.

CRITICAL THINKING BOX 11-5

TRY THIS...

As you go about your work, take note of the various people you interact with and your reactions to them. Write them down so that you can reflect on them. What kinds of thoughts come to mind when you see a female executive, an older woman, or a handsome man dressed in a suit? What kind of thoughts come to mind when you see people of ethnic origins that differ from your own? How do your initial impressions impact on the way you communicate with each of these people?

Picture yourself in the homes of five of your clients. Choose people from different cultural backgrounds. How are their homes different? In what ways do their homes reflect their culture? What do you need to know about each culture so that you can provide care effectively while avoiding any stereotyped beliefs?

Within the work culture, people often communicate using jargon, inside jokes, or slang unique to the work setting. Acronyms are an example of jargon that health care workers understand but patients may not. It may seem to patients and their families that we are speaking in a code or foreign language. To interact effectively, we need to speak clearly, avoiding jargon or slang, and to keep our communication short and to-the-point. Long explanations can be confusing to people who are not familiar with the health care culture.

Differences in the cultural backgrounds of workers can be a real asset. Sometimes we may have to provide care to patients who speak languages other than English, and we may need the skills of co-workers to translate or interpret, especially when cultural values influence the interpretation of the patient's behavior. We need to understand and respect cultural differences in patients. We can learn how to do this by learning about the differences among our co-workers. Respect and empathy enhance communication with people from other cultures, whether those people are patients or co-workers (Dochterman & Grace, 2001).

COMPONENTS OF WRITTEN COMMUNICATION

HOW CAN I COMMUNICATE EFFECTIVELY IN WRITING?

Communication takes place not only when words are spoken, but also when they are written and then read by someone else. A big part of a nurse's overall effectiveness depends on the ability to write effectively. This includes written treatment plans, progress notes, job descriptions, consultation requests, referrals, and memos. Some of you may even write articles for nursing journals or chapters for textbooks!

Mindell provides some guidelines for writing (2001). Determine whether you need to write in a formal way. Most upward communication needs to be formal, which means you should use proper titles, format, grammar, spelling, and punctuation. Never allow something you have written to be sent without careful proofreading. Nothing creates a negative impression faster than sloppy work, misspelled words, or poor grammar. If you need to, ask someone else to do this proofreading; be sure it is done well. Take the time to make necessary revisions before sending your written work on.

Decide what your purpose is before you write (Marquis & Huston, 2000). This will help you to organize your thoughts so that everything you write helps you to meet your purpose. Learn to write exactly what you mean. Choose words that are clear and specific. Often this means simple, small words. Be careful to use technical words only when you are sure you are choosing the correct words and your reader will understand you. Keep your sentences short and simple, with only one idea in each sentence.

Try using the KISS principle: Keep It Short and Simple.

When you learn to be clear and concise, you will write the essential information without many flowery phrases. Your readers will be very grateful if they can follow your thoughts easily. Make your first sentence in each paragraph identify the key point for that paragraph. The reader should not have to guess what you are trying to say. Use a format that guides the reader. This means that visually on each page, main points are easy to locate, and concepts are identified by headings or titles. Remember, how well you write strongly influences how you are evaluated. What you put down on paper makes a lasting impression, and people will make judgments about your credibility and professionalism for a long time after you have actually written the words.

HOW CAN I LEARN TO SPEAK EFFECTIVELY?

From giving a report at the change-of-shift to explaining your plans for a new approach on the unit to the organization's administration, you will have many opportunities to make presentations.

The first step in making effective presentations is to develop a positive attitude. ACCENTUATE the POSITIVE!

Many of us let our anxiety intimidate us. However, public speaking can be a great chance to show off our skills, our ability to be creative, and our willingness to be a star entertainer. Think of your presentation as a wonderful opportunity to have the attention of others on just you, even if only for a few minutes (Arredondo, 2000).

The second guiding principle in making good presentations is practice. PRACTICE makes PERFECT!

A well-planned rehearsal gives you a chance to see how long it will take you to say what you want and will help you feel more comfortable saying the words easily. Here are some tips on presentation preparation from Kushner (1997) and Peoples (1992).

Analyze Your Audience. What do they already know, and what do they need to know? Have an objective or two for what you want your audience to get out of your presentation.

Do Your Homework. Know enough about your subject to make your talk clear and believable. Make sure you can answer at least a few questions.

Plan the Presentation. This includes making an outline of the content and the teaching strategies you might use. Visual aids or activities may be used to involve the audience in active participation. Visual aids should keep the presentation focused and organized. They help you hold your audience's attention. *(Plus you are more likely to persuade with visual cues.)*

Add Spice to the Presentation. The more active your audience's participation, the longer they will pay attention. Choose at least one presentation strategy that involves them, such as question/answer, role playing, or small-group discussion. Key points you want your audience to remember should be highlighted visually on slides or other types of media. *Use an attention grabber at the beginning* to make sure your audience is listening. This may be a friendly greeting, a stimulating question, a startling statistic, a relevant story, or a quote by an expert. Then tell your audience the purpose of the presentation and what it will cover in brief and concise words.

Create Cheat Sheets. Cheat sheets are your clues—the first couple of words around a topic to help you remember what to say or what questions to ask, or small pictures or drawings to jog your mind during the presentation in case you stumble and fumble with your thoughts and words. If the speech or presentation is an important one and fairly formal, you may want to prepare a script. *(Memorize the first 2 minutes of what you are going to say!)* This means you write out exactly what you will say and have it typed double-spaced, with a wide margin on the left side. Here you can write notes to yourself about when to use your visual aids or when to pass out materials for the audience.

The Closing. In your closing, review what you have said, summarize the benefits or implications of what you have said, and reiterate any action you want taken. *(Design your closing FIRST, as it is the most important part of the formal presentation. It may sound crazy to work backwards, but the closing is what the audience will hear last and remember. Write it out and memorize it!)*

Final Details. Be sure to be familiar with the room and equipment you will be using. Determine that everything you need is there before you begin. Make sure the spelling is correct on your visual aids and handouts. Speak with confidence, energy, and enthusiasm. Make as much eye contact as you can. Use your hands and arms to make dramatic gestures. They add energy and interest.

WHAT LISTENING SKILLS DO I NEED TO DEVELOP?

Listening effectively is one of the most powerful communication tools you can have. It is more than just hearing the words of others. Listening involves concentrating all your energy on understanding and interpreting the message with the meaning the sender intended. Of the four verbal means of communication—writing, reading, speaking, and listening—listening requires most of our communication time. Yet we often pay the least attention to our listening skills (Mindell, 2001). It has been estimated that people actually remember only one third of the messages they have heard, although they spend 70% of their time listening (Marquis & Huston, 2000).

Did you know? People speak at 100 to 175 words per minute, but they can listen intelligently at 600 to 800 words per minute (Fowler, 2005).

There are reasons that people are not good listeners (Arredondo, 2000). We simply do not pay enough attention; we hear what we want to hear and filter out the rest. Listening requires concentration, and that means doing nothing else at the same time. Some people think of listening as a passive behavior; they want to be in control by talking more. We think a lot faster than people speak, so we often think way ahead or think about other things or daydream. It may be that there are too many distractions that interfere with listening, such as background noises or movements.

One of the most problematic reasons for ineffective listening is that people allow their emotions to dictate what they hear or do not hear. We pay more attention to people we like or respect and less attention to people or messages that make us feel uncomfortable. If the message is making demands on us to do more, change what we do, or do better, we may stop listening to deal with our own feelings of anger, guilt, or anxiety. We may start planning our own defensive response while the other person is still talking.

Think about situations you've been in where you've had difficulty listening, understanding, or remembering what was said. Consider these examples:

- A psychiatry patient who has recently been admitted displays acutely psychotic thought processes by talking rapidly in pressured speech, using words and phrases so loosely connected that the whole conversation is disorganized and incomprehensible.
- A head nurse spends 5 minutes screaming at her team leader, criticizing everything she has done that day, and then asks the team leader to carry out a very specific and detailed change in the physician's orders for a patient.
- Another nurse asks you to hang an intravenous solution for the patient in room 1253 while you are writing some progress notes on a patient's chart. When you finish, you cannot remember the room number where you agreed to hang the intravenous solution.

It becomes essential to develop effective listening skills (Arredondo, 2000). Here are some tips:

Make sure you can hear what is being said. Move closer, eliminate distracting noises, and, most of all, do not talk. You cannot hear someone else when you are talking.

Focus your attention on what is being said. Actively concentrate by analyzing the key points as they are being said. Take notes. Do not do anything else while you are listening except to concentrate on hearing and understanding what is being said.

Recognize and control your emotional response to what is being said. Focus on hearing and seeing accurately what is being communicated. You will have time to ask questions and explore feelings after the other person finishes.

Decide in the beginning that you will listen and accept the other person's needs and feelings, whatever they are. Improved understanding of the other person is gained through listening, and this understanding will help you to be more effective in solving problems and eliminating negative feelings.

Pay attention to nonverbal communication as you listen to the words. Much of the meaning comes through in the tone of voice, facial expressions, and body movements. You must listen with your eyes and your ears.

Fight off distractions. Do not let the speaker's style of communicating, his or her mannerisms, telephone calls, or other interruptions break your concentration.

Take notes. If a lot of factual, important information is being given, take notes—but just jot down key words or numbers or the note-taking itself will become a distraction. You may also ask the speaker to put in writing what he or she has said.

Let the speaker tell the whole story. Make it a point not to interrupt. Try not to assume you know what is going to be said. Withhold formulating criticisms as you listen.

React to the message, not the person. Ask yourself, "Are my feelings or biases interfering with my listening?" Seek feedback of your understanding by verifying what you have heard.

Respond positively to the feelings being communicated. Empathy and acceptance will make it easier for the communication to continue. Maintain a positive attitude about listening. Recognize that listening is necessary for success. Allow yourself to hear all sides of an issue.

Identify the characteristics of your listening skills in Critical Thinking Box 11-6.

HOW CAN I USE NONVERBAL COMMUNICATION EFFECTIVELY?

Nonverbal communication uses movements, gestures, body position, and voice tone to transmit messages (Arredondo, 2000). To convey confidence and leadership ability, it is necessary to learn to use certain nonverbal signals effectively. Here are some tips:

Make eye contact with the person with whom you are talking. This helps the person interpret your message more favorably and says that you are giving your full attention to the conversation.

Stand up straight, with shoulders back. You may want to lean slightly forward toward the other individual to convey your interest. Stand with your toes pointed slightly outward and slightly apart and approximately 18 inches to 4 feet from the person you are talking to so that you do not invade personal space. Avoid personal contact unless you know the person well and it is a casual conversation.

CRITICAL THINKING BOX 11-6

TRY THIS...

Develop a listening action plan.

1. I listen most effectively when
2. I have difficulty listening when
3. My best listening skills are
4. I need to improve on my skills at
5. In order to improve my listening skills, I will

Use a forceful voice without pauses to suggest confidence. Avoid a whining, nagging, or complaining tone. You may need to listen to your tape-recorded voice to get some insight into how you sound to others.

Watch for distracting behaviors. Avoid negative behaviors that detract from your verbal messages: nodding constantly, yawning, playing with your hair, scratching yourself, cracking your knuckles, or twiddling your thumbs. When you use your hands in gestures, keep your forearm up and the palm of your hand open. Avoid making a fist or shaking a pointing finger at the other person.

WHAT SKILLS DO I NEED TO USE THE TELEPHONE EFFECTIVELY?

Many nurses spend time on the telephone talking with physicians, patients and their families, and other health care workers. Here are some tips for making telephone communication productive. It is always polite to ask the person you are calling if this is a convenient time to talk. You may encounter difficulties reaching people by telephone. If this "telephone tag" problem persists after two attempts, leave a message stating exactly when you will be available to talk (and then be there).

If you anticipate your conversation will involve complex information, make notes ahead of time so you can keep your conversation as focused and brief as possible. With detailed, critical information that is discussed over the telephone, it is wise to follow up with a written communication to that person. Important telephone calls should also be followed up in writing. This helps clarify and confirm the information discussed. If your telephone conversation requires a follow-up action, you need to keep a written record.

It is difficult to focus on the telephone conversation if you are attempting to do something else. Your communication will be more effective if you do one thing at a time. (How many times have you been irritated by a driver who is also talking on a cellular telephone?) Once you have finished your discussion, get off the phone; do not chit-chat or gossip once the information has been communicated. Communicating with physicians on the telephone presents a challenge to recent graduates. Box 11-1 highlights some helpful tips.

HOW CAN I COMMUNICATE EFFECTIVELY BY USING TECHNOLOGY?

Many of us are learning to use the technology that is changing our workplace and making communication easier. Although cellular telephones, fax machines, portable

BOX 11-1 Tips for Communicating with Physicians on the Phone

1. Say who you are right away.
2. Do not apologize for phoning.
3. State your business briefly but completely.
4. Ask for specific orders when appropriate.
5. If you want the doctor to assess the patient, say so.
6. If the doctor is coming, ask when to expect him or her.
7. If you get cut off, call back.
8. Document attempts to reach a doctor.
9. If a doctor is rude or abusive, tell him or her so.
10. If you cannot reach a doctor or get what you need, always tell your manager.

personal computers, modems, and voice mail may be conveniences, they must be used thoughtfully to make a positive contribution to your overall image as an effective communicator. Deep and Sussman (1995) give the following tips for the successful use of communications technology:

Do not misuse or overuse fax machines. Remember that the person on the other end must read every page faxed to him or her, so be brief. If you need to send a long document, use the mail. Send faxes only when you do not mind if the quality of the copy is not first-rate, because many people have fax machines that print less clearly than computers or even copying machines.

When you leave someone a voice-mail message, speak slowly and distinctly. This is especially important when you are leaving your telephone number so that the other person can return your call. It is frustrating to receive a message but not be able to understand the name or have to replay the message to get all of the digits in the phone number. Make your voice-mail message brief but complete, saying when you called, what you want the other person to do, and when you can be reached.

Do not leave callers on hold if you are using call waiting. Explain to the first caller that you must briefly answer another call, then take the number of the second caller, with the assurance that you will call back as soon as you finish your first call. This interruption should take no more than 10 seconds. Be sure to write down the telephone number of the second caller so that you do not forget it by the time you finish the first call.

When you call people, ask if they have time to talk and offer to call back at a more convenient time if necessary. People appreciate the courtesy and will be more likely to have a positive conversation with you if it is conveniently timed and is respectful of their busy schedules.

If you are conducting a conversation or a meeting with a speaker telephone or by means of a teleconference, make sure that each party to the call is introduced to the other people. Do not use the speaker telephone unless you are including a group in the conversation. Even with a conference call, there should be some structure to the discussion, including an agenda or a specified purpose and time for the call.

When you have business cards printed, include your e-mail address and your fax number. If you are sending messages by e-mail, be sure to read your words carefully before sending them. Because you are sending words without the benefit of clarifying nonverbal communication, the likelihood of being misinterpreted is greater. Make sure your messages are as clear as they can be. Include your name and subject in the e-mail note.

Do not send an emotional outburst in an e-mail. These messages can seem more hostile than you intended, and you can alienate or anger many people. If you cannot state your message in person, then do not send it by e-mail (Box 11-2).

Learn to use basic computer software. Most people can effectively use fewer than half of the programs to which they have access. Know how to use word-processing software. This is especially helpful in making your communication easier and more credible.

When you need to send a personal message, especially a reminder or a thank-you, the most powerful way is to send a handwritten note. This conveys the importance you connect with the message and continues the interpersonal aspect of the communication. If you need to communicate something that you expect will have

BOX 11-2 Tips on Using E-Mail Effectively

1. STOP, THINK ABOUT WHAT YOU WANT TO SAY, *THEN* WRITE.
   Be sure to determine if an e-mail is the appropriate communication medium. E-mail is meant for quick, simple communication. Ask yourself would a phone conversation be more appropriate.
2. INCLUDE A DESCRIPTIVE SUBJECT LINE.
   Place in the subject line of the e-mail note, a description of what the e-mail is about—be specific, (i.e., Quarterly QA Report or Case Study Assignment—Informatics).
3. MAKE YOUR E-MAIL NOTE EASY TO READ.
   - Use short paragraphs, usually no more than 4 or 5 paragraphs at most—get to the point, quickly. Consider that most people have a limited attention span with e-mail, especially if they are receiving a lot of e-mail.
   - Have ample white space on the page. Usually 5 to 7 lines of text are best for a paragraph.
   - Use bullets or numbers to guide the reader.
   - Carefully choose your font size, type, and color. Using a bright color (such as purple) may not convey a professional tone like a standard black or navy font would. Very large fonts (14 point) might make your message seem shouting and accusatory. A sans serif font, such as Arial or Tahoma 10-12 point, is easier to read on the computer screen than a serif font, such as Times Roman.
4. BE PRECISE, CONCISE, AND CLEAR.
   - Use a conversational writing style.
   - If responding to multiple questions embedded in a large e-mail, copy the questions into your e-mail and write your answers next to them.
   - When replying to a message, include enough of the original e-mail note to provide context to your response.
   - If in doubt, spell it out—watch using jargon or abbreviations.
   - Always use spell-check and proof your e-mail before you send it out.
5. DEMONSTRATE NETIQUETTE—BE PROFESSIONAL AND MAINTAIN GOOD ONLINE TONE.
   - Do not type in all CAPS! Capitals can be used for emphasis, but ALL CAPS LOOKS LIKE YOU'RE YELLING AT THE PERSON. If you emphasize everything, then nothing is taken as important.
   - Do not type in all lower case, as this violates the rules of English grammar and usage.
   - If a note is upsetting, keep calm and collected. Your emotional state can slip into an e-mail without notice, in the form of curt sentences, skipped pleasantries, and blunt comments.
   - Remember, unlike telephone and personal conversations that fade with time, impulsive e-mail responses have "staying power"—meaning the e-mail is readily available in e-mailboxes, can be printed out, distributed to others, and attain a level of importance that was never intended.
   - A word about **flaming**—which is the expression of extreme emotion or opinion in an e-mail message, often derogatory. Be polite and pleasant and consider whether you want to respond to a "flaming" e-mail.
6. BE CAREFUL WITH ATTACHMENTS.
   - Only open attachments if you trust the source, as attachments can contain executeable files that can spread e-mail viruses and slow down processing.

Continued

BOX 11-2 Tips on Using E-Mail Effectively—cont'd

- Consider the size of the attachments, as large files (greater than 1000KB or 1MB) can clog up networks and rapidly fill your Inbox. Many servers prohibit the sending and receiving of large e-mail file attachments.
- Use spam filters and delete chain e-mails or other scams—do not open the document or have the viewing pane open, as it can perpetuate the spam.

7. WATCH HUMOR.
   - Find different ways to express emotion, body language, and intonation. Use smileys (☺ Emoticons) to convey feeling in message.
   - As in any setting, humor can be misconstrued, so be extra careful and use taste and discretion with any humor that is transmitted.
8. INCLUDE A SIGNATURE.
   - Include a signature with your e-mail, usually no more than 4-6 lines of text. Remember, this part of your message is the last thing the receiver will read.
   - Include your name, title, contact information, and e-mail address or URL. Many e-mail programs can be set up to automatically attach a default signature or signature file to the end of all your outgoing messages (including replies).
9. REVIEW YOUR MESSAGE BEFORE SENDING.
   - Remember e-mail is not confidential—do not send personal or sensitive e-mail, as there is no "secure" e-mail system.
   - Review and proof your message before clicking "Send."
10. RESPOND TO E-MAIL.
    - Make an effort to respond to e-mail within 24 hours. Otherwise, use the auto-reply function to inform the person when you will respond.

a real emotional impact, do it face-to-face. This communication style has more force, too, but it also allows you an opportunity to read the other person's nonverbal communication and offers a chance to negotiate a comfortable understanding following your message delivery.

GROUP COMMUNICATION

WHAT IS GROUP PROCESS?

When we discuss the dynamics and communication patterns in groups, it is important to note that there are personality conflicts that tend to develop during the different cyclical phases of the group. In **forming** the group, think back to orientation day for nursing school. There you sit surrounded by some people you have never seen before and some you have known from your prenursing classes. A common bond is that you are all there for well-defined reasons, including finding out who is in your clinical group and who the instructors will be. Of course, the orientation is mandatory. You sit in the auditorium or classroom talking, listening, and watching those around you, playing your part in a form of controlled pandemonium. The pandemonium can actually be considered the **storming** phase. In the storming phase, you begin to act out the roles you normally portray in the presence of your peers, as you discussed your fears, fantasies, and hopes for a successful outcome to your nursing program (Tuckman, 1977).

Next, you are divided into clinical groups. You now begin to reevaluate the personality composition of the new groups. As you begin to react to your new relationships, you begin to exhibit personality traits to establish the role you would like to be identified with in the group setting. Unfortunately, your unconscious defense mechanisms surface in the form of competitive conflict or one-upmanship within the group, with your hope that your response will secure the desired role in the group. It is at this time that **norming** begins to develop among members of the group, with the help of the clinical and lecture instructors. Norming occurs during the development of mutual goals and guidelines that help to redefine your behavioral roles in the group. This can allow agreement in performing activities to help establish a purposeful clinical experience that involve interdependence and flexibility.

During the **performing** phase, everyone knows each other, is able to work together, and trusts each other. The group works together and makes changes in a seamless way, as there is a high degree of comfort among the group members that funnels all of the energy of the group toward the tasks at hand—getting through nursing school. Later Tuckman added the final stage, **adjourning,** which has been called deforming and mourning by others. This phase is about completion and disengagement, both from the tasks and the group members. Many of you have or will experience the adjourning phase as you move from one clinical group to another or during the transition from student to graduate, as you are nearing completion of your nursing program.

Groups can be multipurpose and multidynamic, as are the basic role choices of each participant in a group. When working in a group, the real fun and excitement start when group members begin responding to and dealing with the unconscious and semiconscious defense mechanisms of the individuals who act them out through the roles they play in the group. The responses of the defensive individual tend to be unproductive, time-consuming, and inappropriate to the harmony and overall function of a group effort. Of course, they do give you something to talk and maybe laugh about later. In my years of nursing and group participation, the following tend to be my favorite dysfunctional group personalities.

The **self-servers** feel that the rules of the group do not apply to them. They show up late. They are usually unprepared to work. At times they will walk in and out of the group when it meets for superficial reasons, while appearing preoccupied with unrelated work or issues from outside of the group. When they do participate, their contributions are of little consequence. If they refuse to be functional members of the group, you may need to ask them to leave the group.

The first response of a **critical conservative** to a creative suggestion is, "No, it won't work" or "But it's always been done this way" and "How can you people succeed if you've never done this before?" They seem to have a criticism for any suggestion other than their own. If it is not done their way, it just is not right. They are obsessively negative and fearful of changes. It may be important to recognize the lessons of experiences and outcomes, but it is equally important to find new approaches to old problems.

The **motor mouths** talk just to hear themselves talk. They interrupt at any given moment to make statements or deliver a verbose response, possibly because they have been quiet for too long. Even when a person is talking, these people will talk over the speaker's words just to be the center of attention. At times, the motor mouth begins to make a statement, only to ramble in and out of the group's issue, and ends up talking about unrelated issues that are usually about himself or herself. I suggest keeping a cloth gag nearby or redirecting their conversation to focusing on the issue and asking them for a short critical assessment of the issues in question.

The **mouse** is the silent observer fearful of voicing an opinion. Usually the mouse sits transfixed watching individuals take risks and responsibility for their input to the group. The mouse nods his or her head at appropriate times and answers questions in one or two words. The mouse may be a real addition to the group, especially if others in the group are able to find ways to engage and encourage the mouse to voice his or her opinions and feelings about the group issues. It is important to remember that they are some of the best observers and listeners; ask them for their input. You may find them to be a valuable asset to your team. Regardless of where you choose to work or the type of care-delivery system you are in, these group members are always there!

HOW CAN YOU IMPROVE COMMUNICATIONS IN GROUP MEETINGS?

Nurses participate in many meetings, from patient care conferences to more formal committee meetings. Communication within a group of people can be an opportunity to influence the quality of care given to patients. When you participate as a member of a group, the following are positive behaviors that will help you to communicate effectively and will also help the group to accomplish its tasks more efficiently:

- Come prepared. Bring all the "stuff" you need.
- Listen. Be open to other viewpoints.
- Keep on track. Do not visit or chit-chat.
- Present your ideas or opinions. Ask other members for theirs.
- State disagreements. Be able to back them up.
- Clarify when needed. Do not assume.

All of us have been to and participated in meetings that were disorganized, confusing, and a waste of time. Critical Thinking Box 11-7 will help you to identify some unpleasant group meeting experiences and give you the opportunity to change future meetings.

CRITICAL THINKING BOX 11-7

TRY THIS...

Think of particularly unpleasant experiences you have had at meetings. You might think about meetings involving your clinical group or your class officers. Develop a list of ideas about what was wrong with those meetings.

WHAT ARE THE RESPONSIBILITIES OF A GROUP LEADER?

If you are the leader of a group meeting, you have additional responsibilities. If you are organized and able to communicate effectively, the meeting is much more likely to run smoothly. This is especially important when you and your group members are busy. You cannot afford to waste time sitting in an unproductive meeting. Nothing is as irritating as time spent arguing with others when you know your work is piling up on your desk. If the irritation continues to build, you and the other group members will be less committed to the goals of the group and some will even stop coming. The key to effective meetings is the planning and organization that occurs before the meeting is actually held. An effective technique using deBono's Six Thinking Hats can spur a group meeting to better productivity and problem solving (Box 11-3). Planning should allow the leader to think through what the meeting is for, who should be there, and how it should run (Huber, 2000). There should be a clear purpose for every meeting

BOX 11-3 Edward de Bono's Six Thinking Hats: Looking at a Decision and Working Through a Problem Considering Six Points of View

Six Thinking Hats is an important and powerful technique created by Edward de Bono that can be used as an effective group process tool in meetings that get bogged down with diverse views and adamant positions. It offers a strategy to "think outside the box" by challenging the group to think or see all sides of an issue. Each "Thinking Hat" represents a perspective or way of thinking. During a meeting, a "different color hat" can be put on or taken off to indicate the type of thinking the person is using. By putting on a different hat in a particular sequence, problem solving is encouraged.

WHITE HAT: NEUTRAL, OBJECTIVE, CONCERNED WITH FACTS AND FIGURES, *THE FACT HAT*

Used to think about facts, figures, and other objective information (think of a scientist's white lab coat).
What facts and data are available?
What facts would help me further in making a decision?
How can I get those facts?

RED HAT: THE EMOTIONAL VIEW, *THE EMOTIONAL HAT*

Used to elicit the feelings, emotions, and other nonrational but potentially valuable senses, such as hunches and intuition (think of a red heart). Encourages people to express their feelings without the need for apology, explanation, or attempt to justify them.
How do I really feel?
What is my gut feeling about this problem?

BLACK HAT: CAREFUL, CAUTIOUS, *THE "DEVIL'S ADVOCATE" HAT*

Used to discover why some ideas will not work, this hat inspires logical negative arguments (think of a devil's advocate or judge robed in black). Helps you to see problems in advance (spot flaws in thinking) prepare for potential difficulties, and prepare contingency plans to counter the issues.
What are the possible downside risks and problems?

Continued

BOX 11-3 Edward de Bono's Six Thinking Hats: Looking at a Decision and Working Through a Problem Considering Six Points of View—cont'd

What is the worst-case scenario?
What are the weak points of the plan? It allows you to eliminate them, alter them, or prepare contingency plans to counter them.

YELLOW HAT: SUNNY AND POSITIVE, *THE OPTIMISTIC HAT*
Used to obtain a positive, optimistic outlook, this hat sees opportunities, possibilities, and benefits of a decision (think of the warming sun). Keeps you going when the going gets tough.
What are the advantages?
What would be the best possible outcome?

GREEN HAT: ASSOCIATED WITH FERTILE GROWTH, CREATIVITY, AND NEW IDEAS, *THE CREATIVE HAT*
Used to find creative new ideas (think of new shoots sprouting from seeds).
What completely new, fresh, innovative approaches can I generate?
What creative ideas can I dream up to help me see the problem in a new way?
Are there any additional alternatives or can we do this in a different way?
Could there be another explanation?

BLUE HAT: COOL, THE COLOR OF SKY, *THE ORGANIZING HAT*
Used as a master hat to control the thinking process (think of the overarching sky, or a "cool" character who's in control).
Review my thoughts—it suggests the next step for thinking.
Sum up what I have learned and think about what the next logical step is—asks for summaries, conclusions and decisions.

From de Bono E: *Six thinking hats*, 1999, MICA Management Resources, *www.debonogroup.com/6hats.htm*. Reprinted with permission of the McQuaig Group.

and every item on the agenda. Every item should require some action by the group. If the purpose could be achieved in another way, such as by making a telephone call or sending a memo, there should be no meeting.

It is the leader's responsibility to send out an agenda ahead of time and to indicate any preparations that members need to make or materials they need to bring. The leader must also be concerned with the room where the meeting will be held. If you are making a formal presentation, some audiovisual equipment will be necessary, and chairs will need to be arranged so that everyone can see the presenter and the audiovisuals. If the meeting is for discussion and decision making, a table at which everyone can sit face-to-face is more effective. Look at Figure 11-4. This type of note-taking clarifies who is responsible for what activities. Ask for a volunteer to keep track of the timeline information. At the conclusion of the meeting, summarize the decisions, and identify the plan of action. Review the timeline information for clarity and understanding regarding group member responsibilities. At the end of the meeting, the time should be established for the next meeting. All members should receive a copy of the timeline information.

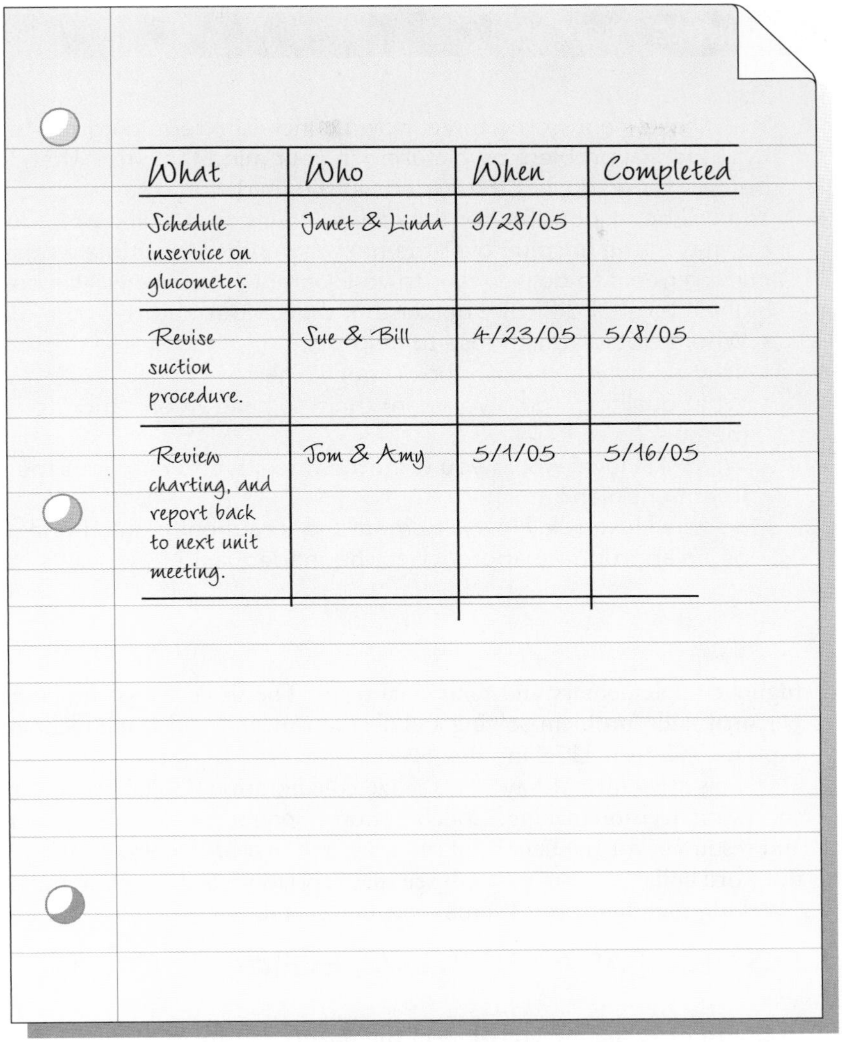

What	Who	When	Completed
Schedule inservice on glucometer.	Janet & Linda	9/28/05	
Revise suction procedure.	Sue & Bill	4/23/05	5/8/05
Review charting, and report back to next unit meeting.	Tom & Amy	5/1/05	5/16/05

FIGURE 11-4
Action timeline for meetings.

TEAM BUILDING

WHAT IS TEAM BUILDING?

Team building is a deliberate process of unifying a group of individuals into a functional working unit, accomplishing specific goals (Farley & Stoner, 1989). Another definition of a team is "a small number of people with complementary skills who are committed to a common purpose in performance of common goals, for which they hold themselves mutually accountable" (Katzenbach & Smith, 1993, p. 45). Katzenbach and Smith state that there needs to be the right mix of attributes in three categories that help ensure a

CRITICAL THINKING BOX 11-8

THINK ABOUT...

Try to assess and come to your own conclusion regarding the following hypothetical problem by picturing in your mind the who, what, and why before you read what the experts in the field would say.

You will be responsible for the care of your critically ill parent during his or her stay in the hospital over the next 2 months. Assemble a team of your nursing peers to deliver care to your parent. The care will be based on the highest level of difficulty because of the serious nature of the diagnosis.

- Whom would you choose to help you?
- Why would you choose those specific nurses?
- What qualities would you want them to have when caring for your family member?
- What skill level would you want them to have to carry out the overall treatment plan?
- If some lacked skill levels to meet the treatment plan criteria, what would be an appropriate approach to this inadequacy?

highly complementary and functional team. The three categories described are interpersonal skills, problem-solving and decision-making skills, and technical or functional expertise (Critical Thinking Box 11-8).

Teams are a formal way to actualize collaboration. Collaboration is at the heart of successful decision making. Collaboration among team members leverages skills, time, and resources for the benefit of the team and that of the organization. If you examine the word collaboration, you will see that "co-labor" is the core of the word—meaning "working together toward some meaningful end."

WHEN NURSES WORK AS A TRUE TEAM, EVERYONE INVOLVED BENEFITS!

In health care, the imperative is in the quality of care and service-oriented teams, as seen by Sovie (1992). It is also clear that teamwork is essential in care delivery outcomes and cost-control (Figure 11-5). Sovie also says that nurse managers and supervisors need to learn how to function in their individual capacity while being effective as team players. It might be argued that there is a difference between the previous concepts of team nursing and the current concepts of team nursing. The differences are not so much the personal mechanics of team nursing but more the constant updating of information in the fields of medicine and technology.

One of the most important ingredients in the team approach to nursing is a positive psychological and emotional bond between members of the team, which helps to develop more cohesiveness between the individuals of the team. Without a positive cohesive bond, there can and will be limits to the overall quality and function of the team. You as nurses are the unknown intervening variables that either make or

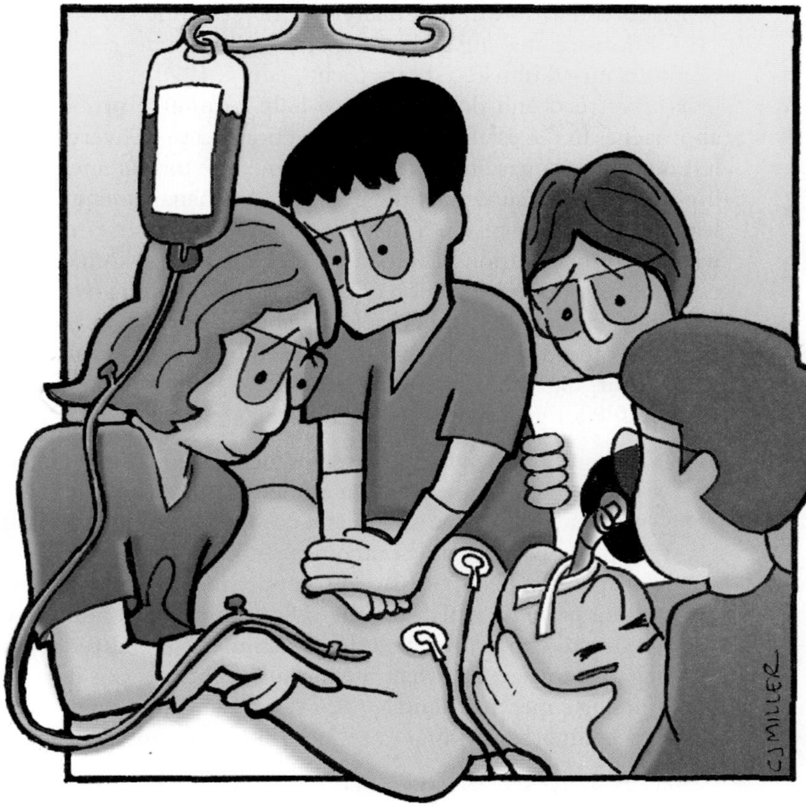

FIGURE 11-5
When nurses work as a team, everyone benefits.

break the quality of the team nursing concept. You and your colleagues, as a professional collective group, have the skills necessary to handle the multitudes of problems associated with care delivery. Questions you may want to ask yourselves are:

- Are you as an individual mentally and emotionally prepared for real-world nursing?
- Do you have and can you maintain a strong positive self-image?
- Is your attitude about yourself and your peers conducive to support team-directed nursing?
- Are you willing to make difficult decisions in directing team care delivery?
- Are you willing to relinquish control of those under your direction when necessary?
- You may want to take the following into consideration:
  - Does management actively and willing support the nursing staff?
  - Is the support constant, measurable, and appropriate to your needs?

Research has shown that many staff nurses prefer to be dependent on their superiors for decision making and are less willing to assume responsibility for care coordination of team-administered care (Schmieding, 1990).

Nurses read and do research to help formulate problem-solving and innovative approaches in the establishment of functional care-delivery models. What is frequently left out of the equation is the extent of the role management is willing to play in helping to ensure the success of the new ideas. Is management willing to share control and leadership to help ensure a successful outcome in nurse-managed teams? I have been witness to the creation of nursing leadership roles—some consisting of team nursing care delivery, decentralization of authority, and shared governance—only to have them fail due to limitations and perceived liabilities placed on the nursing staff by management. At other times, failures were caused by the last-minute intervention of management, usurping the managerial authority of the nursing teams. Some other factors responsible for group or team failure are:

- Nursing staff being unprepared or lacking the intrapersonal skills needed to work with other staff members in a unified team setting.
- Nurses unwilling to move in and out of leadership roles to ensure the unity of the group and best possible outcomes.
- Management being pressured by upper management for faster adaptation to cost-cutting policies, which usually causes communication between management and nursing to consist of veiled threats, innuendoes, mixed messages, and other subtle negative forms that affect the morale of the nursing staff.
- Nursing supervisors and administrative staff who appear to support shared governance but are unwilling to relinquish actual control of the nursing staff.

Action always speaks louder than words. Work toward open and honest communication with administrators. Try to meet them halfway and find out what they are willing to do to support your teams or groups. How much interest do they have in the actual quality of health care delivery? Are they interested in learning the dynamics of your role as a nurse or the role of the nursing team? Let them know what type of support you need from them. Explain to them the importance of mutual respect and support in the overall quality of nursing care.

When forming teams, realize that perfection is an illusion created in the mind of a critic. All of us have different skill levels. To function as a unified team, you will need to work with peers whose skills may need enhancing. You can help your peers by working side by side with them to build confidence while sharing in learning situations. Find ways of making the learning situations enjoyable, show a sense of humor, and give positive reinforcement whenever possible. Fear and guilt undermine confidence and destroy the cohesiveness of a team or group.

In the forming of any team or group, the mental and emotional stability of the individuals who make up the team or group will be reflected in the quality of their work under stress and their ability to focus during care delivery and to establish a working rapport with the other team members. It is important for the stronger team members or group members to involve themselves by giving support and guidance as needed. The attitude of the stronger members of the team can go a long way in building confidence in the other team members. The level of quality for any team is increased substantially by the level of comfort and camaraderie among the individuals who make up the team.

BOX 11-4 Basic Roles of Group Members

The following are some roles that individuals adopt when participating in a group. Each member may adopt more than one role.

- Opinion giver—states beliefs or values
- Opinion seeker—asks for clarification of beliefs or values
- Information giver—offers facts or personal experience
- Information seeker—asks for facts pertinent to what is being discussed
- Initiator—proposes new ideas on how the goal can be reached or how to view the problem
- Elaborator—expands on the idea of another; takes the idea and works out what would happen if it was adopted
- Coordinator—brings together ideas and suggestions
- Orientor—keeps the group focused on goals or questions the direction taken by the group
- Evaluator of critic—examines possible group solutions against group standards and goals
- Clarifier—checks out what someone said by restating or questioning
- Recorder—acts as the group's memory (e.g., takes notes)
- Summarizer—pulls together related ideas, restates suggestions, and offers decisions or conclusions

From Sullivan EJ, Decker P: *Effective leadership and management in nursing*, ed 4, Menlo Park, Calif, 1997, Addison-Wesley, p 144.

The mix of complementary skills and experience also can help to give strength to the overall group. Taking inventory of technical and communication skills helps identify where weakness and strengths need to be addressed or pointed out before assigning individual duties to the team members. The weaker team members should have learning opportunities, support, and guidance in order to strengthen the cohesiveness of the team.

Leadership roles in the team may be rotated to each member of the team. This allows the sharing of responsibilities and a chance to experience and test themselves in a leadership role. Most people will gravitate to their roles in a short period of time. It will be important for the team members to be able to communicate with each other, to ensure the quality and continuity of care to be delivered (Box 11-4, Critical Thinking Box 11-9, and Figure 11-6).

CRITICAL THINKING BOX 11-9

THINK ABOUT…

How is leading a group like the nursing process? The management process?

What motivates an individual to join a group? Stay in a group?

What group role do you adopt when participating in a group?

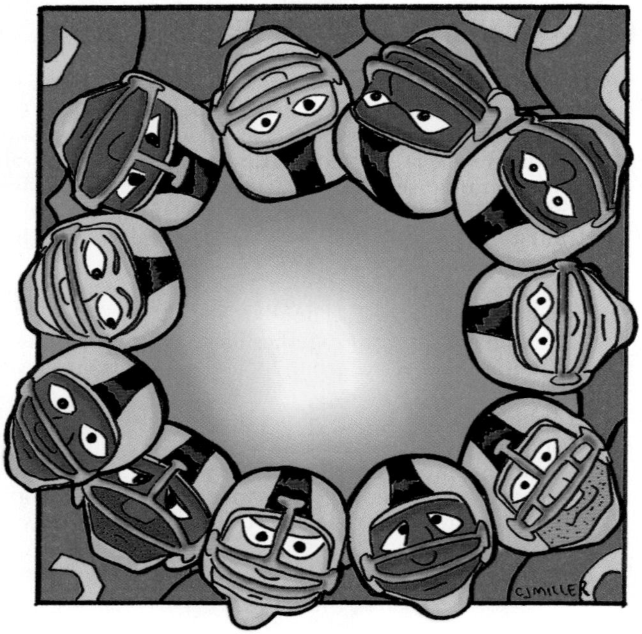

FIGURE 11-6
We win as a team!

ASSERTIVE STYLES OF COMMUNICATION

All of us have a style or way of communicating with others that is often based on our own personality and self-concept. In other words, the kind of person we are and the way in which we see ourselves influence the process of communication. This style can be divided into three common types: passive or avoidant, aggressive, and assertive (Marquis &Huston, 2000). The following are some characteristics of each style:

Passive or avoidant behavior means that a person lets others push him around; does not stand up for himself; does what he is told, regardless of how he feels about it; is not able to share his feelings or needs with others; has difficulty asking for help; and feels hurt, anxious, or angry at others for taking advantage of him.

Aggressive behavior means that a person puts his or her own needs, rights, and feelings first and communicates that in an angry, dominating way; attempts to humiliate or "put down" other people; conveys a righteous, superior attitude; works at controlling or manipulating others; is seen by others as punishing, threatening, demanding, or hostile; and shows no concern for anyone else's feelings.

Assertive behavior means that a person stands up for himself or herself in a way that does not violate the basic rights of another person; expresses true feelings in an honest, direct manner; does not let others take advantage of him or her; shows respect for others' rights, needs, and feelings; sets goals and acts on those goals in a clear and consistent manner and takes responsibility for the consequences of those actions; is able to accept compliments and criticism; and acts in a way that enhances self-respect.

See if you can match the person with his or her style by using the descriptions you have just read.

JANE

Jane is a very shy, quiet senior nursing student who can't think straight when her instructor asks her questions in the clinical area. She wishes she could be more like her classmates, who seem to find it easy to talk about their experiences during clinical conference. During her evaluation, her instructor says she doesn't know enough theory and can't handle the pressures of the clinical unit. Jane says nothing and signs her evaluation. When she gets back to her room alone, she cries uncontrollably.

SUSAN

Susan is a senior nursing student who is highly verbal with her classmates. She is known to be opinionated and in every conference with her clinical group finds a chance to criticize someone. She blames the nursing staff on the clinical unit for making her look bad by giving her too much work to do and not enough time or help. When her instructor tells her she has not used enough theory in her written assignments, she says, "It's not my fault; you should have told me sooner."

MARK

Mark is a senior nursing student who is described by his clinical group as goal-oriented and confident. He wrote learning objectives for himself at the beginning of the last clinical experience and brought them with him, along with a self-evaluation, for his final evaluation conference. He listened to his instructor's suggestions, thanked her, and said, "I appreciate your concern for the quality of my nursing skills. I'm aware now of what I need to pay attention to in my first few months in my new job."

If you decided that Jane used a passive or avoidant style, Susan used an aggressive style, and Mark used an assertive style, you were right. Congratulations!

WHY ARE NURSES NOT MORE ASSERTIVE?

It seems as though many nurses do not consistently act or communicate in an assertive way. Some have a hard time believing in their own rights, feelings, or needs. This difficulty may have gotten its start in childhood through exposure to many negative statements or experiences. It is important to recognize that communication style is learned and reinforced over time. While in nursing school and working in the nursing profession, additional experiences or comments may reinforce those negative messages about self-worth. It can be very difficult to change behavior, especially when risk-taking is necessary. The first step is to recognize what the barriers are. What is it that prevents you from being more assertive? Is it previously learned behavior, or are you afraid of the repercussions of assertive communication? Check the list in Box 11-5. If this list

BOX 11-5 Barriers to Assertiveness

- Assertive communication should not threaten others.
- If you do not have anything nice to say, do not say anything at all.
- If you feel uncomfortable when presenting your position or stating your feelings, then you are nonassertive.
- Assertiveness should come easily and spontaneously.
- Health care facilities do not promote or support assertive behavior.
- You cannot be assertive and consider another person's feelings and behavior.
- Assertive behavior is just another way of complaining.
- If I am assertive, I will lose my job.
- There is no difference between assertiveness and aggressiveness.

includes statements you feel are true, then you have identified some roadblocks to your ability to develop more assertive communication.

Look over this list of barriers to assertive communication and think about yourself. Do any of these explain your feelings? Assertiveness takes self-awareness and practice. It will help you to identify and accept your position right now with regard to assertiveness so that you can make a plan to develop this skill.

WHAT ARE THE BENEFITS OF ASSERTIVENESS?

Assertive communication is the most effective way to let other people know what you feel, what you need, and what you are thinking. It helps you to feel good about yourself and allows you to treat others with respect. Being assertive helps you to avoid feeling guilty, angry, resentful, confused, or lonely. You have a greater chance to get your rights acknowledged and your needs met, which leads to a more satisfying life.

WHAT ARE MY BASIC RIGHTS AS A PERSON AND AS A NURSE?

As an adult human being, you have some legitimate rights. You may have to do some work to allow yourself to believe in your rights. You may have learned other values that make it difficult to accept the validity of these rights. But belief in your own value as a separate individual and confidence in the positive concepts associated with assertiveness as a communication style will help you to believe in your rights.

Consider the rights and responsibilities of the nurse. The issue of rights can become one-sided. When nurses consider rights, responsibilities must also be included. These rights are yours as a registered nurse; acquiring them and holding them are your responsibility (Chenevert, 1988).

HOW CAN I BEGIN TO PRACTICE ASSERTIVE COMMUNICATION?

There are a variety of ways to learn to be more assertive in your communication style, but they all involve self-awareness and practice. It may not feel totally comfortable at first, but as you work at it, assertive communication will come more naturally.

Changing one's behavior requires a conscious decision.

You should practice being assertive in a situation where there is minimal risk to you, so that you can experience success. If sharing your feelings with your instructor or head nurse makes you extremely uncomfortable, set the situation aside. You can work on it after you are more confident. Share your feelings and practice being assertive with someone with whom you are comfortable. Personal risk should be at a minimum.

It is helpful to practice being assertive by yourself at first. Rehearse what you might say by talking to yourself while looking in a mirror. Once you feel more comfortable, ask a friend to help you practice. The two of you can role-play some assertive conversations. You may even want to videotape or audiotape your practice so you can get an idea of how you look and how you sound. When you are ready, try out your new assertive communication skills in a mildly uncomfortable situation you would like to change. Pay attention to how you feel. Ask for feedback from the other person. You will then be able to evaluate your progress and decide what other information you want to practice.

WHAT ARE THE COMPONENTS OF ASSERTIVE COMMUNICATION?

When you communicate assertively, you are able to describe your own feelings and needs, listen to and acknowledge the other person's feelings and needs, define the problem clearly and nonjudgmentally, use body language confidently, and negotiate a workable compromise (Mindell, 2001).

Following are two ways to think about expressing your feelings and needs:

STRATEGY 1:

I think…

I feel…

I want…

STRATEGY 2:

I feel… about… because…

Let us look at an example for each of these.

- I think we've been working every evening for 2 weeks on that report for the nursing office.
- I feel tired and cranky because I'm not paying enough attention to my family's needs.
- I want to ask someone else to write a section of the report.
- I feel hurt and angry about Dr. Jones yelling at me in front of you because I need to feel competent and respected at work.

These statements can be successful when you maintain direct eye contact, stand up straight, and speak in a clear, audible, firm tone of voice. After expressing your own feelings and needs, it is helpful to seek clarification of the other person's feelings or needs. This can be done with the following questions:

"How do you feel about that?"

"What were you thinking and feeling at that time?"

"How would that affect you?"

With skillful listening and clear communication, the problem can be defined without placing blame or "putting down" the other person. Notice the use of "I" messages. That indicates willingness to accept responsibility for the process of defining the problem and negotiating a workable solution. To find a compromise, you have to be willing to meet the other person halfway. You may agree to try it your way one time and the other person's the next. Or you may both agree to change or give up something. You may do something for him or her if she does something else for you. Remember that in the work setting you cannot always have things exactly as you want them. You must be willing to change and compromise (Elgin, 2000).

WHEN TO USE ASSERTIVE COMMUNICATION

Let us look at some examples of situations in which assertive communication would be helpful.

Communicating Expectations

Supervisor: "You're being pulled to the orthopedic unit today because they're short-staffed."

Nurse: "I expect to be oriented into the unit and the equipment before I give nursing care because I haven't worked on that unit in more than a year."

Saying No

Physician: "Come with me right now. I need some help doing a procedure on Mr. Smith."

Nurse: "No, I can't come with you right now. I'm doing a nursing assessment on Mrs. Anderson. I'll be finished in 20 minutes and will help you then."

Accepting Criticism

Head Nurse: "It seems to me that you aren't very good at doing care plans, and they're never done on time."

Nurse: "I have been falling behind on my care plans. I would like to look at some examples of good care plans. Do you think you could help me with that? I'd be willing to spend some time at home reviewing them."

Accepting Compliments

Home care patient's spouse: "You give really thorough care. It's obvious you know what you're doing."

Nurse: "Thank you. Your feedback is important to me."

Giving Criticism

Nurse: "I want to talk with you about your care of Mrs. Samuelson. I found her sitting in a wheelchair alone in the hallway. It is your responsibility to make sure that she is not left alone, so that nothing happens to her."

Aide: "I do not think that's my job."

Nurse: "We talked about your responsibilities this morning when you got your assignment. I expect you to complete your assignment as directed or ask for help."

Providing Feedback

Head Nurse: "I wanted to tell you that I have noticed an improvement in your relationship with Dr. Turner. He has not complained about his patients' care for 2 weeks, and yesterday he told me that he had a satisfying discussion with you about home health care options for Mrs. Atkins."

Nurse: "Thank you. I have been working very hard at not responding angrily to his sarcastic comments and criticisms."

Asking for Help

Nurse: "It is hard for me to do this because I expect myself to care for all patients without difficulty. But I am having a hard time with Mr. Jones. He seems to have a way of pushing my buttons so I get angry."

Community Health Nurse Supervisor: "Are you asking me for something?"

Nurse: "Yes. I need help in understanding why I get so angry at him, and I want to know how to handle him in a more positive way."

Remember that you need to evaluate how your assertive communication feels to you and you need to seek feedback from other people about how you are being interpreted. You need to know whether people perceive you as aggressive rather than assertive. It may mean modifying your communication to make sure you are standing up for yourself without violating the rights of others.

It should also be noted that some situations will not get resolved just because you communicated assertively. Finding a workable solution is a process involving other people who must take responsibility for their own feelings and needs. When others are unable to acknowledge their feelings, to listen, or to negotiate a compromise, your assertive communication may make you feel better about yourself but may not produce an immediate solution. But keep trying. Persistence pays off.

Remember, too, that there are some situations in which you must simply follow orders. You cannot always meet your own needs; you must do what a physician or your head nurse tells you to do. Sometimes you must put aside your own needs to meet the needs of the patients you are caring for. However, your judgment will increase as you gain experience, and you will recognize ways to communicate your needs and feelings, with the goal of improving the processes and procedures used in your work setting.

CONCLUSION

Interpersonal skills, effective communication, group process, and team building are important to the nurse, as they form the foundation for creating an effective working environment. Well-planned, well-executed, and well-validated communication, along with caring and a positive attitude will foster motivation, success, and satisfaction for the nurse in both the student role and as a new graduate.

Now that you have learned a lot about communicating effectively, try doing the student exercise in Critical Thinking Box 11-10. And happy communicating!

CRITICAL THINKING BOX 11-10

COMMUNICATION EXERCISE

Directions: Use the following situations to reflect on key points covered in this chapter. Think of a way to communicate effectively in each situation. You may want to consider your own individual solutions and then role-play or discuss your ideas with a group of your classmates.

1. Develop a list of 10 patients who are hospitalized on your unit. Give for each patient some personal information, a diagnosis, and some data about his or her progress during the last 24 hours. Use the information you have listed to give a change of shift report to the four staff members who will be caring for these patients during the next 8 hours.
2. You have asked to speak to Dr. Sanders about your concerns in caring for one of her patients who has required much physical care since she has gone home from the hospital. Dr. Sanders has a reputation for being cold, aloof, and sarcastic. You have never spoken directly to her alone before.
3. You are a member of the home health care agency's procedures committee. After attending the last meeting, you have been given the responsibility for drafting a revision to the procedure used when administering controlled substances. You know that you need more information before you can begin your work. Send a memo to at least three different members of the agency staff identifying what information you would like them to provide for you. Make a follow-up phone call to make sure.

REFERENCES

Arredondo L: *Communicating effectively*, New York, 2000, McGraw-Hill.

Chenevert M: *Pro-nurse handbook*, ed 3, St Louis, 1988, Mosby.

de Bono E: *Six thinking hats*, 1999, MICA Management Resources, *www.debonogroup.com/6hats.htm.*

Deep S, Sussman L: *Smart moves for people in charge*, Reading, Mass, 1995, Addison-Wesley.

Dochterman J, Grace H: *Current issues in nursing*, ed 6, St Louis, 2001, Mosby.

Dowling E: *10 Tips for effective e-mail*, 2005, MindTools, *www.mindtools.com/email.html.*

Elgin S: *The gentle art of verbal self-defense at work*, Paramus, NJ, 2000, Prentice Hall.

Farley MJ, Stoner MH: The nurse executive and interdisciplinary team building, *Nurs Adm Q* 13(2):24-30, 1989.

Fowler, K: *Active Listening*. Mindtools, 2005, *www.mindtools.com/CommSkll/ActiveListening.htm.*

Huber D: *Leadership and nursing care management*, Philadelphia, 2000, Saunders.

Katzenbach JR, Smith DK: *Wisdom of teams*, New York, 1993, Harper Business.

Kushner M: *Successful presentations for dummies*, Foster City, Calif, 1997, IDG.

Marquis B, Huston C: *Leadership roles and management functions in nursing: theory and application*, ed 3, Philadelphia, 2000, JB Lippincott.

Mindell P: *How to say it for women: communicating with confidence and power using the language of success*, Paramus, NJ, 2001, Prentice Hall.

Northouse P: *Leadership theory and practice*, ed 2, Thousand Oaks, Calif, 2001, Sage.

Peoples DA: *Presentations plus*, New York, 1992, John Wiley & Sons.

Schmieding NJ: A model for assessing nurse administrators' actions, *West J Nurs Resh* 12(3):293-306, 1990.

Sovie MD: Care and service teams: a new imperative, *Nurs Econ* 10(2):94-100, 125, 1992.

Strayhorn JM Jr: *Talking it out: a guide to effective communication and problem solving*, Champaign, Ill, 1977, Research.

Sullivan EJ, Decker PJ: *Effective leadership and management in nursing*, ed 4, Menlo Park, Calif, 1997, Addison-Wesley.

Tuckman B, Jensen M: Stage of small group development revisited, *Group Organiz Stud* 2:419-427, 1977.

Vengel A: *The influence edge: how to persuade others to help you achieve your goals*, San Francisco, 2000, Berrett-Koehler Communications.

CHAPTER 12

CONFLICT MANAGEMENT

JOANN ZERWEKH, EdD, RN, FNP, APRN, BC

Everything that irritates us about others can lead us to an understanding of ourselves.
—*Carl Jung*

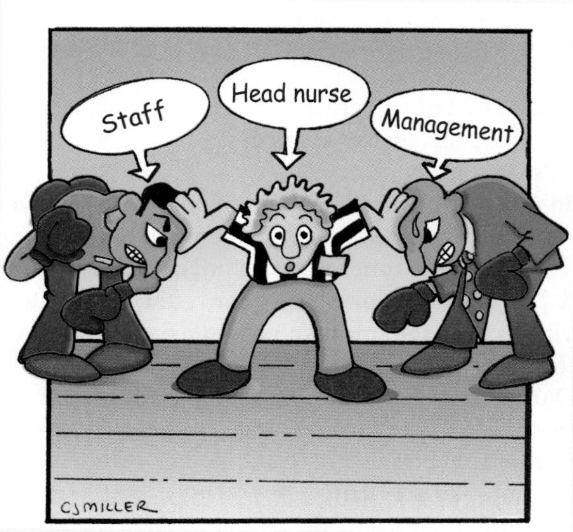

There is a better approach to conflict resolution than fighting it out.

After completing this chapter, you should be able to:

- Identify common factors that lead to conflict.
- Discuss five methods to resolve conflict.
- Discuss techniques to use in dealing with difficult people.
- Discuss solutions and alternatives in dealing with anger.
- Identify situations of sexual harassment in the workplace and discuss possible solutions.

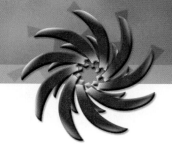

Can you imagine a world without conflict? Why, it would be a world without change! Conflict is inevitable wherever there are people with differing backgrounds, needs, values, and priorities. The presence of conflict in a situation is not necessarily negative but may, in fact, have some positive results. As a process, conflict is neutral. Following are some possible outcomes of conflict:

- Disturbing issues are brought out into the open, which may avert a more serious conflict.
- Group cohesiveness may increase as individuals resolve issues.
- New leadership may develop as a consequence of resolution.
- The results of conflict can be constructive, which occur when productive outcomes are achieved; or destructive, leading to poor communication and creating dissatisfaction.

CONFLICT

WHAT CAUSES CONFLICT?

Let us look at some common factors of conflict as they relate to nursing.

Role Conflict When two people have the same or related responsibilities with ambiguous boundaries, the potential for conflict exists. For example, a nurse on the 11 PM to 7 AM shift may be uncertain whether he or the nurse on the 7 AM to 3 PM shift is responsible for administering enemas until clear on a patient scheduled for a barium enema.

Communication Conflict Failing to discuss differences with one another can lead to problems with communication. Communication is a two-way process; when one person is unclear in a communication, the process falls apart. A recent graduate may find that with a busy schedule, numerous patient demands, and a shortage of time, it is easy to forget to notify a patient's family of a change in visiting hours—a great annoyance to the family members who cannot visit when they arrive.

Goal Conflict We all have unique goals and objectives for what we hope to achieve in our places of employment. When one nurse places his or her personal achievement and advancement above everyone else's, conflict can occur.

Personality Conflict. Wouldn't it be great if we got along with everyone? Of course we all know that there are just some people with whom we have a difficult time. The situation is all too familiar, and many times we may find ourselves with such thoughts as "I'll try and overlook her negative, lousy behavior; after all she doesn't have much of a family life." Trying to change another person's personality is like guaranteeing an unhappy ending to a story.

Ethical or Values Conflict During a cardiac arrest, a young graduate nurse has difficulty with the physician's order of "No Code," on a young adolescent patient. She has difficulty taking care of the adolescent because he reminds her of her younger brother who died tragically in an automobile accident.

Conflicts in nursing may fit into one or more of the aforementioned categories. Consider some common areas of conflict among nursing staff, including scheduling days off, determining vacation leave, assigning committees, patient care assignments, and performance appraisal, to name just a few.

WHAT ARE COMMON AREAS OF CONFLICT BETWEEN NURSES AND PATIENTS—AND BETWEEN NURSES AND PATIENTS' FAMILIES?

Guttenberg (1983) identifies five common areas of conflict among nurses and their patients and families.

1. Quality of care. This is by far the most common area of conflict and the easiest to remedy. Families typically are concerned with how well their loved one is being attended to, how friendly the nurses are, how well the hospital or home health services are provided and coordinated, and how flexible the hospital is with visiting hours and meeting their special needs.

2. Treatment decisions. This area of conflict often arises between the family of an elderly adult and the nurse. A physician may order a treatment with which the family does not agree. In this situation it is very important that the nurse not defend the physician's orders or attempt to persuade or establish with the family that the physician or nurse knows what's best for the patient. In these situations the issue is rarely the treatment itself but rather the family's desire to decide what is right for their loved one. Be sure to clarify the orders and explain to the family that you are supposed to carry them out unless the family negotiates directly with the physician to change them.

3. Family involvement. The situation of a young adult diagnosed with cancer illustrates numerous issues that may arise concerning the presence of family members during procedures and the extent of their involvement in the overall care. Such issues are based on the family's real need to feel significant and adequate in meeting the young adult's needs.

4. Quality of parental care. This can become an issue when nurses are unhappy with how the parents are participating in their child's care. It is helpful to offer parenting classes, to encourage parents to meet other parents, and to model positive parenting techniques.

5. Staff inconsistency. This is another easily preventable issue. Make sure that each shift is consistent in enforcing hospital policies and that they notify other shifts of any attempts at manipulation by family members or patients.

CONFLICT RESOLUTION

WHAT ARE WAYS TO RESOLVE CONFLICT?

Unresolved conflicts waste time and energy and reduce productivity and cooperation among the people with whom you work. In contrast, when conflicts are resolved, they strengthen relationships and improve the performance of everyone involved. The key to successfully managing conflict is tailoring your response to fit each conflict situation instead of just relying on one particular technique. Each technique represents a different way to achieve the outcome you want and to help the other person achieve at least part of the outcome that he or she wants. How do you know which technique to use? That depends on the following:

- How much power do you have in this situation compared with the other person?
- How much do you value your relationship with the person with whom you are in conflict?
- How much time is available to resolve the conflict?

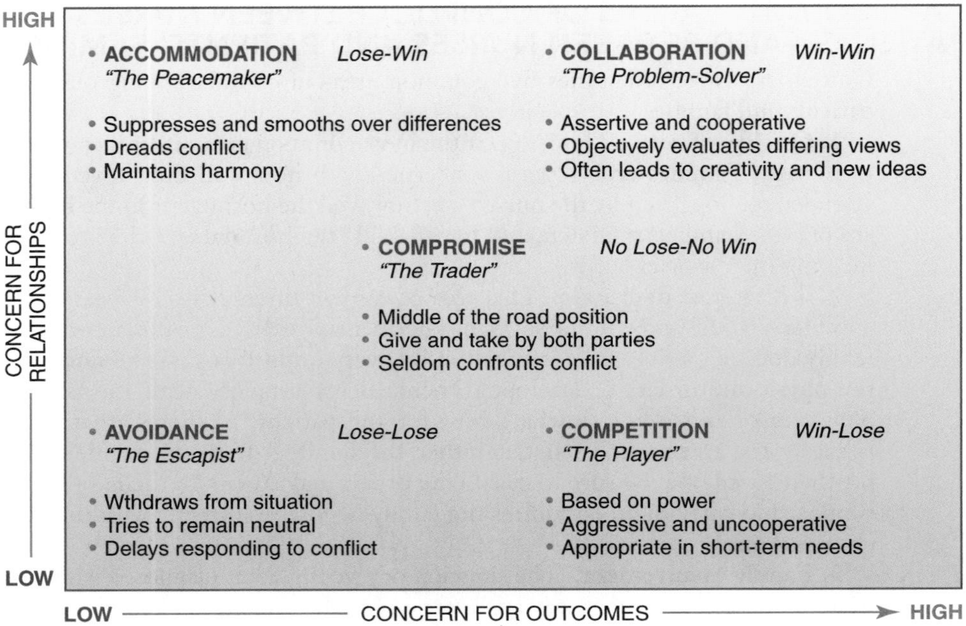

FIGURE 12-1

Model for conflict resolution. *(Modified from Douglas E, Bushardt W: Interpersonal conflict: strategies and guidelines for resolution,* J AMRA *56[18], 1988; and Sullivan E, Decker P:* Effective management in nursing, *Menlo Park, Calif, 1988, Addison-Wesley.)*

An example of a model for conflict resolution can be found in Figure 12-1. This model incorporates several views on conflict resolution. Filley (1975) described three basic strategies for dealing with conflict according to outcome: win-win, lose-lose, and win-lose. Various others have identified five responses to resolve conflict. They are as follows: competition, accommodation, avoidance, compromise, and cooperation. Let us look at an example and apply the model.

Suppose the head nurse on your unit has posted the vacations for the month of December. You, as a recent graduate, have requested to be off during the week of Christmas so that you can be with your family. You notice on the schedule that none of the recent graduates has received the Christmas holidays off. You feel that this is unfair because you will not have an opportunity to be with your family during the Christmas holidays. How can you resolve this conflict?

Competition. This is an example of the *win-lose* situation. In this situation, force—or the use of power—occurs. It sets up a type of competition between you and your head nurse. Typically, competition is used to resolve conflict when one person has more power in a situation than the other. *In the given situation, the head nurse refuses your request for Christmas vacation, explaining that the staff members with more seniority have priority for vacation at Christmas time.*

Avoidance. Avoidance is unassertive and uncooperative, and leads to a *lose-lose* situation. In some situations, avoidance is not considered a true form of conflict resolution because the conflict is not resolved and neither party is satisfied. *In the given situation, you would not have approached the head nurse with the Christmas schedule issue.* Usually both persons involved feel frustrated and angry. There are some situations in which avoiding the issue might be appropriate, such as when tempers are flaring or when strong anger is present. However, this is only a short-term strategy; it is important to get back to the problem after emotions have cooled.

Accommodation. In the given situation, the head nurse would basically put her own concern aside and let you have your way, possibly even working in the scheduled slot for you. Accommodation is the lose-win situation, in which you accommodate the other person at your own expense but often end up feeling resentful and angry. The head nurse loses and the graduate nurse wins in this situation, which may set up conflict among staff and other recent graduates. When is accommodation the best response? Is it when conflict would create serious disruption, such as arguing, or when the person you are in conflict with has the power to resolve the conflict unilaterally? Basically, in this response to conflict, differences are suppressed or played down while agreement is emphasized.

Compromise. Compromise or bargaining is the strategy that recognizes the importance of both the resolution of the problem and the relationship between the two people. Compromise is a moderately assertive and cooperative step in the right direction in which one creates a *modified win-lose* outcome. *In the given situation, the head nurse compromises with you by allowing you to have Christmas Eve off with your family, but not the entire week. The problem lies in the reduced staffing that will occur for a short period of time. The compromise may not be totally satisfactory for either party, but it may be offered as a temporary solution until more options become available.*

Collaboration. Collaboration is the strategy that involves a high level of concern for the problem, the outcome, and the relationship. It deals with confrontation and problem solving. The needs, feelings, and desires of both parties are taken into consideration and reexamined while searching for proper ways to agree on goals. Collaboration is a *win-win* solution, a commitment to resolve the issues at the base of the conflict. It is fully assertive and cooperative. *In the given situation, you and the head nurse discuss the week of Christmas vacation and the staffing needs and agree that you will work the first three days of that week and the head nurse will work the second half of that week. You also agree to be there the first part of the week to complete the audit on the charts from the previous week for the head nurse. In this situation both persons are satisfied, and there is no compromising what is most important to each person. That is, the head nurse gets her audit completed and the recent graduate gets to spend half of the Christmas week with her family.* What is your particular style for resolving conflict (Critical Thinking Box 12-1)?

WHAT ARE SOME BASIC GUIDELINES FOR WHICH TECHNIQUE TO USE?

In some situations, certain techniques and responses work best. You may have to use accommodation or avoidance when you lack the power to change the situation. When you have conflict in a relationship that you value, it might be more helpful to use accommodation, compromise, or collaboration. When there is no immediate, pressing sense of time to solve an issue, then any of the five techniques can be used. However, when you are facing an emergency situation or a rapidly approaching deadline, your

CRITICAL THINKING BOX 12-1

CONFLICT QUESTIONNAIRE

Directions: Consider situations in which you find your wishes differing from those of another person. For each of the following statements, think how likely you are to respond in that way to such a situation. Check the rating that best corresponds to your response.

	Very Unlikely	Unlikely	Very Likely	Likely
1. I am usually firm in pursuing my goals.	______	______	______	______
2. I try to win my position.	______	______	______	______
3. I give up some points in exchange for others.	______	______	______	______
4. I feel that differences are not always worth worrying about.	______	______	______	______
5. I try to find a position that is between others and mine.	______	______	______	______
6. In approaching a negotiation, I try to consider the other person's wishes.	______	______	______	______
7. I try to show the logic and benefits of my position.	______	______	______	______
8. I always lean toward a direct discussion of the problem.	______	______	______	______
CRITICAL				
9. I try to find a fair combination of gains and losses for both of us.	______	______	______	______
10. I attempt to work through our differences immediately.	______	______	______	______
11. I try to avoid creating unpleasantness for myself.	______	______	______	______
12. I might try to soothe the other's feelings and preserve our relationship.	______	______	______	______
13. I attempt to get all concerns and issues immediately out.	______	______	______	______
14. I sometimes avoid taking positions that create controversy.	______	______	______	______
15. I try not to hurt the other's feelings.	______	______	______	______

Continued

CRITICAL THINKING BOX 12-1—cont'd

SCORING: Very Unlikely = 1; Unlikely = 2; Likely = 3; Very Likely = 4.

	Item:	Item:	Item:	
COMPETING:	1 _____	2 _____	7 _____	TOTAL _______
COLLABORATING:	8 _____	10 _____	13 _____	TOTAL _______
COMPROMISING:	3 _____	5 _____	9 _____	TOTAL _______
AVOIDING:	4 _____	11 _____	14 _____	TOTAL _______
ACCOMMODATING:	6 _____	12 _____	15 _____	TOTAL _______

From Thomas KW: Toward multidimensional values in teaching: the example of conflict behaviors, *Acad Manage Rev* 2:487.

best bet is to use competition or accommodation. Just remember the following key behaviors in managing conflict:

- Deal with issues, not personalities.
- Take responsibility for yourself and your participation.
- Communicate openly.
- Listen actively.
- Sort out the issues.
- Identify key themes in the discussion.
- Weigh the consequences.

Suppose that you follow all of these suggestions and you still are confronted with that difficult situation or that difficult person. Read on.

DEALING WITH DIFFICULT PEOPLE

WHAT ARE SOME TECHNIQUES FOR HANDLING DIFFICULT PEOPLE?

Now that we have discussed types of conflict management techniques, we are ready to look at techniques for handling difficult people. How do you deal with an abusive physician or supervisor? How do you react when someone constantly complains and gripes about something? How do you deal with the know-it-all who will not even listen to your thoughts on an issue?

I am sure, if you have not by now, you will in the near future run into a Sherman tank (Figure 12-2). According to Bramson (1981), Sherman tanks are the *attackers*. They come out charging and are often abusive, abrupt, and intimidating. But more importantly, they tend to be downright overwhelming.

Remember Dr. Smith, who flew into a tirade because you forgot to have a suture removal set at his patient's bedside at 8 AM sharp? Remember how you felt? "My heart was beating so loud I could hear it, and I was sure everyone else around could hear it, too. I was so furious at him for the comments he made."

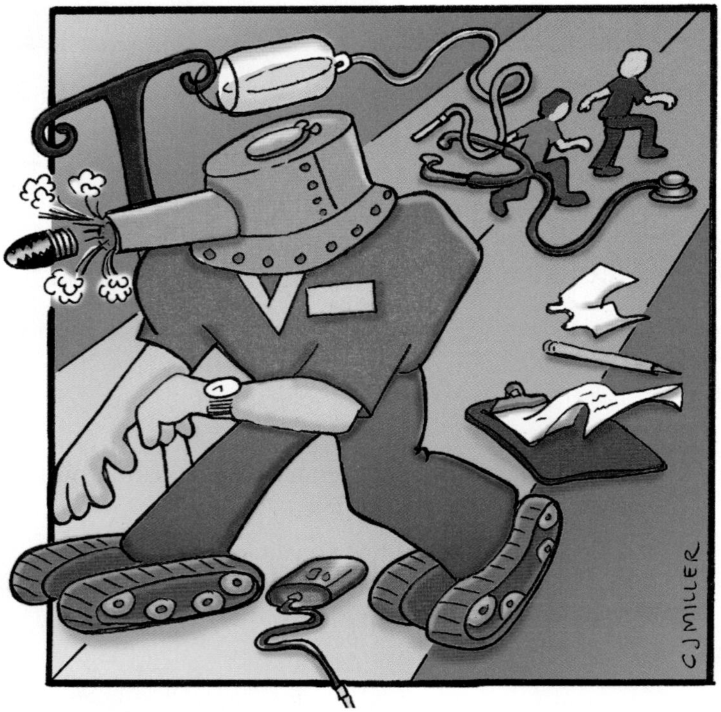

FIGURE 12-2
Sherman Tank.

In understanding Sherman tanks, it is important to realize that they have a strong need to prove to themselves and to others that their view of the situation is right. They have a very strong sense of what others ought to do but often lack the caring and the trust that would be helpful in getting something done. They usually achieve what they want, but to do so causes them a lot of disagreements, lost friendships, and uncomfortable relationships with their co-workers. Sherman tanks are often very confident and tend to devalue those who they feel are not confident. Unfortunately, they demean others in a way that makes them look very self-important and superior. How do you cope with a Sherman tank? The most important thing is to keep your fear and anger under control and avoid an outright confrontation about who is right and who is wrong. Following are some specific things you should do:

- Do not allow yourself to be run over; step aside.
- Stand up for yourself. Defend yourself, but without fighting.
- Give them a little time to run down and express what they might be ranting about.
- Sometimes, it is necessary to be rude; get your word in any way that you can.
- If possible, try to get them to sit down. Be sure to maintain eye contact with them while you are stating your opinions and perceptions very forcefully.

- Do not argue with them or try to cut them down.
- When they finally hear you, be ready to be friendly.

Next to the Sherman tanks are the *snipers* (Figure 12-3). The snipers are the pot-shot artists. They are not as openly aggressive as the Sherman tanks. Their weapons are their innuendoes, their digs, and their nonplayful teasing, which is definitely aimed to hurt you. Snipers tend to choose a hidden rather than a frontal attack. They prefer to undercut you and make you look ridiculous. So, when you are dealing with a sniper, remember to expose the attack, that is, "smoke them out." Ask them very calmly:

"That sounded like a put-down. Did you really mean it that way?" Or you might say,
"Do I understand that you don't like what I'm saying? It sounds as if you are making fun of me. Are you?"

When a sniper is giving you criticism, be sure to get group confirmation or denial. Ask questions or make statements such as, "Does anyone else see the issue this way?" "It seems as though we have a difference of opinion," or "Exactly what is the issue here?

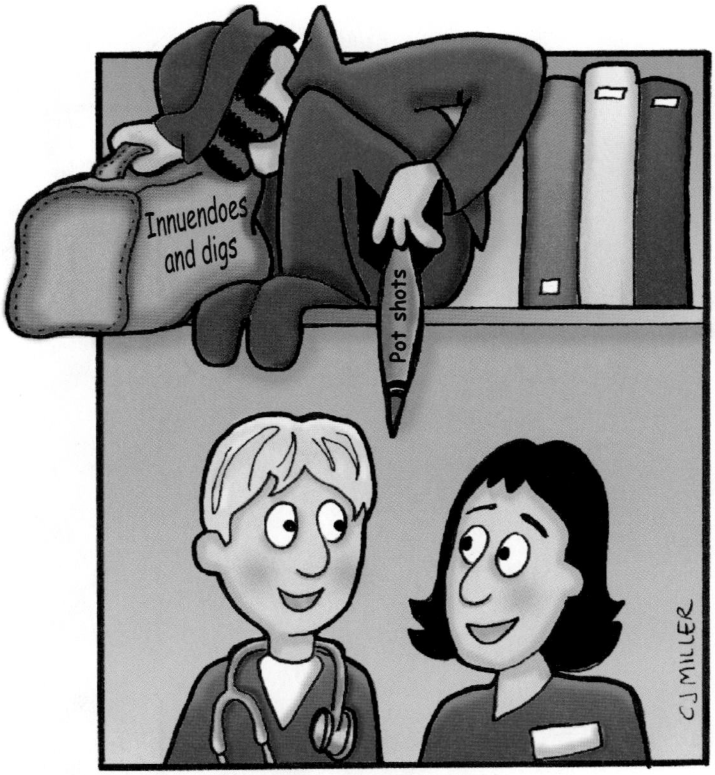

FIGURE 12-3
The Sniper.

What is it that you don't like about what occurred?" One way to prevent sniping is by setting up regular problem-solving meetings with that person.

Another difficult person to cope with is the constant complainer. They often feel as though they are powerless and get attention—but seldom action—on their problem. A complainer points out real problems but does it from a very nonconstructive stance. Coping with a complainer can be a challenge. First, it is important to listen to the complaints, then acknowledge them and make sure you understand what the person said by paraphrasing it or checking out your perception of how the person feels. Do not necessarily agree with them; with a complainer, it is important to move into a problem-solving mode by asking very specific, informative questions and encouraging them to submit complaints in writing. For example, try communicating with the constant complainer in the following manner:

"Did I understand you to say that you are having difficulty with your patient assignment?"

"Would it be helpful if I went to the pharmacy for you, so that you could complete your chart on your preoperative patient?"

Next are the maddening ones: the *clams* (Figure 12-4). The clams have an entirely different tactic from the previous three. They just refuse to respond when you need

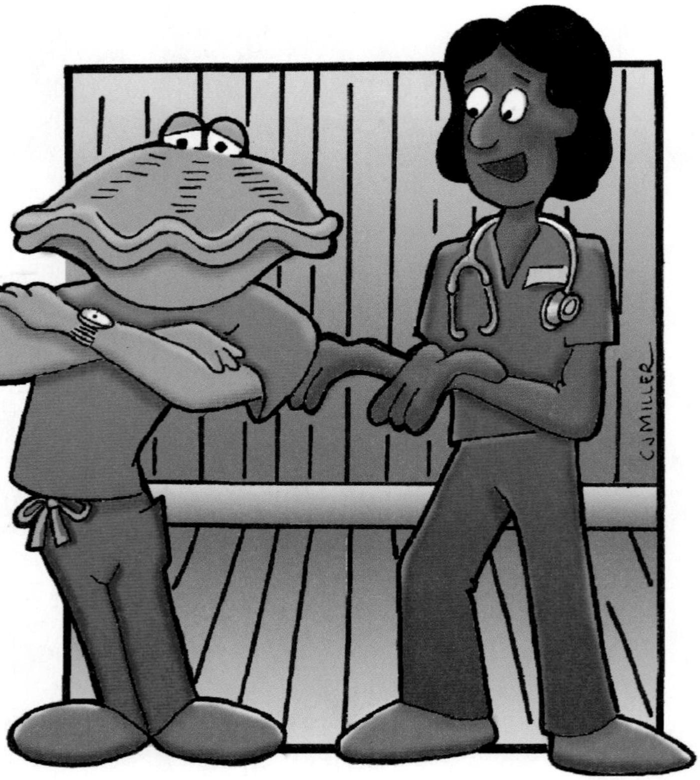

FIGURE 12-4
The Clam.

an answer or want conversation. It might be helpful to try to read a clam's nonverbal communication. Watch out for wrinkled brows, a frown, or a sigh. How to deal with a clam? Try to get them to open up by using open-ended questions and waiting very quietly for a response. Do not fill in their silence with your conversation. Give yourself enough time to wait with composure. Sometimes a little "clamming" on your own part might be helpful by using the technique called the "friendly, silent stare," or FSS. The way to set up the FSS is to have a very inquisitive, expectant expression on your face with raised eyebrows, wide eyes, and maybe a slight smile—all nonverbal cues to the clam that you are waiting for a response. When clams finally open up, be very attentive. Watch your own impulses—do not bubble over with happiness that they have finally given you two moments of their time. Avoid the polite ending; in other words, get up and say,

> **"This was important to me. I'm not going to let this issue drop. I'll be back to talk to you tomorrow at 2 o'clock." Do not be the nice guy and say, "Thanks for coming in. Have a nice weekend. I'll see you tomorrow."**

Be very direct, and inform the clam what you are going to do, especially if the desired discussion did not occur.

WHAT IS ANGER?

Anger is something that we feel. Usually when we get angry, we assume it is because we are upset about what someone has done to us. Often we want to pay them back or take out our rage on them. Usually when anger occurs, it is hard to see beyond the moment because most people are consumed with thoughts of revenge or the wrongdoing that has occurred to them. Weiss and Cain (1991) state that "Anger is often a cover-up emotion… that disguises what is really going on inside you." But, anger is a signal, and according to Lerner (1997), it is "one worth listening to." She goes on further to say that:

> Our anger may be a message that we are being hurt, that our rights are being violated, that our needs or wants are not being adequately met, or simply that something is not right. Our anger may tell us that we are not addressing an important emotional issue in our lives, or that too much of ourselves—our beliefs, values, desires, or ambitions—are being compromised in a relationship. Our anger may be a signal that we are doing more and giving more than we can comfortably do or give. Or our anger may warn us that others are doing too much for us, at the expense of our own competence and growth. Just as physical pain tells us to take our hand off the hot stove, the pain of our anger preserves the very integrity of our self. Our anger can motivate us to say "no" to the ways in which we are defined by others and "yes" to the dictates of our inner self.

No matter what, when feelings of frustration, disappointment, or powerlessness take over, there is no doubt anger is in the making. Anger seems to begin in situations fraught with threats and anxiety.

Anger has two faces. One is *guilt*, which is anger aimed inward at what we did or did not do, and the other is *resentment*, which is anger directed toward others at what they did or did not do.

> The following is true about both guilt and resentment: They both accumulate over time and lead to a cycle of negative energy that poisons our relationships and stifles our personal growth.

However, there is another side of the coin. If feeling angry signifies a problem, then ventilating anger does not necessarily solve it. Actually, ventilating anger may serve to maintain it if change and successful resolution do not occur. Tavris (1984) suggests that we teach two things about dealing with anger: first, how to think about anger and second, how to reduce the tension. More about this later in the chapter.

Lerner (1997) gives some helpful advice on how to determine your characteristic style of managing anger. Box 12-1 has a summary of five different anger styles. Just think about anger from a cardiovascular point of view. Most authorities consider anger one of the most damaging and dangerous emotions because your pulse and blood pressure become elevated, sometimes to dangerous heights.

BOX 12-1 Characteristic Styles of Managing Anger

PURSUERS

- React to anxiety by seeking greater togetherness in a relationship.
- Place a high value on talking things out and expressing feelings.
- Alone or away from the relationship.
- Tend to pursue harder and then coldly withdraw when an important person seeks distance.
- May negatively label themselves as "too dependent" or "too demanding" in a relationship.
- Tend to criticize their partner as someone who cannot handle feelings or tolerate closeness.

DISTANCERS

- Seek emotional distance or physical space when stress is high.
- Consider themselves to be self-reliant and private persons—more "do-it-yourselfers" than help-seekers.
- Have difficulty showing their needy, vulnerable, and dependent sides.
- Receive such labels as "emotionally unavailable," "withholding," and "unable to deal with feeling" from significant others.
- Manage anxiety in personal relationships by intensifying work-related projects.
- May cut off a relationship entirely when things get intense.
- Open up most freely when they are not pushed or pursued.

UNDERFUNCTIONERS

- Tend to have several areas in which they just cannot get organized.
- Become less competent under stress, thus inviting others to take over.
- Tend to develop physical or emotional symptoms when stress is high in either the family or the work situation.
- May become the focus of family gossip.
- Earn such labels as the "patient," the "fragile one," "the sick one," the "problem," or the "irresponsible one."
- Have difficulty showing their strong, competent side to intimate others.

OVERFUNCTIONERS

- Know what is best not only for themselves but for others as well.
- Move in quickly to advise, rescue, and take over when stress hits.
- Have difficulty staying out and allowing others to struggle with their own problems.

Continued

BOX 12-1 Characteristic Styles of Managing Anger—cont'd

- Avoid worrying about their own personal goals and problems by focusing on others.
- Have difficulty sharing their own vulnerable, underfunctioning side, especially with those people who are viewed as having problems.
- May be labeled the person who is "always reliable" or "always together."

BLAMERS
- Respond to anxiety with emotional intensity and fighting.
- Have a short fuse.
- Expend high levels of energy trying to change someone who does not want to change.
- Engage in repetitive cycles of fighting that relieve tension but perpetuate the old pattern.
- Hold another person responsible for one's own feelings and actions.
- See others as the sole obstacle to making changes.

Modified from Lerner H: *The dance of anger: a woman's guide to changing the patterns of intimate relationships*, New York, 1985, HarperCollins.

WHAT IS THE SOLUTION FOR DEALING WITH ANGER?

Change the image of it!

Stop. Appraise the situation. Do not do a thing. You are at a pivotal point. You have two ways to go: One is to get angry, the other is to reappraise the situation. Try to look at a way to reinterpret the annoying comment. Consider the following example:

> "Who does that head nurse think he is to treat me like I'm a dummy!" or "How could someone be so thoughtless as to not remember my birthday!" You can reinterpret these and say to yourself, "Maybe if they weren't so unhappy, they wouldn't have considered doing such a thing" or "Maybe that person's having a rough day." The important thing here is to empathize with the person and to try to find justifications for the behavior that was so annoying to you.

Look. What image (*shoulds*, *musts*, or *need tos*) about yourself or another is about to be or has been breached? In other words, what has just occurred that has led you to feel angry at yourself or another?

> After receiving the end-of-shift report and making rounds to her patients, a recent graduate goes into a patient's room to take vital signs. Within moments the patient has a cardiac arrest. Two hours later while completing her chart, the recent graduate states guiltily, "I should have taken those vital signs earlier. It just needs to be the first thing I do when I get on the unit. I should have been on top of this. I must do better." Notice the self-criticism in the recent graduate's comments. Guilt, like resentment, can be a habit. It demonstrates—too clearly—how we respond to a situation in a negative manner. To help you get in touch with these feelings, try eliminating the words "must" and "should" from your vocabulary for just an hour. It is quite surprising to find out how frequently we use these terms.

Change. How do you change the image? One of the ways is to use humor. Humor makes the anger (guilt and resentment) tolerable. Remember that it is difficult to laugh and frown at the same time. (It only takes 15 facial muscles to laugh, but twice that many to frown.) If reappraising the situation and humor both fail as ways to deal with your anger, some suggest venting the anger—for example, by getting mad, yelling, shouting, telling someone off, or breaking things. Although this might make us feel better momentarily, in the long run such outbursts make us feel worse.

Why does this method of venting anger, that is, letting it all hang out, make us feel worse? First off think of all the physiologic changes that are occurring in your body: blood pressure, pulse, and respirations increase; the muscles contract; and adrenalin is released. Sound familiar? It is the "fight or flight" adrenal response. Can it be healthy to maintain a constant state of stress and readiness to respond? Another disadvantage of an uninhibited outburst of anger is that it may lead the other person to retaliate.

It might be important to recognize the difference between venting and acknowledging our anger. A typical expression of anger might be something such as the following:

> "Hey, you turkey, what do you think you're doing? Don't you know how to put that catheter in? Are you stupid or something? Either you figure it out, or you get out of here. You hear me?"

This approach is insulting, demeaning, and accusatory. It is also likely to lead to some type of provoking comment. In contrast, when we acknowledge our feelings, we make statements such as "*I feel angry about …*," "*I feel hurt about …*," *and* "*I feel guilty about …*." The use of "I" statements is our first step toward taking responsibility for ourselves by owning up to our own feelings instead of blaming others.

Venting anger simply does not work unless you want to intimidate those around you, coerce them into submission with a hot temper, or, better yet, look childish while ranting, raving, and beating the floor or each other with foam bats. So, what does work?

- First, acknowledge the anger *(face it)*: Ask "What am I feeling? Anger? Guilt? Rage? Resentment?"
- Second, identify the provoking or triggering situation *(embrace it)*: Ask "What caused this feeling? Whose problem is it?"
- Third, determine what changes need to occur *(erase it)*: Ask "What can I change? Can I accept what I cannot change?" Then take action and let go of the rest. Other ways to deal with anger and get out of the vicious cycle of guilt and resentment include the following:

Move.

Get Active. Try exercise or anything involving physical activity, such as walking, aerobics, and running. Clean out the garage or a kitchen drawer. If you are sitting, get up. If you are in bed, move your arms around. Just get up and do something!

Focus.

Refocus on Something Positive. Think of your cup as half full, not half empty. Look at the provoking situation: "My head nurse won't give me Christmas off. However, I am not scheduled to work either Christmas Eve or New Year's Eve. So, by working Christmas Day, I'm assured the other days off."

Breathe.

Pay Attention to Your Breathing. Slow it down. Take deep, slow breaths, feeling the air move through your nose and down into your lungs. Check out your body for areas of tenseness. Often anger can be felt as tightness in the chest and abdomen.

Conflict is an inevitable part of our day-to-day experience. How we negotiate and handle conflict and anger may not always be easy. You might be thinking right now "This looks good on paper, but in real life, it is not that easy to put into practice." If you are feeling this way, take a risk at changing your approach and viewpoint.

The important thing is learning about yourself.

How do you deal with conflict? How do you handle difficult people? How do you respond when angry?

SEXUAL HARASSMENT IN THE WORKPLACE

In today's world, sexual harassment as a source of conflict has been taken seriously, as evidenced by the widespread visibility and increased recognition of the issue. The potential impact of harassment on nursing students both in the classroom and in the practice area is significant. According to Dowell (1992), nursing administrators and educators must be proactive in writing and implementing policies regarding sexual harassment. In a study by Libbus and Bowman (1994), 70% of female staff nurses surveyed reported sexual harassment by male patients and co-workers, with the most common complaint being sexual remarks and inappropriate touching. In addition, in a survey of nursing administrators, 68.8% of those who responded reported sexist attitudes among employees in their organizations, and 47.7% reported observing instances of sexual harassment (Blancett & Sullivan, 1993). These studies reflect the prevalence of sexual harassment in health care settings.

The issue of sexual harassment came to the forefront during the 1991 confirmation hearings of Supreme Court Justice Clarence Thomas (Allen, 1992). Now a once-feared and secretive problem is openly discussed in newspapers and by the media. As awareness about sexual harassment increased, we all realized how little we knew about it and what we could do about it. The majority of cases involve women who report being harassed by men. In nursing, the stereotypical situation of sexual harassment involves a nurse (i.e., a woman) and a doctor (i.e., a man) because of the large number of nurses who are women. However, with the increase in the number of men entering the nursing profession, as well as the increase in the number of women entering medicine, there is the potential for men to experience sexual harassment by women in the workplace (Figure 12-5).

WHAT IS SEXUAL HARASSMENT?

According to Friedman (1992, p. 9), "sexual harassment refers to conduct, typically experienced as offensive in nature, in which unwanted sexual advances are made in the context of a relationship of unequal power or authority." He goes on to explain that victims of sexual harassment are subjected to sexually oriented verbal comments, unwanted touching, and requests for sexual favors. The typical problem, known as quid pro quo harassment, arises when unwelcome sexual advances have been made and an employee is required to submit to those demands as a condition either of employment or of promotions. "Hostile work environment" has been used as a legal claim to show that "the atmosphere in the work (or other) environment is so uncomfortable or offensive by virtue of sexual advances, sexual requests, or sexual innuendoes that it amounts to a hostile environment" (Friedman, 1992, p. 16). Let us look at hypothetical examples of how sexual harassment can affect nursing.

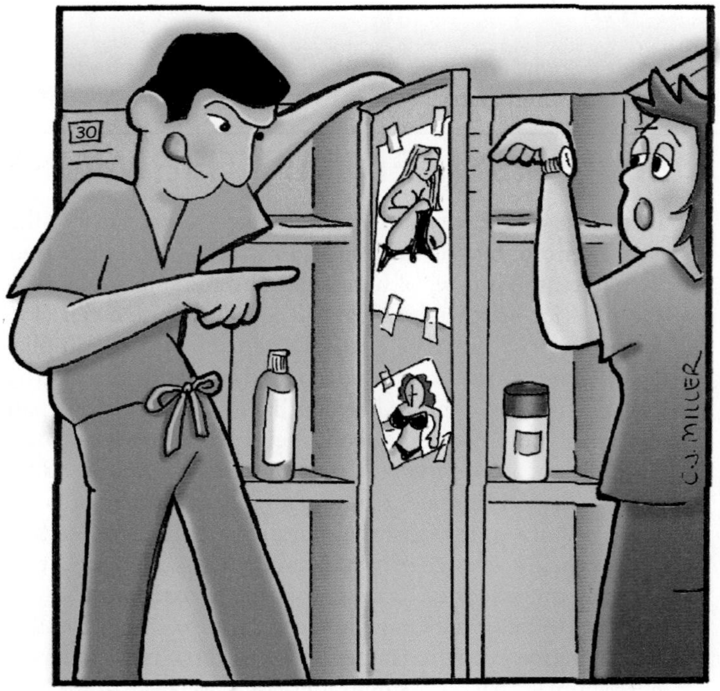

FIGURE 12-5
Sexual harassment.

Tracey, a recent graduate working in the surgical area of the hospital, had been receiving compliments from the chief of surgery. Eventually he asked her out and told Tracey that if she would have an affair with him, he would make certain she was promoted to shift supervisor as soon as the position became vacant.

Lisa, the evening charge nurse, was quite excited that Tom, a recent graduate, was going to work on her unit. Lisa pursued Tom by repeatedly asking him for assistance with patient care and when she called him into her office, she would touch him.

WHAT CAN I DO ABOUT IT?

There are two ways to deal with this type of workplace conflict: informally and formally through a grievance procedure. Start with the most direct measure. Ask the person to STOP! Tell the harasser in clear terms that the behavior makes you uncomfortable and that you want it to stop immediately. Also, you might want to put your statement in writing to the person, keeping a copy for yourself. Tell other people, such as family, friends, personal physician, or minister, what is happening and how you are dealing with it. Friedman (1992) suggests keeping a written journal of harassing events, along with all attempts the victim has used to try and stop the harassment. The need to exercise power and control, rather than sexual desire, is frequently the motive of the sexual harasser (perpetrator). If sexual harassment is occurring as a result of miscommunication and misinterpretation of actions and is primarily sexually driven, not power-driven, then telling the perpetrator to stop will often clear up any misconceptions. However, if the perpetrator is power-driven, the harassment will continue as long as he or she views the victim as passive, powerless, and frightened. What may be most difficult for the recent graduate is facing the fear that surrounds threats of job insecurity or public embarrassment (Friedman, 1992).

If a direct request to the perpetrator to stop does not work, then an informal complaint may be effective, especially if both parties realize a problem exists and want it to be solved. The goal of the informal method is to stop the harassment but not punish the perpetrator. This method assists the person filing the complaint in maintaining some type of harmonious relationship with the perpetrator. "A formal grievance usually requires filing a written complaint with an official group such as a hearing" (Friedman, 1992, p. 65). This is a legal procedure that is guided and regulated by federal and state laws specific to this type of grievance. Before a 1991 amendment to the Civil Rights Act (Title VII), the means of correcting this bad situation—making it right or compensating the victim for difficulty encountered—were quite restricted. What has occurred as a result of this act is that victims of intentional discrimination may now seek compensatory and punitive damages. Each state has an Equal Employment Opportunity Commission, which has as its specific charge the enforcement of Title VII.

Sexual harassment may be one form of conflict you are faced with in the workplace. Learning to deal with your feelings and being aware of actions to take should this unpleasant situation occur are important. When this type of situation is resolved in a constructive, positive manner, it allows you an opportunity to feel better about your ability to deal with conflict.

CONCLUSION

Most of us have experienced conflict. Building effective conflict management skills are key to dealing with clients, staff, and physicians. Various models exist to provide a framework for effective conflict resolution; the "win-win" model of *collaboration* is the strategy that aims for the highest level of resolution and is fully assertive and cooperative in approach. It takes creative nursing management and understanding to recognize and acknowledge that conflict will exist whenever human relationships are involved. This needs to be tempered with open, accurate communication and active listening by maintaining an objective, not emotional stance, as conflict resolution strategies are utilized.

REFERENCES

Allen A: Equal opportunity in the workplace, *J Post Anesth Nurs* 7(2):132-134, 1992.

Blancett SS, Sullivan PA: Ethics survey results, *J Nurs Admin* 23(3):9-13, 1993.

Bramson R: *Coping with difficult people*, New York, 1981, National Press Publications.

Dowd S, Davidhizar R, Davidhizar R: Sexuality, sexual harassment, and sexual humor: guidelines for the workplace in health care, *The Health Care Manager* 22(2):144, 2003.

Dowell M: Sexual harassment in academia: legal and administrative challenges, *J Nurs Educ* 31(1):5-9, 1992.

Filley AC: *Interpersonal conflict resolution*, Glenview, Ill, 1975, Scott Foresman.

Friedman J: *Sexual harassment: what it is, what it isn't, what it does to you, and what you can do about it*, Deerfield Beach, Fla, 1992, Health Communications.

Guttenberg RM: How to stay cool in a conflict and turn it into cooperation, *Nurs Life* 3(3):25-29, 1983.

Lerner H: *The dance of anger: a woman's guide to changing the patterns of intimate relationships*, New York, 1997, Harper & Row.

Libbus MK, Bowman KG: Sexual harassment of female registered nurses in hospitals, *J Nurs Admin* 24(6):26-31, 1994.

Tavris C: Feeling angry? Letting off steam may not help, *Nurs Life* 4(5):59-61, 1984.

Wagner M, Hartman T: *Supreme Court ruling on harassment places premium on employer sexual harassment policies*, Enterprise/Salt Lake City, 34(4):11, 2004.

Weiss L, Cain L: *Power lines: what to say in problem situations*, Dallas, 1991, Taylor.

CHAPTER 13

TIME MANAGEMENT

SHARON DECKER, RN, CS, MSN, CCRN

Gain control of your time, and you will gain control of your life.

—*Anonymous*

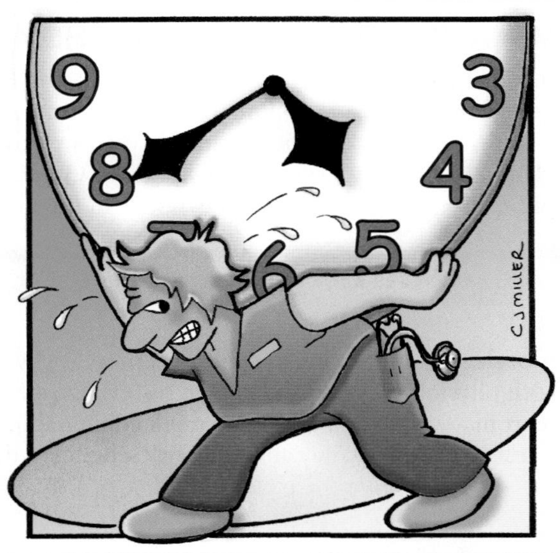

Is time managing you, or are you managing time?

After completing this chapter, you should be able to:

- Identify and describe your individual time styles.
- Discuss strategies that increase organizational skills.
- Describe time-management strategies.
- Discuss principles of priority-setting.

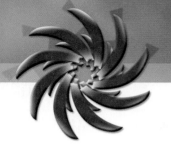

There are so many activities that individuals need to accomplish at any one time that deciding "how to get it all done" and "what to do when" is a daily challenge that is sometimes overwhelming. Nursing school complicates the daily routine. This relentless competition for our attention is described by the term *timelock* (Keyes, 1991).

MANAGING TIME

Regrettably, there is no way to alter the minutes in an hour and the hours in a day. Although we cannot create more actual time, we can alter how we use the time we have available. When employers of recent graduates were asked to identify behaviors seen as being deficit in the graduate, lack of organizational and time-management skills were noted as concerns. The methods and strategies identified by time-management experts can help you cope with timelock.

This section introduces you to the principles of effective time management. You will learn how to gain control of your time, increase your organizational skills, and reduce time waste. You will learn strategies for using the newly acquired hours to achieve your personal and professional goals.

BALANCE IS THE KEY

Making time to meet your individual, family, and professional needs and goals is vital to your overall success. If you neglect your health maintenance needs, completing school may be jeopardized. Putting off assignments until the last minute can lead to extreme anxiety and stressful behavior, which negatively affects personal health and interpersonal relationships. Integrating the principles of time management into your daily life can help you achieve both your personal and professional goals.

WHAT ARE YOUR BIOLOGIC RHYTHMS, AND HOW DO YOU USE THEM?

Individuals have different biorhythms that affect their energy levels during the day and even in different seasons. Rest and sleep are essential for optimal health and emotional and physical responsiveness. Some individuals function best when they go to bed by mid-evening and awake at the "crack of dawn," ready to tackle difficult tasks. Others are more energetic in the mid-afternoon, early evening, or even in the middle of the night.

Whenever possible, schedule difficult activities at your high-energy times.

When possible, get 8 solid hours of sleep. Maintaining a regular sleep–wake rhythm with adequate hours of sleep has both physiologic and psychologic restorative effects. Disruption of this rhythm causes chronic fatigue and decreases one's coping abilities and performance. Factors affecting rest and sleep include anxiety, work schedules, diet, and the use of alcohol and nicotine.

Engage in a relaxing activity 1 hour before going to bed; for example, take a warm bath, read an interesting novel, or learn to initiate progressive relaxation techniques.

Motivate yourself in the morning by reading an inspiring quote, listening to upbeat music, or doing stretching exercises. Take time for a balanced breakfast and visualize your day. Take periodic breaks or switch activities throughout your day to maintain a high energy level. Tension can be released by simple stretching exercises and even laughter.

Alternate mental and physical tasks. This strategy includes taking periodic breaks from studying to engage in a short game of basketball or a short run with the vacuum cleaner.

WHAT IS MEANT BY RIGHT- AND LEFT-BRAIN DOMINANCE, AND WHERE IS MY BRAIN?

People use time in relation to their characteristic brain dominance; left, right, or both (Figure 13-1).

Left-brain–dominant people process information and approach time in a linear, sequential manner. Their thinking structures time by minutes and hours. They tend to

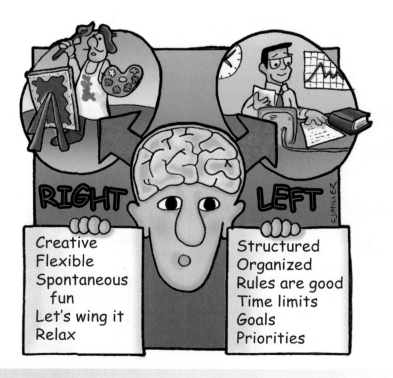

FIGURE 13-1
Are you right-brain or left-brain dominant?

schedule activities in time segments and carry them out in the sequence ordered. Left-brain–dominant people like to know the rules and play by them. They are usually able to meet their goals, but if this behavior is carried to an extreme, the individual is in danger of overwork at the expense of creative, artistic, and relaxing activities.

Right-brain–dominant people resist rules and schedules. They prefer looking at a project as a whole and completing it in their own way and time. These are creative, flexible thinkers. However, if their behaviors are taken to an extreme, they can fail to meet needed completion times, which can induce guilt.

Some people are neither left-brain–dominant nor right-brain–dominant and, thus, are more mixed in their behaviors. Everyone uses both sides of the brain to some extent and thus has the benefits of their full capacities. The use of lists and calendars engages the left brain, whereas techniques such as the use of colored folders and whimsical office supplies help individuals to use right-brain holistic thinking to solve problems.

Which are you? (Check out The Brain-Dominance Questionnaire at *www.scs.sk.ca/cyber/prest/brain.htm*.)

- I am left-brain–dominant.
- I am right-brain–dominant.
- I am left-brain–dominant and right-brain–dominant.

In addition to assessing your own dominant time style, it is helpful to be aware of the time styles of the people with whom you live and work. Heaping rigid rules on a right-brain–dominant person will lead to increased resistance and frustration for everyone. Better to assign them clean-up of the kitchen or utility room to be completed by a specific time; inform them of the consequences of it not being done. It would be appropriate to have some right-brain–dominant persons on the recruitment and retention committee and some left-brain–dominant persons on the policy and procedures committee.

Knowing your time style can help you maximize your strengths and modify your weaknesses. Individual time styles can be modified, but it is wasted energy to fight or work against natural inclination. Once you are aware of your time style, you can begin to create more time for what you want and need to do by increasing your organizational skills.

HOW CAN I MANAGE MY PHYSICAL ENVIRONMENT?

A place for everything and everything in its place.

Organizing and maintaining your physical environment at home, school, and work can dramatically reduce hours of time and the emotional frustration associated with "looking for stuff."

At home, set up a specific work area for such things as school supplies, papers, and books. A separate area or corner should be set up where you can pay bills, send letters, order take-out food, and take care of other household chores. At school and at work, a locker with extra supplies is also helpful. If none is available, use a compartmentalized carrier of some sort for essential items.

When studying or working on major projects, find a space that provides a comfortable, but not cozy, area. This area should be as free from distractions as possible, with adequate lighting. If you are studying, break your time into 50-minute segments followed by 10-minute breaks. Prior to beginning each study session, gather the appropriate tools—textbooks, paper, pens, highlighters, and reference material—to avoid wasting time once you begin your work.

Compartmentalize. When practicing nursing, have a pen, notebook, personal data assistant (PDA), and/or other reference materials along with your pencil, notepaper, scissors, penlight, for example, in a designated holder or closed notebook. At work, validate that supplies are organized and stocked by the type of procedure for quick access. An intravenous start tray or carts with needed equipment for insertion of central lines or chest tubes are examples of such time-savers.

Color-code files, keys, socks, and whatever you can. Office supply stores are good sources of color-coded items. Color-coding keys with a plastic cover enables you to immediately pick out your car key, house key, or locker key. Drug syringes are color-coded for accurate and rapid identification in a resuscitation situation. One clinical research team copies their material on purple paper so that all nurses gathering the data can easily identify the correct forms.

Convenience. Move and keep frequently used items nearest to where they are used. If your agency is still doing paper charting, keep extra nurse's notes in the area where you chart. Store infrequently used items farther away. A work team needs to agree on where essential items are to be stored in consistently designated places.

Declutter the clutter. At work as well as at home, designate one person to regularly clear work areas.

WHAT ABOUT ALL THE PAPERWORK—HOW CAN I MANAGE IT?

Handling each piece of paper only one time is a great time-saver. Whenever possible, spend 30 seconds filing an important paper in the appropriate folder. This technique can save you 30 minutes of searching time when you need to use the information again. Following are five ways to deal with paper:

- File it.
- Forward it.
- Respond to it—on the same sheet if possible.
- Delegate it.
- Discard it.

Use the A-B-C system when items cannot be handled at once because of your time commitments. Sort mail and messages by relative importance. The A pile will require action as soon as possible. The B pile will wait until you can get to it (i.e., B items may become A items later, especially if they have time-dates). The C items can wait until you can "get around to doing them." Because of their relative unimportance, most of the C-pile items can usually be discarded at some point.

A—Do it now (i.e., as soon as possible).
B—Necessary, but do it later.
C—When I get to it.

In a nursing setting, pace your paperwork by charting throughout the day instead of at the end of the shift. Waiting until the last hour of the shift, when you are likely to be fatigued, reduces accuracy and completeness. Standardized, preprinted change-of-shift reports and other kinds of flow charts also help to document objective data effectively and efficiently. There is now "light at the end of the tunnel": Bedside and other computers are likely to become the major method of communication in your professional lifetime.

Remember, chart as you go; do not wait until the end of the shift.

WHAT ABOUT MANAGING THE TELEPHONE?

Polite comments at the beginning and end of a telephone conversation are necessary to maintain positive interpersonal communications. However, when time limits are necessary, focus the conversation on the business at hand. Some possible phrases include "How can I help you?" or "I called to ... " To end the conversation, summarize the actions to be followed through: "I understand, I am to find out about ... and get back to you by the end of the week. Thanks for calling." Professional courtesy demands you turn off your cellular phone while in the classroom, during clinical, and while attending a workshop.

Having conversations to maintain friendships, to touch base with a relative, to relax yourself, to vent your emotions, or to serve similar social purposes can be combined with routine housekeeping duties. Who has not swept the floor, put away dishes, sorted mail, or cleaned out a drawer while chatting with a friend?

One time-management principle is, "Don't agonize. Organize!"

WHAT ABOUT ALL THAT E-MAIL?

Restrict work or school-related e-mail to one account with another account for personal communication. Turn off the notification chime, and set aside time during the day to read and answer your e-mail instead of answering each one as it arrives. This could be one of your first tasks in the morning while you are enjoying your coffee. Do not let e-mail pile up in your Inbox. Read it, answer it, and, if important, transfer it to a designated folder or delete it. When you are communicating with your instructor by means of e-mail, be sure that you include your class number or title in the subject line. Many instructors manage their e-mail by sorting it with respect to class, so a standardized subject line helps with their time management. Your e-mail program may have parameters that allow you to designate specific messages to be sent directly into a special file. This helps move information out of the Inbox and keeps you organized. Spend some time in your e-mail program. Look at all of the functions and what they do. Use your e-mail program to your best advantage—it can become your best friend in terms of helping you organize your e-mails in folders. Specific tips for effective use of e-mail are provided in Box 13-1.

Use your delete key aggressively, and eliminate junk e-mail without reading it.

BOX 13-1 Tips for Effective E-Mail

Before committing—THINK.
If it is in writing, you are accountable.
E-mail is not necessarily confidential.
Use that "SUBJECT" line.
Proofread before you send.

HOW CAN I DEAL WITH ALL THE INTERRUPTIONS?

Interruptions are one of the major threats to effective time management. Not only is time taken away from goal-directed activities but additional time is needed to get refreshed and back on track. Of course some interruptions are inevitable, but they can be minimized. Begin by recognizing when you are interrupting yourself. Do you start one task and then begin another rather than concentrating on completing the first? Do you respond to added distractions (television, ringing telephones, chatty friends) at times when task completion is required? In these instances, you are cooperating with the interruption and allowing yourself to be interrupted. When possible, in nonemergency situations, use your time-management strategies and communication skills to remain focused on the task at hand. People will accept that you may need to get back to them when you have finished what you are doing. Write down when and where you can reach them and then follow through. Turn off your telephone's ringer and let the message service or answering machine pick up the calls, but check it every hour or so. This way you can return the calls you want to respond to and at your convenience.

Responding to interruptions can also mean you are doing your job. For example, when you are interrupted to answer a patient's call light or answer a physician's telephone call, you are doing your job. These activities are part of your nursing responsibilities. They may not be of an urgent nature and can be delayed a short time, or they may be urgent and necessitate immediate response; either way, you will need to deal with them eventually. Rather than feeling that you have been interrupted, remind yourself that what you are doing is accomplishing part of your job. There are many aspects of your job that you cannot control, but you can always choose how you respond.

Everyone needs some totally uninterrupted time in which to relax, refocus, and reenergize. During clinical experience, at work, or at home, spend a few minutes in a quiet place by yourself (e.g., the nurses' lounge, the chapel, an empty patient room, a bedroom at home) to evaluate what is happening or what needs to happen next. Take several deep, slow breaths, read, meditate, relax, or get in touch with yourself. (Parents with small children can take turns watching their children so each adult can have some uninterrupted private time.) Again, taking a break from fast-paced activity and relaxing will reenergize you and result in more productive use of time. (If now is a good time to take a break from this chapter, we will proceed when you get back!)

HOW CAN I MANAGE MY CALENDAR?

Calendars are available to schedule to-do activities by the month, week, and day. You gain control of your life by completing a schedule (Tables 13-1 and 13-2).

TABLE 13-1

Weekly Personal Calendar

Monday	Tuesday	Wednesday	Thursday	Friday
Cleaners 9 AM workout	Pick up health insurance forms 3:30 PM carpool	4 PM workout	4-7 PM professional organization meeting	9 AM workout

Scheduling provides you with a method to allocate time for specific tasks and is a constant reminder of your tasks, due dates, and deadlines. Schedule only what can realistically be accomplished and leave extra time before and after every major activity. Tasks, meetings, and travel can take longer than anticipated, so give yourself some time to transition from one project to another. Schedule personal time in your calendar. If someone wants to meet with you during this time, just say, "I'm sorry, I've got an important appointment. When would be another convenient time?" Color code your appointments according to priorities to stimulate the right side of your brain.

Leave white space (nothing) in your schedule so you will have time for yourself and family, or schedule uninterruptible time for both.

TABLE 13-2

Daily Nursing To-Do List

(A) IMMEDIATE ACTIVITIES			
A-1		Check IV tube	Mr. D, Room 20
A-2		Assess chest tube	Mrs. B, Room 15
A-3		Suction ET tube	Ms. F, Room 12
(A) SCHEDULED ITEMS			
A-4	9:00 AM	Dressing change	Ms. P, Room 10
A-5	10:00 AM	Medications	Ms. B, Ms. P, Ms. J
A-6	12:00 PM	CT scan	Ms. W, Room 25
A-7	2:00 PM	Medications	Mr. D, Ms. P
A-8	3:00 PM	Change-of-shift report	
(B) TO BE DONE WHEN TIME ALLOWS			
B-1		Diabetic teaching	Mr. X, Room 17
B-2		Social service consultation	Mr. X, Room 17
(C) IF TIME AVAILABLE			
C		Access Web-based continuing education program	
C		Reorganize reference materials on unit	

CRITICAL THINKING BOX 13-1

Develop your time calendar—will it be a week-at-a-glance or a month-at-a-glance? Think about what works the best for you.

At the beginning of each week, review the activities scheduled for the week to avoid unexpected "surprises." Overscheduling of more tasks than any human being can do in 1 day inevitably leads to frustration. Build in some flexibility. It will not always be possible to follow your exact schedule. However, when you do get "derailed," having a plan will help you get back on track with a minimum of time and effort (Critical Thinking Box 13-1).

Strategy: Leave some extra time before and after every major event to allow for transition.

MANAGING TASKS

HOW DO I DEAL WITH PROCRASTINATION?

Everyone procrastinates, especially when a task is unpleasant, overwhelming, or cannot be done perfectly. Procrastination can lead to last-minute rushes that cause unnecessary stress. The time spent stressing about doing something takes more time than actually doing it! The anticipation itself can also be worse than the actuality, draining your energy and accomplishment. Here are some tips for getting started.

Consider the Consequences. Ask yourself what will happen if you do something and what will happen if you do not do it. If there are no negative outcomes of not doing something, there is no point in spending time doing it. You can eliminate that activity!

If something will happen because you don't do it, then, of course, you need to get started.

The Earlier, the Better. Most projects take longer than planned, and glitches happen; for example, coffee spills all over your study notes the night before the test, your computer crashes, or your dog eats your notes. To compensate for the inevitable delays and avoid crises, start in advance and plan for your project to take three times longer than you think. Be realistic and use your common sense in scheduling this time frame.

Schedule times to work on your project, and track your progress on a calendar.

"By the Inch, It's a Cinch." Break projects into small, manageable pieces; gather all the resources required to finish the project; and plan to do only the first step initially.

For example, to study for a test, first collect all the related notes and books in one place. Next, review the subjects likely to be tested. If you are having difficulty getting started, plan to work on these steps for only 5 to 10 minutes. (Anybody can do just about anything for 5 to 10 minutes, eh?) Frequently, this will create enough momentum to get you going. When you have to stop, leave yourself a note regarding what the next steps should be. Here are some hints for effective studying.

- Study difficult subjects or concepts first.
- Study in short "chunks" of 50 minutes time.
- Take a brief 10-minute break after every 50 minutes of studying.
- Schedule study time when you are at your best.
- Use waiting times. (Compile and carry 3 × 5 notecards wherever you go. They should contain information you need to review and can be pulled out anywhere—even when you are standing in that long line at the checkout counter.)
- Keep a calendar for the semester that includes all of your assignments, tests, and papers. Use a different color for entering deadlines for each course.
- Make a weekly to-do list. Prioritize this list, and cross off each task as you complete it.
- Before beginning a project, know what you are doing. Determine the goals, benefits, costs, and timetable for the endeavor. If you are working in a group, at the beginning of the project, make sure everyone understands their responsibilities; you should also designate who is in charge of organizing group meetings. Leave time during the project for unexpected delays and to revisit and modify your goals. Be flexible.

Reward Yourself. Bribing yourself with a reward can help you get started and keep you going. "If I concentrate well for 1 hour on reading the assigned chapter, then I can watch my favorite television show guilt-free." Often, the stress reduction that comes from working on the project that has been put off is a reward in itself (Critical Thinking Box 13-2)!

Schedule a time for celebration and self-reward with all of your projects.

Avoid the Myth of Perfection. Many of us were brought up with the well-intentioned philosophy that "Anything worth doing is worth doing well." What is usually meant is "worth doing perfectly." The fear of not doing something well enough or perfectly also feeds the tendency to procrastinate.

Certainly, everyone needs to make the best effort they can, but not everything needs to be done perfectly. Consider what the standard needed is—not the standard of perfection possible—and how you can meet it with a minimum amount of time and effort. Effective procrastination (i.e., procrastination that is used appropriately) is recognizing

CRITICAL THINKING BOX 13-2

What do you do to reward yourself for a job done well?

when a task should be purposefully postponed. This technique is a conscious decision and is used when time is needed to accomplish a task with a higher priority. Here are some hints for managing procrastination.

- Set priorities.
- Eliminate wasted time by avoiding excessive social telephone calls.
- Break a task into separate small steps.
- Establish multiple, specific, and realistic short-term goals.
- Get started by taking one step at a time.
- Periodically review your progress.
- Reward yourself as you accomplish each short-term goal.
- Avoid doing the work of others.
- Delegate tasks when possible.
- Be realistic.

MANAGING OTHERS

Communicating and getting along with other people are always a challenge. Most people are easy to be with and are straightforward and supportive. They add to your energy and ability to function effectively, and they contribute to your goal attainment. However, if you experience a phone call or visit from someone who just wants to talk when you are busy, you need to avoid being trapped. Tell them, "Now is not a good time. Could we discuss this later?" or even "I've got another appointment. Could we postpone this conversation until tomorrow?" Some individuals drain energy from others and from organizational accomplishment through their whining, overcriticizing, negative thinking, chronic lateness, poor crisis management, overdependency, aggression, and similar unproductive behaviors. Occasional exhibitions of such behavior in relation to personal crises that happens to everyone can be dealt with easily. It is the people who use these behaviors as their everyday *modus operandi* (method of operating) who interfere with attainment of individual and organizational goals. Even in the best of human relationships, conflict and extreme emotions are inevitable. To protect your time and achieve your goals, it may be necessary to limit your time with such individuals. Avoidance is one strategy. Learning to say "no" and assertive communication can help as well. The content and skills mentioned in Chapter 11, Effective Communication, and Chapter 12, Conflict Management, provide assistance in learning these skills. Box 13-2 provides some hints for managing others.

BOX 13-2 Tips for Managing Time and Others

1. Make use of "mini" time periods.
2. AVOID PERFECTIONISM.
3. Take "mini" vacations throughout the day to refresh your brain.
4. Minimize the time spent with individuals who constantly complain and criticize.
5. Use assertive communication with individuals with whom you are having a problem.
6. Develop rituals (such as changing clothes) when you get home that say "I'm off duty."

WHAT ABOUT DELEGATION AND TIME MANAGEMENT?

You do not have to handle everything personally. Use your delegation skills at home to identify tasks and activities that can be completed by others, leaving you more time to study and concentrate on important projects.

> Delegate the laundry, and save yourself 1 to 2 hours per week. With this strategy, you could gain 4 free hours in a month.

MANAGING YOUR GOALS

Goals are the incremental steps required to achieve long-term success. Personal and professional goals are critical to lifestyle management. Keeping your goals in mind enables you to plan and carry out activities that contribute to your goals and eliminate or reduce those that do not. Be realistic when setting your goals: Allow enough time to complete them appropriately. Activities that contribute to goals are your high-payoff, high-priority activities and those that do not are low-payoff, low-priority activities. Your goals should be demanding enough that completion provides a feeling of satisfaction.

Many goal-directed activities need to be scheduled with completion times. This is sometimes called *deadlining* the to-do list; the use of the term *completion times* may seem less stress-producing than the use of *deadlines*. All kinds of calendars are available to schedule to-do activities by the month, week, and day. There are organizer notebooks and computerized organizers. It is also easy to make your own forms. Knowing your goals and priorities promotes flexible rescheduling, resulting in more effective time management and successful accomplishment.

BEGIN BY LISTING

It will be helpful to list all your goal-related activities on a master to-do list. Another approach, which is also a useful learning exercise, is to record all your activities in a time log as they occur (e.g., record them every day for several days or a week). This will give you an overview of how you are using your time and provide a baseline for a to-do list. Either way, decide the order in which to do the activities in your list. You will have to decide the order in which your activities need to be completed—in other words, you will have to prioritize.

Cross out items on your to-do list, cards, and schedule as you do them. This will give you immediate, positive feedback—an instant reward for your efforts and progress. When the inevitable interruptions occur, scan the to-do list and reevaluate your priorities in relation to your remaining time.

> Reward yourself as you cross out items on your to-do list.

PRIORITIZE WITH THE ABCD SYSTEM

Others are constantly demanding your time and energy; therefore, you need to establish priorities but be flexible. Being flexible will allow you to change your priorities

BOX 13-3 Prioritization using the ABCD System

A Absolute (Immediate priority)
B Better (as-soon-as possible)
C Can wait until later
D Don't worry about it

throughout the day as situations change. Additionally, as you work, always try to combine activities (multitask) or delegate tasks in an effort to manage your time appropriately.

Scan your to-do list and decide which are A, B, C, or D items (Box 13-3). The activities that are most closely related to your goals are the high-payoff ones; these are A priorities. Effective use of your time-management skills demands that you focus most of your energy on A-priority items. List these according to the urgency of the time limits. Train yourself to do the hardest task first. Attending to the hardest activity first reduces the nagging anxiety that you "should be . . ." and helps you make progress early to identify, gain control of, and possibly prevent additional problems. This is an example of the classic time-management principle, Pareto's 80/20 Rule.

According to Pareto, an early 1900s economist, 20% of the effort produces 80% of the results. For example, spending 20% of your time studying the hardest course can produce 80% success. In your home, 80% of what needs cleaning is in the kitchen and bathroom; spend 20% of your cleaning time on these two rooms and 80% of the cleaning will be done. Eighty percent of your nursing care will be with 20% of your patients. This illustrates that there are proportionally greater results in concentrating at least 20% of your efforts on higher-payoff priorities. You will need to balance your priorities because it is impossible to achieve our best at all times.

The B items also contribute to goal achievement and, so, are high-payoff, but they are generally less urgent and can be delayed for awhile. Eventually many B items become A items, especially as completion times approach. It is also possible to do some B items in short periods of time, reading an article as you wait in a long line or "waste" time waiting for someone.

Items that do not substantially contribute to goals or do not have to be accomplished within a specific timeframe are C items. These activities really can wait until you get around to them. Keep a list of things to be done when time permits. Some C items may never be accomplished. Of course, some C items become B or A priorities. However, many C items will fit the "nothing will happen if you do not do something" category for the D items. D items are those "nice to do" but not necessary. Some of these items could be classified as time wasters and can be ignored when you have limited time.

Remember to develop daily (or time) benchmarks, which allows you to assess your daily progress in relation to the time spent on a specific project.

KEEP IT GOING

Continuously review your lists, schedules, and outcomes, and reward yourself for achieving your goals. As you evaluate and revise accordingly, ask yourself: "Did I have a plan with priorities in writing?" "Was I doing high-payoff activities that pertain to my goals?" "Was I doing the right job at the right time?"

No one is perfect. Omissions and errors will occur and are good learning experiences. Do not waste time regretting failure or feeling guilty about what you did not do; consider these learning experiences of "what not to do" and opportunities for learning "what to do." Remind yourself that there is always time for important things and that if it is important enough, you will do it.

MANAGING TIME IN THE CLINICAL SETTING

One of the main sources of job dissatisfaction reported by nurses is too little time. This "limited time" to provide patient care has been accelerated by the nursing shortage and the increase in numbers of patients and the acuity of these patients. In response to this issue, nurses must develop competent skills in time management and priority-setting. Nurses can use several techniques to maximize the time spent providing patient care. Remember the 80/20 Rule discussed earlier in this chapter? Here is another example—20% of your patients will require 80% of your time! Those 20% should be the sickest patients; when their care and needs are met first, then the rest of the assignment is much easier. It will be important to determine which patients require the most time (the 80%): do they require time that can be delegated to someone else, or do they require the time because they are the most unstable and ill patients (Figure 13-2) and (Critical Thinking Box 13-3)?

GET ORGANIZED BEFORE THE SHIFT REPORT

Develop your personal flow sheet, or use one provided by the agency to write down information you need to begin coordinating care for a group of patients. Modify this form as you discover areas needing improvement. Make several copies so you will always have one handy. Avoid gossiping and other distractions as you receive a report and begin to fill out your time-management (or work organization) form. Get the information needed to plan the care for your patients, and begin to organize your shift activities (Figure 13-3).

PRIORITIZE YOUR CARE

Setting priorities has become difficult in relation to the dichotomy between the expected outcomes of efficiency and effectiveness and the perceived limitation of resources, including "time." Priority-setting is not only based on patient needs, but it is influenced by the needs of the organization and the accountability of the nurse. Priorities are established and reprioritized throughout the day according to patients' assessed needs and unscheduled interruptions, both minor and emergent. Plan your day around the patient you perceive to be the sickest. This is the patient who is at the greatest risk of harm if you do not address his needs first.

Prioritize your patients after you receive report and immediately proceed to the patient whom you have placed highest on your priority list. Remember, this prioritization may change as you complete your initial assessments. Additional modification

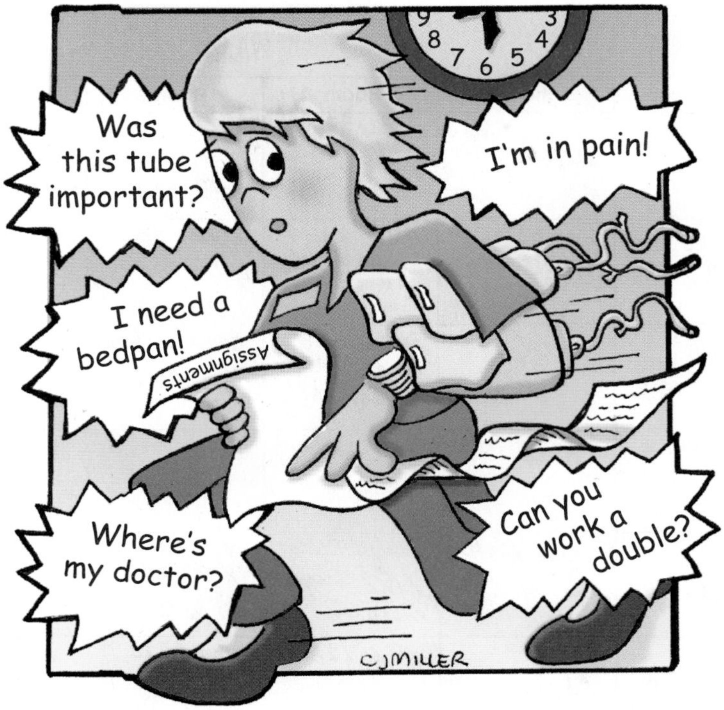
Was this tube important?
I'm in pain!
I need a bedpan!
Assignments
Where's my doctor?
Can you work a double?
CJMILLER

FIGURE 13-2
Time management and work organization can be challenging.

will be made according to the placement of patient's rooms to avoid wasted time and movement. When you first enter the patients' rooms, introduce yourself as you wash your hands and complete a quick environmental assessment. Think about any supplies you will need when returning to the room. Complete the focused assessment, validate the safety of your patient, and proceed to your next patient. Once you have completed your initial rounds, reassess your initial prioritization, modify according to your assessments, and plan your day.

CRITICAL THINKING BOX 13-3

Develop a flow sheet to organize your time and patient care for your clinical schedule. Obtain an assignment for an RN on one of the units to which you are assigned for clinical. Can you prioritize and delegate this RN's assignment appropriately?

Name: Susan

Time	Activities	Room 416	Room 417	Room 418
7-8	✓MAR Shift report ✓ Vitals	✓ Bld sugar 7:30 insulin	IV @ 125/hr. turn ✓ pulses	7:45 pre-op NPO ✓ consent form
8-9	assessments meal trays	meds x3-9 up for meals	meds x2-9 lf leg dsg. assist c̄ meal	To OR
9-10		Shower Chg bed ✓ pain meds	Complete bath ✓ pulses turn	
10-11	Chart			Chg bed
11-12	meal trays lunch	up for meals ✓ Bld sugar insulin?	turn ✓ pulses assist c̄ meal	
12-1	Chart Assessment	meds x2 -12	IVPB-12	Return fm. OR? N.G. suction I.V.
1-2		diabetic teaching	turn ✓ pulses lf. leg dressing change	
2-3	I+O's IV's report info			

FIGURE 13-3
Work organization sheet.

> Prioritize patients by using the ABCD system or Maslow's Hierarchy of Needs. Of highest priority are the patients with problems or potential problems related to the airway, next are those having any difficulty with breathing, and then circulation. When using Maslow's Hierarchy of Needs to assist with prioritization, you need to meet physiologic needs first: that is, resolve any difficulty with oxygenation first. Again, remember to be flexible and reprioritize as emergencies occur.

For example, a characteristic assignment for the day could be:

A patient who is 1 day postoperative and wants something for pain.

A geriatric patient who is vomiting.

CRITICAL THINKING BOX 13-4

How do the efficient nurses on your clinical unit prioritize their time and their patients?

A patient with diabetes who is angry about the care from the last shift.

A geriatric patient who has soiled the bed with urine.

Which of these patients needs your immediate attention? Most likely the one who is vomiting because he is at increased risk for aspiration, then probably the patient who is in pain, then the angry patient, and so on. With each patient, you may spend less than 5 minutes in the room before you move on to the next patient. But you will have a good idea of what each patient's immediate needs are.

Identify the busiest times on the unit; do not schedule a dressing change when medications need to be given. Plan on preparing medications at least 30 to 45 minutes before the hour they are due. This will provide time to research any medications with which you are unfamiliar. Do not procrastinate; start early. If you have dressing changes for several patients, start with the cleanest and progress to the more contaminated wounds. If you have diabetic teaching for three patients, maybe you can get them together and do it at one time (Critical Thinking Box 13-4).

PLAN TIME FOR CHARTING

Do not put charting off until the end of the shift. On a busy unit, you will forget half of what you have done for all your patients by the end of the day. How many times have you seen staff nurses staying late so they can complete their charting? Make notes for charting on your work organization form, and cross through it when it is charted. Plan on stopping about three to four times a shift to make charting entries. Do not obliterate anything on your form because you will need the information for an accurate shift report (Critical Thinking Box 13-5).

Watch those nurses who always seem to get everything done, done well, and still enjoy nursing. Ask them about their "secrets" of time management, and try out some of their tips.

CRITICAL THINKING BOX 13-5

When would you schedule charting time in your current daily clinical schedule?

REQUEST CONSISTENT PATIENT ASSIGNMENTS WHENEVER POSSIBLE

This allows you to develop relationships with your patients and their families and promotes time management as you become familiar with the special needs of these patients.

ORGANIZE YOUR WORK BY PATIENT

By using this technique, the nurse maximizes the number of tasks that can be accomplished with each visit to the patient. The nurse thinks strategically about "How can I multitask or accomplish several objectives in one visit to the patient?" By using this technique, the nurse would combine the assessment, administration of medications, and teaching during one patient visit (see Figure 13-3).

DEVELOP AND USE ASSERTIVE COMMUNICATION

Assertive communication is a technique used to get one's needs met without purposely hurting others. It incorporates the principles of therapeutic communication, active listening skills, and a willingness to compromise. When you use these skills, you will be able to express yourself more effectively during challenging situations and handle confrontation in a professional manner. When you are confronted by a situation that provokes anger, take a deep breath, pull yourself away, get your emotions under control, and then approach the individual privately in a nonthreatening manner. Following are some hints for using assertive communication:

- Use I statements: "I am really upset. . . . "
- Describe the behavior that has upset you and focus on the present: "You have been having excessive personal telephone calls over the past 2 days. . . . "
- Discuss the consequences of the behavior: "This behavior is contrary to the agency policy and could result in. . . . "
- State how the behavior needs to be modified and the time for this change: "You must immediately stop this interruption to your work and request that only emergency phone calls be. . . . "

WHAT ABOUT DELEGATING AND TIME MANAGEMENT?

Many studies have demonstrated that approximately 50% of nursing time is spent on nonnursing activities. These include cleaning, running errands, clerical duties, and stocking supplies. Appropriate delegation of nonnursing tasks can provide the nurse with additional time to dedicate to patient care. Some patient care tasks can be delegated once the training and competence of unlicensed personnel have been verified. These requirements vary in different states and institutions.

Delegation includes more than asking someone to do something. Delegation has been defined by the American Nurses Association (ANA) as "the transfer of responsibility for the performance of an activity from one individual to another, with the former retaining accountability for the outcome" (ANA, 1995). This definition emphasizes that delegation increases the responsibility and accountability of the registered nurse (RN). Be sure you know the delegation rules and regulations of your state's nursing practice act. Check out Chapter 14 for a quick review of the five rights of delegation according to the National Council of State Boards of Nursing (NCSBN, 1997).

Additionally, you will also need to know the delegation policies and job descriptions of nursing team members in your employing agency.

In general, women have more difficulty delegating than men do because of their socialization. Women are socialized to please others and to anticipate and meet the needs of others. Because the majority of the nursing profession remains female, you can understand the magnitude of the problem. In today's society, women, men, and nurses have so many responsibilities that sharing and delegating some of them are essential.

To increase delegation skills, it is sometimes necessary to overcome the myth of perfection. In teaching or training someone else to do a delegated task, initially they may or may not be able to perform the activity as well as you can; however, it is not important that they do this perfectly, in the way you do it, or even as well as you do. What is important is that they meet the standards required to complete the task adequately. As long as safety is not compromised, it is more effective time management to delegate to others. With experience, most people will improve (and may even surpass you) (Critical Thinking Box 13-6).

HOW DO I KNOW WHAT AND WHEN I CAN DELEGATE?

As previously stated, knowing the nurse practice act of your state, in addition to the policies for each institution, is critical in delegating appropriately and safely. Once that has been established, consider some general guidelines regarding what and when to delegate.

You should not delegate to anyone other than another RN the task of assessment to determine changes in a patient's condition. Licensed practical nurses or vocational nurses perform patient assessment (gathering data), but it is the RN who must confirm and interpret these findings. Assessment should not be delegated when a decision needs to be made regarding patient care, the patient's condition is changing, or there is a new patient the RN has not previously assessed.

According to the nursing process, after assessment and analyzing comes planning. This is another role of the RN. Data can be gathered from a number of sources, including input from a vocational nurse or unlicensed assistive personnel (i.e., a patient care attendant or nursing assistant). Ultimately it is the responsibility of the RN to determine the immediate plan of care and the comprehensive plan of care for the patient.

Another area of the nursing process that is reserved for the RN is the area of evaluations. It is the RN's responsibility to determine the patient's response to procedures, medications, nursing care, and so forth. Nursing judgment based on the assessment and evaluation of the patient must also remain the responsibility of the RN. It all comes down to the RN's responsibility in implementing the nursing process. Time management with delegation can help the RN more effectively implement the nursing process.

CRITICAL THINKING BOX 13-6

On your clinical unit, how many levels of personnel provide patient care? How are the patients or nursing care delegated?

CRITICAL THINKING BOX 13-7

Determine how and to whom patients are delegated on your current clinical unit. What guidelines are implemented?

Determine which patients are the most stable and whose positive progress can be anticipated. The stable patients with predictable progress should be the first to be delegated. The unstable, unpredictable patient should only be delegated to an RN. An RN should be assigned to any patient who is undergoing a procedure or treatment that may cause them to become unstable.

When you are dealing with unlicensed assistive personnel, you can delegate to them those activities that are standard with specific guidelines that are unchanging. For example, feeding, dressing, bathing, obtaining equipment for the nursing staff, picking up meal trays, refilling water containers, straightening up cluttered rooms—all of these activities should have guidelines according to the institution policies, fit within the job description, and be followed by the unlicensed assistive personnel.

Patient teaching and discharge planning are also the responsibility of the RN. It is the RN's responsibility to determine the patient's learning needs and to establish a teaching plan. It is also the RN's responsibility to coordinate and implement the discharge planning. The RN should request input from all nursing personnel who have assisted to provide care for this patient or who are involved (e.g., dietary, physical therapy) in the care of the patient. It is important that once the RN implements the teaching plan, the other RNs, licensed practical nurses, vocational nurses, and unlicensed assistive personnel are aware of what the patient has been taught so they may follow-up and report any pertinent observations to the RN (Critical Thinking Box 13-7).

Nursing care makes a difference in patient outcomes. This care is more than providing tasks. It incorporates assessment, care planning, initiation of interventions, interdisciplinary collaboration, and outcome evaluations. It includes patient and family teaching, therapeutic communication, counseling, discharge planning, and teaching. To maximize the impact nursing care can have on patient outcomes, nurses must develop and integrate multiple strategies to promote effective time management.

CONCLUSION

When you get your personal life organized, you will become effective in getting priorities accomplished at home. When you get your school activities organized, you will study more effectively, be less stressed, and be able to prioritize more effectively. With these two areas organized, there will be more time for you to spend on yourself! You will find that once you get organized with your clinical schedule, you will become a more effective nurse and begin to have the time to perform the type of nursing care that you were taught. Often you will hear nurses complain about not having enough time in clinical to provide the type of bath or teaching they would like to do because of the lack of time. Check them out; most often they are the most guilty of wasting time (e.g., taking time to gossip after report, wasting time complaining that they do not have enough time, not delegating effectively, allowing unnecessary interruptions, not organizing their patient care, or not delegating when appropriate). Wow, all the things that this chapter is all about!

REFERENCES

The American Nurses Association basic guide to safe delegation, Washington, DC, 1995, American Nurses Association.

Keyes R: *Timelock : how life got so hectic and what you can do about it*, 1991, HarperCollins.

National Council of State Boards of Nursing: *Nursing regulation: delegation and UAP issues*, 1997, *www.ncsbn.org/regulation/uap_delegation_documents.asp*.

CHAPTER 14

Delegation in the Clinical Setting

RUTH HANSTEN, PhD, MBA, BSN, FACHE
MARILYNN JACKSON, PhD, MA, BSN

Let whoever is in charge keep this simple question in her head (NOT how can I always do the right thing myself but) how can I provide for this right thing always to be done?

—*Florence Nightingale*

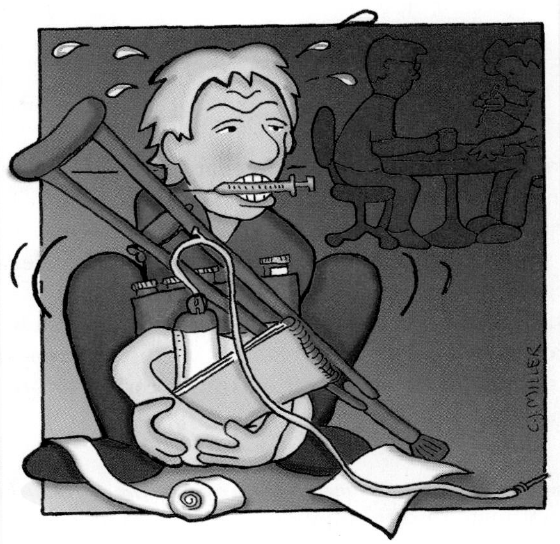

Nurses need to recognize when to delegate.

After completing this chapter, you should be able to:

- Define the operational terms delegation, supervision, and accountability.
- Delegate tasks successfully on the basis of outcomes.
- Select the right person for the right task.
- Apply the "four *Cs*" of initial direction for a clear understanding of your expectations.
- Provide reciprocal feedback for the effective evaluation of the delegate's performance.

Unless you are practicing on a deserted island with only one patient and you as the health care provider, chances are great that you will be working with other members of the health care team. How do you make best use of the resources they have to offer? What is your role as the registered nurse (RN) on the team in terms of making these decisions? Your ability to effectively delegate tasks that need to be done, on the basis of desired outcomes will go a long way in determining the success of the efforts of your work.

WHAT DOES DELEGATION MEAN?

We begin where we always must, with an understanding of the terms under discussion. Fortunately, there have been many people hard at work for years, creating operational definitions of the term delegation to assist us in standardizing our approach. It helps if everyone is talking about the same thing when in the heat of controversy! Clinical delegation has been with us since the dawn of team nursing, but in the past years it has taken on new meaning, as we have seen the addition of many types of assistive personnel in our care-delivery models. Many RNs are uncomfortable with the idea of someone "practicing on their license," or at the very least, taking away the tasks they like to do best. Let us take a look at delegation and accountability to clarify the issue that many RNs perceive as someone practicing on their license. It helps to clear the air by beginning with the vocabulary and achieving an understanding of the basic concepts we are talking about.

Delegation: "Transferring to a competent individual the authority to perform a selected nursing task in a selected situation. The nurse retains the accountability for the delegation" (NCSBN position paper, 1995).

As you can see, this is a very generic definition, used as a standard across the country; most states have incorporated similar definitions into their nurse practice acts. (Have you reviewed your state nurse practice act lately?) A good deal of decision making is left to you as the RN. You will be selecting what task and in what situation to delegate. You will make a decision to delegate on the basis of your assessment of the desired outcome and the competency of the individual delegate. This is certainly more involved than a simple process for time management! In the pages ahead, we discuss steps that use the "four rights" that will assist you in this practice, making it easier for you to maximize the work of your team in a safe manner.

Supervision: "The provision of guidance or direction, evaluation and follow-up by the licensed nurse for accomplishment of a nursing task delegated to unlicensed assistive personnel" (NCSBN position paper, 1995).

Nurses are often confused regarding supervision. This responsibility does not belong to only the one with the title of manager or house supervisor; rather, the expectation by law is that any time you delegate a task to someone else, you will be held accountable for the initial direction you give and the timely follow-up (periodic inspection) to evaluate the performance of the task. See Figure 14-1 for the Delegation Decision-Making Tree.

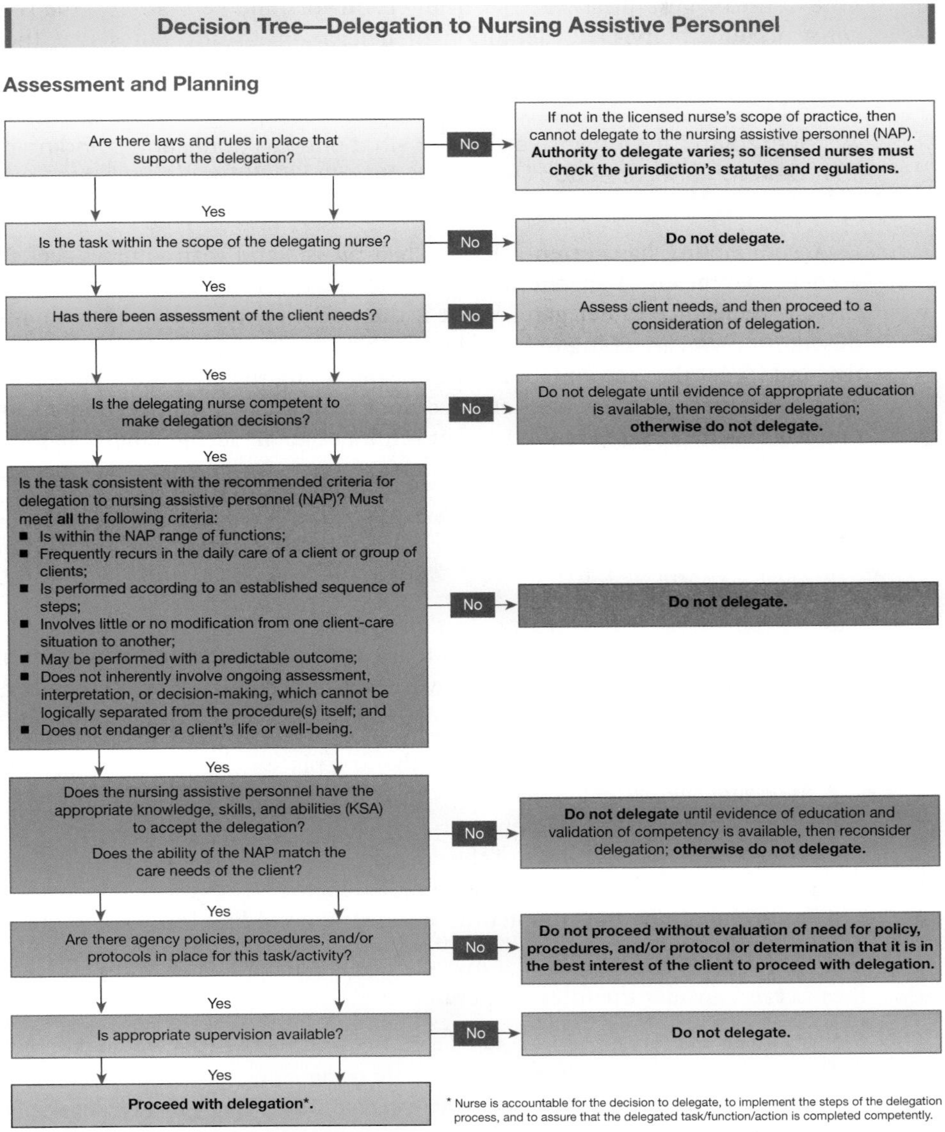

FIGURE 14-1
Delegation decision-making tree.

Delegation and supervision are integrated processes: Once you delegate, you must supervise.

WHO IS ACCOUNTABLE HERE?

One of the biggest questions concerning teamwork and delegation is the issue of personal accountability. The definition of delegation already notes that the nurse is accountable for the total nursing care of the individuals. What does this really mean?

Accountability: "Being answerable for what one has done, and standing behind that decision and/or action" (Hansten & Jackson, 2004).

Accountability has gotten a lot of "bad press," and many nurses feel that being accountable means "I am the one to blame." With that kind of attitude, no wonder there is reluctance to delegate! What is the point if someone else is going to make a mistake and you are going to be taking the blame? (Notice how we focus on the negative and forget that accountability also means taking the credit for the positive results we achieve through the actions and decisions we make, and our freedom to act because of our licensure.) Here is an important reminder about accountability before you take the weight of the world on your shoulders:

"The delegate is accountable for accepting the delegation and for his/her own actions in carrying out the task" (NCSBN, 1995, p. 3).

It is important to focus on what you are accountable for in this process and to let the delegate also assume his or her own level of accountability. Remember, you are accountable for the following:

- Making the decision to delegate in the first place.
- Assessing the patient's needs.
- Planning the desired outcome.
- Assessing the competency of the delegate.
- Giving clear directions and obtaining acceptance from the delegate.
- Following up on the completion of the task, providing feedback to the delegate.

What if the delegate makes a mistake doing the task? What are you accountable for? Let us consider the following example:

It is 7 AM on your busy medical-surgical unit. You scan your assignment quickly, reviewing the high points with your nursing assistant before going into report. With trays coming at 7:30, you remind your assistant that your patient in room 210 will be going to surgery this morning and is to have nothing to eat or drink. Coming out of report, you make brief rounds, only to

find that (you guessed it!) your patient in room 210 is happily drinking her morning coffee and eating a bagel.

What are you accountable for?

Did you delegate correctly?

What do you do now?

In your review of the previous guidelines, you identified that you did indeed delegate appropriately. Your communication may or may not have been as complete as it needed to be (more about that later). You are accountable for correcting the clinical effects of this error: Did the patient eat or drink too much, requiring that surgery be canceled or delayed? You will call the operating room and make the appropriate adjustments in this patient's care on the basis of the decision regarding her surgery time. What about the nursing assistant? You are also accountable for following up with her regarding her performance, giving the appropriate feedback so that she understands her level of personal accountability as well. For more on the "how-to's," read on as we discuss the four rights of clinical delegation.

THE FOUR RIGHTS OF CLINICAL DELEGATION*

Right task	Right communication
Right person	Right feedback

THE RIGHT TASK

The first part of any decision regarding delegation is the determination of what needs to be done and then the assessment of whether this is a task that can be delegated to someone else. Many nurses, unfortunately, suffer from "supernurse syndrome" and believe that no task should be delegated because no one can do it better, faster, or easier than they can (Figure 14-2). In comparison, other nurses may be all too eager to delegate the least desirable tasks to someone else. A word of caution is necessary here: If we focus only on making task lists for people to do, we eliminate the very core of our purpose. Remember, your role as the RN on the team involves the coordination and planning of care, with your primary focus on identifying with the patient and the physician the desired outcomes for your patients. Once determined, interventions will be readily apparent, and the decision regarding possible delegation of these tasks must be made.

*The National Council of State Boards of Nursing describes the "Five Rights of Delegation," discussing the "right circumstance" as an additional consideration for the nurse. "Right Circumstances—appropriate client setting, available resources, and consideration of other relevant factors," suggests that the staffing mix, community needs, teaching obligations, and the type of patients being cared for should also be considered (NCSBN, 1995).

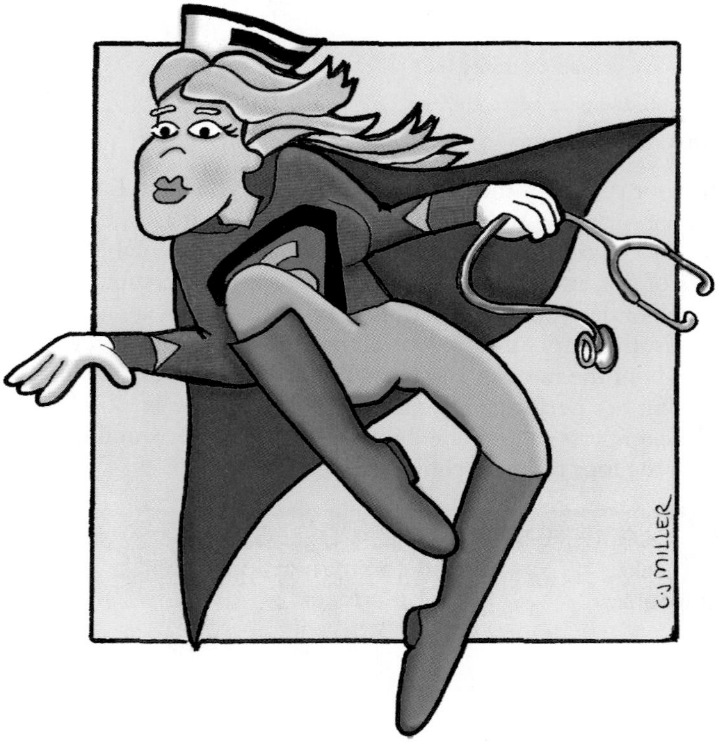

FIGURE 14-2
Many nurses suffer from "supernurse syndrome."

WHAT CAN I DELEGATE?

Fortunately, there are several references to assist you in making this determination. The first place we recommend looking is in the nurse practice act for your state. At this point, the majority of state boards have addressed the issue of delegation and have developed rules that may offer specific guidelines regarding who can do what. The scope of practice for each level of care provider usually includes a description of the tasks that may be performed at that level.

The next place to look is in your organization, getting a copy of the job description and the skills checklist for each care provider. This will give you a very specific list of tasks to work from, but remember, there are other considerations. Simply because the skills checklist includes ambulation of patients, it may not be advisable to delegate the first ambulation of a postoperative total hip replacement patient to the new patient care assistant (Critical Thinking Box 14-1).

IS THERE ANYTHING I CANNOT DELEGATE?

Again, your first resource is the law. Many states are very specific in their description of what cannot be delegated and therefore belongs only to the RN's scope of practice. The National Council of State Boards of Nursing (NCSBN) reminds us that

CRITICAL THINKING BOX 14-1

IN YOUR ORGANIZATION, CAN YOU DELEGATE THE FOLLOWING TASKS?

YES	NO	
________	________	Bladder retention catheter insertion
________	________	Taking vital signs
________	________	Feeding a patient
________	________	Hygienic care
________	________	Medication administration
________	________	Discontinuing an IV line
________	________	Teaching insulin administration

IV, Intravenous.

> Nursing is a knowledge-based process discipline and cannot be reduced solely to a list of tasks. The licensed nurse's specialized education, professional judgment and discretion are essential for quality nursing care....While nursing tasks may be delegated, the licensed nurse's generalist knowledge of patient care indicates that the practice-pervasive functions of assessment, evaluation and nursing judgment must not be delegated. (NCSBN, 1995)

According to nurse-attorney Joanne P. Sheehan, nurses cannot delegate the following:

- Assessments that identify needs and problems and diagnose human responses.
- Any aspect of planning, including the development of comprehensive approaches to the total care plan.
- Any provision of health counseling, teaching, or referrals to other health care providers.
- Therapeutic nursing techniques and comprehensive care planning. (Sheehan, 2001, p. 22)

If you have questions and need clarification for your state, call the board of nursing for assistance. You can get their information on the NCSBN website at *www.ncsbn.org* or from the list in Appendix B. Be aware that your state may have introduced or passed a bill that may affect your practice with residents of neighboring states. As of August 2005, states had passed or are in the process of approving interstate compact licensure regulation legislation designed to allow nurses to practice across state lines because of Internet consultation, telenursing, or other technology that would broadcast nursing practice across state borders (NCSBN, 2005). If you have questions and need clarification in your state, call the board of nursing for assistance (Critical Thinking Box 14-2).

Beyond the law, your employer will have job descriptions and skills checklists that should clearly define the role of the caregiver. If you have not seen these items, be sure to review them soon. This is the baseline for determining "who does what" and selecting the right task to delegate. As many organizations develop creative assistant roles to leverage the professional judgment of scarce registered nursing personnel, the scope of practice of each role is defined first by law. If the organization extends the

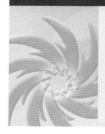

CRITICAL THINKING BOX 14-2

WHERE TO LOOK FOR DETERMINATION OF THE RIGHT TASK

Nurse practice act
Employee job description
Skills checklist
Demonstrated competency

role of a patient care technician to include preoperative teaching, you want to be aware that this is clearly an RN function and not allowed by law to be delegated to the technician. A job description and a policy would not override the legal limits of the scope of practice.

With the right task selected according to the scope of practice, the policies in your agency, and your assessment of the situation, there is still work to be done. Who will do this task? (Figure 14-3)

THE RIGHT PERSON

Matching a task that can be delegated to the right person involves that definition of delegation once again. Nurses must select the right task for a competent person in

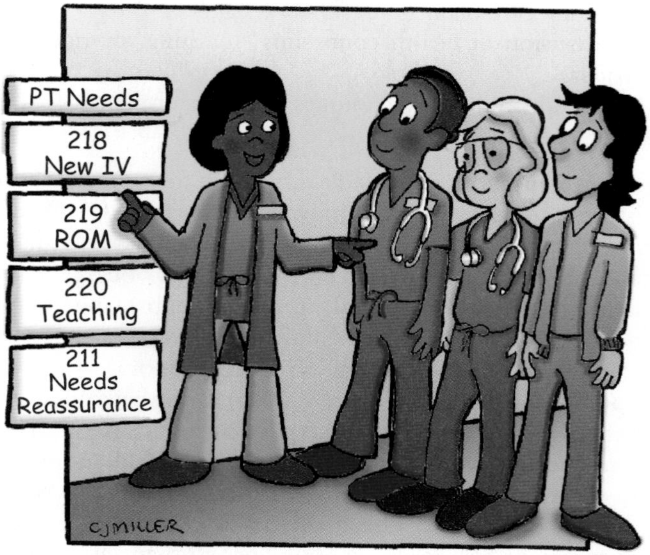
PT Needs
218 New IV
219 ROM
220 Teaching
211 Needs Reassurance
CJMILLER

FIGURE 14-3
It can be difficult to know who is the best person to handle a given situation.

CRITICAL THINKING BOX 14-3

TALKING ABOUT OUTCOMES: WHAT'S IN IT FOR ME?

- Provides a method to decide appropriate assignments: who should be doing what task
- Gives you a sense of purpose for the shift (short term) and long term
- Enhances your ability to motivate co-workers along a track to achieving the outcomes
- Clarifies your role as leader of the team
- Verifies and clarifies patient/family expectations when outcomes are discussed and planned with them
- Promotes job satisfaction for the whole team

a *selected* situation. We have already discussed how you would determine the correct task. But how do we select the right person in the right situation?

HOW CAN I USE OUTCOMES IN DELEGATING?

In planning for the right person to do a task, focusing on outcomes is essential (Critical Thinking Box 14-3). For example, two patients can be admitted to a hospital. Each of these individuals will need a bath today (task), but who will do the bath is related to the outcome you are trying to achieve. For Mr. Peterson, who has been homeless and is in dire need of hygienic care so that you can perform a complete and accurate skin assessment, the priority outcome you and your patient desire is that Mr. Peterson will be clean. With Ms. Ibutu, who is a paraplegic, today is the day that her caregivers and she will demonstrate how they will assess the skin for areas of breakdown and how to perform range of motion to her lower extremities. The RN's decision about who will do the task is dependent on the plan of care and the goals that the team has established in the discussion with the patient or family (Table 14-1).

This same logic applies when you have heard in report that a patient is unstable. In your current care-delivery system on your unit, the licensed practical nurse (LPN) (or licensed vocational nurse [LVN]) may carry out the initial vital sign data-gathering in your postoperative intensive care unit (ICU). Suppose, for example, that the report you received stated that there had been increasing cherry red drainage in the chest tube and that the patient's cardiac monitor showed supraventricular tachycardia, with increasing respiratory rate. On the basis of the outcome for the shift, Mr. Handelsky will maintain cardiorespiratory homeostasis and continue on critical path for first day post-thoracotomy. Using your insight that his condition may be deteriorating, you may make a different decision regarding who will be there for initial patient contact. If the assistant working with you today is an experienced team member, you may choose to send him in to see the patient immediately while you check on another critical patient. Or if the assistant is a float from an agency, known to you only by initial questioning, you may immediately make a visit to see Mr. Handelsky and begin

TABLE 14-1

Using Outcomes in Delegating

Patient	Outcome	Task/Process	Who will perform it?
Mr. Peterson	Patient will be clean	Bath	Nursing assistant or other care associate
Ms. Ibutu	Patient and caregivers will know how to perform skin assessment and range of motion	Bath with education regarding home care	RN: teaching plan; OT, PT, or rehabilitation aide may also assist
Mr. Handelsky	1. Patient will maintain cardiorespiratory homeostasis and continue on care path day 1 2. Patient will be free of pain and comfortable for this shift. Long-term outcome, pain-free death	Initial baseline vital signs and assessment, close monitoring Pain assessment and treatment, comfort measures (repositioning skin care)	RN: assessment and interpretation of data LPN: data-gathering and reporting RN: initial plan for comfort measures and pain assessment Assistant: comfort measures, report of progress

LPN, Licensed practical nurse; *OT*, occupational therapist; *PT*, physical therapist; *RN*, Registered Nurse.

to set up the plan for the data-gathering and schedule for reporting that you will expect from your assistant. This would be a very different process if the outcome you wanted to achieve was pain relief and comfort for a terminal patient.

Take a moment to consider the outcomes for a particularly difficult patient you have been dealing with lately. Were you clear on outcomes? If so, have you shared them with colleagues? Focusing on outcomes takes time. But, as many have often said, "If you fail to plan, you plan to fail." Why should an RN focus on outcomes? Discussion of goals not only establishes who should be doing what task, but also allows RNs to motivate others. How many of us jump on a train if we do not know where it is going? A purpose and a destination allow all of the team members to function more effectively. When assistive personnel are given the same assignment daily, without variation, without any understanding of why they are doing what they are doing, it is similar to being an assembly line worker putting widgets in a machine. Satisfaction and motivation of co-workers generally come from the feeling that they are making a difference in the lives of their patients.

In a similar manner, you as the leader of the team would feel much better at the end of your shift or assignment if you could feel comfortable with the outcomes you have assisted the patient in achieving. You could actually verify the outcomes and plan with the patients, much as you were always told to do by the teachers in your nursing program! Much time is saved by streamlining the care to the patient's expectations.

Again, the RN is accountable for the patient, for determining the situation in which delegation will be used, and for the selection of the right person to do the right task, in addition to the periodic inspection and follow-up of those they supervise.

THE RIGHT CIRCUMSTANCES

The NCSBN describes "Five Rights of Delegation," discussing the "right circumstance" as an additional consideration for the nurse. "Right Circumstances—appropriate client setting, available resources, and consideration of other relevant factors" suggests that the staffing mix, community needs, and teaching obligations, in addition to the type of patients being cared for, should also be considered (NCSBN, 1995). Different rules for delegation may apply regarding what and how an RN must delegate in home care, long-term care, or in community homes for the developmentally disabled or group boarding homes for assisted living (Hansten, Washburn, and Kenyon, 1999, p. 316).

HOW CAN I DETERMINE THE STRENGTHS AND WEAKNESSES OF TEAM MEMBERS?

Often motivated by the fear that a delegate may make a mistake in an assigned task, nurses focus on the potential weaknesses of their team members. As nurses, we are educated to anticipate the worst so that we can prevent accidents, adverse drug reactions, and negative sequelae to disease processes and treatments alike. Prudent as this approach may be for the safety of all concerned, it is worthwhile to discuss the need to be clear on the strengths of the team members as well.

Recall the last time you were given specific, positive feedback about your performance as an RN. (We hope this occurs often!) How did you feel? Most of us are energized and restored by the reinforcement that our hard work has been recognized. When working with assistive personnel or any other colleague, the recognition of strengths will begin to get us on the right track in our relationship.

Assigning tasks on the basis of the strengths of the person will allow the individual and the patient to experience the very best care. Now, as a supervising RN, you are in a new position with respect to the long-term performance of delegates. If assistive personnel are assigned only those tasks they are good at, they may not grow in their abilities and skills. This mistake is exemplified by a hospital that had created a new multiskilled patient care assistant (PCA) role with certified nursing assistants (CNAs). These CNAs had been trained to do phlebotomies as well, as authorized by the state board. Phlebotomists had been eliminated but were given the option of training for the new PCA role. When all of the PCAs worked together, the lab tests were drawn by those who had been phlebotomists because they were more comfortable with that skill. You can certainly imagine the chagrin of the supervising nurses when all the PCAs who were former phlebotomists were off on vacation and maternity leave. None of the PCAs who were formerly CNAs had become proficient at this skill! Recognize strengths, and encourage the best patient care possible by using them, but challenge delegates to grow too.

The dreaded weaknesses in performance of team members can often be prevented by asking the right questions before delegation. Nurses can be reticent about asking personnel such as float or agency replacement staff about whether they feel comfortable in completing the assignment they have received. Float and temporary personnel tell us that they would prefer being asked about their competency at the beginning of a shift or assignment, with the offer of help and clarification, rather than having to locate an RN to request information. The American Nurses Association (ANA) Code of Ethics states, "The nurse is responsible and accountable for individual nursing practice and determines the appropriate delegation of tasks consistent with the nurse's obligation to provide optimum patient care" (ANA, 2001). Be assured that although it is the responsibility of the RN to assess the competency of those they supervise, the delegate must be "accountable for accepting the delegation and for his/her own actions in carrying out the task" (NCSBN, 1995). The RN who is familiar with the situation, however, must ask the correct questions to determine whether the person is competent.

For example, if an RN were planning to ask a nursing assistant to feed a baby with respiratory difficulties, based on the outcome that the baby would be able to ingest 12 ounces of formula this shift, what questions might the RN ask to determine the potential strengths and weaknesses? If the individual has not had experience in this procedure, how could the nurse ensure future competency? In this situation, an RN would certainly ask questions about past experiences with feeding babies with difficulty swallowing. If the delegate assures the RN that she is competent, the RN may go further in asking what the CNA would do if coughing or choking occurred. Depending on the situation, the RN would probably want to demonstrate feeding techniques and observe the skills to ensure the competency of the delegate.

WHAT ARE THE CAUSES OF PERFORMANCE WEAKNESSES?

Let us take a look at an example of a performance weakness and try to determine what the potential causes may be.

In this scenario, you are an RN working a night shift on a hematology-oncology unit, and an agency nursing assistant, Pam, comes to work with you this shift. Pam is excited about the possibilities of interviewing for a regular night shift position and would love to work extra on holidays and weekends. As you begin to discuss her assignment for the night, she states, "Oh, I forgot to tell you, I do not ever take patients who are HIV-positive! Ever!"

There are some potential costs and benefits to your response to this statement. As the charge nurse, you could ignore this statement and continue with your work. You may decide this person has problems, and you may elect to deny her request for an interview. Or you may determine there is something behind her refusal. How you respond may cost you a potentially valuable staff member and could upset the other members of your staff and the patients. Avoiding the problem or accommodating her refusal could become a terrible headache for making assignments and would be contrary to the mission of your organization.

Experience has shown that there are several potential causes of performance inadequacies (Critical Thinking Box 14-4). One of the most common causes is that the employee is not aware of what is expected of him or her. Does Pam know that at this facility it is part of your policy that everyone takes care of all patients, whether or not they are known to be HIV-positive? Perhaps being aware of this expectation would assist Pam in making her decision about whether to apply for work on this unit.

Often, being clear about expectations is not enough. Each of us has some blind spots in his or her own performance. Perhaps we think we are doing just fine, meeting performance competencies and beyond, but colleagues have noted that we are not performing procedures according to policy. If these observations are not shared,

CRITICAL THINKING BOX 14-4

POTENTIAL SOURCES OF PERFORMANCE WEAKNESS

- Unclear expectations
- Lack of performance feedback
- Educational needs
- Need for additional supervision and direction
- Individual characteristics: past experiences, motivational or personal issues

we will blithely believe we are doing great. Another common cause of performance difficulties is that no one has shared their perceptions of our performance with us. Pam may have adopted this attitude regarding other patients in other work settings, and because of the desperation for her help, no one had shared the fact that this behavior falls short of competencies in her job description.

Another common origin of performance weakness is an educational need. Does Pam need more education about how HIV infection is transmitted and how it is prevented? Surely she had to complete some content regarding this in her CNA certification course, but it seems she did not internalize this content. Or is there a personal problem? She may have just witnessed the death of a loved one from AIDS and feel unable to cope with seeing others with this disease for the short term.

The amount of supervision needed can be another source of performance problems. As an RN, you must determine the degree of "periodic inspection" needed by the delegate. Some people require additional direction but are still able to do the job competently. In the absence of that direction, they will be unable to create positive patient outcomes. Nurses tell us they wish that the assistive personnel on their staff would be "self-directed and take initiative without being told." We question whether an RN's hope that all will do their jobs without interaction or supervision on his or her part fits with the definition of supervision! Again, as leader, the RN must determine how much supervision is needed for the individual delegate, just as we determine the degree of observation needed for each patient on the basis of our assessment of their needs. In Pam's case, her reluctance to work with patients with HIV may have nothing to do with supervision but may reflect a need for guidance, education, or a frank discussion of expectations.

As the RN who is supervising Pam, what steps would you take to determine the cause of Pam's performance weakness, the assertion she refused to care for patients with HIV? What questions would you ask? How would you respond so that you could continue to use Pam's services this shift, maintain the integrity of your mission, and preserve the potential for hiring a new employee?

Matching the right person with the right task is the second step in the circular process of delegation. This process includes planning and articulating priority patient outcomes, assessing the competency of the delegate to perform the task, determining the potential strengths and weaknesses of the assistive personnel, and planning how much supervision is needed. To ensure that the right task will be done by the right person, additional clarification of expectations, performance feedback, and planning for education needs may be necessary; these steps will promote the long-term success of the team. The right communication will begin that clarification process, bringing us to the next step in the four rights of delegation.

THE RIGHT COMMUNICATION

HOW CAN I GET THE DELEGATE TO UNDERSTAND WHAT I WANT?

No matter what, it always comes back to communication. How clear you make your initial direction will be the cornerstone in determining the success of your delegated task and, ultimately, the performance of your team. The bottom line, whether the patient outcome was achieved, hinges on your ability to give initial direction that clearly defines your expectations of the delegate in performing the assigned task. It is not surprising that this is a step that is often done poorly or left out entirely because the assumption is made that the individual "knows what the job is and should just do it."

The first component of supervision, according to its definition, is the provision of initial direction. Achieving a balance in which we provide enough information for the person to understand the request without overstating the case and risking confusion or condescension requires that we tread a fine line. The use of the "four Cs" of initial direction will help you to plan your communication (Critical Thinking Box 14-5).

Let us assume that you are working in a home health agency and you are planning the care for a patient with congestive heart failure. You have made your initial visit, assessing the patient and planning the outcomes you and the team will work toward in the next 3 weeks. Your patient is taking diuretics and antihypertensives, in addition to potassium supplements and being on a restricted diet. She is frequently short of breath and requires an assistant three times per week for hygienic care. In addition to providing hygienic care, you would like that assistant to monitor the blood pressure on the days you are not making a visit and to notify you if the blood pressure is outside of the range of 120 to 170 systolic and 50 to 90 diastolic. Using the four *C*s listed, you can evaluate your communication.

CRITICAL THINKING BOX 14-5

THE FOUR *C*s OF INITIAL DIRECTION

CLEAR: Does the team member understand what I am saying?

CONCISE: Have I confused the direction by giving too much unnecessary information?

CORRECT: Is the direction according to policy, procedure, job description, and the law?

COMPLETE: Does the delegate have all the information necessary to complete the task?

"Mrs. Jones has a heart condition and high blood pressure that requires medication and constant monitoring. One of our goals is to help Mrs. Jones have a stable blood pressure, in a range that is normal for her. On the days that you are visiting and giving the patient her bath, I would also like you to take her blood pressure. If it is outside the range of 120 to 170 systolic and 50 to 90 diastolic, I would like you to let me know. We may need to adjust her medication, change her diet, or call her physician for different orders."

Clear: Does the home health aide understand what is being asked of her? This direction is fairly straightforward: an easily understood instruction of taking the blood pressure.

Concise: Have you confused the assistant by giving too much information? Or is it enough for her to complete the task? Only the assistant can help you with this determination. You will need to ask directly, "Am I confusing you, or do you have enough information to do the job?" Every individual has different needs. However, you will want to make certain to check this out; some people will not be honest or accurate in their assessments of their understanding or abilities, leading to trouble later. Many of us are reluctant to ask questions, being afraid to admit our need for additional information. (We do not want to look like we do not know what we are doing!) This reluctance can ultimately result in harm to the patient because assumptions are made that the direction was understood when, in fact, it was not.

Correct: Can a home health aide monitor blood pressures? Where would you look for additional information if you were not sure?

Complete: Does the assistant have enough information to fulfill your expectations? Once again, you will need to ask the delegate for clarification of his or her understanding of what you are asking. If you expect this assistant to also note the respirations and alert you to increased effort of breathing, have you shared that in your initial direction? Or did you assume she would naturally observe all vital signs because you alerted her to the patient's condition (and besides, she is a good assistant)? In our attempts not to appear condescending (I do not want to insult this assistant by reminding her to note the respirations—she might think I do not trust her to think!), we may often choose not to be as complete as we should be in giving initial direction.

Another common pitfall is the rationale that comes from working with someone over a period of time. A working relationship develops, and a routine or pattern of performance is established. When this happens, we start talking less and less to the other individual, believing that "she knows what I expect her to do." Consider the following situation:

You are working on a surgical unit in a partnership with Sam, an LPN you have been working with for the past year. Your easygoing style has led to a comfortable reliance on each other and the feeling that each knows what the other expects. On this particular evening shift, you are traveling down the hall, intent on medicating one of your patients. You also see a postanesthesia care unit (PACU) nurse bring one of your patients back from surgery. Seeing Sam coming your way, you state, "Sam, the postop is back in room 103." Evaluate your initial direction.

Did you believe that Sam just knew you wanted him to check on the patient, get the first set of vital signs, position the patient, check the dressing and the drains, and note the status of the intravenous tube?

Thirty minutes later, you are standing at the nurses' station, noting an order. Sam is charting. You ask him, "Sam, how's the patient in room 103 doing?" Expecting a brief report, you are surprised when Sam says, "I don't know. I thought you were going to take him." What went wrong?

No matter how long you have been working with someone, the right communication is essential to ensure the success of teamwork. Sam did not *accept* the delegated task (remember what the delegate is accountable for?) because he did not understand what you meant. Be sure that you check the delegate's understanding of what you are saying. Failing to do this may result in unmet expectations, which lead to anger and frustration. More importantly, the patient will not receive the optimal care that both of you want to provide.

You have carefully assessed the patient, determined your plan on the basis of outcomes, and selected the right task to delegate to the right person. You have even given clear initial direction as part of the right communication. Now what? The final right of delegation is also a part of supervision: the periodic inspection of the actual act. Read on as we continue with a discussion of the right feedback.

THE RIGHT FEEDBACK

HOW CAN I EFFECTIVELY GIVE AND RECEIVE FEEDBACK?

Many nurses have shared their discomfort with giving and receiving feedback from co-workers. Few of us enjoy telling co-workers how they are doing or hearing about how we may have missed the mark (Figure 14-4)! When supervising others, it is absolutely necessary to give feedback during your "periodic inspection." By following a formula for giving and receiving feedback and practicing it daily, RNs are assisted in the difficult job of correcting the performance of others. The reciprocal feedback process also permits you, as supervising RN, to hear how your own supervisory performance and communication affected the outcomes of the team (Critical Thinking Box 14-6).

Let's look at how this process can be used in a situation in which positive feedback is intended.

An RN (Pat) is working with a float RN (Julia) for the first time. Julia is new in the pool but is an experienced nurse. Pat is so pleased with Julia's experience and performance that she has gone off to have a nice long break and lunch with an old friend from the third floor. She has also taken time to meet with a colleague from the evening shift regarding a unit problem. Unfortunately, she has not been present on the unit much today. When Pat is having lunch with her friend, she exclaims, "That new float Julia is just excellent! If it weren't for her, I couldn't be here having lunch with you. I hope that she knows how organized and valuable she is!" Her friend, Alex, states, "Well, you know you should tell her, not just me, about this." When Pat returns to the floor, flushed with good intentions of making Julia's day with effusive praise, she tells Julia about how lucky she has been to work with her today.

Because all of us crave positive feedback, and Julia is new to your organization, will Julia tell Pat that she's been trying to find her for hours? Probably not. But she *may* tell others that "Pat is one of those 'dump and run' nurses. I don't want to work on that floor again!" What if Pat asked *first*, "How have things been going for you today, Julia? I know this is your first day on the unit." Julia may have determined it was possible

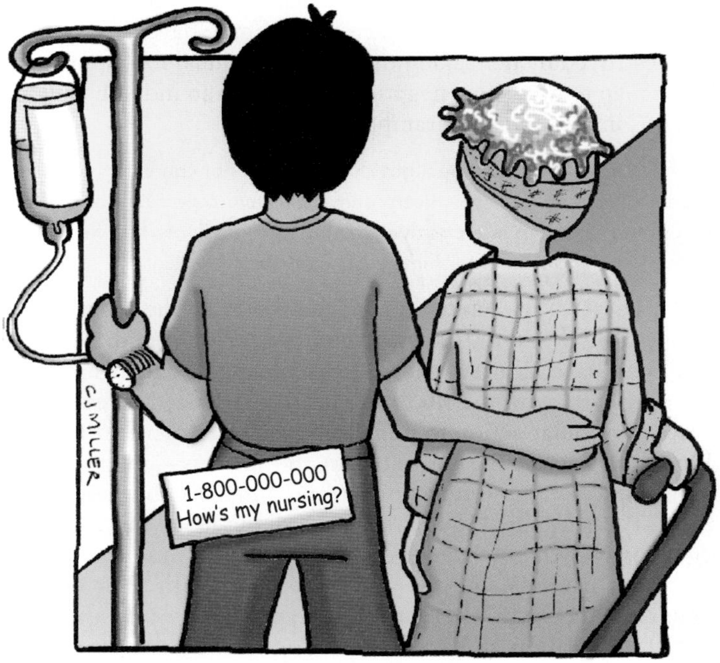

FIGURE 14-4

Providing feedback to the people you supervise does not have to be intimidating.

CRITICAL THINKING BOX 14-6

FEEDBACK FORMULA

- Ask for the other individual's input first!
- Give credit for effort.
- Share your perceptions with each other.
- Explore differing points of view, focusing on shared outcomes.
- Ask for the other individual's input to determine what steps may be necessary to make certain desired outcomes are achieved.
- Agree on a plan for the future, including timeline for followup.
- Revisit the plan and results achieved.

Modified from Hansten R, Jackson M: *Clinical delegation skills: a handbook for nurses*, ed 3, Sudbury, Mass, 2004, Jones & Bartlett.

(and expected) to give reciprocal feedback: "I've been trying to find you! I have completed everything, but it hasn't been easy. Where have you been?" The best intentions can be destroyed by not asking the other individual for input first.

If you plan to give some negative feedback to an individual, you will also need to ask for her/his input first. For example:

> **You have just noted that the night shift CNA did not chart the intakes and outputs (I & O's) on three patients on your telemetry unit. You have called him and are thinking about how to discuss this with him in a positive manner, yet you know that he is not going to want to chat because it is about time for him to get some rest.**

If you said, "Why didn't you put the I & O's on the charts!?" the CNA would react defensively. If you state, "How was your night? I noted that the I & O's are not on the charts," you have allowed the person to respond with what happened. If this CNA went home early with the flu or the unit experienced three codes, it would not be an effective or popular action to pounce on the team member for missing data.

This brings us to the next step in the process—giving credit for what has been accomplished. Let us return to Pat and Julia. At this point, Julia's input has been received. Pat can state, "Well, I can see I didn't help you as much as I should have and I forgot to give you my beeper number. But I do want you to know that I've checked on all of our patients, and they are very happy with their care today." After hearing input and giving credit where it is due, exploration of the gaps in the relationship and their communication and initial direction at the beginning of the shift can now be undertaken with open and frank discussion.

The discussion of differences will progress most smoothly if each party recognizes that they share common objectives: safe, effective care of the patients on their unit, as reflected in the fulfillment of shared, planned outcomes or goals determined by collaborative discussion among patients and care team members. When difficulties or conflicts occur, remember the reason you are both there: the patients.

Julia and Pat may clarify what happened and what actions each may take to ensure that the missed communication does not happen again in the future. Do not try to "fix" the situation for the other individual or prescribe what you will do for them. The other individual will know what he or she needs to do to achieve your shared outcomes. For example, Pat may have decided that what would fix it for Julia would be to convene an hour before shift tomorrow and go through the unit manuals and read procedures. However, the most Julia may need is a beeper number and some more discussion and planning about assignments at the beginning of the shift.

Why wait for the other individual to come up with ideas when we can solve it for them? RNs who lead teams throughout the nation tell us that their work lives would be much better if everyone were behaving in an accountable manner. When we ask others for their step-by-step plan to prevent the problem in the future, it helps them determine that they are accountable for their own performance. In our scene with the missing I & O data, the RN will ask, "How can you make sure those I & O's are charted before you leave in the future? What will work for you?" This type of statement confers the necessary respect for the delegate's ability to determine how to adapt his work performance.

Do not miss the final steps in the formula. The individuals must agree on how they will proceed in the future and when they will revisit the problem or issue again.

Julia may determine that she'll remind Pat in the future when she gets to the unit that she will need her beeper number and a plan for the day. When the next shift is completed, they will want to compare notes about how the shift has proceeded and whether patient outcomes have been achieved. The CNA may decide to ask the RN next week whether she has noted any missing I & O's. The pair will be able to evaluate whether the CNA's charting plan has been effective and can proceed to celebrate the success of the plan or to try other interventions.

Practice using the feedback formula. Remember the following three most important points:

- Ask for the other person's input first.
- Give credit for accomplishments and efforts.
- Ask the other individual to come up with steps for resolving the issue.

How would you use this formula to tell a supervisor that you are concerned about how long it has been since you have heard about your intershift transfer and you are getting worried about whether it will take place? How would you give positive feedback to an individual on your team who has been improving his ability to get out on time? What about a delegate who is "missing in action," the person you cannot seem to locate when you need her?

CONCLUSION

We often hope for an exact prescription for what to delegate, when, and how. Because nursing assessment and professional judgment are necessary for clinical delegation, each situation will be different. Whether you work in an intensive care unit in a large tertiary hospital or a rural long-term care facility, the template of the delegation process—*matching the right task with the right delegate, communicating effectively, and offering and receiving feedback*—will be similar. To judge your comfort and assess your ability to integrate this process in your daily work life, complete the exercise in Critical Thinking Box 14-7. Good luck!

CRITICAL THINKING BOX 14-7

ASSESSING YOUR DELEGATION SKILLS

Assemble these documents:

- Your state nurse practice act
- Your job description and those of co-workers and delegates
- Skills checklists
- The patient list or assignment form from your unit
- A list of the usual staffing complement for your shift

1. Using the above, determine the short-term outcomes for an average patient assignment based on the information you have been

Continued

CRITICAL THINKING BOX 14-7—cont'd

given in a report. What tasks could be delegated to the individuals you have on staff? When will you complete further assessment of the patient situations?

2. Based on the outcomes and job descriptions, how will you determine the competency of individuals to complete the tasks you have determined could be delegated?
3. How will you communicate the team's plan using outcomes in your discussion?
4. How often will you communicate with the delegates, based on their need for supervision and patient complexity and dynamics? Have you used the four Cs?
5. How will you evaluate the effectiveness of your plan? How will you give positive feedback to the team?
6. A mistake was made by a delegate. You determined the person was competent, but the procedure was done improperly. For what are you accountable? How will you give feedback to the individual, encouraging his or her growth and accountability?
7. Have you implemented the Four Rights of Delegation?

REFERENCES

American Nurses Association: *Code of ethics for nurses*, 2001, *www.ana.org/ethics/chcode.htm*.

Hansten R, Jackson M: *Clinical delegation skills: a handbook for professional practice*, ed 3, Sudbury, Mass, 2004, Jones & Bartlett.

Hansten R, Washburn M, Kenyon V: *Home care nursing delegation skills: a handbook for practice*, Gaithersburg, Md, 1999, Aspen.

National Council of State Boards of Nursing: *Concept paper on delegation*, Chicago, 1990, NCSBN.

National Council of State Boards of Nursing: *Delegation: concepts and decision making Process.* Chicago, 1995, NCSBN.

National Council of State Boards of Nursing: *Nursing regulation: mutual recognition*, 2004, *http://ncsbn.org/nlc/rnlpvncompact_mutual_recognition_state.asp*.

Sheehan JP: UAP delegation: a step-by-step process, *Nurs Manage* 32(4):22-24, 2001.

UNIT V

Current Issues in Health Care

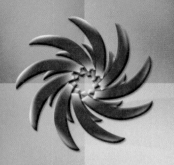

CHAPTER 15

The Health Care Organization and Patterns of Nursing Care Delivery

SUSAN SPORTSMAN, RN, PhD

Every patient needs a nurse.

—*American Nurses Association*

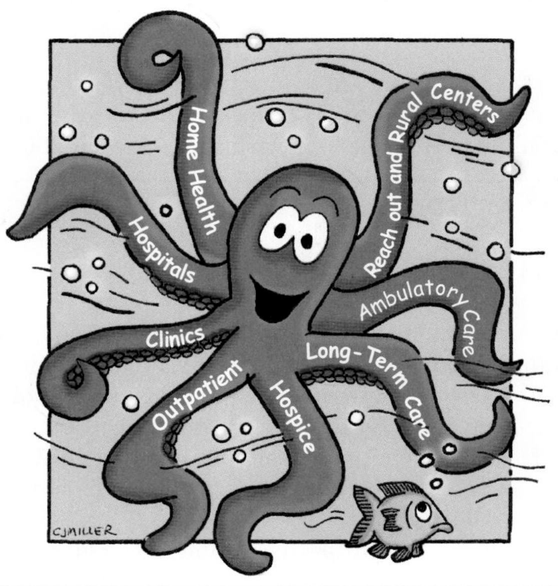

Health care organization should all be within reach.

After completing this chapter, you should be able to:

- Describe challenges facing health care that impact the delivery of nursing care, including:
  - Reduction of costs
  - Evidence-based care
  - Shortage of health care professionals
  - Patient/workplace safety
- Trace the history of the use of nursing care delivery models.
- Consider ways to structure nursing services to improve care while reducing costs.

The United States health care delivery system has been rapidly changing over the last 25 years. The first decade of the new millennium is half over, and these changes seem to be escalating, making the health care environment even more complex. Nurses practicing in such an environment must be comfortable with change and be willing to embrace the challenges that change will bring. A first step to ensuring that your nursing practice evolves in a positive direction is to be knowledgeable about these changes.

WHAT ARE SOME IMPORTANT CHALLENGES CURRENTLY FACING HEALTH CARE?

REDUCTION IN COSTS

There is general consensus by society that health care in the United States costs too much. For example, growth in Medicaid spending, which can be used as a marker of overall costs in health care, averaged a 10.2% per year growth between 2000 and 2003 (Holahan & Ghosh, 2005). The escalating cost of care and its influence on the cost of all goods and services during the past 25 years has set the stage for employers and consumers to demand that care be less expensive and/or more effective (Sportsman & Hawley, 2002). The strategy that has been used to reduce costs can be described in broad terms as **managed care**.

The ultimate goal of managed care can best be illustrated by the following formula (Sportsman & Valadez, 2001):

$$\text{Value} = \frac{\text{Access} + \text{Quality}}{\text{Cost}}$$

A good value is achieved when (1) costs of care are reduced, (2) the effectiveness of the care is improved so that less care is required, or (3) care is provided earlier in the patient's disease so that less care is ultimately needed (Sportsman & Hawley, 2002).

HOW DOES MANAGED CARE CHANGE REIMBURSEMENT PATTERNS?

In an effort to reduce costs, while maintaining or improving access and quality, many payers (insurance companies and governments) have changed the way they pay hospitals and providers for services. In the early 1900s, patients or their families paid the physician directly for the care they received. As health care insurance became an employment benefit, third-party payers became more common. These third party payers paid the provider an agreed-upon fee for each service provided. The more the provider charged, the more the payer paid.

In the early 1980s, Medicare introduced the prospective payment system as a way of reimbursing hospitals. This marked the beginning of a movement to control health care costs. Under this system, which other insurance companies soon adopted, a fixed fee was paid to the hospital according to a preset reimbursement rate for the diagnosis given at discharge. A hospital could treat a patient so that a shorter length of stay is necessary, reducing the consumption of resources. This would allow the hospital to show a greater profit or smaller loss for caring for this patient with a particular diagnosis. This practice began the trend to pay for health care at a prearranged rate rather than as billed.

In the most extreme type of managed care, called capitation, employers pay a set fee each month to an insurance company for each covered employee and dependent. That amount does NOT vary based on the care given. Potential patients may never need any health care or may require extensive hospitalizations. Regardless, the costs of care must be taken out of the set fee. Under this arrangement, there is incentive for the insurance company to work aggressively to keep employees healthy, because prevention and/or early intervention are likely to be less expensive than hospitalization. Conversely, if patients do not stay healthy and overuse hospitalization, the health care provider may actually lose money.

As a part of the managed care trend, health maintenance organization (HMO) plans have become very popular as a form of insurance. In HMOs, an annual payment is made on behalf of the members to a group of providers who deliver all of the health services covered under the plan, including physician and hospital services. HMOs have grown in the past few years because they provide a strong incentive to avoid hospitalization, which consequently reduces costs. HMO members often like the ease of utilizing health care with an HMO, because there are fewer uncovered services and forms to fill out. However, the choice of providers is limited; members must use physicians that are part of the HMO and they may not see specialty physicians without a referral from their primary care provider.

The preferred provider organization (PPO) is another type of insurance plan designed to meet the goals of managed care. To avoid out-of-pocket expenses, members must use physicians who have agreed to provide services at a lower price to the insurer. However, members may use an "out-of-network" provider without a referral, if they are willing to pay more for that service.

WHAT IS THE IMPACT OF MANAGED CARE ON HEALTH CARE ENTITIES?

To achieve large economies of scale, thereby reducing costs, the corporatization of health is taking place. Small operating facilities, such as individual hospitals or physician's offices, are merging into large-scale organizations, so that duplicate processes and redundant facilities, equipment, and procedures can be eliminated and costs reduced (Critical Thinking Box 15-1).

There has also been a shift from nonprofit hospitals to those that have for-profit status. Nonprofit organizations do not pay taxes; instead, they return their earnings to the community through support of the organization. In contrast, for-profit organizations pay taxes and return their earnings to stockholders. Regardless of whether or not the hospital has nonprofit status, the nurse's work environment is likely to involve a corporate culture, in which there is an increased emphasis of the business aspect of health care (Critical Thinking Box 15-2).

CRITICAL THINKING BOX 15-1

How will the merging of small hospitals into larger regional hospitals affect the accessibility of health care for rural communities?

CRITICAL THINKING BOX 15-2

Should a hospital be allowed to operate as a for-profit organization? Are for-profit hospitals managed more efficiently?

WHAT IS MEANT BY INTEGRATED HEALTH CARE DELIVERY SYSTEMS?

As a part of corporatization of health care, individual health care organizations that merge into systems to provide all needed services under one corporate umbrella are known as integrated health care delivery systems (IHS). These systems may offer prevention services, acute- and long-term care facilities, home health care and hospice services. The system may own the individual entities or may contract to provide specialty services. With integrated health care systems, employers and insurance companies have the ability to contract with one system to meet all the health care needs of their employees or members rather than negotiating multiple contracts with many organizations.

Integrated health care systems may offer a high degree of continuity of care among the various health care entities within the organization. This allows patients to enjoy a sense of seamlessness in care, as they move from hospital to the nursing home, hospice, or rehabilitation center. However, this requires that staff from the various entities work collaboratively instead of in a competitive way, which has been typical in the past.

HOW DOES CASE MANAGEMENT SUPPORT MANAGED CARE?

Case management is one of the strategies suggested to ensure coordination of care while reducing costs. Although case management in acute-care hospitals is relatively

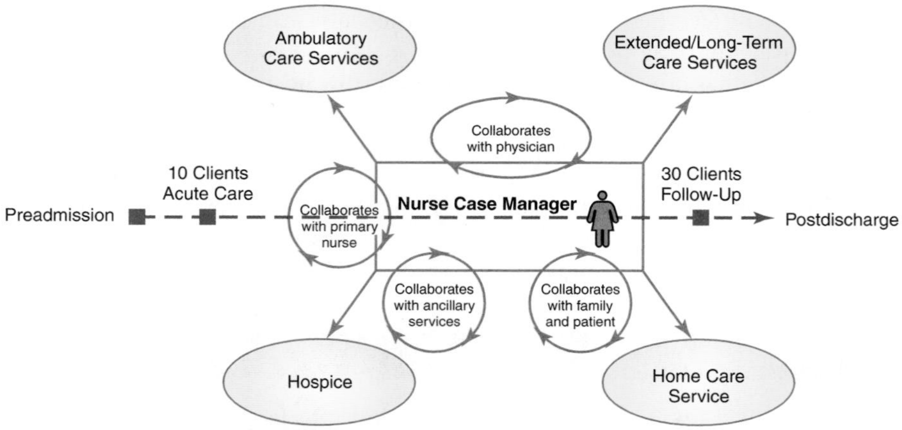

FIGURE 15-1
Case management structure.

new, it has been used for many years in long-term or community-based care as a way to make sure that health care services were coordinated (Figure 15-1). According to the Case Management Society of America (CMSA), case management is a collaborative process that assesses, plans, implements, coordinates, monitors, and evaluates options and services to meet a person's health needs. The case manager uses communication and available resources to promote quality, cost-effective care (CMSA, 2005). Case management, like the nursing process, is based on circular steps. Figure 15-1 illustrates this process. Table 15-1 outlines the components of the case management process.

TABLE 15-1
Case Management Process

Components of the Case Management Process		
Steps in the Process	**Definition**	**Activities to Be Accomplished by Case Manager**
Assessment	Process of collecting pertinent information about a person's situation to identify needs and develop a plan.	• Identify factors likely to affect treatment or recovery (e.g., age; identified chief complaint; other medical conditions; mental, social, psychosocial, or emotional problems; use of medications; financial status; lifestyle; occupational issues; support systems). • Determine what social and community resources are available to patient. • Determine patient's financial resources, including available insurance benefits. • Identify patient's/significant other's expectation and understanding of the problem.
Reassessment	Occurs periodically as new information becomes available or as changes occur.	• Identify abnormal coping patterns, unusual family dynamics, or potential barriers to recovery. • Gather information regarding abnormalities from multiple sources (e.g., patient record, other providers, patient, significant other). • Organize and classify data collected, identifying patterns to determine what is pertinent.
Planning	Process of setting goals and objectives and determining actions necessary to them. The plan must be time-specific, and steps to the plan should include the sequence, duration, and frequency of the actions. Care maps, critical paths, and/or disease-management protocols may be used to develop the plan.	• Develop goals, objectives, and actions in collaboration with other caregivers, the patient, significant other, insurance companies, or employers and other interested parties. • Determine the costs and benefits of available resources. If patients need treatment for which they have no coverage, look for alternative sources of care.

Continued

TABLE 15-1

Case Management Process—cont'd

Components of the Case Management Process		
Steps in the Process	**Definition**	**Activities to Be Accomplished by Case Manager**
Implement	Process through which the agreed-on plan is enacted.	• Refer patient/significant other to services. • Help patient to self-refer. • Educate patient regarding options.
Coordinate and monitor	Process by which the resources are secured and integrated to accomplish the goals/objectives of the plan. Case manager is responsible for smooth implementation of care. Care maps, critical pathways, and disease-management protocols and checklists may be used to document this process.	• Communicate the results of referrals and treatment to other caregivers. • Monitor issues that affect the patient's recovery or integration back into the community (e.g., home support, physical and environmental barriers, occupation, educational level). • Maintain communication with insurance plans or others paying for services. • Follow-up with patient and others periodically throughout episode of care. • Evaluate possible barriers to care or patient compliance (e.g., lack of understanding, lack of transportation, family support, scheduling conflicts).
Evaluation	Process of measuring quality and outcomes of products and services to determine whether the activities have produced the desired effect. Evaluation data may also be used to modify existing programs, plan new ones, or develop clinical benchmarks.	• Evaluate the frequency and the duration of treatment for appropriateness. • Compare actual outcomes with expected ones. If goals/objectives have not been reached, determine why not. • Revise the plan on the basis of feedback gathered from the evaluation.

Modified from Ling C: Why and what you should know about case management, *Health Week*, February 2, 1998.

Case managers work in all types of health care organizations (acute-care, subacute-care, rehabilitation, psychiatric/substance abuse, and a variety of community service agencies). In addition, they may work for insurance or utilization review companies, in employee health for large businesses, or to ensure coordination of care in integrated health care delivery systems. Registered nurses, social workers, and therapists may all be case managers; although how they perform their role depends on the scope of practice of their discipline. All case managers must be skilled at communication, critical thinking, negotiation, and collaboration. They must be knowledgeable about resources available to patients. The case manager not only deals with individual patients, but also with family and other support systems of the patient.

Case management is effective in providing care, but all patients do not need this intensity of interaction. To provide such care to all patients would be wastefully expensive. Patients should only be assigned a case manager if they:

- Have complicated health care needs
- Are receiving care that is expensive as well as complicated
- Pose discharge-planning problems
- Receive care from multiple providers
- Are likely to have significant physical or psychosocial problems.

WHAT TOOLS ARE USED TO SUPPORT CASE MANAGEMENT?

Clinical pathways and **disease-management protocols** are similar strategies that support the work of the case manager to reduce expensive variations in care.

Clinical pathways, also known as care maps, are multidisciplinary plans of "best" clinical practice for groups of patients with a specific medical diagnosis.

These pathways support the coordination and delivery of high-quality care. There are four essential elements of a clinical pathway:

- A timeline outlining when specific care will be given
- The categories of care or activities and their interventions
- Intermediate and long-term outcomes to be achieved
- A variance record

The variance record allows caregivers to document when and why the progress of individual patients varies from that outlined in the pathway. Clinical pathways differ from practice guidelines, protocols, and algorithms, because they are used by the multidisciplinary team and have a focus on quality and coordination of care for individual patients (What are Clinical Pathways?, 2005). Table 15-2 is a schematic representation of a clinical pathway that takes into account the number of days allocated by the patient's diagnosis, in addition to information for teaching and discharge.

Disease management is a system of coordinated health care interventions and communications for persons with conditions in which self-care is important in controlling the disease.

Disease management:

- Supports the physician or practitioner/patient relationship and plan of care
- Emphasizes prevention of exacerbations and complications by using evidence-based practice guidelines and patient empowerment strategies
- Evaluates clinical, humanistic, and economic outcomes on an ongoing basis, with the goal of improving overall health (DMAA, 2005)

Managed care organizations often enroll members who have a specific disease, such as diabetes, in a program tailored for the needs of patients with that condition. The program focuses on prevention and educational activities when members are NOT in the acute stage of the disease, so that they will be prepared to understand and manage

TABLE 15-2

Clinical Pathway Major Chest Procedures—4-Day Recovery

Time Frame	1	2	3	4	Discharge
Location	**TCI →OR →CVICU → RNF**	**POD #1**	**POD #2**	**POD #3**	**POD #4**
Date/Unit	**Date Unit**	**Date Unit**	**Date Unit**	**Date Unit**	**Date Unit**
Patient satisfaction	What can we do to enhance your stay with us?	What can we do to enhance your stay with us?	What can we do to enhance your stay with us?	What can we do to enhance your stay with us?	What can we do to enhance your stay with us?
Discharge planning	Patient verbalizes expected LOS and postop activity. PERS initiated. Patient's primary support person identified.	Verbalizes understanding of progress. Patient's needs identified and notify as needed for D/C.	Verbalizes understanding of progress. Patient's needs identified and notify as needed for D/C.	Verify all medications, supplies, services are arranged for discharge.	Discharge instructions given to patient.
Patient education	Instruct family to go to surgical waiting room. Orient patient during emergence from anesthesia.	Reinforce IS, C & DB exercises, pain management, and ambulation. Provide patient/family with information R/T discharge needs.	Provide patient/family with information R/T discharge needs/procedures and progress.	Provide patient/family with information R/T discharge needs/procedures and progress.	Discharge instructions R/T medications, activity, diet, treatments, and incisional care.
Tests/procedures/consults	CXR, CBC, KP6; ABGs, BPH/Ventolin q6; respiratory therapy; pain management; CHIRP.	CXR, oximetry. Radiation oncology prn. Hemo/oncology prn. Home health care prn.	CXR, oximetry. Respiratory therapy.	Oximetry. Pulmonary rehab prn	
Allied health interventions		Respiratory Tx per respiratory consult algorithm.	Respiratory Tx per respiratory consult algorithm.	Wt qd; VS routine; IS 10x/hr w.a.; pain control with PO.	VS routine; IS 10x/hr WA

Nursing/medical interventions	Monitor rhythm; VS routine; I & O; wt qd; O_2 N/C; chest tubes to suction; Foley; wean from vent.	Telemetry; I & O; wt qd; VS routine; IS 10x/hr w.a.; C & DB; D/C 1 CT; epidural pain control, D/C Foley.	D/C telemetry; D/C I & O; wt qd; VS routine, IS 10x/hr; C & DB; epidural pain control (to be D/C when last CT out); D/C CT; wean O_2 to room air; remove incisional dressings and begin wound care.	UAL. Preop diet.	UAL. Preop diet.
Mobility	BR; turn q2, HOB ↑ 30; up in chair after extub.	OOB with assistance and chair 1 qs.	Chair qs and ambulate hall TID.		
Nutrition	NPO; ice chips; clear liquids D5½NS+ 20 KCl.	Clear liquids → full liquid diet; IV to HL if tolerating liquids.	Advance diet as tolerated.		
Outcomes criteria	Admission assessment completed. Anesthesia consult documented. Patient assessment completed and WNL. Patient premedicated. Patient/family satisfaction addressed.	Patient with adequate oxygenation per pulse oximetry; hemodynamically stable; alert and oriented × 3. Adequate pain control. Patient/family satisfaction addressed.	Tolerate diet. Has BM normal for patient. Comfort level maintained. Ambulate W/O SOB. Patient/family satisfaction addressed.	Tolerate diet. Has BM normal for patient. Comfort level maintained. Ambulate W/O SOB. Breath sounds and secretions clear. Patient/family satisfaction addressed.	Breath sounds and secretions clear. Ambulates independently W/O SOB. Infection free. Patient/family satisfaction addressed.

From Phipps W, Sands J, Marek J : *Medical-surgical nursing: concepts and clinical practice*, St Louis, 1997, Mosby.
4/1/97 (1:\cct\thoracic\75a-fdr) Thoracic FDR – 4 Day Recovery, Courtesy The Cleveland Clinic Foundations, 1997. This is a general guideline to assist in the management of patients. This guideline is not designated to replace clinical judgment or individual patient needs.
C & DB, Cough and deep breathe; *CHIRP*, rehab program; *CT*, chest tube; *CXR*, Chest radiograph; *D/C*, discharge; *HL*, heparin lock; *HOB*, head of bed; *IS*, incentive spirometry; *OOB*, out of bed; *prn*, as needed; *qs*, quantity sufficient; *R/T*, routine; *SOB*, short of breath; *UAL*, up ad lib; *WA*, when awake; *W/O*, without.

symptoms throughout their lives. Nurses, often employed by health plans, are frequently involved in this component of disease management. Disease-management protocols also outline standard interventions to be implemented during the acute stage of the illness, although physicians or other providers may make modifications to provide individualized care. Disease-management programs are primarily for patients with chronic diseases that occur frequently, those that vary widely in treatment options, and those that are very expensive to treat (Finkelman, 2000).

Both critical pathways and disease-management protocols are generally based on clinical guidelines that incorporate nationally acceptable ways to care for a specific disease. Clinical guidelines are specific practice recommendations that come from a rigorous review of the best evidence on a specific topic (Melnyk & Fineout-Overholt, 2005). These guidelines are typically developed by government agencies, such as the Agency for Healthcare Research and Quality (AHRQ), or an organization devoted to a specific disease, such as the American Health Association. A website developed by AHRQ, in collaboration with the American Medical Association (AMA) and the American Association of Health Plans, provides a resource for clinical practice guidelines at *www.guideline.gov.*

EVIDENCE-BASED PRACTICE

HOW DO WE KNOW THAT CRITICAL PATHWAYS AND DISEASE-MANAGEMENT PROTOCOLS REFLECT THE LASTEST AND BEST PRACTICE?

In 2000, the Institute of Medicine (IOM) released a report, "Crossing the Quality Chasm: A New Health System for the 21st Century" (IOM, 2000). This report noted that it takes 17 years for the results of research in health care to be transmitted consistently into practice.

> Evidence-based practice is one strategy to reduce the amount of time required to integrate new health care findings into practice.

Evidence-based practice is the conscientious use of current best evidence in making decisions about patient care (Sackett et al, 2000). It flows from clinicians asking, "What is the best way to manage a particular situation?" Melnyk and Fineout-Overholt (2005) believe that evidence-based practice uses the following steps to answer clinical questions:

- A systematic search for the most relevant evidence to the question
- Critical evaluation of the evidence found (Is the evidence logical and valid?)
- Your own clinical experience (Does your experience fit with the evidence?)
- Patient preferences and values (Will your patients accept the recommendations drawn from the evidence?)

The answer to the questions can then be implemented in practice or incorporated into critical pathways and disease-management processes.

Most nurses use their own clinical experience and patient preferences and values in planning nursing care. However, searching for the evidence to the question at hand and critically evaluating it may be more difficult. Table 15-3 outlines a rating system to

TABLE 15-3

Evaluation Criteria for Evidence for Clinical Questions

Level	Definition
Level I	Evidence comes from a review of a number of randomized controlled trials (RCTs) or from clinical practice guidelines that are based on such a review
Level II	Evidence comes from at least one well-designed RCT
Level III	Evidence comes from well-designed controlled studies that are not randomized
Level IV	Evidence comes from well-designed case-controlled and cohort studies
Level V	Evidence comes from a number of descriptive or qualitative studies
Level VI	Evidence comes from a single descriptive or qualitative study
Level VII	Evidence comes from the opinion of authorities and/or reports of expert committees

From Sackett D, Straus S, Richardson W, et al: *Evidence-based medicine: how to practice and teach EBM*, London, 2000, Churchill Livingstone.

help you know how strong the evidence from research or other sources might be. (See Chapter 24 for more information on how evidence-based practice affects economics.)

There are at least three centers in schools of nursing in the United States that can serve as resources regarding evidence-based practice in nursing. These include:

- The Academic Center for Evidence-Based Nursing (ACE) at the University of Texas Health Science Center at San Antonio: *www.acestar.uthscsa.edu*
- The Center for Research & Evidence-Based Practice (CREP) at the University of Rochester School of Nursing in New York: *www.urmc.rochester.edu/son/ebp/*
- The Sara Cole Hirsch Institute for Best Nursing Practice Based on Evidence at Case Western Reserve School of Nursing: *http://fpb.cwru.edu/HirshInstitute/* (Critical Thinking Box 15-3).

SHORTAGE OF NURSES

Although hospitals and other health care organizations have experienced nursing shortages over the past 50 years, the most recent shortage, which began in 1998, seems to be the most long lasting (Buerhaus, Staiger, & Auerbach, 2004).

In 2002, the Health Resources and Service Administration (HRSA) reported that the current nursing shortage will deepen because the numbers of nurses who are retiring will not be replaced by those entering the profession.

CRITICAL THINKING BOX 15-3

What are the advantages to using evidence-based nursing care? What are the barriers? How might these barriers be overcome?

Thirty states experienced a nursing shortage in 2000; however, by 2012, the crisis will intensify, with 44 states, plus the District of Columbia, expected to experience RN shortages (HRSA, 2002). This trend is made more severe because of the growing number of older patients, the advances in technology, the aging of nursing faculty, and the wide range of career options now available to young people.

In 2002, employment and earnings of RNs working in hospitals increased sharply, suggesting that the shortage might be easing. A closer analysis of this trend, however, found that two thirds of the increase in employment in 2002 came from older RNs. The remainder was RNs born in other countries (Buerhaus, Staiger, & Auerbach, 2004). This migration, coupled with wage increases, relatively high national unemployment, and widespread private sector initiatives aimed at nursing recruitment explains the increase. Unfortunately, the American College of Healthcare Executives (ACHE) reported in 2004 that 72% of hospital CEOs were still experiencing a nursing shortage in their facilities (ACHE, 2004). In January 2004, the Hodes Group released the results of a poll of 151 health care recruiters designed to determine turnover rates, cost-per-hire, and vacancy rates for RNs. The survey found that the average RN turnover rate in U.S. hospitals was 15.5%, and the vacancy rate was 13.9% (Hodes, 2004).

WHAT CAN BE DONE TO RECRUIT NURSES TO THE PROFESSION?

Since 1999, several groups have focused on nursing recruiting. For example, the Johnson & Johnson Campaign for Nursing's Future included national television; print and interactive advertising; a public relations component; and recruitment materials distributed to hospitals, high schools, nursing schools, and other organizations to encourage nursing as a career field for a diverse population. In February 2004, Johnson & Johnson also launched a new public awareness campaign to generate interest in careers as nurse educators (*www.nursesource.org* and *www.discovernursing.com*). There has also been work done to improve the work environment for nurses as a means of enhancing the image of nursing as an attractive career (Box 15-1).

HOW CAN HEALTH CARE ORGANIZATIONS RETAIN NURSES?

Retention of nurses in the work environment is as important as effective recruitment. Certainly, adequate compensation and flexible staffing are two strategies that make nurses want to continue their employment within an organization. However, maintaining a positive work environment is equally important. A review of literature regarding job satisfaction of nurses consistently found eight factors that can encourage nurses to remain in their jobs.

These factors included:

- An environment that allows professional autonomy
- Good communication and interpersonal relationships
- The structure of the department and/or prevalent leadership style
- Work recognition (both internal and external to the employment site)
- Working conditions
- Professional practice
- Pay/benefits
- Staffing/scheduling issues (Kuhar et al, 2004)

BOX 15-1 Can the Shortage Be Fixed?

Question posed to nurses: "If you had the power, a magic wand, to solve the nursing shortage, what is the first thing you would do and why?

- **Nursing dean:** "The first thing I would do is change the public perception to make nursing's image more accurate. It's that public perception that nursing is an assistant to medicine…I think it is one of the major stumbling blocks to having very talented, smart men and women choose nursing today."
- **Assistant hospital administrator:** "Everybody thinks the solution is marketing and advertising. I think it's mentoring and coaching and encouragement. There are too many barriers."
- **Staff nurse:** "Working conditions would be so much better if you had the supplies available to take care of the patients, and you weren't so overworked that when you left at the end of the day you felt like you didn't provide adequate care to anybody."
- **Former nurse recruiter:** Nurse recruiters in hospitals are recruiting. "Pull out the stops, do the sign-on bonuses, basically bribe them in some way to get them in the door. But until you can stop the bleeding, they're coming in the front door and leaving out the back door. It's not a quick fix, but I would provide leadership training in every facility." Within the top ten reasons that nurses leave positions, "More than half of them have to do with their direct supervisor."

"Recruitment is sales, retention is leadership."

From McPeck P: Can we fix it?, *NurseWeek (South Central edition)* 5:17-19, 2004.

Recognizing that these characteristics influence a positive work environment is not new. In the early 1980s, during a previous nursing shortage, the American Academy of Nursing conducted research to identify organizational attributes of hospitals successful in recruiting and retaining nurses. American Academy of Nursing Fellows nominated 165 hospitals throughout the nation that had reputations for successfully attracting and retaining nurses and delivering high-quality nursing care. Ultimately 41 hospitals were distinguished by high nurse satisfaction, low job turnover, and low nurse vacancy rates, even when hospitals located in the same area were experiencing nursing shortages. These hospitals were called "magnet" hospitals because of their successes in attracting and keeping nurses. The core organizational attributes that were common to these "magnet" hospitals included:

- The nurse executive was a formal member of the highest decision-making body in the hospital.
- Nursing services were organized in a flat organizational structure with only a few supervisory personnel.
- Decision-making was decentralized to the unit level, giving unit nurses as much discretion as possible in providing care.
- Administrative structure supported nurses' decisions about patient care.
- Good communication existed between nurse and physicians. (Havens & Aiken, 1999)

Since the early 1980s, significant research about magnet hospitals has documented that having these factors in place in hospital nursing services has produced positive benefits for patients and staff. Hospitals that organize their nursing services around

CRITICAL THINKING BOX 15-4

What are the factors that YOU think result in a great working environment? What factors result in an unacceptable environment?

these characteristics are associated with lower Medicare mortality rates, higher levels of patient and nurse satisfaction, lower levels of nurse emotional exhaustion, and fewer nurse-reported needle-stick injuries (Aiken, Smith, & Lake, 2002).

Ten years after the identification of the original magnet hospitals, the American Nurses Credentialing Center (ANCC) established a new magnet hospital designation process, similar to accreditation by the Joint Commission on Accreditation of Healthcare Organizations (JCAHO). Recently, the recognition program has been expanded to provide national recognition for excellence in long-term care nursing services. In the current competitive environment, receiving the magnet status may serve as a recruiting and marketing tool for hospitals, attesting to a professional work environment and quality nursing care (Sportsman, 2005) (Critical Thinking Box 15-4).

PATIENT SAFETY

Patient safety is a large issue in the current health care environment. In 1996, the IOM initiated a concerted, ongoing effort to assess and improve the quality of care in the United States. The first phase documented the seriousness of the quality problems. In the second phase (1999-2001), two reports were released. "To Err is Human: Building a Safer Health System" (IOM, 1999) focused on how tens of thousands of Americans die each year because of medical errors. "Crossing the Quality Chasm: A New Health System for the 21st Century" (IOM, 2000) defined six aims to improve health care quality, including that care is:

- Safe
- Effective
- Patient-centered
- Timeny
- Efficient
- Equitable

The third phase, which is going on now, focuses on determining ways that the future health care delivery system described in earlier reports can be realized. Box 15-2 outlines some of the more recent IOM reports from this initiative. Visit *www.iom.org* for more information.

One of the IOM reports, "Keeping Patients Safe: Transforming the Work Environment of Nurses," suggests that the work environment of nurses needs to be changed to better protect patients. The report makes recommendations in the areas of (1) nursing management, (2) workhorse deployment, and (3) work design and organizational culture (IOM, 2003). For example, restructuring of hospital organizations in

BOX 15-2 Recent Reports of Health Care Quality from the Institute of Medicine

Leadership by Example: Coordinating Government Roles in Improving Health Care
Crossing the Quality Chasm: A New Health System for the 21st Century
Ensuring Quality Cancer Care
Envisioning the National Health Care Quality Report
To Err is Human: Building a Safer Health System
Fostering Rapid Advances in Health Care
Health Professions Education: A Bridge to Quality
Priority Areas for National Action: Transforming Health Care Quality
Key Capabilities of an Electronic Health Record System
Patient Safety: Achieving a New Standard for Care
Keeping Patients Safe: Transforming the Work Environment of Nurses
1st Annual Crossing the Quality Chasm Summit: A Focus on Communities

From *www.iom.edu.*

response to managed care often has undermined the trust between nurses and administration. The report urges health care organizations to involve nurse leaders in all levels of management in decision-making and to ask nursing staff their opinions about care design, because nurses are very effective in detecting processes that contribute to errors.

A report, "Health Care at the Crossroads: Strategies for Addressing the Evolving Nursing Crisis" released by JCAHO in 2002, concurs with the IOM recommendations. This report suggests that nurse executives should delegate decision-making authority to nurse managers and other nursing unit leaders about how units should be run and how scarce resources should be spent. This demonstrates the confidence that the nurse executive has in the competency of the managers. In turn, the authority to make real-time, critical decisions at the point of care should be delegated from the unit leaders to the nursing staff. In the middle of the night, when administrators are not present, the decisions of nurses control patient outcomes (JCAHO, 2002).

This concern about patient safety extends to other areas within JCAHO. In 2004, the JCAHO Board of Commission established National Patient Safety Goals, which have been revised for 2005. (See Table 22-1 on p. 528 for the 2005 Hospitals' Patient Safety Goals.)

One of the 2005 JCAHO Hospitals' Patient Safety Goals is to improve the effectiveness of communication among caregivers (see Table 22-1 on p. 528). Although the requirements of this goal deal with clear communication regarding physician orders and test results, there are other issues surrounding communication that may reduce patient safety and job satisfaction of nurses. A national study, "Silence Kills," sponsored in part by American Association of Critical-Care Nurses (AACCN), describes interviews with more than 1700 nurses, physicians, clinical-care staff, and administrators, and found that fewer than 10% of them speak to colleagues about behaviors that could result in errors or other types of harm to patients. These behaviors may include trouble following directions, demonstration of poor clinical

TABLE 15-4

AACN Standards for Establishing and Sustaining Healthy Work Environments

Category	Standard
Skilled communication	Nurses must be as proficient in communication skills as they are in clinical skills.
True collaboration	Nurses must be relentless in pursuing and fostering true collaboration
Effective decision making	Nurses must be valued and committed partners in making policy, directing and evaluating clinical care, and leading organizational operations
Appropriate staffing	Staffing must ensure the effective match between patient needs and nurse competencies
Meaningful recognition	Nurses must be recognized and must recognize others for the value each brings to the work of the organization
Authentic leadership	Nurse leaders must fully embrace the imperative of a health work environment, authentically live it, and engage others in its achievement.

From American Association of Critical Care Nurses: *AACN standards for establishing and sustaining healthy work environments: a journey to excellence*, 2005, *www.aacn.org*.

judgment, or taking dangerous shortcuts. The results are often broken rules, mistakes, lack of support, incompetence, poor teamwork, disrespect, and micromanagement. When clinicians speak up, these conversations are called "crucial conversations" (AACCN, 2005).

The authors believe that having "crucial conversations" should result in significant reductions in errors, improved quality of care, reduction in nursing turnover, and marked improvement in productivity (Patterson et al, 2005). In an effort to address the issues identified in "Silence Kills," the AACCN has established Standards for Establishing and Sustaining Healthy Work Environments. Table 15-4 identifies these standards. (Also see Critical Thinking Box 15-5.)

CRITICAL THINKING BOX 15-5

WHAT DO YOU THINK?

How many hours are too long to work?

Is there an increase in errors made by nurses working 12 hours or longer?

How would you handle it if the supervisor asked you to work 6 more hours after your 12-hour shift because the floor is short?

What is your responsibility as a professional when it comes to overtime?

WHAT ARE THE EFFECTS OF VARIOUS PATTERNS OF NURSING CARE DELIVERY?

Over the years, nursing care has been delivered in many ways, including total patient (private duty model), functional, team, primary, and relationship-based care (Figure 15-2). Although we often talk about these systems as distinct from one another, in the real world, you seldom find pure forms of these systems. Consequently, you must be prepared to work in systems that may be a combination, tailor-made to fit the needs of a specific organization.

WHAT IS THE TOTAL PATIENT CARE OR PRIVATE DUTY MODEL?

Originally nursing was organized around the total patient care or private duty model. Registered nurses were hired by the patient and provided care to one patient, typically in their home. In the 1920s, 1930s, and again in the 1980s, this approach was used in which one nurse assumes responsibilities for the complete care of a group of patients on a 1:1 basis, providing total patient care during the shift.

The quality of care in the total patient care model is considered to be high, because all activities are carried out by RNs, who can focus their complete attention on one

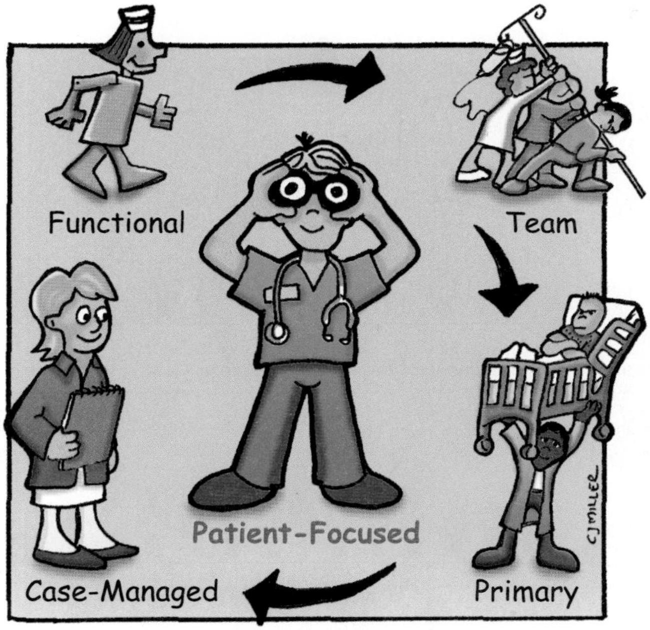

FIGURE 15-2
Evolving patterns of nursing care delivery.

patient. Tiedeman and Lookinland (2004) suggest that this model is efficient because it (1) decreases communication time between staff caring for a patient, (2) reduces the need for supervision, and (3) allows one person to perform more than one task simultaneously. Some nurses prefer this model because they can focus on patients' needs without the work of supervising others; others feel that their skills and time are wasted doing patient care activities that could be done by others with less skill and education. Patient satisfaction tends to be high with this model if continuity of care and communication are maintained among nurses (Tiedeman & Lookinland, 2004).

WHAT IS FUNCTIONAL NURSING?

The movement to use RNs as employees of hospitals came with the outbreak of World War II. RNs took over the work in the hospital and that, coupled with the war effort, stimulated the nursing shortage of that period. This forced hospitals to develop alternative models of nursing. The positions of aides and licensed vocational/practical nurses came into being, and in some states, they were allowed to perform functions such as administration of medications and treatments. This functional kind of nursing, which broke nursing care into a series of tasks performed by many people, resulted in a fragmented, impersonal kind of care (Figure 15-3). Fragmentation of care caused patient problems to be overlooked, because they did not fit into a defined assignment.

Tiedeman and Lookinland (2004) note that this assembly-line approach provided little time for the nurse to address psychosocial or spiritual needs. They cite a number of studies, which found that errors and omissions increased when functional nursing was used. This approach would seem to be cost efficient, because it can be implemented

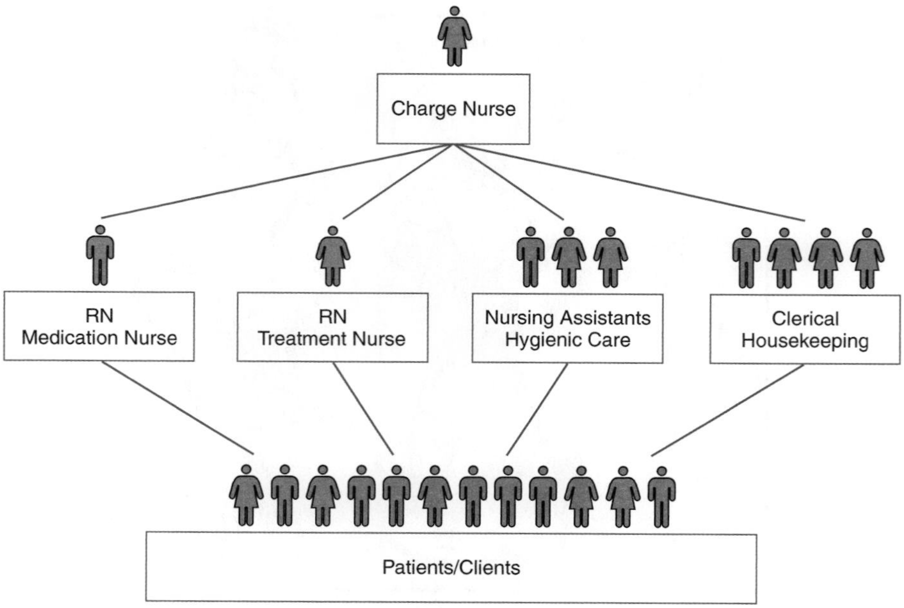

FIGURE 15-3
Lines of authority: functional nursing.

with fewer RNs. However, there are studies that suggest that the functional method, in fact, costs more than primary nursing care. In addition, patients, nurses, and physicians have been critical of this approach because of the fragmentation and the lack of accountability for the total patient (Tiedeman & Lookinland, 2004).

WHAT IS TEAM NURSING?

In the 1950s, team nursing evolved as a way to address the problems with the functional approach. In this type of nursing, groups of patients were assigned to a team headed by a team leader, usually an RN, who coordinated the care for a designated group of patients (Figure 15-4). The team leader determines work assignments for the team on the basis of the acuity level of the group of patients and the ability of the individual team members. The following is an example of the components of a team:

- An RN who is the team leader
- Two licensed vocational nurses/practical nurses assigned to patient care
- Two unlicensed assistive personnel (UAP)

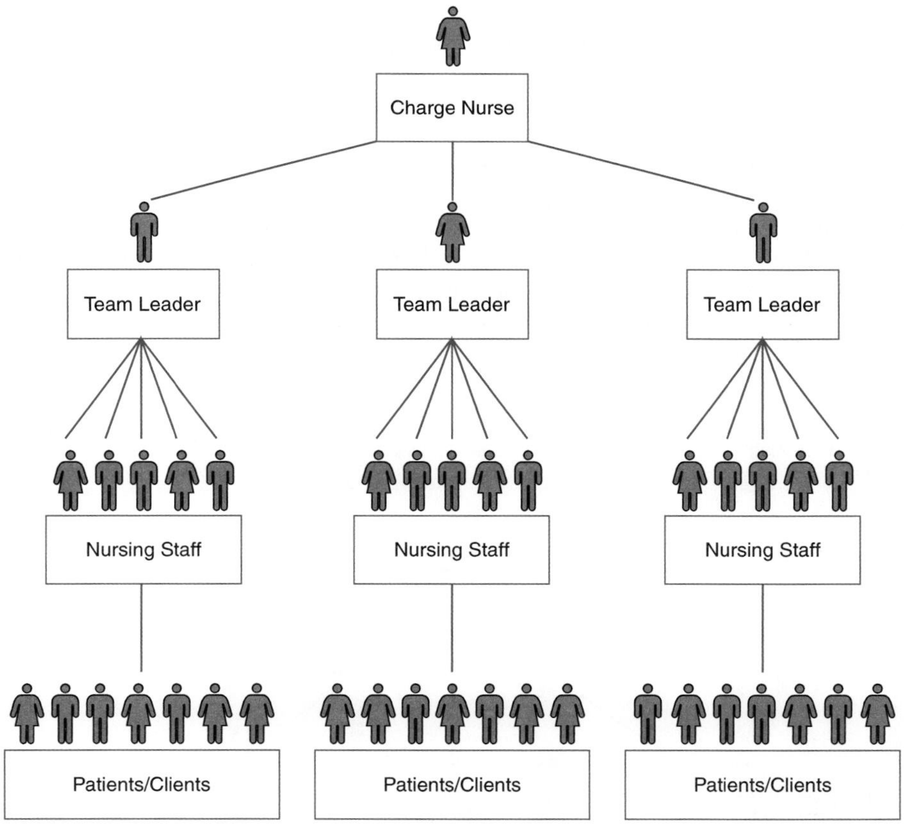

FIGURE 15-4
Lines of authority: team nursing.

The success of team nursing centers on good communication among the team members. It is imperative that the team leader continuously evaluates and communicates changes in the patient's condition to the team members. The team conference is a vital part of this approach, allowing the team to assess the needs of their patients and revise their individual plans of care on an ongoing basis.

Tiedeman and Lookinland (2004) suggest that the team model allows the nurse to know patients well enough to make assignments that best match patient needs with staff strengths. Patient needs are coordinated, and continuity of care may improve, depending on the length of time each member stays on the team. However, care can be fragmented and the model ineffective when staff is limited. In addition, the amount of time required to communicate among team members may decrease productivity (Tiedeman & Lookinland, 2004).

WHAT IS PRIMARY NURSING?

In the 1960s and 1970s, primary nursing evolved. In this system, a nurse plans and directs the care of a patient over a 24-hour period. This approach is designed to reduce or eliminate the fragmentation of care between shifts and nurses, because one nurse is accountable for planning the care of the patient around the clock. Progress reports, referrals, and discharge planning are usually the responsibility of the primary nurse. When the primary nurse is off duty, an associate nurse continues the plan of care. An RN may be the primary caregiver for some of the assigned patients and an associate nurse to others. Some forms of primary nursing evolved into an all-RN staff (Figure 15-5). You may also find primary nursing being mixed and modified with nurse extenders, such as paired partners, or partners in care. Although team nursing took the RN away from bedside care, primary and modified primary care puts the nurse back in close contact with the patient.

Relationship-based practice is the new name for primary nursing. The RN, who may be called the care coordinator, the responsible nurse, the principal responsible nurse, the case manager, or the care manager, manages and coordinates patient's care

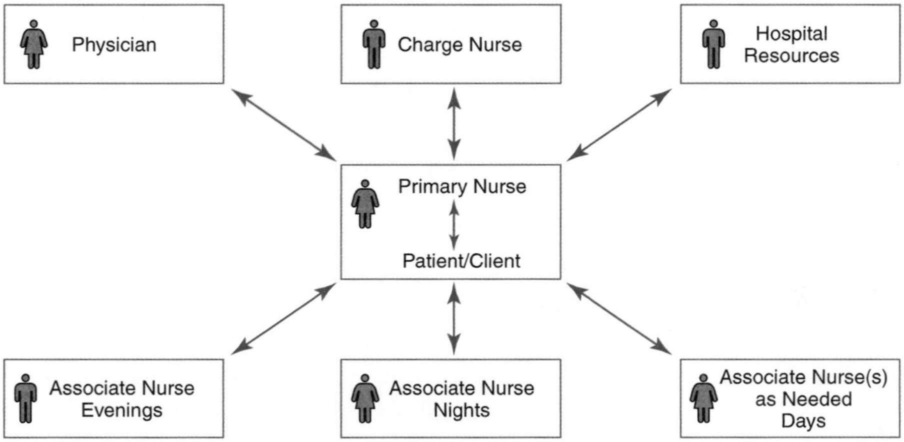

FIGURE 15-5
Lines of authority: primary-care nursing.

in the hospital and the discharge plan. This nurse develops a relationship and can be identified by the patient, their families, and the health care team as having the responsibility and authority for planning the nursing care the patient is to receive.

WHAT IS PATIENT-FOCUSED CARE?

Patient-focused care is another delivery system that has evolved during the last 15 years. Because of earlier nursing shortages, some traditional nursing interventions, such a phlebotomy and diet instruction, have been given to members of departments that do not report to nursing. These ancillary workers spend a great deal of time in transit from one unit to another. Time is also lost when there is not work for this single-function member to do. These tasks can be centralized on the unit under the direction of the RN. UAP are cross-trained to perform more than one function, thus increasing the level of productivity. In this system, the patient comes into contact with fewer people, and the RN, who is familiar with the patient's plan of care, supervises the delivery of care. This model also moves RNs to a higher level of functioning, because they are now accountable for a fuller range of services for the patient. Tasks that do not require an RN can be delegated to UAP under the supervision of the RN.

WHAT IS THE MOST EFFECTIVE MODEL OF NURSING CARE?

There has been a great deal of literature about models of care delivery. However, there is a lack of systematic evaluation regarding the use of the various models, often because of the lack of similarity in staffing and patient populations on comparison units (Tiedeman & Lookinland, 2004). As a result, it is impossible to determine the impact models of nursing care have on patient outcomes, costs, or job satisfaction. It may be that the model of nursing care delivery is less important than other factors, including the nurse-to-patient ratios, use of overtime, and the organizational culture in which the nurse works, in influencing outcomes (Critical Thinking Box 15-6).

WHAT IS THE IMPACT OF STAFFING PATTERNS ON THE QUALITY OF CARE?

In 2004, the AHRQ released a report that summarized the latest findings of AHRQ-funded and other research on the relationship between nurse staffing levels and adverse patient outcomes. This report concluded that:

- Lower levels of hospital nurse staffing are associated with more adverse outcomes.
- Patients in hospitals today are more acutely ill than in the past, but the skill levels of the nursing staff have declined.
- Higher acuity patients have added responsibilities that have increased the nurse workload.
- Avoidable adverse outcomes, such as pneumonia, can raise treatment costs by up to $28,000.

CRITICAL THINKING BOX 15-6

What factors influence the patterns of nursing care delivery?

- Hiring more RNs does not decrease profit.
- Higher levels of nurse staffing could have positive impact on both quality of care and nurse satisfaction (AHRQ, 2004).

The largest of these studies found significant associations between too few nurses on a unit and higher rates of pneumonia, upper gastrointestinal bleeding, shock/cardiac arrest, urinary tract infections, and failure to rescue. Other studies in the review found associations between lower staffing levels and pneumonia, lung collapse, falls, pressure ulcers, thrombosis after major surgery, pulmonary compromise after surgery, longer hospital stays, and 30-day mortalities (AHRQ, 2004).

JCAHO data confirm the effect of insufficient staffing on the outcomes of nursing care. As of September 2004, insufficient staffing levels were listed as a cause in 64% of the sentinel events that were entered into the JCAHO database. *Sentinel events* are any unexpected occurrences involving death or serious physical or psychological injury, or the risk thereof. Serious injuries specifically include a loss of limb or function. The phrase "risk thereof" includes any variation in the process of care for which a recurrence would carry a significant chance of a serious adverse outcome (JCAHO, 2005).

Determination of the number of nursing staff needed relative to the number and acuity of patients on a unit is the challenge of staffing. In the past 20 years, patient classification systems (or acuity systems) have been used to determine the number of nurses needed on a unit at any one time. Patient acuity is the measure of a patient's need for nursing care in a 24-hour period, considering the extent of each patient's illness. Patient classification systems, particularly with increased computerization and the ability to access the system online, provide many benefits. Not only do they determine acuity (patient mix) and workload for patient care units or specific clinical populations, they also (1) help managers determine how and where staff spend time; (2) identify trends in patient population; (3) document staffing patterns and workload and care practices; (4) effectively allocate limited resources; and (5) benchmark units to support financial decisions (Hader & Claudio, 2002)

HOW ARE NURSING WORK ASSIGNMENTS DETERMINED?

Once appropriate staffing levels for a unit are determined, specific nurses must be scheduled. How work assignments are given vary with individual institutions.

> A major problem in scheduling nurses is the fact that patient acuity fluctuates dramatically from day to day and from season to season.

For example, over the Christmas holidays there is often a significant decrease in the number of elective surgeries. In response, some hospitals may close units or reduce the number of staff on any given unit. By contrast, in the middle of the influenza season, the hospital might be full and understaffed.

Nursing has tried a variety of approaches to anticipate the number and qualifications of nurses that will be needed for a specific period of time for a specific group of patients. Regulatory agencies such as JCAHO require that staffing be based on some sort of organized system. Staffing in organizations may be based on budgeted nursing hours per patient per day. Hours per patient per day are calculated by the number of patient care staff working during a 24-hour period and divided by the number of patients served in a day.

Whether nursing resource requirements are defined by nursing hours per patient days or as nurse-patient ratios, the underlying assumption is that all patients, patient days, and nursing staff are equal. However, the need for nursing care varies significantly among patients and over the length of each patient's stay in the hospital. As the intensity of patient care increases and length of stay decreases, hours per patient day or nurse-patient ratio may not adequately express the resources needed (Graf et al, 2003). The competencies of the staff also influence the numbers and types of staff needed. The most accurate way of determining optimal staffing is through the judgment of an experienced nurse who is knowledgeable about quality and fiscal management.

There were two approaches to document that the organization has a minimum number of nurses to ensure safety in any given acute care unit: (1) establishment of a hospital-specific written staffing plan, which typically uses computerized patient acuity systems as a basis and (2) identifying and mandating fixed staffing ratios. A written plan should include the following critical factors:

- Establishing initial staffing levels that are recalculated at least annually or more often as necessary
- Setting staffing levels on a unit by unit basis
- Identifying ways to adjust staffing levels from shift to shift, based on intensity of patient care
- Using outcomes and nurse-sensitive indicators to evaluate the adequacy of the plan

Written staffing plans should be developed by an advisory committee composed of a number of registered nurses, a significant portion of whom are involved in direct patient care at least part of the time. Some states, such as Kentucky, Virginia, Texas, and Oregon, have incorporated the need for a written staffing plan into legislation (Spetz, 2004) (Critical Thinking Box 15-7).

CRITICAL THINKING BOX 15-7

How might you handle a staffing crisis? What are the advantages and disadvantages to each of the following:

- What are the unit census, acuity, and patient-classification systems?
- Does your organization have a float pool within the staff, or an agency or outside staff available?
- Check on your part-time staff to work an extra shift.
- Will another staff member cover the extra shift for a day off later in the schedule?
- Can you do with partial-shift coverage during the "peak" shift hours?
- Ask a staff member to work a double shift—either stay late or come in early.
- Work the shift yourself.
- What other solutions can you think of?

In 1999, California was the first state to pass comprehensive legislation to establish minimum nurse-to-patient ratios for RNs and LP/VNs in acute care, acute psychiatric and specialty hospitals. Once the bill was passed, the California Department of Health Services was charged with determining what the ratios in various patient care areas should be (Spetz, 2004). For example, the Department of Health Services (DHS) wrote regulations requiring hospitals to maintain a one-nurse-to-6-patients ratio in medical-surgical units, which would decrease to a one-nurse-to-5-patients ratio in January 2005. However, in November 2004, DHS gave hospitals a 3-year reprieve from meeting the stricter nurse ratio level, because of concerns about hospital closings and delays in critical patient care (California Department of Health Services, 2004).

WHAT ABOUT SCHEDULING PATTERNS?

Nursing has also always been concerned about scheduling practices and options because in many health care environments, nursing care must be provided 24 hours a day, 365 days per year. That is why there are numerous scheduling patterns other than the typical 8-hour shift 5 days a week. From working 10 hour days 4 days a week to the weekend alternative (known as the Baylor plan) of two 12-hour weekend shifts for 36 hours of pay, nurses have tried numerous patterns and combinations of shifts.

WHAT ABOUT THE USE OF OVERTIME?

With the current shortage of health professionals, employees are also encouraged and sometimes required to work overtime. Golden and Jorgensen (2002) looked at the cost of overtime in all sectors of the U.S. economy. They describe studies that find that accident rates begin to increase at the ninth hour of work and to double that of the ninth hour after the twelfth. In addition, job stress from overwork is estimated to be responsible for costs of $150 billion per year in absenteeism, health insurance premiums, diminished productivity, compensation claims, and direct medical costs among U.S. industries (Golden & Jorgensen, 2002).

According to the National Sleep Foundation (NSF), a deficit of sleep can result in decreased alertness, problems with completing tasks, reduced concentration, irritability, and unsafe action and decision making (Tabone, 2004). These problems, known as "the fatigue factor," have an impact on the care delivered by health care providers. Gaba and Howard (2002) found that 41% of medical residents reported a fatigue-related error. They also noted that being awake for 24 hours was equivalent to having a blood alcohol level of 0.10 %. In a review of several studies, Jha, Duncan, and Bates (2002) found that when adults, who typically require 6 to 10 hours of sleep, get less than 5 hours of sleep over a 24-hour period, their peak mental abilities decline. After two nights without sleep, cognitive performance can fall to nearly 40% of baseline. Lack of sleep can also result in slower response times, altered mood and motivation, and reduced morale and initiative.

The review of sleep studies in nurses found that self-reported alertness, performance, and job satisfaction lessen with longer shifts. For example, in a 2004 study, nurses were asked to keep log books for a month documenting the number of hours they worked each day, their overtime, and the errors, including the "near-misses," they made. The risk for making an error greatly increased when nurses had to work shifts that were longer than 12 hours, when they worked significant overtime, or when they worked more than 40 hours per week. The likelihood of making an error was three times greater when nurses worked shifts that lasted at least 12.5 hours. Working overtime also increased the odds of making at least one error, regardless of how long the shift was originally scheduled (Rogers et al, 2004). JCAHO has recognized problems associated with overtime, and in the 2002 white paper on the nursing shortage, stated that mandatory overtime should only be used in emergency situations.

CONCLUSION

The emphasis on cost control and managed care has changed the way that nursing care is delivered. New models of health care delivery are being developed in which we look at the desired outcome and manage backwards to achieve that outcome at the lowest level of expenses. Because some of the unexpected negative consequences of managed care, there is a renewed emphasis on evidenced-based care to enhance patient safety. We are continually challenged to develop more innovative and creative ways to ensure excellence in patient care with limited dollars. Nurses can meet this challenge.

REFERENCES

Agency for Healthcare Research and Quality: *Hospital nurse staffing and quality of care: research in action*, 2004, *www.ahrq.gov*.

Aiken L, Smith H, Lake E: Lower Medicare mortality among a set of hospitals known for good nursing care, *Medical Care* 59:215-222, 2002.

American Association of Critical Care Nurses: *AACN standards for establishing and sustaining healthy work environments: a journey to excellence*, 2005, *www.aacn.org*.

American Association of Critical Care Nurses and VitalSmarts: *Silence kills: the seven crucial conversations for healthcare*, 2005, *www.silencekills.com/UPDL/PressRelease.pdf*.

American College of Healthcare Executives Research Publications: *Top issues confronting hospitals:* 2004, 2004, *www.ache.org/pubs/research/ceoissues.cfm*.

Buerhaus P, Staiger D, Auerbach D: New signs of a strengthening U.S. nurse labor market?, *Health Affairs*, 2004, *http://content.healtaffairs.org/cgi/content/full/hlthaff.w4.526/DCl*.

California Department of Health Services: *California nurse patient ratios*, 2004, *www.dhs.ca/gov*.

Case Management Society of America: *Definition of case management*, 2005, *www.csma.org*.

Disease Management Association of America: *Definition of DM*, 2005, *www.dmaa.org/definition/html*.

Finkleman A: *Managed care: a nursing perspective*, Upper Saddle River, NJ, 2000, Prentice-Hall.

Gaba DM, Howard SK: Fatigue among clinicians and the safety of patients, *N Engl J Med* 347(16): 1249-1255, 2002.

Golden L, Jorgensen H: Time after time, (briefing paper), Washington, DC, 2002, Economic Policy Institute.

Graf C, Millar S, Feilteau C, et al: Patients' needs for nursing care, *J Nurs Admin* 29(2):258-266, 2003.

Hader R, Claudio T: Seven methods to effectively manage patient care labor resources, *J Nurs Admin* 33(2):76-81, 2002.

Hall L, Doran D, Pink G: (2004) Nursing staffing models, nursing hours, and patient safety outcomes, *J Nurs Admin* 34 (1):41-45, 2004.

Havens D: Comparing nursing infrastructure and outcomes: AACC magnet and non-magnet hospitals, *Nurs Econ* 19(6):258-266, 2001.

Havens S, Aiken L: Shaping systems to promote desired outcomes: the magnet hospital model, *J Nurs Admin* 29(2):14-20, 1999.

Health Resources and Services Administration: *The Registered Nurse population: findings from the 2000 National Sample Survey*, 2002, National Center for Health Workforce Analysis, U.S. Department of Health and Human Services, Health Resources and Services Administration, Bureau of Health Professions, *http://bhpr.hrsa.gov/healthworkforce/reports/rnsurvey/default.htm*.

Holahan J, Ghosh A: *Understanding the recent growth in Medicaid spending*, 2000-2003, Health Affairs, 2005, *http://content.healtaffairs.org/cgi/content/abstract/hlthaff.w5.52*.

Institute of Medicine, The National Academies: *Crossing the quality chasm: a new health system for the 21st century*, 2000, *www.iom.edu*.

Institute of Medicine, The National Academies: *Keeping patients safe: transforming the work environment of nurses*, 2003, *www.iom.edu*.

Institute of Medicine, The National Academies: *To err is human: building a safer health system*, 1999, *www.iom.edu*.

Jha A, Duncan B, Bates D: *Evidence report/technology assessment, No. 43: Making health care safer: a critical analysis of patient safety practice*, 2002, *www.ahcpr.gov/clinic/ptsafety/index.html*.

Joint Commission on the Accreditation of Health Care Organizations: Facts about the sentinel event policy, 2005, *www.jcaho.org/accredited+organizations/sentinel+event/sefacts.htm*.

Joint Commission on the Accreditation of Health Care Organizations: National patient safety goals for 2005 and 2004, 2005, *www.jcaho.org/accredited+organizations/patient+safety/index.htm*.

Joint Commission on the Accreditation of Health Care Organizations: *Health care at the crossroads: strategies for addressing the evolving nursing shortage*, 2002, *www.jcaho.org/about+us/public+policy+initiative/health+care+at+the+crossroads.pdf*.

Kuhar P, Miller D, Spear B, et al: The meaningful retention strategy inventory: a targeted approach to implementing retention strategies, *J Nurs Admin* 34(1):10-18, 2004.

McPeck P: Can we fix it?, *NurseWeek* 11(5): 17-19, 2004.

Melnky B, Fineout-Overholt E: *Evidence-based practice in nursing and health care: a guide to best practice*, Philadelphia, 2005, Lippincott Williams & Wilkins.

Patterson K, Grenny J, McMillan R, Switzler A: *Crucial conversations: tools for talking when stakes are high*, New York, 2005, McGraw-Hill.

Rogers AE, Hwang WT, Scott LD, et al: The working hours of hospital staff nurse and patient safety, *Health Affairs* 23(4):202-212, 2004.

Sackett D, Straus S, Richardson W, et al: *Evidence-based medicine: how to practice and teach EBMh* London, 2000, Churchill Livingstone.

Spetz J: *California's minimum nurse-to-patient ratios: where are we, how did we get here and where do we go next?*, San Franscisco, 2004, California Health Workforce Studies, The Center for Health Professions, University of California, *www.futurehealth.ucsf.edu/cchws/ratios.html*.

Sportsman S: Human resource practices and management in hospitals. In Leiyu S (Ed.): *Human resources practice and management in the health care sector*, 2005, Jones and Bartlett.

Sportsman S, Hawley L: *Critical practice management strategies for nurse practitioners: a guide to business principles and practices in primary care practice*, Washington, DC, 2004, American Nurse Association Publishing Company.

Sportsman S, Valadez A: Managed care and the law. In O'Keefe M: *Nursing practice and the law: avoiding malpractice and other legal risks*, Philadelphia, 2001, F.A. Davis.

Tabone S: Nurse fatigue: the human factor, *Texas Nursing*, 8-10, June-July, 2004.

The Bernard Hodes Group: *The health care metrics survey*, 2004, *www.hodes.com/aboutus/dsp_press_template.asp?ID=5600*.

Tiedeman M, Lookinland S: Traditional models of care delivery: what have we learned?, *J Nurs Admin* 34(6):291-297, 2004.

What are clinical pathways?, 2005, *www.svh.stvincents.com.au/qi/Clin_Pathways/cp_what.htm*.

CHAPTER 16

ECONOMICS OF THE HEALTH CARE DELIVERY SYSTEM

MARY ELLEN MURRAY, PhD, RN

By identifying the forces pushing the future, rather than those that have contained the past, you possess the power to engage with your reality.

—*Megatrends 2000, John Naisbitt and Patricia Aburden*

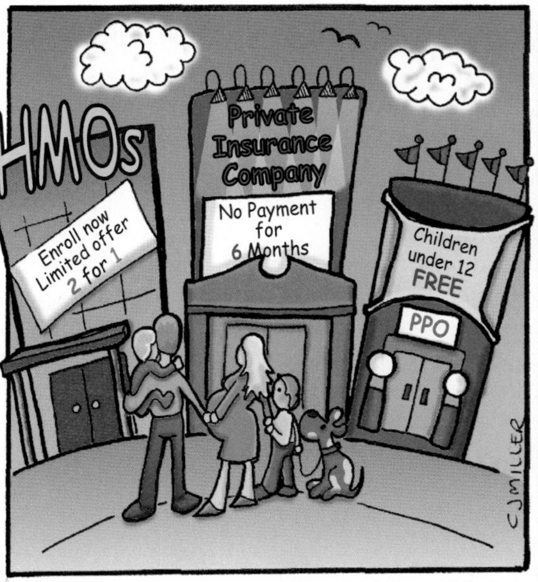
HMOs
Enroll now
Limited offer
2 for 1
Private
Insurance
Company
No Payment
for
6 Months
Children
under 12
FREE
PPO
CJMILLER

Health care consumers are going to be shopping around to get the most for their health care dollar.

After completing this chapter, you should be able to:

- Define economics and health care economics.
- Compare the market for health care to a normal market for goods and services.
- Use a basic knowledge of health care economics to analyze trends in the health care delivery system.
- Describe what is meant by operating budget, personnel budget, and capital budget.
- Describe what is meant by the term fiscal responsibility in clinical practice.
- Discuss strategies you will use to achieve fiscal responsibility in your clinical practice.

Costs in the American health care system are out of control—bad and getting worse! In 1995, national health care expenditures (NHCE) topped $1 trillion dollars for the first time. By the year 2012, those expenditures are projected to exceed $3 trillion dollars. Currently, health care expenditures consume more than 14% of the gross domestic product (GDP, the value of all the goods and services produced in the United States annually), an amount predicted to exceed 17% by 2012 (NHCE projections, 2002-2012). The outcome of this investment, in terms of the public health of the population, is a nation lagging behind many comparable industrialized nations. There are currently, in the year 2005, an estimated 40 million persons without health insurance. There is very limited prescription drug coverage under Medicare. There are great disparities in access to health care among racial and ethnic populations. There are vast differences in the reimbursement for the treatment and care of physical and mental illness (Murray, 2002). All of these statistics have implications for the clinical practice of nursing.

WHAT ARE THE TRENDS AFFECTING THE RISING COSTS OF HEATH CARE?

Both intrinsic and extrinsic factors contribute to rising costs of health care. Intrinsic factors include characteristics of the population, the demand for health care, and employer-paid health insurance. Extrinsic factors include the availability of technology, prescription drug costs, and workforce costs (Figure 16-1).

INTRINSIC FACTORS

The United States population grew by 32.7 million people during the period 1990-2000, the largest increment in American history (U.S. Census Bureau, 2001). The Annual Demographic Supplement to the 2002 Current Population Survey reported 59.6 million persons over the age of 55 years. Of those, 9.8% have incomes below the poverty level, with the number increasing to more than 10% at ages over 65 years. This is important information because older people typically utilize increased health care resources and may not have the income to purchase them.

There is also an increasing demand for health care in the United States. Demand, in the economic sense, is the amount of health care a consumer wishes to purchase. Part of the increased demand has to do with the widespread availability of health insurance that has the effect of lowering the cost of health care to individuals. The need for health care is defined (Feldstein, 1999) as the amount of health care that the experts believe a person should have to remain as healthy as possible, based on current medical knowledge. The question then arises, should the amount of health care provided be based on need or demand?

EXTRINSIC FACTORS

The availability of new medical technology has contributed to the rising costs of health care. If an institution does not offer technology that a competitor offers, it is likely that the market share (percentage of persons in an area selecting that institution) of the

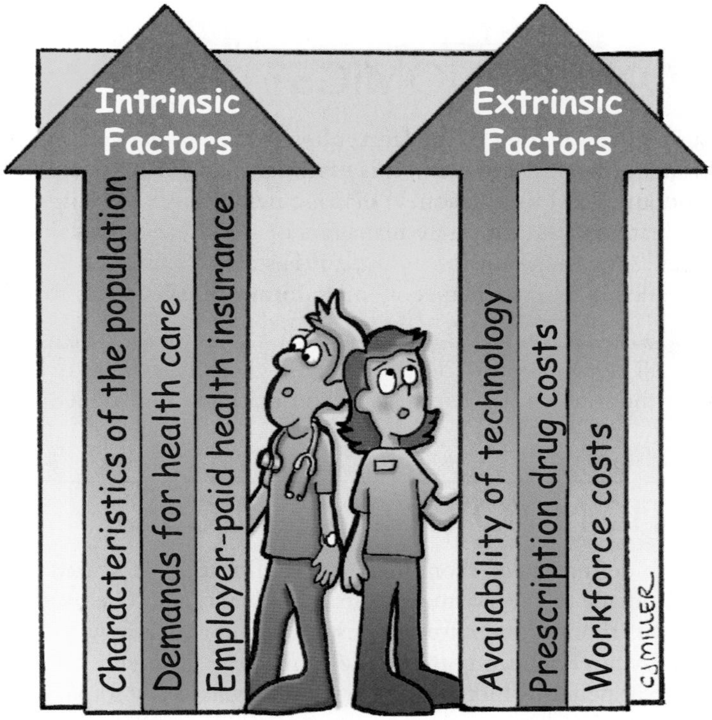

FIGURE 16-1
Trends affecting the rising cost of health care.

institution will decline. To attain a competitive edge, an institution needs to be an early adopter of expensive, new technology. Then, thinking sequentially, someone has to pay for the technology, and this cost will be passed on to consumers in the form of higher health care costs.

Prescription drug care costs are projected to continue to rise in an amount exceeding 10% per year through 2008. This is an increase from the actual amount of $140.6 billion dollars in 2001 to a projected $309.7 billion in 2008 (Heffler et al, 2004). This is another factor that will continue to drive health care costs. In evaluating the importance of this factor, it should be noted that these data were projected before the passage of the Medicare prescription coverage plan. Although the plan offers limited coverage, the additional expenditures will drive these projected costs higher.

A final factor driving health care costs is the increase in hospital spending growth (Heffler et al, 2004) that is expected to rise from an actual amount of $451 billion dollars in 2001 to a projected amount of $860 billion by the year 2012. One of the main factors contributing to these increases is rising labor costs. Although this is good news for the nursing profession, it is part of a national problem.

WHAT IS THE EFFECT OF CHANGING CLINICAL PRACTICE ON ECONOMICS?

Because nurses belong to the largest health care profession and are thus in a position to influence health care costs, it is essential that all nurses understand basic concepts of economics and fiscal (money) management. This knowledge was previously taught in graduate courses for nurse managers or nurse executives. However, the world has changed! One nurse author (Hunt, 2001) states, "Clinical competency is not the only tool needed in an era when economics dominates the health care arena."

Today all nurses need to couple their clinical skills with business skills that enable them to be full participants in designing and delivering health care.

INTRODUCTION TO ECONOMICS

A simple definition of economics is the allocation of scarce resources. An analogy might be made to the income that an individual earns. The paycheck is a limited, finite amount of money, and choices must be made about how to spend, or allocate, the money. Such choices might include rent, a car payment, food, clothing, and health insurance payments. Individuals may not be able to pay for all of the goods or services that they wish to have, so decisions must be made and priorities established.

Similarly, health care is a limited resource, and choices have to be made. The choices about health care that concern economists are made at the national level. These choices include: how much does the country wish to spend on health care, what services does the country wish to provide, what is the best method for producing health care, and how will health care be distributed (Feldstein, 1999).

WHAT ARE THE CHOICES ABOUT AMOUNT OF SPENDING?

Currently, the United States is spending approximately 14% of its income on health care. As the payor for Medicare (the national health insurance program for people aged 65 years or older, some people under age 65 with disabilities, and people with end-stage renal disease) and Medicaid (a joint federal and state program that pays for medical assistance for certain individuals and families with low incomes and resources), the federal government is the nation's largest purchaser of health care. Yet this amount does not fully meet the needs of the populations served under these programs, let alone provide for the health care needs of persons without any insurance. The United States has repeatedly elected not to establish a system of national health insurance. This represents a choice made about the allocation of health care resources. Box 16-1 summarizes the benefits of the Medicare standard plan, although many other options are available.

WHAT ARE THE CHOICES ABOUT SERVICES TO PROVIDE?

Oregon State passed legislation between the years 1989 and 1995 that provides an example of choices about the services provided to persons with Medicaid coverage.

BOX 16-1 Original Medicare Insurance Coverage

Medicare provides coverage to approximately 40 million Americans. Medicare is the national health insurance program for:

- People aged 65 years or older
- Some people under age 65 with disabilities
- People with End-Stage Renal Disease (ESRD), which is permanent kidney failure requiring dialysis or a kidney transplant

MEDICARE PART A (HOSPITAL INSURANCE)

What It Covers

Medicare Part A helps cover inpatient care in hospitals, and skilled nursing facilities (not unskilled or long-term care). It also covers hospice care and some home health care. Certain conditions must be met to qualify for these benefits. For Days 1 to 60, the patient pays a deductible of $912. Inpatient mental health care is the same deductible but there is a lifetime limit of 190 days. For skilled nursing home care, there is no payment for days 1 to 20 if the stay follows a 3-day covered hospital stay. There is no co-payment for *covered* home health visits. For hospice care, the patient must pay part of the cost for outpatient drugs and inpatient respite care.

Costs

Most people do not have to pay a monthly payment, called a premium, for Medicare Part A. This is because they or a spouse paid Medicare taxes while they were working.

MEDICARE PART B (MEDICAL INSURANCE)

What It Covers

Medicare Part B helps cover doctors' services, outpatient hospital care, and some other medical services that Medicare Part A does not cover, such as some of the services of physical and occupational therapists, and some home health care. Medicare Part B helps pay for these covered services and supplies when they are medically necessary. It also covers some preventive services. For doctor office visits, durable medical equipment, ambulance service, the patient must pay 20% of the Medicare-approved amount.

Costs

Most people pay the monthly premium of $78.20 in 2004 for Medicare Part B. There is a $110 Part B deductible each year before Medicare starts to pay its share.

What Is Not Covered

Dental services, hearing examinations and hearing aids, routine eye examinations and glasses, routine physical examinations, health and wellness education.

Be aware that there are several options available to persons who enroll in Medicare. These data reflect the original plan and reflect 2004 benefits.
From Center of Medicare and Medicaid Services, *www.medicare.gov/Basics/*.

Consumers and providers of health and social services were charged with developing a ranked list of health care services in order of their benefit to the entire population being served and to reflect community values. Coverage for all conditions at a certain level would be set by the state legislature dependent on budget constraints. In the listing of services, treatment of, for example, premature infants, cleft palate, hip fracture, or stroke was covered, whereas radial keratotomy, cosmetic dentistry, and treatment of

CRITICAL THINKING BOX 16-1

What implications does the Oregon plan have on the health care industry? Have you encountered this type of "rationing system" in your own state's programs?

varicose veins were not included (Oregon Health Policy and Research [OHPR] Home Page, 2004). Although this is one type of rationing of health care, and Americans are typically opposed to any type of rationing system, it must be noted that the services denied under the Oregon plan are consistent with those denied reimbursement under other private and public insurance plans (Critical Thinking Box 16-1).

WHAT ARE CHOICES ABOUT METHODS TO PRODUCE HEALTH CARE?

One informal definition of managed care is: the right care, in the right amount, by the right provider, in the right setting. This definition implies that there are several ways to produce health care. For example, a woman may choose to have an annual physical examination by a nurse practitioner, a certified nurse-midwife, a gynecologist, or a family practice physician. Each provides care from a different perspective and at a different price. In another example, certain procedures that were once done only in hospitals are now done in an outpatient setting, many with the addition of home health nursing. Lumpectomy and simple mastectomies are surgical procedures that are now done in an outpatient setting and that illustrate a different method of producing health care. Deciding the best method is subject to research and must include an analysis of the costs.

WHAT ARE CHOICES ABOUT ALLOCATION?

These decisions involve "who gets what." The underlying question is: Is health care a right or a commodity (like cars or clothing) to be allocated by the market place? The World Health Organization (WHO) states in its constitution that the enjoyment of the highest attainable standard of health is one of the fundamental rights of every human being (WHO, 2004). Although it does not declare health care to be a basic human right, the *Code for Nurses* (American Nurses Association [ANA], 2001) does state that nurses should provide care without consideration of the patient's social or economic status. However, even if one believes that health care is a right, challenging questions remain. How much health care is a right? Who pays for all the health care of people who cannot afford health care? When teaching senior nursing students, who universally agree that health care is a right, one faculty member asks the students how much of their paycheck they would be willing to forfeit in taxes so that everyone could have health care. It is rare that students are willing to subsidize others' health care at a cost of more than one third of their salary.

Even beyond the costs of care is the question of allocation decisions; that is, who decides who gets what health care. Several responses are possible: the government, payors of health care, individuals, and the market place.

Government Allocation Decisions. Through its funding of Medicare, the government has made multiple allocation decisions. The United States government has decided it will pay for inpatient health care and some outpatient care for patients older than 65 years of age and selected others (see Box 16-1). Unfortunately, many of the persons covered by Medicare have come to believe that Medicare covers "everything," and this is not so. There are many limits to the services reimbursed by Medicare and many requirements that must be met before the government will make payment (Critical Thinking Box 16-2).

Payor Allocation Decisions. All insurance companies have rules about the services that will be covered and the requirements that must be met under their policies. One rule might involve the presence of "pre-existing patient conditions." If, for example, a patient has been diagnosed with AIDS or has been treated for mental illness, they may be denied coverage for treatment of that particular condition, or denied coverage all together. When the insurance is a benefit of employment, this is less likely to occur. At other times, if an individual is applying for insurance, she/he may be required to fill out a questionnaire about health history or submit to a physical examination. The results of these may be used to deny or limit coverage.

Once the insurance is in effect, there are additional rules regarding the services that will be covered. Most policies require preauthorization, or pre-approval of services before the patient receives care, except in cases of emergency. For example, a physician's office will typically communicate the need for a surgical procedure to the insurance company and obtain this approval. If the patient is admitted to the hospital in an emergency, the hospital has a limited amount of time to gain the approval, or reimbursement for the care may be denied.

Another restriction on resource allocation involves the process of concurrent utilization review (UR). This is a strategy used by managed care companies to control both costs and quality. The process requires that hospital staff, typically registered nurses, communicate the plan of care for a hospitalized patient to the payor or their representative. The payor then determines if the care is appropriate, medically necessary,

CRITICAL THINKING BOX 16-2

A Hospice is reimbursed $75 per visit by Medicare B for home visits. For one particular group of patients, it costs the Hospice an average of $98 per day to provide care.

What are the implications for the hospice?

What options should the Hospice nurse manager and nurses consider?

and covered under the terms of the policy or the contract with the provider (Murray & Henriques, 2003). For example, if a patient is admitted to the hospital the day before elective surgery, the day will almost certainly be denied reimbursement. Preoperative patient teaching and surgical preparation can be done on an outpatient basis at a much lower cost than a day in the hospital.

Marketplace Allocation Decisions. A final alternative for the allocation of resources is the marketplace. This decision making implies that health care is a normal good, like a car or a piece of clothing, where an increase in income leads to an increase in demand for the good (Parkin, 2000), and the rules of supply and demand apply. However, the market for health care has some significant differences from the market for normal goods.

Unpredictability of demand. The first difference in the market for health care is the unpredictability of demand. There is a great demand for health care when a person is ill, and the timing of illness is, of course, uncertain.

Consider for example, the case of a patient needing a heart transplant. A patient does not wait until the price comes down. Rather, the surgery is purchased at any price if a donor heart is available.

Consumer knowledge. Another difference in the health care market involves the knowledge of the consumer. If an individual is purchasing a coat or a car, they know a good deal about what they are purchasing. This is not the case in health care, about which patients have imperfect knowledge.

Barriers to entry to the market. Even if patients had sufficient knowledge to treat their own illnesses, the health care market is fraught with barriers. All providers must pass examinations and be licensed by appropriate boards. Prescriptive authority is heavily regulated and closely controlled.

Lack of price competition. Finally, the health care market, unlike the market for clothing and automobiles, does not engage in price competition. When, for example, have you heard of a sale on appendectomies or "2 for the price of 1" hip replacements? Of course, it does not happen. But more concerning is the fact that health care consumers frequently do not know the cost of their care, if it is being paid for by insurance. In fact, many consumers indicate that they "never saw a bill" for their hospitalization, and this is considered to be a measure of the quality of their insurance. Is there another product that would be routinely purchased without knowledge of its price? The lack of this knowledge leads to predictable consumer health care purchasing behavior.

The classic Rand Health Insurance Experiment (Keeler & Roth, 1983) was a controlled research study that examined the effect of different co-payments on the utilization of health care. Participants in the study either received free care, or paid co-payments of 25%, 50%, or 95%. Economic theory would predict that as price increases, the purchase of goods or services would decline. That is exactly what happened. With a co-payment of 25%, there was a decline in utilization of health care of 19% compared to a free plan. There were even greater declines in utilization of health care services at the higher rates of co-payments. This consumer behavior is so predictable that health care economists have a term for it: *moral hazard*. It refers to a situation in which a person uses more health care services because the presence of insurance has lowered the price to the person.

BUDGETS

A *budget* is a tool that helps to make allocation decisions and to plan for expenditures. It is important that staff nurses understand budget processes because these decisions directly impact their clinical practice. For example, staff nurses working on a patient care unit may feel that there is not enough time to care for acutely ill patients on the unit. A clinical manager may respond that the "budget will not allow" additional staff. Savvy staff nurses will understand the budget process and be able to relate patient acuity to staffing needs. To engage in these discussions, all nurses need to understand basic concepts of budgets as well as different types of budgets: capital budgets, operating budgets, and personnel budgets (Figure 16-2).

WHAT ARE THE BASIC CONCEPTS OF BUDGETS?

When preparing a budget, one must first consider the unit the document will serve. It could be an entire hospital, a department, or an individual patient care unit. This discussion will focus on the budget of a patient care unit, because that is the work environment of most registered nurses.

The basic terms that nurses must know are:

Revenue: All the money brought into the unit as payment for a good or service. Some departments in the hospital are defined as revenue centers. Examples might

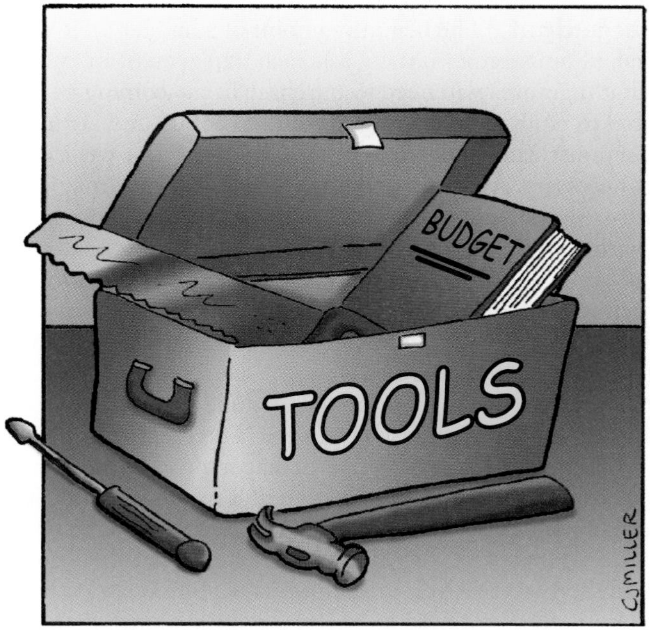

FIGURE 16-2
Budget—a tool that helps make allocation decisions.

include radiology or surgery. Typically, these departments generate a great deal of income for the larger organization.

Expense: All the costs of producing a product. Patient care units are typically labeled as cost centers; that is, they do not directly generate revenue. Most hospitals have a fixed room rate that includes nursing care. Nurse leaders have questioned the appropriateness of nursing care being lumped into the room rate, but few have been able to effect a change. Some exceptions to this include nursing care to patients in the recovery room, intensive care, or labor and delivery, where there is a separate charge for nursing care.

Margin (or profit): Revenue minus expenses equals margin or profit. Nurses may cringe at the thought of hospitals making a profit but every hospital, whether it is defined as a *not-for-profit hospital* or *for-profit hospital*, must make a profit. Profits are needed to replace equipment, purchase new technology, and, in some cases, provide care for indigent patients. In addition, for-profit hospitals must pay stockholders a return on their investment. The necessity of making a profit is so crucial to the continued existence of an organization, that there is an old adage that states, "No margin, no mission." This means that if an organization does not make a profit, it is unable to fulfill the purpose or mission of the organization, no matter what it might be.

WHAT ARE THE TYPES OF BUDGETS?

The budget process involves the development of three budget types that are combined to make an overall budget for the patient care unit: the capital budget, the operating budget, and the personnel budget. The budget covers a 12-month time period that may begin January 1, July 1, or October 1, depending on the institution.

Capital Budget. The beginning point of a budget cycle is usually the *capital budget*. Hospital administrators usually ask each department or patient care unit for a list of items that their area will need to purchase in the coming year. These items are usually restricted to equipment costing more than $5000 and lasting more than 1 year. Each manager must rank such requests for the unit and write a justification of why the item is necessary. At a unit level, the nurse manager may request replacement beds, telemetry equipment, or computers, for example. Most managers will discuss unit needs with staff nurses and seek their input. Staff nurses do the work of the organization and are in the best position to know what is needed for patient care. Next, all of the organization's needs are summarized and prioritized according to the funds available. Rarely is there sufficient capital to fund all the requests, and difficult decisions and choices must be made.

Operating Budgets. This budget includes a statement of the expected expenses of the unit for a time period, usually 1 year. The budget process begins with a statement of volume projections. The nurse manager projects how much patient care will be given in the coming year. The volume that nurses are concerned with is measured in patient days, and, therefore, the question is, "How many patient days of care will be provided in the coming year?" The manager would first look at past data to examine how many days were given in the previous year. It is also helpful to look at monthly data, so that one could determine if there was a month that exceeded projections, perhaps due to a flu epidemic or a month that had a very low number of patient days, perhaps due to vacations of medical staff who admit patients. Knowledge of these trends helps the manager to project volume for the next year. The manager would next consider any changes in the patient care unit that might effect volume projections. For example, if two new surgeons are added to the staff, if the unit would begin to provide care for a new clinical population of patients, or if the unit is to be designated as the overflow unit for same-day surgery patients, all of these would increase the volume projections.

In addition to projecting the patient day volume, nurse managers also examine the activity of the unit and the acuity (the intensity of care required by patients) of patients. The activity is usually described as *admissions, discharges, and transfers* (ADTs). One measure of activity is the average daily census, how many patients are occupying beds on the unit at midnight. However, this measure by itself results in underestimating the work of the unit. A more accurate picture is gained by the addition of the ADT data, because these patients may not be counted in a midnight census, but they require many hours of care by registered nurses (Critical Thinking Box 16-3).

Managers must also consider the acuity of the patients on the unit. In an intensive care unit, patients are extremely ill and require many hours of care per day. The number of care hours decreases as patients are moved to general patient care units. Each institution considers the acuity of patients, but may use different methods of arriving at measurements. There are several computerized software packages available, whereby nurses enter patient data, and the software program produces estimates of the staffing needs of the unit. Programs are designed for each clinical population of patients, obstetrics, pediatrics, psychiatry, and the like. Nurses enter data concerning many factors, including numbers of patients, functional abilities, telemetry monitoring, and postoperative day. These factors help to define how much care patients need and thus can be used to project staffing needs. At the time the budget is created, the nurse manager can review the data to see if the staffing planned for the unit was adequate to meet patient care needs.

The *operating budget* also includes all of the items necessary for care on the unit. These are called *line items* in a budget and include such things as supplies, telephones, small equipment (such as wheelchairs, nurse pagers, and fax machines), postage, and copying costs. Some of these are *variable costs*—that is, costs that change with the volume of patients cared for in a year. Some institutions would include a factor for the variable costs of housekeeping or laundry. There may be a line item for travel for staff nurses to attend clinical conferences or to pay for specialty certification of nurses. These are expenses frequently paid by employing institutions. Other costs, such as heat and

CRITICAL THINKING BOX 16-3

In most hospitals, nursing care is "lumped" in with the room charge and thus nursing care is an expense in the budget and not a revenue center. All patients (except ICU, step-down) pay the same amount for nursing care. What are the advantages/disadvantages of this for nursing?

CRITICAL THINKING BOX 16-4

As a staff nurse, you have been asked to serve on your unit's financial management committee. You have been told to reduce expenses by 3% overall—in any way you choose to do it.

Given the definition of fixed and variable costs—where do you think you could begin to look for cost reductions. Give some ideas of possible cost reductions. Remember that your commitment is to preserve the high quality of patient care.

electricity, are considered *fixed costs*, and do not change with volume of patients. A nurse manager considers all these things when planning an operating budget (Critical Thinking Box 16-4).

Personnel Budget. The *personnel budget* for a nursing unit is the largest part of unit expenses, and nursing is the largest part of personnel expense. This has caused some hospital administrators, who need to reduce expenses to quip:

"Follow the dollars, and they will lead to nursing."

Staff nurses need to understand how a nurse manager determines the number of nurses required to care for patients. As discussed, beginning considerations are acuity and volume. Next, the manager engages in a series of calculations, all of which are easily understood by staff nurses.

Hours per patient day (HPPD). Each patient-care unit will have a designated number of hours of care per patient day. In an intensive care unit, this might be as high as 22 hours per day; on a general surgical unit, it might be 6 to 8 hours. However, nurses need to be aware that these hours must be spread over three shifts (if the institution uses 8-hour shifts) or two shifts (in the case of 12-hour shifts). Nurse managers typically derive *staffing patterns*, that is, combinations of staff (RN, LPN, nursing assistants) that are needed for each shift. These may vary for weekends, night, and even days of the week. For example, if Monday is a day when many surgical procedures are performed, staffing must include higher numbers of registered nurses to assess and monitor postoperative patients.

Full time equivalent (FTE). An FTE represents the number of hours that a nurse employed full-time is available to perform all of the employment activities. This is calculated to be 2080 hours (52 weeks times 40 hours), but is usually split into productive and nonproductive time (Hunt, 2001).

Productive time. This figure reflects the amount of time the nurse is available to give care to patients. One work day (8 hours) is usually considered to be 7.5 productive hours.

Nonproductive time. This time reflects the amount of time that is not available for patient care. Some examples of nonproductive time include vacations, days off, holidays, time at educational seminars, time for committee work, such as quality improvement, breaks, and lunch. If these factors are not calculated into the budget, staffing needs may be seriously underestimated. Savvy nurse managers know their staff and can project nonproductive time. For example, if a unit has a very senior staff that accrues annual vacations of 4 to 6 weeks, this must be considered in the budgeting process.

What are the Economics of Caring? As clinicians, many nurses are reluctant to incorporate a knowledge of health care economics into their clinical practice, feeling that it makes them somehow less compassionate or less caring. However, it can be argued that the reason nurses must understand health care economics is that they can bring the values of nursing to the decision-making process for patient care. For example, an administrator with a master of business administration degree may examine the budget of a patient care unit and make a decision to decrease staffing. A nurse who understands the budgeting process can argue persuasively about the ADTs on the unit and the increasing acuity of patients receiving care.

At the level of providing care for individual patients, staff nurses must understand fiscal responsibility for clinical practice. *Fiscal responsibility* concerns a twofold responsibility: first to the patient and second to the employing institution. It is defined as: the duty/obligation of the nurse to allocate (1) financial resources of the patient to maximize health benefit to the patient and (2) financial resources of the employer to maximize organizational cost-effectiveness (Figure 16-3).

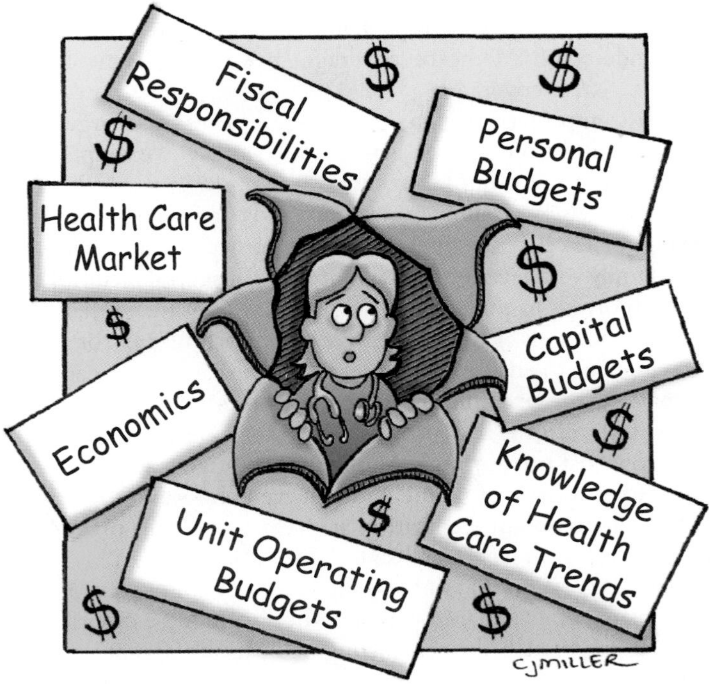

FIGURE 16-3
Nurses play an important role in the economics of health care.

FISCAL RESPONSIBILITY TO THE PATIENT

The primary fiscal responsibility the nurse has is always, and most importantly, to the patient. This means that a nurse uses the most cost-efficient combination of resources to maximize the health benefit to the patient. A nurse needs to understand the costs of care and different reimbursement systems because this will effect the development of a plan of care. It is important that nurses assess the resources that a patient has available to dedicate to health care. These may include insurance coverage, but also the availability of family members or others to aid in care.

For example, many churches team up to provide transportation to treatment for patients receiving chemotherapy. Communities vary widely in the resources they offer to patients and families. There may be free support groups, online chat rooms, or meals on wheels available. All of these are valuable community health care resources that are not monetary.

In another example, when creating a discharge plan for a patient, it is essential that a nurse understand the health care resources the patient requires and how they will be paid. A physician may write orders for prescription medications that are not covered by the patient's insurance.

Often patients are reluctant to admit that they cannot afford these medications, and they may either not have the prescription filled, or they may go without other necessities to purchase the medication. Sometimes patient even resort to cutting medications in half to make them "last longer," thereby receiving only a partial dose of the medication. If nurses understand patients' insurance coverage and include this in assessment data, they can make better plans of care. It is especially important that nurses understand Medicare coverage, because in some hospitals almost 50% of patients have this coverage.

It is also important that nurses engage in early discharge planning, beginning the process on admission or even before admission. For example, if a patient is to have a scheduled surgery for hip replacement, the nurse in the orthopedic surgery clinic may talk with the patient about convalescence and continued physical therapy in the rehabilitation unit of a skilled nursing facility. If this process is done before admission, the patient and the family will have the opportunity to visit several facilities and make a selection.

It is important to understand that this does not mean that patients will not receive care or medications if the patient cannot afford to pay for it. It does mean that the nurse will work to ensure that patients get the care they need, regardless of their ability to pay. In the example of a patient who is to be discharged with a prescription he/she cannot afford, it is possible that there are programs within the hospital that provide low cost medications. Another alternative is to determine if a generic drug is available at a lower cost. Some patients even choose to mail order their prescriptions from Canada to obtain medication at lower costs. This practice is legal in Wisconsin, although it is not in legal in all states.

It is also important that nurses understand that fiscal responsibility for clinical practice is a responsibility shared with all other health care disciplines. Nurse practitioners and physicians write orders requiring medications, diagnostic procedures, and laboratory tests. Therefore, they share fiscal responsibility. Clinical social workers have a great knowledge of health care resources available to patients both in the hospital and in the community. All members of the interdisciplinary team share this responsibility

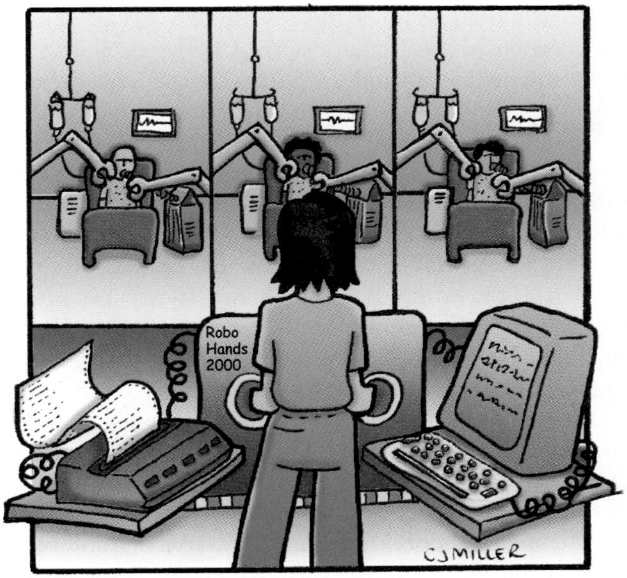

FIGURE 16-4
Advances in computer technology continue to assist the nurse, but technology cannot replace the humanistic aspect of nursing care.

and contribute to the goal of maximizing the benefit of health care resources for patients (Figure 16-4).

FISCAL RESPONSIBILITY TO THE EMPLOYING INSTITUTION

Nurses also have a responsibility to the institution or agency where they are employed. The most important way a nurse is fiscally responsible is by providing quality patient care. For example, thorough hand washing and the use of sanitizing gels prevents infections that may increase patient costs. Similarly, the prevention of falls and decubiti are clinical practices that have significant cost implications.

> Nurses who continually improve their clinical practice by using evidence-based practice or "best practice" guidelines are also engaging in quality practice that is cost-effective.

Nurses also have an obligation to use the resources of the institution wisely. The most costly health care resource that nurses allocate is their time. The nurse considers patient care needs and prioritizes how professional nursing time shall be allocated. Although it would be ideal for nurses to have sufficient time with each patient, it is rarely possible. As a beginning point, the nurse knows that the most important reason that a patient is hospitalized is to receive assessment and monitoring by a registered nurse. If a patient does not need this assessment, it is likely that they can be safely cared for in a less expensive health care setting, such as a skilled nursing facility. The care planning the nurse does includes prioritizing the needs of unstable patients. At other times, the nurse may make a decision the patient and family require teaching from a professional nurse. It may also be that the patient and family require psychosocial support, a nursing intervention that requires a high level of nursing expertise.

Nurses also need to understand *prospective payment systems*. Under prospective payment, the hospital is paid a set amount for the care of a patient with a certain condition or surgery. If the hospital engages in efficient clinical care practices, the organization makes a profit. If the hospital is not efficient, it may lose money. Medicare reimburses under this prospective system (called *Diagnostic Related Groups* or *DRGs*) as do many private insurance companies. This system has had a large impact on nursing practice. For example, if the nurse does not have a discharge plan in place on the day a discharge decision is made, perhaps due to the lack of planning for transportation for a patient, it may be that the patient will remain in the hospital for an additional day while arrangements are made. This incurs unnecessary costs for the hospital. From another perspective, an unnecessary hospital day is a quality issue. Patients in the hospital are subject to the possibility of infection, the hazards of immobility and bed rest, and even the potential for malnutrition.

Another way that nurses practice fiscal responsibility is by accurately documenting the patient's condition. This must include the severity of the patient's illness as well as the plan of care. If this is not documented, it may be that insurance companies will not reimburse for the care. For example, if the nurse documents "up and about with no complaints," it is very likely that the hospital day will not be covered. However, if the nurse documents the assessments and monitoring that are being done at frequent intervals, the care will likely be reimbursed.

There are other ways in which nurses recognize institutional fiscal responsibility. For example, the nurse should be aware of bringing only the needed supplies into a

BOX 16-2 Strategies for Fiscally Responsible Clinical Practice

The nurse:

- Makes conscious decisions about the allocation of professional nursing time.
- Understands Medicare and Medicaid insurance coverage.
- Engages in evidence-based practice and follows best practice guidelines.
- Shares information with patients and families about the costs of care and alternatives.
- Assigns assistive personnel (nurse aides, certified medical assistants) appropriately to help with care.
- Works with the members of other health care professionals to promote fiscal responsibility for clinical practice.
- Documents patient condition accurately.
- Begins discharge planning on admission.
- Completes charge slips for patient supplies, if required.
- Avoids burnout by taking scheduled breaks, meal times, and vacations.
- Engages in safe clinical practice that will avoid personal injuries.

BOX 16-3 Questions for the New Graduate to Consider Asking During Interviews

How are financial concerns of patients dealt with? For example, if a patient is unable to afford needed medications on discharge, what resources are available to nurses to help the patient?
How is acuity of patients assessed and factored into staffing?
What are the budgeted hours per patient day for the unit?
What is the turnover rate on this unit? Why do nurses stay/leave this unit?
How do staff nurses have input into capital budget requests for the unit?
How are data about unit financial indicators communicated to the staff?
What percentage of salary is used as an estimate of fringe benefits?
What is the overtime rate on this unit?
Can you tell me about the discharge planning process for patients on this unit?

patient room, because any unused supplies cannot be returned to stock. Some supplies are to be charged to patients upon use. The fiscally responsible nurse makes this a part of practice, if required.

Another example involves breaks and meal times. The nurse takes breaks and meal times as scheduled, to remain healthy and fully functioning on the job. An occasional shift may be hectic, and it may not be possible to take breaks, but if this is the norm, it is a situation that creates burnout and should be resolved.

Box 16-2 summarizes some strategies to help achieve fiscally responsible clinical practice. Box 16-3 summarizes some questions that a new graduate of a nursing program might want to ask during a job interview to assess how a prospective employer views fiscal responsibility.

CONCLUSION

Given the dire predictions about health care costs that are forecast in the next 10 years, it is imperative that nurses consider the economics of clinical practice. Throughout most of nursing history, nurses have not wanted to learn about the costs of care, placing such knowledge in about the same category as unnecessary paper work. Nurses proclaim that they want to be caregivers, not accountants. However, nurses humanize health care institutions. They bring the values of caring and compassion to the workplace. In the turbulent years to come, incorporating fiscal responsibility into clinical practice will be seen as another way of caring (Murray, 2002).

REFERENCES

American Nurses Association: *Code of ethics for nurses with interpretive statements*, Washington, DC, 2001, American Nurses Publishing.

Centers for Medicare & Medicaid Services: *National health care expenditure projections: 2002–2012, www.cms.hhs.gov/statistics/nhe/projections-2002/proj2002.pdf.*

Centers for Medicare & Medicaid Services: *National health care expenditure projections: 2002-2008, www.cms.hhs.gov/statistics/nhe/projections-2002/t2.asp.*

Feldstein PJ: *Health care economics*, ed 5, New York, 1999, Delmar.

Heffler S, Smith S, Keehan S, et al: *Health spending projections through 2013*, Health Affairs Web exclusive, 2004, 4-79-93, *http://content.healthaffairs.org/.*

Hunt PS: Speaking the language of finance, *AORN J* 73(4):774-787, 2001.

Keeler EB, Rolph JE: How cost sharing reduced medical spending of participants in the health insurance experiment, *JAMA* 249(16):2220-2222, 1983.

Medicare information resource, www.cms.hhs.gov/medicare/.

Murray ME: Another way of caring, *RN Newsletter Madison District Nurses' Association* 4(1):2-3, 2002.

Murray ME, Henriques JB: A test of mental health parity: Comparisons of outcomes of hospital concurrent utilization review, *J Behav Health Serv Res* 31(3):66-78, 2004.

Murray ME, Henriques JB: Denials of reimbursement under managed care, *Manag Care Interface* 16(4): 22-27, 2003.

Oregon Health Policy and Research (OHPR) Home Page: *Prioritized list*, 2004 *www.ohppr.state.or.us/index.html.*

Parkin M: *Microeconomics*, ed 5, New York, 2000, Addison-Wesley.

U.S. Census Bureau: *Annual demographic supplement*, 2002, *www.bls.census.gov/cps/ads/sdata.htm.*

U.S. Census Bureau, U.S. Department of Commerce: *The older population in the United States: March 2002*, 2003.

Welcome to Medicaid, www.cms.hhs.gov/medicaid/whatis-medicaid.asp.

World Health Organization basic texts, ed 44, 2004, *www.who.int/governance/en/.*

CHAPTER 17

Political Action in Nursing

MICHAEL L. EVANS, PhD, RN, CNAA, FACHE

One of the penalties for refusing to participate in politics is that you end up being governed by your inferiors.

—*Plato*

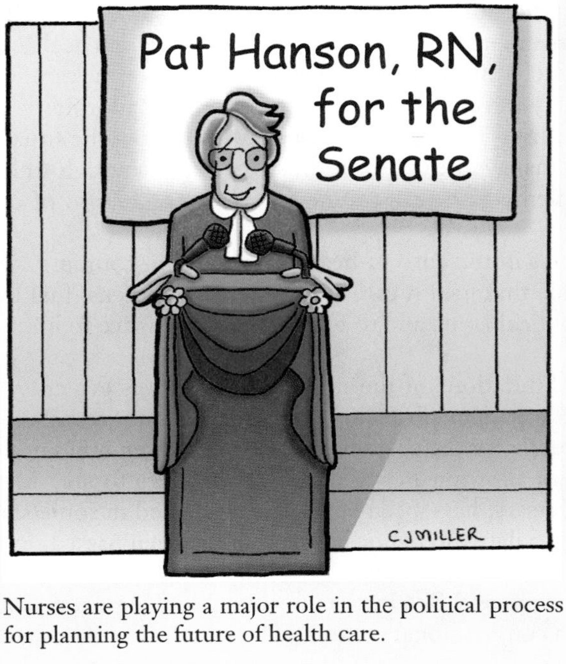

Nurses are playing a major role in the political process for planning the future of health care.

After completing this chapter, you should be able to:

- Define politics and political involvement.
- State the rationale for individual nurse's involvement in the political process.
- List specific strategies needed to begin to affect the laws that govern the practice of nursing and the health care system.
- Discuss different types of power and how each is obtained.
- Describe the function of a political action committee.
- Discuss selected issues affecting nursing: multistate licensure, nursing and collective bargaining, and equal pay for work of comparable value.

Too often nurses feel the legislative process is associated with wheeling and dealing, smoke-filled rooms, and the exchange of money, favors, and influence. Many believe politics to be a world that excludes people with ethics and sincerity—especially given the controversies in past presidential administrations. Others think only the wealthy, ruthless, or very brave play the game of politics. It seems that most nurses feel that the messy business of politicking should be left to others while they (nurses) do what they do best and enjoy most: take care of patients.

Today, however, nurses are coming to realize that politics is not a one-dimensional arena, but a complex struggle with strict rules and serious outcomes. In a typical modern-day political struggle, a rural health care center may be pitted for funding against a major interstate highway. Certainly, both projects have merit, but in times of limited resources not everyone can be victorious. Nurses now know that to influence the development of public policy in ways that affect the way we are able to deliver care, we must be engaged in the political process.

Leavitt and colleagues (2002) wrote that "the future of nursing and health care may well depend on nurses' skills in moving a vision. Without a vision, politics becomes an end in itself—a game that is often corrupt and empty" (p. 86). To demonstrate these skills, nurses must elect the decision-makers, testify before legislative committee hearings, compromise, and get themselves elected to decision-making positions. Nurses realize that involvement in the political process is a vital tool that they must learn to use if they are to carry out their mission (providing quality patient care) with maximum impact.

Based on research, there is "an estimated 14.0 percent of the population without health insurance coverage during the entire year in 2000" (U.S. Census Bureau, 2000). These uninsured individuals (approximately 38.1 million) receive virtually no health care while countless other inadequately insured individuals receive health care only sporadically. Rural and inner-city residents have alarmingly high morbidity and mortality. Health care for rural citizens is virtually nonexistent. Although the situation is improving in some ways with managed care, even those fortunate enough to have insurance often experience problems accessing the care they need because of cost-cutting strategies.

Nurses' recognition of problems in the current health care system, combined with their commitment to the principle that health care is a *right* of all citizens, fuel their desire to become active in the political arena and to form a collective force to improve the health care system.

An example of the force and limitations of the nursing collective is evidenced in organized nursing's efforts to get a patient protection act through Congress. Similar legislation has been introduced yearly for the past several years; however, it has not yet passed. Several initiatives, such as allowing newly delivered mothers to stay in the hospital overnight if deemed necessary, have been successfully enacted in some states and local jurisdictions. However, to date, no major legislation has been passed on the federal level.

The legislation used in this example is S.B. 6 by Senator Daschle (Democrat, South Dakota) as presented in the 106th congressional session (1999-2000). This legislation, although oversimplified in this description, would, among other provisions: (1) provide access to individuals needing emergency care regardless of the specific terms of their health care coverage, such as preauthorization; (2) require that quality-assurance measures be instituted to collect uniform quality data; and (3) establish certain parameters concerning the coverage information available to patients about the insurance plans and ensure the privacy of individual health data.

In the course of this bill's progression through the Senate, the American Nurses Association (ANA) President (at that time) Dr. Beverly Malone testified before the Senate Committee on Health, Education, Labor and Pensions (ANA, 2001). She eloquently addressed nursing's commitment to a broad-based patient protection act. Knowing that compromise language may need to be drawn, she spoke to nursing's support of specific points included in the bill and, at the same time, delineated our areas of disagreement. For example, she spoke of the importance of language that prohibited retaliation for health care professionals who advocate for their patients. Furthermore, she spoke of the importance of language that prohibits discrimination against any health care provider on the basis of type of licensure. That is, a patient protection bill must protect the consumers' right to choose any type of provider based on the service needed, not just medically provided care. On several occasions during the lobbying process, notices were sent through the association's legislative action network Nursing Strategic Action Team (N-STAT), instructing grass roots nurses to inform their senators of their views. Although the bill did not garner the support necessary to be enacted that session, nursing was part of the process to shape the act and will see this policy enacted in the future. Note Figure 17-1, which shows that the final draft of the law may be totally different from the original intent.

Nursing will continue to lobby for new federal and state legislation that improves the quality and availability of nursing and health care.

WHAT EXACTLY IS POLITICS?

Politics, described as "the process of influencing the allocation of scarce resources" (Mason et al., 2002, p. 9), is a vital tool that enables the nurse to "nurse smarter." Involvement in the political process gives an individual nurse a tool that augments his or her power—or clout—to improve the care provided to patients. Whether on the community, the hospital, or on the nursing unit level, political skills enable the nurse to identify needed resources, gain access to those resources, and overcome obstacles, thus facilitating the movement of the patient to higher levels of health or function. Let us look first at the nursing unit level:

Your hospital is in the process of selecting a new supplier of widgets. You and the other nurses on your unit want to have input into that decision, because widgets are essential to the care of your patients and you have a definite opinion about the type of widget that works best. But the intensive care unit nurses, who are thought to be more important and valuable because the nursing shortage has made them as rare as hen's teeth, have the only nurse position on

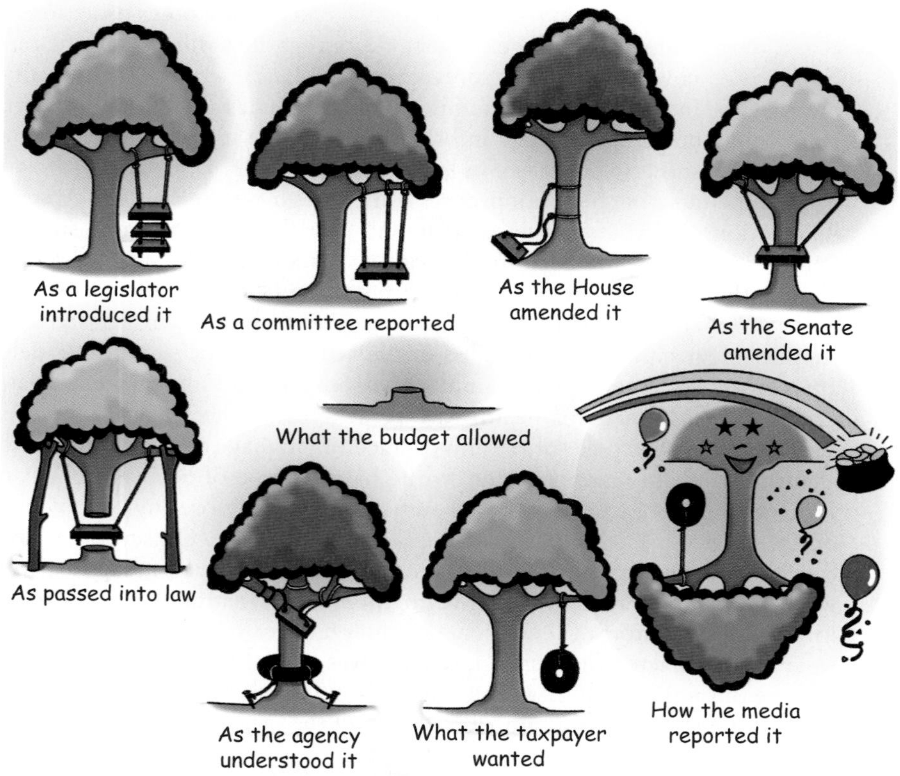
As a legislator introduced it
As a committee reported
As the House amended it
As the Senate amended it
As passed into law
What the budget allowed
As the agency understood it
What the taxpayer wanted
How the media reported it

FIGURE 17-1
How laws grow.

the review committee (and therefore, the director's ear!). You and the nurses on your unit strategize to secure input into this important decision.

Your plan might look like this:

- Gather data about widgets—cost, suppliers, possible substitutes, and so on.
- Communicate to the head nurse and supervisor your concern about this issue and your plans to get involved in the decision (by using appropriate channels of communication).
- State clearly what you want—perhaps request a seat on the committee when the opportunity arises.
- Summarize in writing your request and the rationale, submitting it to the appropriate people.
- Establish a coalition with the intensive care unit nurses and other concerned individuals.
- Recall that the vice president for purchasing's mother was a patient on your unit and needed widgets in her care and be sure to include this example in your written request.

- Get involved with other hospital issues and contribute in a credible fashion (i.e., do not be a single-issue person).

WHAT OTHER STRATEGIES WOULD YOU SUGGEST?

This vignette illustrates what a politically astute nurse would do in this situation. Although the example applies to a hospital setting, the strategies are comparable to those necessary for getting involved on a community, state, or even federal level. Practicing at the local level will provide good experience for larger issues—one has to start somewhere. Furthermore, a nurse involved on the local level will be able to hone her or his skills—gaining confidence in her or his ability to handle similar "exercises" in larger forums.

In the above example, the nurse was able to formulate several "political" actions to influence the outcome of the widget decision (Critical Thinking Box 17-1).

WHAT ARE THE SKILLS THAT MAKE UP A NURSE'S POLITICAL SAVVY?

Ability to Analyze an Issue (Those Assessment Skills Again!). The individual who expects to "influence the allocation of scarce resources" must do the homework necessary to be well informed. She or he must know all the facts relevant to the issue, how the issue looks from all angles, and how it fits into the larger picture.

Ability to Present a Possible Resolution in Clear and Concise Terms. The nurse must be prepared to coherently frame and present arguments in support of his recommendation. Preparation includes anticipating questions and objections so that a rebuttal will be logical and well developed.

Ability to Participate in a Constructive Way. Too often, a person disagrees with a proposal being suggested to a hospital unit (or city council), but only gripes about it. The displeased individual seldom takes the time to study the problem or to understand its connection with other hospital departments (or city programs in a broader issue). Most important, the displeased person seldom suggests an alternate solution.

In short, if an individual's concern is not directed toward solving the problem, she/he will not be seen as a team player, but as a troublemaker. Constructive responses, perhaps something as simple as posing a single question such as "What solution would you suggest?" may help those involved think in positive terms and redirect energy to a more productive mode. Positive action can produce the kind of creative brainstorming that results in a solution.

Ability to Voice One's Opinion (Understand the System). Once the homework is done, let the *right* person know the determined opinion or solution. For example, the nurse might communicate concern and knowledge about the issue to the head

CRITICAL THINKING BOX 17-1

What are some issues in your school or hospital that are examples of political issues or the result of politics?

nurse and supervisor. Of course, it is important to make an intelligent and well-informed decision about to whom it is best to voice one's opinion.

Having a confidant or mentor who knows the environment is one way to acquire this information. Another strategy is to use your listening skills. Simply standing back and listening are assets that will come in handy! Whatever the technique, studying the dynamics of the institution with all senses will help the nurse decide on the best person and the most appropriate way to communicate the proposed solution.

Ability to Analyze and Use Power Bases. While discussing issues with colleagues and studying the organization, be alert to the various power brokers. In the widget vignette, the nurse notes the VP of Purchasing is an obvious source of power in the hospital. She (the VP of Purchasing) will certainly concur with, if not make, the final decision. However, be aware that power does not always follow the lines on the organizational chart. The power of the nurse aide on the oncology unit who just happens to be the niece of the newly appointed member of the Board of Trustees may escape the notice of some. This person could be used to influence a decision if necessary. Similarly, the fact that the VP of Purchasing's mother was on the unit should be filed in your memory for future use.

Facts may be facts, but where one gets information can sometimes make a statement as powerful as the information itself. Having the ability to use many different channels of information will give the nurse the power to choose among them.

WHAT IS POWER, AND WHERE DOES IT COME FROM?

Sanford (1979) describes five laws of power. She recommends that these laws be studied to identify strategies to develop power in nursing. The laws are as follows:

LAW 1: POWER INVARIABLY FILLS ANY VACUUM

When a problem or issue arises, the prevailing desire is for peace and order. People are willing to give power to someone interested in restoring order to situations of discomfort. Therefore, someone will eventually step forward to handle the dilemma. It may be some time before the discomfort or unrest grows to heights sufficient for someone to take the lead. Even then, a poorly thought-out solution may be brought forward.

Nonetheless, a person exerting power will step forward to offer a solution. In some situations, this person may be the previously identified leader, the head nurse, or the chair. More often there is an official power broker influencing the action. Know that there are opportunities to exert influence—for example, by taking the leadership role (i.e., stepping forward to fill the vacuum).

LAW 2: POWER IS INVARIABLY PERSONAL

In most instances, programs are attributed to an organization. For example, a fictitious program, ImmunEYEs, was proposed by the state and national children's and health associations. If one investigated, however, it might be found that the program began with a small group of friends talking over a pizza one evening, lamenting the number of infants still not immunized. In the course of their conversation, one might have said,

"If we were to create a media blitz that would get the need for immunizations in the consciousness of parents—get the need for immunizations in their face!" And the next person might have said—in their eyes! "Yea, ImmunEYEs. Let's do it!"

Initiatives such as this start with one person creating a new approach to a problem. That person exercises power by providing the leadership or spark to create the strategy to carry out such an initiative, thus inspiring people to contribute to the effort.

LAW 3: POWER IS BASED ON A SYSTEM OF IDEAS AND PHILOSOPHY

Behaviors demonstrated by an individual as she or he exerts power reflect a personal belief system or a philosophy of life. That philosophy or ideal must be one that attracts followers, gains their respect, and rallies them to join the effort. Nurses have the opportunity to ensure that a patient's right to health care (versus privilege), access to preventive care, and similar values are reflected in policies and procedures.

LAW 4: POWER IS EXERCISED THROUGH AND DEPENDS ON INSTITUTIONS

As an individual, one can easily feel powerless and unable to deal with the complex problems facing a hospital, community, or state. But through a nursing service organization, a state nurse association, or a similar organization, that individual can garner the resources needed to magnify her power. The person-to-person network, the communication vehicle (usually an organization's newsletter or journal), and the organizational structure are established for precisely this function—to support and foster changes in the health care system.

LAW 5: POWER IS INVARIABLY CONFRONTED WITH AND ACTS IN THE PRESENCE OF A FIELD OF RESPONSIBILITY

Actions taken speak to the other nurses for whom nurses act and, most important, the patients for whom nurses advocate. The individual in the power position is acting on behalf of the group. Power is communicated to observers and is reinforced by positive responses. If the group thinks that its ideals are not being honored, the vacuum will be filled with the next candidate capable of the role and supported by the organization.

ANOTHER WAY TO LOOK AT POWER AND WHERE TO GET IT

In a classic, much-referenced work, French and Raven (1959) describe five sources of power. They are (in order of importance): reward power, coercive power, legitimate power, referent or mentor power, and expert or informational power. These descriptions of power were presented in the discussion of nursing management in Chapter 10. The discussion there described the use of power within the ranks of nursing. Here, the use of power is presented as it applies to the political process, especially through political action in nursing.

The strongest source of power is the ability to *reward*. The best example of making use of the reward power base is the giving of money. If, for example, one gives a decision-maker financial support for a future political campaign, the recipient will feel obligated to the donor and may, from time to time, "adjust opinions" to repay these obligations! Today, because caps have been placed on campaign contributions, the misuse of this type of reward has been reduced.

An additional source of reward-based political power is the ability to commit voters to a candidate through endorsements. This illustrates the importance of having a large number of members in an organization; in other words, a large voting bloc.

Second in importance is the power to *coerce* or "punish" a decision-maker for going against the wishes of an organization. The best example of this power, the opposite of *reward*, is the ability to remove the person from office at election time.

Third in importance is *legitimate* power, or the influence that comes with role and position. Influence derives from the status that society assigns individuals as a result of, for instance, old family money, membership in a respected profession, or a prominent position in the community. The dean in a school of nursing has a certain amount of influence just because of who she or he is. Right? A nurse's commitment to enhancing nursing's influence explains why we encourage and assist each other to achieve key decision-making positions—to build nursing's legitimate power base.

The fourth power base is that of *referent* or *mentor* power. This is the power that "rubs off" of influential persons. When representatives of the student body talk with the faculty about a problem they are having with a course and receive her or his support, the curriculum committee or dean is more likely to listen sympathetically than if the students were arguing only for themselves. The faculty, joining with the students to solve their problem, adds to the students' power. The wish to build this type of power encourages nurses to join coalitions, especially those including organizations with greater power than our own.

The last and weakest of the power bases is that of *expert* power. Nurses know about health and nursing care and are, therefore, able to impart knowledge in this area with great confidence and style. Typically, nurses communicate this authority through letters written to legislators, testimonies presented in hearings, and through other contacts made on behalf of nursing and patients. Nurses do this well, but remember that this is the weakest source of power.

In summary, power is derived from various sources. Nurses use, with the greatest frequency and ease, the weakest of the power bases—that deriving from their expertise. Although this is an important power base, we must develop and exercise the other types as well. Only then will nurses realize the full extent of our potential (Critical Thinking Box 17-2).

NETWORKING AMONG COLLEAGUES

It has been said that one should never be more than two telephone calls away from a needed resource, whether it be a piece of information, a contact in a hospital in another city, or input into a decision one is about to make. The key to successful networking is

CRITICAL THINKING BOX 17-2

Who are the people in positions that reflect the different power levels in your school, hospital, and community?

consciously building and nurturing a pool of associates whose skills and connections augment your own.

As a recent graduate, one should begin the important task of networking by selecting an instructor from nursing school, one who is able to speak to your performance during nursing school. Ask this person if they would be willing to write a letter of reference for your first job. If she or he agrees, nurture this contact from now on. Keep this individual apprised of your whereabouts, your successes, and your plans for the future. This person will be an important link not only to your school, but also to your future educational and career undertakings. Then, at each future work site, find a head nurse or supervisor willing to write a reference and with whom to maintain contact. Keep building the network over your career.

Remember that this network must be nourished. Constant use of one's resources without reciprocation will exhaust them and make them unreliable sources of assistance in the future. But if properly cared for, this network will provide support for the rest of your career.

BUILDING COALITIONS

A *coalition* is a group of individuals or organizations who share a common interest in a single issue. Groups with whom nurses might form coalitions are as diverse as the topics about which nurses are concerned. For example, nurses are concerned about and lobby for adequate, safe childcare, a safe environment, and women's issues. The numerous organizations interested in these diverse issues are potential candidates for a coalition with nursing organizations. It is not unusual, however, for two organizations to be in a coalition on one issue but adversaries on another. Indeed, this is common in the political arena, where negotiations and compromises are the norm.

A warning: *the selection of coalition partners should strengthen your cause or organization.* Forming coalitions is a strategy to empower oneself. Therefore, build coalitions with organizations enjoying greater power than nursing, not less (Critical Thinking Box 17-3 and Figure 17-2).

WHAT ABOUT TRADE-OFFS, COMPROMISES, NEGOTIATIONS, AND OTHER TRICKS OF THE TRADE?

Politics is not a perfect art or science. In the heat of battle, nurses are often called on to compromise, but if they are unwilling to give on some principle; they sacrifice all. To hold out for the ideal typically means that no progress toward the ideal will be realized. Often, changes in health care policies are achieved in incremental steps. However, the decision to compromise a value or principle must be carefully made with full realization of the implications—not an easy decision!

CRITICAL THINKING BOX 17-3

What are examples of nursing coalitions in your community or state?

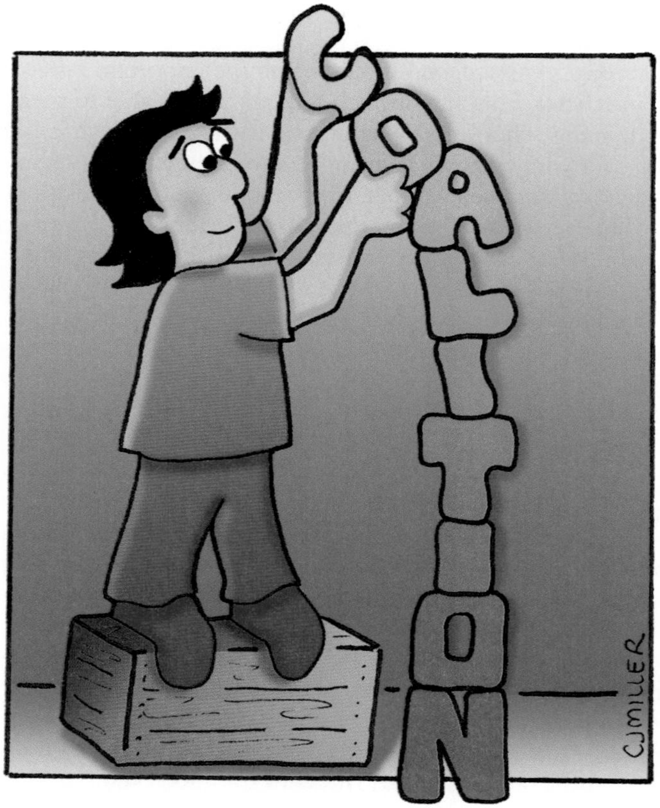

FIGURE 17-2
How do we build a coalition?

The political skills discussed so far apply to any situation, whether in a family, a hospital unit, or a community. The next part of the chapter is focused on skills that apply specifically to the governmental process.

HOW DO I GO ABOUT PARTICIPATING IN THE ELECTION PROCESS?

One key to successful political activity is involvement in the election process. This is the stage where one can get to know the candidates; they also get to know you. In addition, it is a time when one makes important contacts for that network (Box 17-1).

Getting involved in a candidate's campaign is simple. First, study the positions to be filled. Then, with the help of the local nurses' association, the local newspaper, or the county or state Democratic or Republican Party, select the candidate whose views on health care most closely match yours. Next, find the candidate's campaign headquarters. After this, contact the candidate's volunteer coordinator and see when volunteer help is needed. Most campaigns are crying for assistance with folding letters and stuffing envelopes, looking up addresses, and preparing bulk mailings. They will welcome

BOX 17-1 How Important Is One Vote?

In 1645 one vote gave Oliver Cromwell control of England.
In 1649 one vote caused Charles I of England to be executed.
In 1776 one vote gave America the English language instead of German.
In 1845 one vote brought Texas into the Union.
In 1868 one vote saved President Andrew Johnson from impeachment.
In 1875 one vote changed France from a monarchy to a republic.
In 1876 one vote gave Rutherford B. Hayes the presidency of the Nazi Party.
In 1941 one vote saved Selective Service—just weeks before Pearl Harbor was attacked.
Author unknown

From Goldwater M, Zusy M: *Prescription for nurses: effective political action*, St Louis, 1990, Mosby, p 31, with permission.

you with great enthusiasm! Be sure to tell the campaign staff that you are a nurse and would be more than willing to contribute to the candidate's understanding of health care issues and to assist in drafting the candidate's positions on these issues (Critical Thinking Box 17-4).

Beware: *involvement in campaigns and party organizations can lead to catching the political "bug."* Victims of the political bug are overcome by a powerful desire to make changes in the system and see a multitude of opportunities to educate people about the health needs of a county, state, and nation. An example of two nurses who caught the bug: During a past national presidential election, the nurses at a state caucus volunteered to write the resolution for the party's position on health care, which, if passed, would become a plank in the platform. After much work drafting the statement and bringing it before various committees, they were ecstatic when it passed and became the health statement for their party! (Review Box 17-2 as an example of the effectiveness of political action by nurses.)

WHAT IS A POLITICAL ACTION COMMITTEE?

Another way that nurses can influence the elective process is through involvement in an organization's political action committee (PAC). Political action committees, or PACs, grew out of the Nixon/Watergate era, when Congress decided that candidates for public office were becoming too dependent on money supplied by special interests—individuals who give large political contributions and thereby exert undue influence over the elected official's decisions.

CRITICAL THINKING BOX 17-4

Who in your state government supports legislature that is pro-nursing and pro–health care?

BOX 17-2 Resolution Against Physician Abuse of Registered Nurses Passed by the 2001 Texas Nurses Association House of Delegates

Submitted by: Committee on Practice Issues
Category: Action
Rationale: Establishes action on issue of nursing shortage

Whereas, surveys and anecdotal information confirm that registered nurses experience verbal abuse as a routine part of their job and,

Whereas, of the thousands of nurses surveyed, it was found that 90% of nurses have experienced verbal abuse and most encounter an average of 5 incidents per month and,

Whereas, physicians are identified as regular perpetrators of verbal abuse and,

Whereas, registered nurses and the physician community recognize that it is a minority of physicians who engage in abuse of registered nurses and,

Whereas, the actions of this minority have negative consequences on the professional relationship between physicians and registered nurses and,

Whereas, verbal abuse is linked to increased turnover rates of nurses and,

Whereas, in professional work environments, registered nurses should not encounter such behavior and,

Whereas, in a nurse shortage environment, the profession cannot afford to lose even a single nurse to abuse and,

Whereas, nurses and physicians are called upon to be colleagues in the daily care of patients and communities and,

Whereas, the development of systems to increase patient safety, and manage chronic illness called for in the most recent Institute of Medicine Reports also require professional collegiality and,

Whereas, Texas Nurses Association is committed to Workplace Advocacy and the improvement of the workplace environment of registered nurses in Texas, therefore be it

RESOLVED, that the Texas Nurses Association make the elimination of physician abuse of registered nurses TNA's Eighth Commitment to Workplace Advocacy.

RESOLVED, that the Texas Nurses Association will advocate no less than a ZERO TOLERANCE of physician abuse of registered nurses.

RESOLVED, that the Texas Nurses Association work with employers of registered nurses in developing model policies against physician abuse of registered nurses.

RESOLVED, that the Texas Nurses Association work with the Texas Medical Association to promote adoption by the physician community of a ZERO TOLERANCE for registered nurse colleague abuse.

RESOLVED, that the Texas Nurses Association research and promote the use of strategies to support registered nurses who encounter abuse in the workplace such as:

- ✓ Code Nurse, a method that encourages nurses to drop what they are doing on a unit and come to silently support nurses who are experiencing physician abuse on the units.
- ✓ Conference calls, a strategy that provides witnesses when nurses make calls at night to physicians who are known to engage in abuse.
- ✓ The implementation of physician and nurse counselors who work with identified abusers of registered nurses.
- ✓ Education for registered nurses and physicians that provide strategies for identifying and managing abusive situations.

Moved by Sandy Oliver, passed. No opposition.

As a result, Congress limited the amount of money an individual may contribute to a candidate, established strict reporting requirements, and created a mechanism whereby individuals can pool their resources and collectively support a candidate.

The ANA National Political Action Committee (PAC) is called ANA-PAC. Through this vehicle, nurses across the country organize to collectively endorse and support candidates for national offices. Likewise, state nurses' associations have state-level PACs to influence statewide elections. There may be PACs in your area that endorse candidates in city elections. All PACs must comply with the state or federal election codes and report financial support given to candidates for public office.

Today, PACs play an important role in the political process, because they provide a mechanism whereby small contributors can act as a collective, participating in the electoral process when otherwise they would feel outmaneuvered by the bigger players.

The ANA's Endorsement Handbook stresses four points regarding PACs:

- **Political focus.** The only purpose of any PAC is to endorse candidates for public office and then supply them with the political and financial support they need to win an election.
- **No legislative activities.** A PAC does not lobby elected officials; that is the job of the state nurse association and its government-relations arm. A PAC simply provides financial and campaign support for candidates whose views are generally consistent with those of its contributors.
- **Not "dirty."** A PAC does not "buy" a candidate or a vote; but the very nature of political life suggests that candidates who recognize an organization's ability to affect their electoral prospects will be inclined to listen to the group's views when considering specific pieces of legislation.
- **Health concerns only.** Nursing PACs evaluate the candidates on nursing and health concerns only. In other words, ANA-PAC might solicit the candidates' ideas about how Congress might address the problem of elder abuse in long-term care facilities. But the organization as a nursing PAC should not include questions, for instance, about the source of funding for the new cabinet on foreign commerce. The organization speaks for members only on issues covered in its philosophic statements, resolutions, position statements, legislative platforms, or other documents that its members as an organization have accepted (Critical Thinking Box 17-5).

CRITICAL THINKING BOX 17-5

How has ANA-PAC affected nursing on a national level? What have been the most recent activities of this organization? How does your state organization communicate or affect nursing and health care legislation in your state?

ANA-PAC, The American Nurses Association's Political Action Committee.

AFTER GETTING THEM ELECTED, THEN WHAT?

Lobbying is the attempt to influence or sway a public official to take a desired action. Lobbying is also characterized as the education of the legislator about nursing and its issues. Educating officials, like educating patients, is an important part of the nurse's role.

As nurses, we can lobby in several different ways. The first and best opportunity to lobby comes when the nurse first meets the candidate and evaluates her or him as a potential officeholder. This is the time to assess the candidate's knowledge of health care issues. Take the time to teach and to learn.

A second opportunity comes when the official needs information to decide how to vote on an issue. Depending on time constraints, the issue, and other considerations, a nurse might decide to lobby the official in person or in writing. If time and financial resources permit, the most powerful type of contact is a face-to-face visit. The only way to ensure time with your senator or representative is to make an appointment. Even then, you may not be successful.

If an unscheduled visit to the Capitol precludes an appointment, the best time to catch your senator or representative is early in the day, before the legislative sessions or committee meetings start; they rarely start before 10 or 11 AM. Contact with the legislator's aid or assistant can be just as effective as time with the official. Busy federal and state officials depend heavily on their staff. Treat staff members with the respect they deserve!

Finally, remember that contact should be made between legislative sessions and during holidays when the official is in her or his home district. The structure and content of the visit should be similar to that of a written contact. That is, know your issue, keep it short, identify the issue by its bill number and title, and communicate exactly what action you want the senator or representative to take. Box 17-3 is a list of specific

BOX 17-3 *Do*'s and *Don't*s When Lobbying

DO:

- Make sure your legislator knows constituents who are affected by the bill; suggest visits to programs in his/her area.
- Clearly identify the bill, using title and number, if possible.
- Be specific and know about the issue or bill before you write or talk.
- Identify yourself (occupation, hometown, member of ANA).
- Use your own words; if writing, use your own stationery. No form letters!
- Be courteous, brief, and to the point.
- Provide pertinent reasons for your stand.
- Show your legislator how the issue relates to his/her district.
- Respect your legislator's right to form an opinion different from yours.
- Present a united front. Keep our internal problems at home.
- Write letters of appreciation to your legislators when appropriate.

Continued

BOX 17-3 *Do's* and *Don'ts* When Lobbying—cont'd

- Write letters at appropriate times, for example, when a bill is in committee, request action that is appropriate for that stage in the legislative process.
- Establish an ongoing relationship with the public official.
- Know issues or problems your legislator is concerned about, and express your interest in assisting him or her.
- Attend functions sponsored by coalition members. Be seen!
- Get involved in your legislator's campaign for reelection—or his or her opponent's, if necessary!

DON'T:

- Write a long letter or one on multiple points; deal with a single bill or concern per letter or contact.
- Use threats or promises.
- Berate your legislator.
- Be offended in the event of a canceled appointment. Things are unpredictable during a legislative session.
- Demand a commitment before the legislator has had time to consider the measure.
- Pretend to have vast influence in the political area.
- Be vague.
- Hesitate to admit you do not know all the facts, but indicate you will find out—and do!

"Do's and Don'ts When Lobbying." As you begin lobbying, add your recommendations to the list.

If you cannot visit your representative because of time or travel restrictions, a well-written letter, electronic message (e-mail), or telephone call can communicate your message. Examine the sample letter in Box 17-4. Note that some pointers are listed at

BOX 17-4 Example of a Letter to a Public Official

Ima Nurse, RN
123 Main Street
Any Town, USA 12345-6789
The Honorable Y. R. Important, Jr.
United States Senate
Washington, DC 20510
Dear Senator Important:

I request your support of SB 101 regarding appropriations for nursing education and research. This bill is vital to the country's efforts to improve the number and quality of registered nurses. As you recall, the 1998 Verimportant Nursing Study demonstrated the growing demand for Advanced Nurse Practitioners to work with the increasing numbers of people older than 65 years of age. This bill will provide

Continued

BOX 17-4 Example of a Letter to a Public Official—cont'd

funding to increase the number of faculty and student slots in the country's schools of nursing and to support nursing research in gerontologic nursing. The expanding numbers of older people in our area of the country are not able to get the health care they deserve. During a trip home, I would like to take you to the Main Street Senior's Clinic. I know that you would be pleased with this service, as are the health care providers and the clients.

Will you support this bill? Do you have any questions about it? If so, please call me or the State Nurses' Association Headquarters.

Thank you for your concern with this issue and your continuing support of health care issues.

Sincerely yours,

Ima Nurse, RN

Points to note:

1. Neat, without typos or grammatical errors
2. Correctly addressed
3. Professional letterhead
4. Covering single topic
5. Refers to the bill by number and content
6. States request in first sentence
7. Brief rationale for request
8. Uses RN in inside address and salutation

the foot of the page. Examples of the proper way to address a public official may be found in Box 17-5.

Letters are common methods of communicating with elected officials; however, a telephone call or e-mail is often necessary to relay your opinion when time is limited before an important vote. The suggested format and content of the electronic message and telephone message are similar to that of a letter or face-to-face interview.

Decisions about the type of contact to make with the decision-maker will vary depending on the situation. For example, if the bill is coming up for the first time in committee, the strategy may be that 10 to 15 people write letters or e-mail messages or call the members of the committee. At this point, the number of contacts with the office is important. The reason is that the legislator's assistant typically answers the telephone or opens the mail, tallies the subject of the contact, and puts a hash mark in the "Pro HB 23" or "Con HB 23" column. Therefore, a greater impact will be realized if the contacts pertain to one bill. Bags of form letters, however, may have a negative impact on a lobbying effort. Make sure your callers/writers understand the issue and are able to individualize their contact with the elected official. People who contact the legislator's office with a script that they do not understand will not further the lobbying efforts of an organization.

The aforementioned efforts are sufficient early in the process; however, if a major, controversial bill is coming up for a final vote in the Senate, activating a statewide

BOX 17-5 How to Address Public Officials

The President
Writing*: The Honorable (Full Name)
President of the United States
The White House
Washington, DC 20500
Dear Mr./Madam President:
Speaking:
"Mr./Madam President"
"President (Last Name)"

The Vice President
Writing: The Honorable (Full Name)
Vice President of the United States
Executive Office Building
Washington, DC 20501
Dear Mr./Madam Vice President:
Speaking:
"Mr./Madam Vice President"
"Vice President (Last Name)"

A Senator
Writing: The Honorable (Full Name)
United States Senate
(will have office building and room address)
Washington, DC 20510
Dear Senator (Full Name):
Speaking: "Senator (Last Name)"

A Representative
Writing: The Honorable (Full Name)
U.S. House of Representatives
(will have office building and room address)
Washington, DC 20515
Dear Mr./Ms. (Full Name):
Speaking: "Representative (Last Name)"
"Mr./Ms. (Last Name)"

A Member of the Cabinet
Writing: The Honorable (Full Name)
Secretary of (Cabinet Agency)
(will have office building and room address)
Washington, DC 20520
Dear Mr./Madam Secretary:
Speaking: "Mr./Madam Secretary"
"Secretary (Last Name)"

*The correct closing for a letter to the president is "Very respectfully yours." The correct closing for all other federal officials noted here is "Sincerely yours."

network and bombarding the senators with letters, e-mail messages, telephone calls, and telegrams—as many as possible—is a typical strategy. The bigger the issue, the bigger the campaign should be.

At several points in a lobbying season, but certainly after contacting the elected official for a major vote, a follow-up thank-you letter will strengthen your contact with the legislator and help establish you in her or his political network. In addition to reinforcing the reason for your original contact, thank the official for her or his concern with the issue and work in solving the problem by writing the bill or voting for it (or whatever) and for paying attention to your concern (Critical Thinking Box 17-6).

In summary, there are specific skills to learn for effective political involvement. But remember that many of the skills needed to be politically savvy are the very ones that will serve you well in everyday professional negotiations (Figure 17-3).

CRITICAL THINKING BOX 17-6

When are the bills that affect nursing and health care going to be presented to your state legislature?

As a recent graduate getting oriented to your first job and beginning to look around at what you and your colleagues need to improve, you will agree that political involvement is necessary to reach your goals.

This author implores you not to wait to be "allowed" to make a difference, not to wait to be invited to join, and not to let someone else do the job. Please step forward! Act like the powerful, informed, influential nurse that you are. There is much that needs to be done; be a part of the action!

Margaret Mead said, "Never doubt that a small group of thoughtful, committed citizens can change the world. Indeed, it's the only thing that ever has." The nursing profession has much to accomplish; I'm pleased you will be joining us.

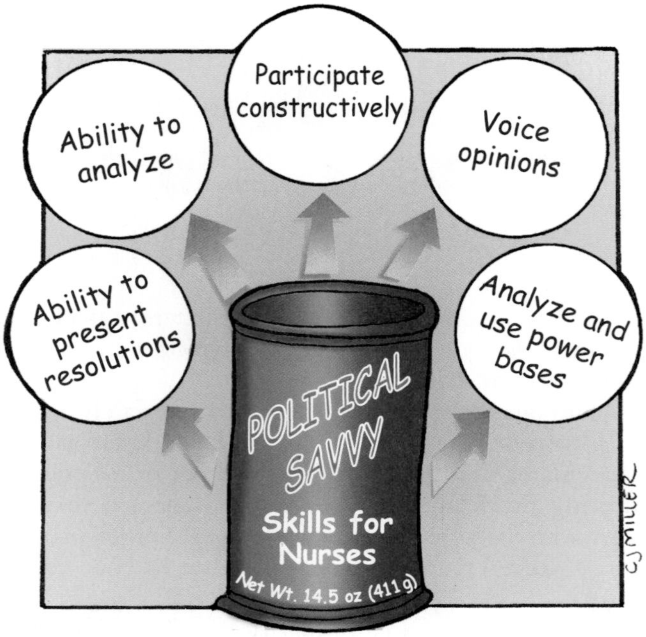

FIGURE 17-3
Skills to make a nurse politically savvy.

CONTROVERSIAL POLITICAL ISSUES AFFECTING NURSING

PROPOSED UNIFORM CORE LICENSURE REQUIREMENTS

What Is It? The National Council's Nursing Practice and Education Committee has proposed the development of core licensure requirements. This was in response to an increasing concern regarding the mobility of nurses and the maintenance of licensure standards to protect the public health, safety, and welfare. With the implementation of Mutual Recognition, it is important that health care consumers have access to nursing services that are provided by a nurse who meets consistent standards, regardless where the consumer lives. The National Council (1999) defines competence as "the application of knowledge and the interpersonal, decision making, and psychomotor skills expected for the nurse's practice role, within the context of public health, welfare and safety" (p. 3).

The competence framework is based on the recommendations from the 1996 Continued Competence Subcommittee. This framework consists of the three following primary areas:

- Competence development: the method by which a nurse gains nursing knowledge, skills, and abilities.
- Competence assessment: the means by which a nurse's knowledge, skills, and abilities are validated.
- Competence conduct: refers to health and conduct expectations, including assurance that licensees possess the functional abilities to perform the essential functions of the nursing role (National Council of State Boards of Nursing, 1999, p. 3).

These proposed requirements are going to cause controversy in the nursing community and will most likely require additional legislation in most states. An interesting question proposed by the committee was: *Do you really think nursing is that much different, that much safer on your side of the state boundary line* (p. 3)? The summary of the proposed competencies may be found in the *Book of Business* from the 1999 meeting of the National Council of State Boards of Nursing. Contact the National Council for the full paper that includes the rationales for the proposed requirements and discussion of how the committee developed the recommendations.

Organized nursing and state boards of nurse examiners have been working on a proposal to address some of the questions that is now ready to pilot. Agreements, known as *interstate licensure compacts*, are being created among several states that will specify the rights and responsibilities of nurses who choose or are required to work across state boundaries and the governing body responsible for protecting the recipients of nursing care (Thomas, 1999).

At press time, Arizona, Arkansas, Delaware, Idaho, Iowa, Maine, Maryland, Mississippi, Nebraska, New Mexico, North Carolina, North Dakota, South Dakota, Tennessee, Texas, Utah, Virginia, and Wisconsin had enacted multistate compacts; however, legislation is pending in several states. New Jersey and Indiana have enacted mutual recognition legislation; however, they will not implement the compact until a later date *(www.ncsbn.org/nlc/rnlpvncompact_mutual _recognition_state.asp).*

CRITICAL THINKING BOX 17-7

How will interstate licensureer compacts affect the licensure and practice of nursing in your state?

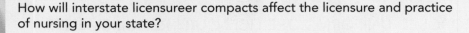

States entering into interstate compacts agree to mutually recognize a nursing license issued by any of the participating states. To join the compact, states must enact legislation adopting the compact. The nurse will hold a single license issued by her or his state of residence. This license will include a "multistate licensure privilege" to practice in any of the other compact states (both physical and electronic). Each state will continue to set its own licensing and practice standards. A nurse will have to comply only with the license and license renewal requirements of her or his state of residence (the one issuing the license), but she or he must know and comply with the practice standards of each state in which she or he practices *(http://www.ncsbn.org/nlc/index.asp)* (Critical Thinking Box 17-7).

As these agreements are established, experience with additional problems arising from the multistate practice of nursing will be identified and solved in amendments to state practice acts.

NURSING AND COLLECTIVE BARGAINING

> March! There are no bunkers, no sidelines for nursing today. We find ourselves the center of attention. As the government and corporate America fight escalating health care costs, AIDS is wreaking havoc and technology swells unchecked. Underpaid, overworked, and overstressed nurses are in the midst of a conflagration. Nursing is in greater demand than ever before. Remember Scutari. We must organize, unite, go on the offensive.
> —Margretta Styles, 1988, as quoted in Hansten and Washburn, 1990, p. 53.

The National Labor Relations Act is a federal law regulating labor relations in the private business sector (extended to voluntary, nonprofit health care institutions in 1974). This law grants employees the right to form, to join, or to participate in a labor organization. Furthermore, the law gives the employee the right to organize and bargain with his or her employer through a representative of his or her own choosing.

Collective bargaining continues to be a point of debate among nurses. Those supporting collective bargaining argue that it is a tool to force positive changes in the practice setting, a method of controlling the practice setting. Many positive changes in the clinical setting are attributed to advances made during contract negotiations.

The major advantage of coverage under a collective bargaining agreement is that it is a contract negotiated and signed by duly authorized representatives of management and nurses and is, therefore, binding and enforceable. Opponents counter that such a written contract, although explicitly delineating terms of employment, can restrict the freedom, flexibility, and, as a result, the professional judgment of an RN.

In addition, opponents feel that as a profession, nurses should not use collective bargaining, but instead should influence the practice setting in ways that mean employee and employer working as a team and not as adversaries. They contend that a strike, the ultimate tool of any labor dispute, should not be used. Opponents further argue that practice standards are not negotiable. The points of disagreement between employer and employee are always economic: pay, vacation, sick leave, and similar issues. Chapter 18 presents a more detailed discussion of collective bargaining issues. Regardless of your opinion on collective bargaining, the process will involve political action.

What do you think? A paragraph in the ANA's publication *What You Need to Know About Today's Workplace: A Survival Guide for Nurses* summarizes the challenge for us:

> In a work environment that is constantly changing, it is imperative that nurses are able to assess the true merits of various labor-management structures, to evaluate the real value of proposals to upgrade compensation packages, to determine appropriate levels of participation in workplace decision-making bodies, and to distinguish between long-range solutions and "quick fixes" to workplace problems (Flanagan, 1995, p. 5).

EQUAL PAY FOR WORK OF COMPARABLE VALUE OR COMPARABLE WORTH?

The concept of comparable worth or pay equity holds that jobs that are equal in value to an organization ought to be equally compensated, whether or not the work content of those jobs is similar. Pay equity relates to the goal of equitable compensation as outlined in the Equal Pay Act of 1963, and "sex-based wage discrimination" is a phrase that refers to the basis of the problems defined by Title VII of the Civil Rights Act of 1964.

As long ago as World War II, the War Labor Board suggested that discrimination probably exists whenever jobs traditionally relegated to women are paid below the rate of common-labor jobs such as janitor or floor sweeper. One of the first cases was that of the *International Union of Electrical Workers v. Westinghouse*. The union proved that male-female wage disparity existed and uncovered a policy in a manual that stated women were to be paid less because they were women. Back pay and increased wages were given in an out-of-court settlement in an appellate-level decision.

It was nurses who initiated the action, in Lemons v. the City and County of Denver. Nurses employed by the city of Denver claimed under the Civil Rights Act that they were the victims of salary discrimination, because their jobs were of a value equal to various better-paid positions throughout the city's diverse workforce. The court ruled that the city was justified in the use of a market pricing system (a form of pay based on supply and demand) even though it acknowledged the general discrimination against women. The court said that the case (and the comparable-worth concept) had the potential to disrupt the entire economic system of the United States. Because of this judgment and the fact that the nurses were unable to prepare a job evaluation program to substantiate their claim, the judge dismissed the case.

Another important concept in this area is "salary compression." That is, at the beginning of a nurse's career, she or he can expect to enter a beginning staff nurse

TABLE 17-1

Salary Data

United States: Averages of All Reporting Hospitals (in Thousands)			
Health Care Provider	**Average Minimum**	**Average Mid**	**Average Maximum**
Staff nurse	31.7	40.4	49.1
Nurse practitioner—general care	47.3	59.6	71.8
Pharmacist	47.8	59.4	70.9
Physician's assistant	47.8	60.3	72.6
Case manager	36.8	46.4	55.9
LPN/LVN	21.7	26.9	32.0

From Watson Wyatt Data Services: *ECS hospital and health care professional, nursing & allied services personnel compensation report*, Rochelle Park, NJ, 2000/2001, Watson Wyatt Data services.
LPN, Licensed practical nurse; *LVN*, licensed vocational nurse.

position earning approximately $31,700. This same nurse can expect to earn a maximum salary of $49,100, or a 54.8% salary progression, over a career (Watson Wyatt Data Services, 2000/2001). Table 17-1 offers a comparison of nursing salary with that of other professions.

One explanation offered for the discrepancy is that the salary system for nurses is based on the assumption that most nurses are temporary workers. Therefore, salary structures are relatively flat, with essentially no allowances for administrative responsibilities and almost no differential for experience.

CONCLUSION

Needless to say, much work continues to be done in this important area. Nurses and women in general must continue to strive for equitable compensation based on the inherent value or worth of the work performed, instead of on the basis of historically depressed pay levels or other discriminatory factors. Changes will be achieved as we educate others about inequities, initiate legal remedies in courts and state legislatures, and effect changes in the workplace.

REFERENCES

American Nurses Association: *ANA cheers Senate passage of Patients' Rights Bill*, 2001, *www.nursingworld.org/pressrel/2001/pr0630.htm.*

Flanagan L: *What you need to know about today's workplace: a survival guide for nurses.* Kansas City, Mo, 1995, American Nurses Association.

French JRP, Raven B: The bases of social power. In Cartwright D (Ed.): *Studies in social power*, Ann Arbor, Mich, 1959, University of Michigan.

Hansten RI, Washburn M: *I light the lamp*, Vancouver, Wa, 1990, Applied Therapeutics.

Leavitt JK, Cohen SS, Mason DJ: Political analysis and strategies. In Mason DJ, Leavitt JK, Chaffee MW (Eds.): *Policy and politics in nursing and health care*, St Louis, 2002, Saunders.

Mason DJ, Leavitt JK, Chaffee MW: Policy and politics: a framework for action. In Mason, DJ, Leavitt JK, Chaffee MW (Eds.): *Policy and politics in nursing and health care*, St Louis, 2002, Saunders.

National Council of State Boards of Nursing: *Map of state compact bill status*, 2001, *www.ncsbn.org/nlc/index.asp*.

National Council of State Boards of Nursing: *Nurse licensure compact*, 2001, *www. ncsbn.org/nlc/index.asp*.

National Council of State Boards of Nursing: Uniform core licensure requirements: a supporting paper. In *Book of business*, Chicago, 1999, NCSBN.

Sanford ND: *Identification and explanation of strategies to develop power for nursing in power: nursing's challenge for change*, Kansas City, Mo, 1979, American Nurses Association.

Texas Nurses Association: Texas moves toward multi-state nurse licensure legislation in 1999, *Tex Nurs* 72(10):4, 11, 1998.

Thomas K: A word from the executive director: multi-state regulation moves forward, *RN Updates XXX(1), Austin*, Tex, 1999, Texas State Board of Nurse Examiners.

U.S. Census Bureau: Health insurance coverage: 2000, *www.census.gov/main/www/cen2000.html*.

Watson Wyatt Data Services: *ECS hospital and health care professional, nursing and allied services personnel compensation report*, Rochelle Park, NJ, 2000/2001, Watson Wyatt Data Services.

CHAPTER 18

Collective Bargaining: Traditional and Non-Traditional Approaches

MARY FOLEY, PhD, RN (TRADITIONAL APPROACH), AND
KATHLEEN WILLIAMS, PhD, RN, AND JO CAROL CLABORN, RN, MS
(NON-TRADITIONAL APPROACH)

It is time for a new generation of leadership to cope with new problems and new opportunities. For there is a new world to be won.

—*John F. Kennedy*

Difficulties are meant to rouse, not discourage. The human spirit is to grow strong by conflict.

—*William Ellery Channing*

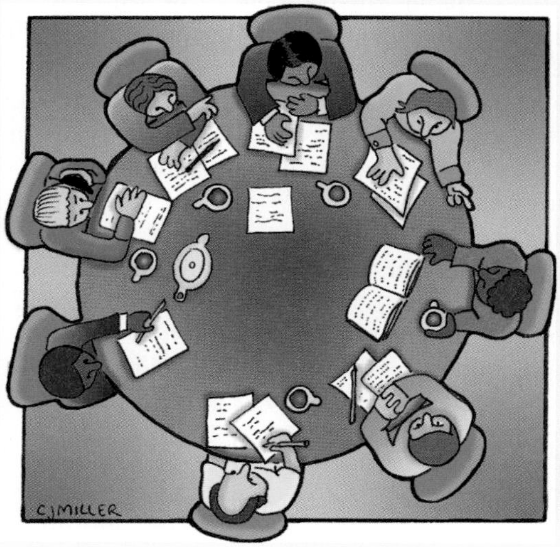

Is there a place for collective bargaining in nursing?

After completing this chapter, you should be able to:

- Identify the milestones in the history of collective bargaining.
- Compare traditional and non-traditional collective bargaining.
- Identify conditions that may lead nurses to seek traditional or non-traditional collective bargaining.
- Identify the positive and negative aspects of traditional and non-traditional collective bargaining.

You will soon be accepting your first position as an RN. You will not only be adjusting to a new role, but to a new workplace. Even in these times of dramatic change in health care, many of you will start your career in a hospital. In fact, the demographics about nurses show that

- Approximately 60% of nurses in practice are providing care in hospitals (Workplace issues, 2005).
- The hospital is also the most common employer of graduate nurses in their first year of practice; more than 84% of new graduates were working in the hospital in their first year of employment (Smith & Crawford, 2003).

As you begin to interview for your first position in your career as a professional registered nurse, there is no doubt you will find yourself both excited and anxious. Your prospective employer will assess your ability to think critically and perform professionally in the health care setting. The potential employer will ask, "Is this applicant a person who will be able to contribute to the mission and quality of health care offered by this organization?"

While the employer assesses your potential to make a contribution within an organization, it is equally important that you remember that an interview is a ***complex two-way street***. You will, of course, be eager to know about compensation, benefits, hours, and responsibilities. These are very tangible and immediate interests. However, they are not likely to be the best predictors of your own satisfaction with your practice in the long run (Upenieks, 2003).

You should be prepared to assess the potential employer's mission and ability to support your professional practice and growth. It is extremely important that you gain essential information about the organization and its culture. It is easy to overlook very significant organizational issues that will ultimately impact your everyday professional practice of nursing. "How and who does the potential employer include in developing solutions and making decisions in the dynamic environment of health care?" "How will you voice your expertise and the challenges you repeatedly encounter? Will your ideas for process improvement be encouraged?"

Hospital structures and governance policies can have a dramatic influence on how effective a nurse is and how he or she can fulfill his or her obligation to patients and families. Nurses have defined themselves as professionals and, as professionals, must have a voice in and control over the practice of nursing. When that voice and control are not supported by the work setting, a conflict will arise. In some states, nurses have chosen to gain a voice in and assume control of their practice by using a traditional collective bargaining model. Most states (Center for American Nurses [CAN], 2005a) have elected to control practice through "interest based bargaining" (IBB) or a non-traditional approach to collective bargaining (Budd et al, 2004) (Box 18-1).

WHEN DID THE ISSUES OF COLLECTIVE BARGAINING BEGIN?

Since World War II, there have been phenomenal advances in medical research and the subsequent development of life-saving drugs and technologies. The introduction

BOX 18-1 Terms

Traditional collective bargaining—A legally regulated collective bargaining unit, or union that assists members to gain control over practice, economics in the health care industry, and other health care issues that threaten the quality of patient care.
United American Nurse (UAN)—The traditional collective bargaining unit affiliated with the American Nurses Association and a member of the AFL-CIO.
Non-traditional collective bargaining—Shared governance, interest based bargaining (IBB), a collaborative based, problem-solving approach to assist nurses to have a voice in the workplace and control over issues that affect their practice.
Center for American Nurses (CAN)—An organizational member of the American Nurses Association that represents the interests of nurses that are not formally represented by a collective-bargaining unit or union (Budd et al, 2004).

of Medicare and Medicaid programs in 1965 provided the driving force and the continued resources for this growth. These health care benefit programs reflected the altruism and social consciousness of the American populace. This initiative opened the access to health care for millions of Americans who were previously disenfranchised from health care.

The explosion in knowledge and technology coupled with an expanded population able to access health care quickly impacted the demands on all health care providers. These advances have required nursing education to adapt as the complexity and volume of patients accessing health care has increased. For example, as cost containment has become the watchword of the hospital industry, staff downsizing and increased nurse workloads have occurred at the same time that the patient population's acuity level has risen. In other words, the patients are sicker—and yet they are moved more quickly through the acute-care setting through such innovations as same-day surgery, same-day admissions, and early discharge. Add periodic shortages of nurses prepared for acute care, long-term care, and home care; the substitution of nurses with unlicensed assistive personnel; and chronic financial pressures on the health system, and tensions are understandably high.

Enormous financial challenges confront health care institutions. As a registered nurse working in the health care industry, you will encounter and use newly developed and very costly health care technologies. At the same time, you will experience first-hand the impact of public and private forces that are focused on placing restraints on cost and reimbursement for a patient's care.

As a professional registered nurse, you are at the intersection of these potentially conflicting forces. For you, these forces will be less abstract and are not just the important concepts and issues facing a very large industry. As a nurse, these concepts and forces are patients with names, faces, and lives valued and loved within a family and a community. You are responsible for the care you provide and for advocating on their behalf and, as you will soon discover, the health of the health care industry.

As a nurse, you will become familiar with how, when, and why events occur that adversely or positively impact the patient and the organization's health. This places you in a unique position to take an active lead in developing solutions. These solutions must be good for patients and for your organization. During your interview, you should be prepared to assess the potential employer's mission and ability to support your professional practice and growth. It is easy to overlook very significant organizational issues that will ultimately impact your everyday professional practice of nursing. Therefore, during your interview, it would be important for you to ask: How and who does the potential employer include in developing solutions and making decisions in the dynamic and potentially conflicted environment of health care? "How will you voice your expertise and the challenges you repeatedly encounter? Will your ideas for process improvement be encouraged?" (Williams, 2004)

THE EVOLUTION OF COLLECTIVE BARGAINING IN NURSING

In the early 1940s, most nurses working in hospitals were subject to arbitrary schedules, uncompensated overtime, no health or pension benefits, and no sick or personal time (Meier, 2000).

In 1946, the American Nurses Association's House of Delegates unanimously approved a resolution that formally initiated the journey of RNs down the road of collective bargaining. This resolution called upon the State Nurses Associations to work actively to secure the general and economic welfare of a membership that had suffered significantly in the workforce (United American Nurse [UAN], 2002). Since that time, nurses have had an expanding right and freedom to organize and bargain as units with employers.

Many formally organized unions have competed for the right to represent nurses. It was the opinion of nurses supporting this precedent that the state nurses associations were not only proper and legal, but also the preferred representatives for nurses in this country for purposes of collective bargaining. During the late 1980s, the demand among nurses for representation continued to grow; yet efforts to organize nurses for collective bargaining were being stymied by a decision from the National Labor Relations Board (NLRB) that stopped approving all-RN bargaining units. A legal battle then ensued with the American Nurses Association (ANA) and other labor unions against the American Hospital Association. The NLRB issued a ruling that reaffirmed the right of nurses to be represented in all-RN bargaining units.

WHO REPRESENTS COLLECTIVE BARGAINING IN NURSING?

NON-TRADITIONAL COLLECTIVE BARGAINING

A relatively new approach is a non-traditional process that is referred to as interest based bargaining (IBB), or shared governance (Brommer, Buckingham, & Loeffler, 2003; Budd et al, 2004). This is a non-traditional style of bargaining that attempts to problem-solve differences between labor and industry. Although this style of bargaining and mediation will not always eliminate the need for the more traditional and adversarial collective bargaining, this nonadversarial approach of negotiation may be closer to the basic fabric of the discipline of nursing and its ethical code.

The organization that represents IBB, or the non-traditional collective voice in nursing, is the CAN, a professional association and an Associate Organizational Member (AOM) of the ANA. The primary responsibility of CAN is to deal with the issues of workplace advocacy. In 2000, the ANA's Commission on Workplace Advocacy was created to address the needs of individual nurses in the workplace who were not represented by collective bargaining. As a result of that commission's work, the membership category of AOM was created, and CAN was accepted as the AOM to address the needs of the nurses. In 2003, the CAN was established. CAN defines its work in workplace advocacy as a multitude of services designed to address the services, products, and programs necessary to support the professional nurse in negotiating and dealing with the challenges of the workplace and in enhancing the quality of patient care (CAN, 2005b).

At a time when competition for nurses was growing, the ANA strengthened its own collective bargaining capacity by creating the UAN in 1999 as the AOM with the responsibility of representing the collective bargaining needs of nurses. In 2001, it was elected as a member of the American Federation of Labor and Congress of Industrial Organizations (AFL-CIO). This provided the benefit of representation by nurses without the fear of distracting competition from other unions who are also members of the AFL-CIO. As Jacob, Cleland, and many other nursing leaders have stated, the professional association has the means and responsibility to represent nurses (Cleland, 1975).

The national professional organization for nursing is the ANA, with its constituent units, the state, and territorial nursing associations. Through its economic security programs, the ANA recognizes state nursing associations as the logical bargaining agents for professional nurses and has been the premier representative for nurses since 1946! These professional associations are indeed multipurpose; their activities include economic analysis, education, nursing practice, research, traditional as well as non-traditional collective bargaining, lobbying, and political action.

Currently, there are 37 states in which the state organization is a member of CAN. There are 27 states represented by the UAN. As these numbers indicate, there are some states that have elected to have dual representation (CAN, 2005a; Workplace Issues, 2005). For example, the Colorado Nurses Association recognizes CAN as the single AOM to handle issues of workplace advocacy, and the UAN as the single AOM to handle workplace issues utilizing collective-bargaining strategies (Colorado Nurses Association, 2005) (Critical Thinking Box 18-1).

CRITICAL THINKING BOX 18-1

What is the status of your state nursing association in regard to workplace issues? Is your state a member of CAN or UAN or both? What is being done on a local basis that reflects the activities of your state association?

> Whether your state is a member of CAN or UAN, or both, it is necessary to recognize that workplace advocacy is a concern that directly affects every practicing nurse. It is going to be critical that nurses support the organizational efforts to address the growing problems regarding the safety of the workplace, as well as safe and competent nursing care.

CAN AND UAN: WHAT ARE THE COMMON ISSUES?

Staffing Issues. Inadequate staff, poorly prepared staff, high patient acuity, and excessive use of registry personnel are all problems that motivate nurses covered by union contracts, as well as those in non-traditional contracts, to submit assignment-despite-objection reports. The same problems should also initiate constructive follow-through by management to improve the situation. Inaction could serve as a basis for a grievance or negotiated change in the union contract. Ideally, the professional performance or professional practice committee (one that is mandated by a contract or established as a shared governance agreement) at the facility will work with nursing administrators to address nurses' complaints and decide whether they reflect a pattern or remain unresolved. A nurse who registers a complaint alerts management to a problem. This act can be constructive in that it can help a nurse vent frustration and anger and help him or her turn a bad experience into a positive one. Better care standards result.

Staffing requirements are mandated by various agencies. For example, Medicare, state health department licensing requirements, and the Joint Commission on the Accreditation of Healthcare Organizations (JCAHO) each publish staffing standards. However, standards that outline nurse-to-patient ratios do not address the issue of what qualifications the nurse must have. For example, a standard that requires one nurse per patient in the intensive care unit does not mandate that the nursing staff needs to have had certain education and experience to work in the intensive care unit. Please refer to Chapter 25, Workplace Issues, for further discussion regarding staffing issues.

Objection to an Assignment. The right and means for a nurse to register objection to a work assignment are considered an essential element in a union contract with professional values. Professional duty implies an obligation to complete an assignment despite the nurse's disagreement with it. Nurses cannot abandon their post without risking disciplinary action. Some contracts and national proposals endorse objection (support nurses who disagree in writing with an assignment) when the assignment could violate the patient protection language of the state nurse practice act. In the traditional collective-bargaining unit, an assignment-despite-objection report is submitted to the nursing administrator and the bargaining agent simultaneously, thus officially registering the complaint. In the non-traditional unit, an assignment-despite-objection report may also be submitted in writing; however, the policies within the institution will dictate who should receive the complaint—the representative nurses and hospital administration that are identified within the shared governance procedures, and/or the participatory management policies would respond to the disagreement.

Concept of Shared Governance. Many facilities are implementing a variety of practice models that they call *shared governance*. This describes a system in which nurses have organizational autonomy; in other words, they have control over their practice (Hinshaw, 2002). Also labeled *self-governance, participative decision making, staff by-laws,* and *decentralized nursing services,* these are structural activities meant to address nurse participation in control of practice. The concept of shared governance has worried unions that represent nurses in collective bargaining. The historical precedents of shared governance in an academic setting mandate caution when applied to heath care settings. It is necessary to avoid a legal finding that the nurses who are part of a shared governance model have become so involved in the governance activities of the facility that they are no longer eligible for representation by a bargaining agent. This is exactly what happened in the Yeshiva University faculty precendent (Yeshiva, 1980).

Some shared-governance models make no effort to hide the fact that their express purpose is to involve nurses in decision making and still maintain the unilateral decision-making authority of managers. That certainly would violate the principles of professional participation in decision making. It is also a major disadvantage to nurses employed by institutions if shared-governance models are adopted in lieu of collective bargaining agreements. In an environment in which collective bargaining already exists, it is probably unnecessary to adopt a totally new model to achieve shared governance if in fact the professional practice committee is involved, as it should be, in providing staff nurse input into decisions that affect the professional practice of nursing.

Health Hazards. Nurses are using collective action to protect themselves against health hazards and unsafe working conditions and to advocate for positive health and safety programs. Right-to-know provisions (knowledge of where and what a hazardous substance is and how to use it safely) and job security in the case of reassignment can be written into contracts as well as an agreement within shared governance. Nationally, the ANA is urging the Occupational Safety and Health Administration (OSHA) to provide hazardous-substance information to health workers. Nursing associations have advocated for inclusion of strict infection control guidelines for health care facilities to protect workers from blood-borne pathogens, including hepatitis B and HIV. An aggressive safe-needle campaign was initiated in November 2000; the ANA and other health care worker advocates were able to celebrate the passage of national legislation that expanded protection from blood-borne diseases through the use of safe needle devices. Nursing has also played a major role in designing and advocating stringent ongoing education and training on universal precautions, postexposure protocol, and latex allergies.

Clinical or Career Ladder. The clinical ladder or career ladder has a place in both styles of collective-bargaining negotiations (Huey, 1982; Wieczorek et al, 1982). The clinical ladder was designed to permit recognition of the long-term career nurse who wishes to remain clinically oriented. The idea to reward the clinical nurse with pay, and status, along a specific track or "ladder" is the result of the contributions of a nurse researcher, Dr. Patricia Benner. Her descriptions of growth and development of nursing knowledge and practice provided the basis for a ladder model that can be used to identify and reward the nurse along the steps from novice to expert (Benner, 1982). Reports issued by the Institute of Medicine (1983) and the U.S. Department of Health and Human Services (USDHHS) Secretary's Commission on Nursing (1988) cited the career ladder as an effective tool for use in the retention of career-minded nurses.

Negotiations. The principles of successful negotiations are difficult to articulate. Nurse negotiators must represent a diverse population (a multiple of specialty areas, educational backgrounds, and practice needs). Nurses have little or no introduction to labor practices or procedures in nursing education programs, so they must learn on the job.

Professional goals and practice needs should be discussed in negotiations, but personnel directors, hospital administrators, and hospital lawyers often seem to have difficulty relating to discussions of nursing practice concerns. The resolution of disagreements about professional issues necessitates a long and thoughtful process. Perhaps the complex issues such as recruitment, retention, staffing, and health and safety, can be better addressed in the more collegial setting of the non-traditional model.

THE DEBATE OVER COLLECTIVE BARGAINING

COLLECTIVE BARGAINING: PERSPECTIVES OF THE TRADITIONAL APPROACH

Is There a Place for Collective Bargaining in Nursing? Should nurses use collective bargaining if they are professionals? Is nursing a profession or an occupation? These are questions nursing has debated throughout its history and continues to debate today.

A profession can be defined as a vocation that requires a long period of specialized education to prepare one for service to society. Because of their expertise and the value of their service, society grants professionals a measure of autonomy in their work. This autonomy permits professionals to make independent judgments and decisions on the basis of a theoretical framework that is learned through study and practice.

Conflict arises as nurse-employees advocate for their professional role in patient care and their health care institutions demand productivity and savings. A study conducted by a Kansas labor-relations consulting firm defined why hospital employees and nurses joined unions and how union organizers garnered their support. Their conclusion confirms what has been suggested again and again.

> A myth widely subscribed to by hospital management is that big, powerful unions organize professional nurses. In fact, unions do not organize nurses; professional nurses organize themselves. They do this because administrators and nursing supervisors fail to recognize and address nurses' individual and collective needs (Stickler & Velghe, 1980, p. 14).

A study from the University of California, Berkeley, found that nurses who engage in traditional collective bargaining believe it is the only solution to a management-employee power struggle. They conclude that nurses decide to unionize because of their "inability to communicate with management and their perception of authoritarian behavior on the part of management" (Parlette, O'Reilly, & Bloom, 1980, p. 16).

Nursing has used collective action to its benefit, achieving professional goals while protecting and promoting public interest through lobbying efforts in the political arena.

Many nurses support collective bargaining in the workplace as a way to control their practice by redistributing power within the health care organization.

"The power bestowed upon the nursing profession should derive not from the hospital administrator's benevolence, but rather from the public's view of the value of services provided by the practitioner" (Cleland, 1975, p. 17).

Ada Jacox (1980) has criticized nursing departments that fail to acknowledge that nurses are professionals. In her view, the authority for nursing practice must rest within the profession. She suggests that collective bargaining through the professional organization may be a way for nurses to achieve collective professional responsibility.

Legal Precedents for State Nursing Associations. The legal precedent that determined that state nursing associations are qualified under labor law to be labor organizations is the 1979 Sierra Vista decision. Many nursing leaders contend that these associations are not only proper and legal, but are the preferred representatives for nurses in this country for purposes of collective bargaining.

The state nursing association is the only safe ground that can be called a neutral turf, on which professional nurses can meet and discuss issues as colleagues, issues that are of a generic and important nature to all nurses, regardless of title.

It is in the nursing associations that staff nurses, educators, advanced-practice nurses, and administrators are able to talk as nurses. Issues associated with clinical ladders, staffing, unlicensed assistive personnel, patient acuity, reimbursement climate, and regulatory matters affect all nurses and benefit from our collective thinking and the application of our collective resources.

Nurse Participation in Collective Bargaining. If the ANA and state nursing associations are logical bargaining agents for professional nurses, why are so few nurses joining associations and even fewer pursuing collective bargaining? Part of the problem is that almost 80% of nurses belong to no association and have no professional affiliation. Most persons join an organization only in response to a particular incentive or when coerced. Otherwise, people will "free ride," or enjoy whatever collective goals are obtained without helping to pay for them (Olson, 1971).

Collective bargaining for nurses usually occurs in states where there is also significant union activity. The climate is very volatile across the country, and unions are trying to organize new categories of workers, with special emphasis on the growing health care sector in states that have not traditionally been active in the labor movement. Some state nursing associations had previously left the arena because of external pressures: challenges from competing unions, excessive resistance by employers, or state policies that make unionization difficult, such as right-to-work laws. (In states with right-to-work laws, it is illegal to negotiate an agency shop requirement; membership and dues collection can, therefore, never be mandatory, even if the workers are covered by a collective bargaining agreement.) Philosophic conflicts regarding the benefits and risks of the professional association bargaining have also led nurses in some states to abandon or avoid union activities.

Rabban (1991) has concluded that when "substantial" and "unambiguous" support for professional values is included in collective bargaining agreements, unionization and professionalism are compatible. How will collective professional goals be achieved if so many nurses depend on the time and finances of so few? There are 2.2 million working nurses, but only a few hundred thousand are organized for collective bargaining. Some believe that the ANA's efforts to address workplace concerns will result in larger membership numbers in the near future, but for now, there are too few nurses involved in the nursing associations.

Where Does Collective Bargaining Begin? Nurses in the private sector are guaranteed legal protection, as stated in the National Labor Relations Act, if they seek a collective bargaining agent. Once a drive for such representation is under way and 30% of the employed nurses in an institution have signed cards signaling interest in representation, both the employer and the union are prohibited from engaging in anti-labor action. Employers are prohibited from firing the organizers, refusing to allow dissemination of union information in the workplace, and ignoring the request for a vote for union representation. After the organizing campaign, a vote is taken; a majority made up of 50% plus one of those voting selects or rejects the collective bargaining agent.

Your employer may choose to bargain in good faith on matters concerning working conditions by recognizing the bargaining agent before the vote. This approach usually occurs only if management believes a large majority supports the foundation of a union. In other cases, your employer may appeal requests for representation to the National Labor Relations Board (NLRB). Before and during the appeal, other unions may intervene and try to win a majority of votes.

Arguments are made before the NLRB regarding why, by whom, or how the nurses are to be represented. For example, the hospital may raise the question of "unit determination." The original policy interpretation of the labor law simultaneously limited the number of individual units an employer or industry would have to recognize, yet allowed for distinct groups of employees, like nurses, to have separate representation. Nurses historically had been represented in all-RN bargaining units, and most bargaining units throughout the country reflected that pattern.

What Can a Contract Do? Generally speaking, what can a union contract do in a hospital setting? A study of 36 hospitals nationwide, all of which had extensive experience with collective bargaining, illustrates the positive effects a union can have:

1. Unions stimulate better hospital management by fostering formal, central, and consistent personnel policies with better lines of communication.
2. Unions "force" improvements in the workplace so that recruitment and retention become easier (Juris & Maxey, 1981).

Wages. Wages are the foundation of a contract. Wages are the remuneration one receives for providing a service and reflect the value put on the work performed. In a 1990 article on the history of nursing's efforts to receive adequate compensation, Brider reaffirmed the need to continue efforts on behalf of nursing salaries. The author correctly stated that "… from its beginnings, the nursing profession has grappled with its own ambivalence: how to reconcile the ideal of selfless service with the necessity of making a living" (p. 77). The article cited the nurses who recorded both their joy in productive careers and their disappointment with the way their work was valued. Nursing has certainly come a long way from the $8 to $12 monthly "allowance" in the early 1900s, but the challenge remains to bring nursing in line with comparable careers.

At the beginning of the 21st century, it is clear that there is another shortage of nurses looming. Whenever the supply and demand favors nursing, wages are evaluated, and there is usually an adjustment of entry level wages (to address recruitment) and wages paid for nurses who remain in practice (for retention).

The larger issues of nurse compensation involve the challenge of addressing the negative effects of "wage compression." This economic concept means that nurses who have been in practice for 10 and 12 years may make less money than recent graduates in their first nursing jobs! Unfortunately, it is not uncommon during times of shortages to see hiring bonuses, or relocation bonuses, to attract nurses into new positions. It would be preferable to see those dollars redistributed for the purposes of building the base. Other innovative approaches would be to use those dollars to support nurses while they learn new skills or advance their career.

Job Security Versus Career Security. It is probably not news to any student enrolled in a nursing program that he or she has entered a field that is undergoing many challenges—both from within and outside nursing. The economic environment in the health care industry, coupled with rapid technologic progress, and a renewed interest in primary and preventive care has dramatically shifted a great deal of health care away from the hospital setting. The 2000 Division of Nursing Sample Survey (USDHHS, 2000) confirmed that nurses have professional opportunities across a diverse continuum, but it also validated that large numbers of nurses, 59% of the 2.2 million working nurses, are still employed in hospital-based care. The health care environment is ever changing. Managed care, managed care reform, shorter lengths of stay, new technologies and pharmaceuticals, limited resources, and a growing demand on all health services by our growing aging population are just a few of the factors that affect the world in which nursing care is delivered. These new paradigms have challenged nurses and their representatives to modify bargaining strategies and turn attention to issues of sustaining quality nursing care in the face of shortages, to overcome negative practices such as mandatory overtime, and to advocate for health and safety initiatives like safer needle devices and ergonomics.

Seniority Rights. Nurses who remain on staff at an institution accrue seniority rights. These rights derive from the idea that permanent employees should be rewarded for their service and viewed as assets. In nursing employment contracts, there are provisions (seniority language) that give senior nurses the right to accrue more vacation time and be given preference when requesting time off, new positions, or relief from shift rotation requirements. In the event of a staff layoff, the rule that states "the last hired become the first fired" protects senior nurses. Seniority rules may be applied to the entire hospital nursing staff or be confined to a unit. Transfers and promotions must reward the most senior qualified nurse in the institution.

Resolution of Grievances. Methods to resolve grievances, which are sometimes explicitly spelled out in a contract, are an important element of any agreement. A grievance can arise when provisions in a contract are interpreted differently by management and an employee or employees. This difference often occurs when issues related to job security (a union priority), job performance, and discipline (a management priority) arise. *Grievance mechanisms* are used in an attempt to resolve the conflict with the parties involved. The employer, the employee, or the union may issue a grievance. Nurses who are covered by contracts should be represented at any meeting or hearing that they believe may lead to disciplinary action being taken against them. Such representation can be provided by a co-worker, an elected nurse representative, or a member of the labor union's staff.

If the grievance mechanism does not lead to resolution of the issue, some contracts allow referral of the issue to arbitration. A knowledgeable—but neutral—arbitrator acceptable to both parties (union and hospital) will be asked to hear the facts in the case and issue a finding. In pre-agreed, binding arbitration, the parties must accept the decision of the arbitrator. For example, some hospital contracts require that when management elects to discharge (suspend or terminate) a nurse, the case must be brought to arbitration. On the basis of the arbitrator's finding, the nurse may be reinstated, perhaps with back pay, remain suspended, or be terminated. If the contract states that the arbitrator's decision is final and binding, there is no further contractual avenue for either party to pursue.

Arbitration. Arbitration has also been used to resolve issues involving the "integrity of the bargaining unit." Arbitrators have been asked to decide whether nurses remain eligible for bargaining unit coverage when jobs are changed and new practice models are implemented.

Mediation, arbitration, and fact-finding have all been used to resolve conflicts in union contracts. There is strong support for use of these methods, but hospital management personnel often resist using them. Nurses usually fare well when contract enforcement issues are submitted to an arbitrator and facts, not power or public relations, determine the outcome.

What Are the Elements of a Sound Contract?

Membership. The inclusion of union security provisions is an essential element of a sound contract and one of the defined goals of collective bargaining (union integrity). *Security provisions* include measures such as enforcement of membership requirements (collection of dues and access by the union staff to the members). A legal modification of the closed shop is the *agency shop*, in which new employees are required to join the union within a given period (Figure 18-1).

Retirement. The usual pension or retirement programs for nurses have been either the Social Security system or a hospital pension plan. Individual retirement accounts, which are transferable from hospital to hospital in case of job change, are relatively rare, and should be a topic of negotiations. The ANA has entered an agreement with a national company to provide a truly portable national plan, unrestricted by geographic location or employment site. Although this plan could be complicated by conflicting state laws governing pension plans, a precedent was set as long ago as 1976, when California nursing contracts mandated employer contributions to individual retirement accounts for each nurse with immediate vesting (eligibility for access to the fund) and complete portability for the participants (meaning that the nurse could take the pension to another hospital and continue to add to it).

One of nursing's most attractive benefits has been a nurse's mobility, the opportunity to change jobs at will. A drawback of this mobility, however, is the loss of long-term

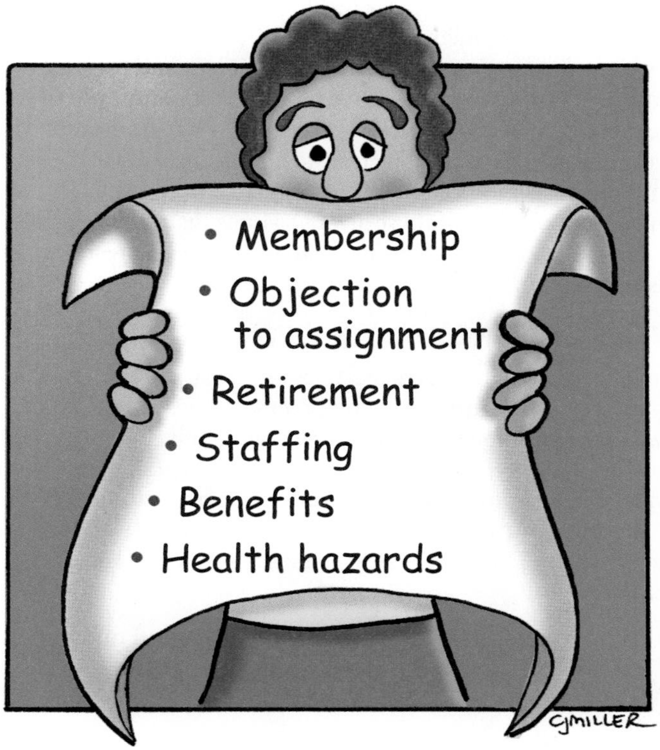
• Membership
• Objection to assignment
• Retirement
• Staffing
• Benefits
• Health hazards
CJMILLER

FIGURE 18-1
Effective elements of a sound contract.

retirement funds. With financial cutbacks in the hospital industry, retirement plans are in danger of being targeted as givebacks in negotiating rights or benefits to be traded away in lieu of another issue or benefit that may be more pressing at the time. Health insurance coverage persists as a key concern of employees and has been at the root of the majority of labor disputes in all industries in the last few years. It is not inconceivable that nurses may be asked to trade off long-term economic security (pensions) for short-term security (e.g., health benefits, wages).

Other Benefit Issues. All employees in the United States have been experiencing a dramatic reduction in their health benefits packages. This trend is reflective of the crisis of the health care system and the escalating costs of health care. Nurses have not been immune to the reduction in health benefits, and access to health care benefits will continue to be a major issue for nurses and all employees until substantial reform is accomplished.

Other issues that have affected nurses as employees are family-leave policies, availability of daycare services, long-term disability insurance, and access to health insurance for retirees. An issue of special concern to nurses involves the scheduling of work hours. Although more men have been joining the nursing profession, nursing remains a 97% female occupation. That reality must be addressed by benefit packages that provide flexibility for women who assume multiple roles in today's society. Women, and nurses in particular, provide care to both children and parents. Nurses are asking nursing contract negotiators to secure leave policies that permit use of sick time for family needs and scheduling that is both flexible and allows part-time employment and work-sharing.

Staffing issues such as objection to an assignment, inadequate staffing, poorly prepared staff, mandatory overtime, nurse fatigue, and health hazards are all issues in a union contract; however, these are also issues that are an ongoing concern of all nurses, regardless of the type of bargaining situation in their respective states. These issues are discussed in Chapter 25, Workplace Issues.

HOW CAN NURSES CONTROL THEIR OWN PRACTICE?

Hospital management representatives often ask staff nurses what they mean when they say their goal is to control nursing practice. These managers seem unclear about what it is we consider appropriate practice issues, and they react negatively to the concept of control. The essence of the professional nurse contract is control of practice. For example, nurse councils or professional performance committees provide the opportunity for nurses within the institution to meet regularly. These meetings are sanctioned by the contract. The elected staff nurse representatives may, for example, have specific objectives to

- Improve the professional practice of nurses and nursing assistants.
- Recommend ways and means to improve patient care.
- Make recommendations to the hospital management when, for example, a critical nurse staffing shortage exists.
- Identify and recommend the elimination of hazards in the workplace.

The importance and relevance of such professional practice committees was documented by a 1986 review of state nursing association contracts. When 381 agreements were analyzed, 424 references to professional practice committees were identified.

Nurse Practice Committees. Nurse practice committees should have a formal relationship with nursing administration. Regularly scheduled meetings with nursing and hospital administrators can provide a forum for the discussion of professional issues in a "safe" atmosphere. Many potential contract conflicts can be prevented by discussion before contract talks begin or grievances arise. Ideally, physicians should be a part of these forums; joint-practice language has been proposed in some contracts.

> Trends have see-sawed between a climate of shortage to one of record layoffs of RNs, and now the shortage that by every indication may be severe and prolonged.

Environments that reduce the number of direct-care nurses, mid-level management nurses, nurse educators, and clinical staff specialists will jeopardize patient care. Numerous studies have confirmed the relationship between the staffing level of RNs and the quality of patient outcomes (Kovner & Gergen, 1998). Since the recognition of magnet hospitals began in 1994, almost 40 hospitals and one long-term care facility have been awarded a magnet credential. Approximately 20% of the facilities awarded the recognition have a collective-bargaining agreement with the nurses.

Strikes and Other Labor Disputes. Just what can nurses do in the face of a standoff during contract negotiations? Nurses' options are quite different than they were before 1968, when nurses felt a greater sense of powerlessness. At that time, despite nurses' threats of sick-outs, walkouts, picketing, or mass resignations, the employer maintained an effective power base. Threats of group action attracted public attention, but nurses' threats had little effect on employers because nurses represented through the ANA had a no-strike policy. As negotiations became more difficult, it was apparent that nurses were in a weaker bargaining position because of the no-strike policy. The ANA responded to the state nursing associations and, in 1968, reversed its 18-year-old, no-strike policy.

> Strikes are used only after every other alternative fails. Nurses who strike take their appeals to the "street," hoping for positive public response.

Strikes remain rare among nursing units, but, as was mentioned previously, when patient care and safety are at risk, nurses may have to strike, as they started to in 2000 to address mandatory overtime. Many nurses are uncomfortable with the idea of striking, believing that they are abandoning their patients. This image may conflict with the service ideal. It is important for nurses who contemplate striking to discuss plans for patient care with nurses who have previously conducted strikes so that they will be assured that plans to care for patients are adequate.

When an impasse is reached in hospital negotiations, national labor law requires nurses to issue a 10-day notice of their intent to strike. Every effort must be made to prevent a strike in the public's interest. Mediation is mandated by the NLRB, and a board of inquiry to examine the issue may be created before a work stoppage. The hospitals are supposed to use this time to reduce the patient census and to slow or halt elective admissions. In the meantime, the nurses' strike committee will develop schedules for coverage of emergency rooms, operating rooms, and intensive care areas. This coverage is to be used only in the case of real emergencies. Planning patient care coverage should reassure nurses troubled by the strike scenario. Nurses who agree to work in emergencies or at other facilities during a strike often donate their wages to funds set up for striking nurses.

The National Labor Relations Act governs labor practices and prohibits certain unfair practices once an organizing campaign has been initiated. An employer cannot engage in interference, domination, discrimination, or refusal to bargain and cannot unjustly discipline an employee simply for union activities.

Business and labor are both in search of more positive ways in which to work together. National grants have been sponsored by the Department of Labor and the Federal Mediation and Conciliation Service to undertake alternatives to traditional bargaining. At least two Midwestern nursing organizations used "win-win" bargaining techniques and found them to be constructive methods of negotiation.

COLLECTIVE BARGAINING: PERSPECTIVES OF THE NON-TRADITIONAL APPROACH

How to effectively address the concerns of the workplace advocacy, higher standards of practice, and economic security are not new issues. These concerns have moved nurses in some areas of the country to organize and use unions and collective bargaining models. This section is designed to provide you with information and rationale for a different approach to the position of the traditional collective bargaining. In the end, it will be up to you and your concept of the professional nurse's role to grapple with this issue during your professional life.

Simultaneous Debates. Nursing today has acquired the generally recognized characteristics of a profession. One of these characteristics is a lengthy period of specialized education and practice preparation. The activities that are performed by professions are valued and recognized as important to society. In addition, a member of a profession has an acquired area of expertise that allows the person to make independent judgment, act with autonomy, and assume accountability. Nurses also have specialty organizations and are eligible in some areas to receive specialty credentialing.

Another professional aspect of nursing is its strongly written and documented ethical code. The 2001 ANA Code of Ethics for Nurses was published (see Chapter 19). It articulates the values, goals, and responsibilities of the professional practice of nursing. The provisions of the Code that outline our duties to care, advocate, and be faithful to those who entrust their health care to us are well integrated into the educational preparation of the registered nurse. They are also widely recognized and respected by the public.

Collective Bargaining: The Debate That Continues. The debate over the appropriateness of collective bargaining continues. The combination of an explosion in knowledge and technology and an expanded population able to access health care quickly brought both public and private sector payers of health care to the inevitable quest to rein in the cost of health care. This gave "birth" and "life" to a growing collection of payment systems. We now have gatekeepers, specific practice protocols, contractual agreements between payers and providers, and provider and consumer incentives that govern the place, provider, type, and quantity of a patient's care.

These developments have impacted the everyday care in a growing number of settings. Nurses are challenged daily in practice environments that have, by necessity, taken on business models and processes to survive financially. The nurses who advocate for CAN feel that this business and financial environment is not conducive to the patient-focused model and ethical values that have been an inherent part of the professional education and practice preparation of nurses.

All too often, the intense clinical education of the registered nurse practicing in today's health care has not prepared the nurse to appreciate the financial and regulatory realities of a large industry. Perhaps even more tragic is that as the professional nurse enters this work environment, he or she may not see the magnitude of his or her potential for leadership and problem-solving within an environment that continues to evolve.

The history of the position of nursing during the first half of the 20th century may, in part, explain our slow journey toward leadership. Some nurses have organized and relied on collective-bargaining units to speak for them. The debate about the fit of union membership and a profession is likely to continue for some time.

It is important to remember that this early journey toward collective bargaining followed a period of unprecedented economic hardship. It also preceded the post World War II knowledge and technology explosion in health care that pushed the time-honored "nurses training" toward a sophisticated professional education.

Although the initial journey began with limited rights, these rights have been expanded in the past 50 years. Budd and colleagues (2004) recently reviewed some of the outcomes of the expansion of these protections and rights. They found that many state nurses associations had successfully negotiated for salary and benefit increases, overtime, shift-differential pay, shortened work hours, formal grievance procedures, and some strategies to improve the patient care environment.

Traditional Collective Bargaining: Its Risks and Benefits. The goal of the traditional collective bargaining model is to win something that is controlled by another. There is a "we versus they" approach. The weapon is the power of numbers. Although a desired contract is achieved, long-lasting adversarial relationships may develop between the nurses and the employer (Budd et al, 2004) (Critical Thinking Box 18-2).

CRITICAL THINKING BOX 18-2

A CASE TO CONSIDER: WHAT DO YOU THINK?

During Spring of 2004, 25 practicing registered nurses participating in a seminar were asked to comment on their thoughts and experiences with collective bargaining. This took place in a region of the country that throughout most of the 20th century had a well-grounded and solid economy that was rooted in industries dominated by traditional labor unions and collective bargaining. The majority of the registered nurse participants were members of collective-bargaining units representing a variety of health care institutions. Two themes dominated the intense conversation. The first theme was the profound commitment of these nurses to their ethical duty to provide quality care to the patients. The second theme was the personal, internal conflict, distress, and tension with the collective bargaining experience.

One of the most interesting aspects of this discussion was that regardless of the outcome, the periods of collective bargaining and contract negotiations were not described with any sense of joy or triumph. None of the seminar participants found the process satisfying. The nurses who had the experience of living through a collective-bargaining process that threatened or resulted in an actual work stoppage described a period that was ripe with animosity, mistrust, and lingering concerns about abandonment of their duty to provide care. Some of the participants

Continued

CRITICAL THINKING BOX 18-2

A CASE TO CONSIDER: WHAT DO YOU THINK?—cont'd

had experienced crossing picket lines and being subjected to harassment and verbal abuse by their colleagues. Both groups of nurses found themselves pitted against not only management but against other nurses.

An unfortunate experience of this group of nurses was a decade of decline and departure of the majority of the heavily unionized industries that were fundamental to the economic life of the region. While nurses were striking for increased wages and benefits, a major corporation in the region announced the layoff of 600 factory workers. Both stories appeared on the front page of the local paper on the same day (Williams, 2004).

With the soaring cost of health care, the changes in health care reimbursement, and the subsequent reining in of health care costs, where does that leave nursing in the collective bargaining process? Does this not further aggravate the already adversarial relationship of nurses and their employers? Traditional collective bargaining held promise and assisted the professional nurse's evolution toward economic stability. These were important gains. However, the power and potency of nursing as an industry leader has not emerged through traditional collective bargaining efforts. This may explain the dissatisfaction of the nurses participating in the seminar with traditional collective bargaining.

As discussed earlier, the 2.2 million registered nurses working in health care are by far the largest component of the professional health care workforce. This is a professional group with a tradition steeped in values and an ethical code that presses the nurse to consider the value of the human as patient, as community member, and as fellow health professional.

Can nursing effectively step away from the adversarial process of traditional collective bargaining into an effective leadership role? IBB may offer nurses a nonadversarial approach, but it will require nursing to demonstrate an understanding of interests and outcomes that are important to other members of the health care industry (Budd et al., 2004). This is a non-traditional style of bargaining that attempts to problem solve differences between the workforce and the employer—or the nurse and the hospital. Although this style of bargaining and mediation will not always eliminate the need for the more traditional and adversarial collective bargaining, this nonadversarial approach of negotiation may be closer to the basic beliefs underlying professional nursing as well as the nursing code of ethics.

The recognition of nonadversarial approach by the ANA is relatively new; the CAN was established in 2003. Box 18-2 lists the primary purposes for CAN.

In considering the IBB approach, it is important to consider state associations that have made significant contributions to their local membership, as well as to the national advances for non-traditional, nonadversarial bargaining for the promotion of workplace advocacy (Box 18-3). Do these commitments sound familiar?

BOX 18-2 Purposes of CAN

The primary purposes of CAN are:

- To offer non-collective bargaining workplace advocacy strategies, programs, and services to nurses.
- To support nurses in personal and professional growth and development in the practice settings to promote positive work-related experiences.
- To collaborate with others to provide services and to develop policies that positively impact the work environment of all nurses.
- To promote and provide leadership and mentoring in the workplace environment.
- To conduct, evaluate, and support workplace-related research.

Reprinted with permission from Center for American Nurses, 2005.

BOX 18-3 Eight Commitments to Workplace Advocacy

Workplace advocacy is a nurse-to-nurse strategy that can give RNs a meaningful voice in their workplace. As a result of Texas Nurses Association (TNA) workplace advocacy efforts in the past, Texas now has one of the strongest Nursing Practice Acts in the country. The following are eight commitments to workplace advocacy. The Texas Nurses Association will:

Work to secure mechanism within health care systems that provide opportunities for registered nurses to affect institutional policies. Mechanisms include:

- Shared governance
- Participatory management models
- Magnet hospital identifications
- Statewide staffing regulations

Develop with stakeholders a conflict resolution process for nurse/nurse employers that addresses registered nurse concerns about patient care and delivery issues.

- Active participation with the Texas Hospital Association and the American Arbitration Association to develop a conflict resolution process that meets the needs of nurses in resolving patient care issues.

Provide legislative solutions to Texas registered nurses by reviewing issues of concern to nurses in employment settings and introducing appropriate legislation. Previous initiatives include:

- Whistle-Blower
- Safe Harbor Peer Review
- Support for Board of Nurse Examiners rules outlining strong nursing practice standards

Explore the development of a legal center for nurses that could provide legal support and decision-making advice as a last recourse to unresolved workplace issues. Its purpose would be to:

- Provide fast legal assistance
- Earmark precedent-setting cases that could impact case law and health care policy

Continued

BOX 18-3 Eight Commitments to Workplace Advocacy—cont'd

Support the RN in practice with self-advocacy and patient advocacy information by providing products that increase knowledge about:
- Laws and regulations governing practice
- Use of applicable standards of nursing practice
- Conflict resolution techniques
- Statewide reporting mechanisms that allow the nurse to report concerns about health care institutions and professionals
- Professional behaviors, core values, and conduct that supports effective negotiation

Promote to RNs those health care institutions in Texas that demonstrate outstanding nurse/employer relations.

Work with Texas schools of nursing to develop materials that incorporate self-advocacy and patient advocacy information into the nursing curriculum.

Advocate for the elimination of physician abuse of RNs with the physician community and employers by:
- Working with physician professional organizations to develop a campaign to end physician abuse of RNs
- Working with health care facilities to establish Zero Tolerance for physician abuse of RNs.
- Developing model policies against physician abuse of nurses
- Encouraging nurse-to-nurse advocacy to stop abusive situations

Reprinted with permission from Texas Nurses Association, *http://texasnurses.org/wkplaceadv/wp_index.htm*.

FUTURE TRENDS

WHAT LIES AHEAD?

The nursing community was struck in the late 1980s with a deeply entrenched, widespread, and possibly permanent imbalance between the demand for nurses and the ability of nursing education to supply adequately prepared RNs to meet future public needs. For about 2 years, it was common to pick up publications or turn on a national talk show, whether on radio or television, and find coverage of the shortage of nurses. As we continue through the 21st century, we are at a similar crossroads, and as the public demand for nurses continues to rise, there may be enduring shortages of nurses prepared for future roles.

The public should be concerned about an inadequate supply of nurses. Building on that concern, and the recent terrorist attacks on America, there is increased interest by the press and the policymakers to be sure nurses are prepared in adequate numbers, and that their working environment supports quality nursing care. That attention is helping nurses achieve better wages and working conditions and must also lead to support for nursing faculty and loans and scholarships to address the educational pipeline for nursing. The question of job satisfaction, however, must not be overlooked.

> In survey after survey, the no. 1 reason nurses are unhappy with their nursing practice environment is their dissatisfaction with the care that they are able to give in that environment.

Nurses throughout the country have felt firsthand the effects of cost containment. Those effects have been detrimental to the quality of care that professional nurses are charged to provide. From a professional practice perspective, mandatory overtime and short staffing are some of the factors that may be contributing to the preponderance of medical errors documented in the Institute of Medicine report on medical errors, "To err is human: building a safer health system" (Institute of Medicine, 2000). The ANA was the sole voice in recognizing these as potential contributing factors and has led the way in pushing research agendas that further quantify what number of work hours is safe, and how patient safety can be ensured. Furthermore, just as occurred during the whistle-blower issue, the ANA and the state nursing associations are in the lead in federal and state legislative efforts to address overtime and state staffing in the context of safe patient care.

What lies ahead for collective bargaining and all forms of collective action for nurses must be viewed within the context of the larger changes occurring in the health care system and in the financing mechanisms.

> There is still a heightened awareness among politicians and the public that something is grievously wrong with not just how we pay for our health care, but what we are receiving at that high cost.

This issue of health access is one that will probably be with us for the rest of our professional lives. As nurses advocate for improved access to health services, we believe those services will, by necessity, be delivered in environments and by providers that have not traditionally been a part of our medical care system. Just as cost containment of the 1980s brought emphasis on home care, early discharge, and alternatives to institutional care, remedies to improve access will include school-based care, workplace-based care, community care, and broader access to nursing care.

The very nature of nursing supply and demand defies prediction. The profession of nursing must and will ensure that adequate numbers of nurses are properly prepared and that the public will demand that nurses are part of any, and all, care structures they use.

CONCLUSION

Nursing has a unique contract with society to promote good health care and, as a natural outcome, promote the health and welfare of the nurse and the profession of nursing. The multipurpose nature of the professional nursing association will preserve the future of nursing. This chapter cannot stand alone, nor can the nurses in the workplace stand alone if they are to offset the forces that negate the contributions of nurses. Political action and lobbying, research, and education are necessary to further the cause of nursing and to meet the public's health care needs. Although nursing works to change the health system and improve citizens' access to care, nurses will continue to depend on collective action and a collective voice through both of the agencies established within the ANA, to advocate for optimal working conditions and standards of practice. Welcome to nursing! Join us in our efforts to unify our skills, knowledge, and voices as we create our vision.

REFERENCES

Benner P: From novice to expert, *Am J Nurs* 82(3): 402-407, 1982.

Brider P: Professional status: the struggle for just compensation, *Am J Nurs* 90(10):77-80, 1990.

Brommer C, Buckingham G, Loeffler S: Cooperative bargaining styles at Federal Mediation and Conciliation Services: a movement toward choices, Federal Mediation and Conciliation, 2003, *www.fmcs.gov/internet/itemDetail.asp?categoryID=35&itemID=15880.*

Budd K, Warino L, Patton M: Traditional and non-traditional collective bargaining: strategies to improve the patient care environment, *Online Journal of Issues in Nursing* 9(1), 2004.

Center for American Nurses (CAN): *Community: CAN member associates*, 2005a, *www.nursingworld.org/can/statesmembers.htm.*

Center for American Nurses (CAN): *Our center: CAN history*, 2005b, *www.centerforamericannurses.org/can/about/history.htm.*

Cleland V: Taft-Hartley amended: implications for nursing. The professional model, *Am J Nurs* 75(2):288-292, 1975.

Colorado Nurses Association: *Workplace issues*, 2005, *www.nurses-co.org?default.sap?PageID=10002243.*

Hinshaw A: Building magnetism into health organizations. In McClure ML, Hinshaw A (Eds.): *Magnet hospitals revisited: attraction and retention of professional nurses*, Washington, DC, 2002, American Nurses Publishing.

Huey F: Looking at ladders, *Am J Nurs* 82(10): 1520-1526, 1982.

Institute of Medicine: To err is human: building a safer health system, ed 1. In Kohn L, Corrigan J (Eds.): *IOM report*, Washington, DC, 2000, National Academy Press.

Jacox A: Collective action: the basis for professionalism, *Superv Nurse* 11(9):22-24, 1980.

Juris H, Maxey C: The impact of hospital unionism, *Mod Healthcare* 11:36, 1981.

Kovner C, Gergen PJ: Nurse staffing levels and adverse events following surgery in U.S. hospitals, *Image* 30:4, 1998.

Meier E: Is unionization the answer for nurses and nursing?, *Nursing Economic$*, 18(1), 36-37, 2000.

Olson M: *The logic of collective action: public goods and the theory of groups*, Cambridge, Mass, 1971, Harvard University Press.

Parlette GN, O'Reilly CA, Bloom JR: The nurse and the union, *Hosp Forum* 23(6):16-17, 1980.

Rabban D: Is unionization compatible with professionalism?, *Industrial Labor Relations Rev* 45(1): 97-110, 1991.

Smith, J, Crawford L: *Report of findings from the 2002 RN practice analysis*, Chicago, 2003, National Council State Boards of Nursing.

Stickler KB, Velghe JC: Why nurses join unions, *Hosp Forum* 23(2):14-15, 1980.

Texas Nurses Association: *Workplace advocacy*, 2005, *http://texasnurses.org/wkplaceadv/wp_index.htm.*

United American Nurse (UAN): *2002 Resolutions*, 2005, *http://nursingworld.org/uan/resolutions_2002_4.htm.*

Upenieks VV: The Interrelationship of organizational characteristics of magnet hospitals, nursing leadership, and nursing job satisfaction, *Health Care Manager* 22(2), 83-98, 2003.

U.S. Department of Health and Human Services, Division of Nursing: *Sample survey*, Washington, DC, 2000, Bureau of Health Professionals, DHHS.

U.S. Department of Health and Human Services Secretary's Commission on Nursing: *Final report*, Washington DC, 1988, USDHHS.

Wieczorek RR, Weissman GK, Hiatt H: A clinical career pathway: the Mount Sinai experience part 1, *Nurs Health Care* 3(10):533-535, 1982.

Williams K: Ethics and collective bargaining: calls to action, *Online Journal of Issues in Nursing*, 2004, *http://nursingworld.org/ojin/ethicol/ethics_15.htm*.

Workplace issues: director of constituent member associations that provide collective bargaining, Nursing World, 2005, *www.nursingworld.org/dlwa/barg/snadir/htm*.

Yeshiva, supra, 103 LRRM at 2553, 1980.

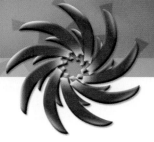

CHAPTER 19

Ethical Issues

ALICE B. PAPPAS, PhD, RN

People of Orphalese, you can muffle the drum, and you can loosen the strings of the lyre, but who shall command the skylark not to sing?

—*Kahlil Gibran, The Prophet*

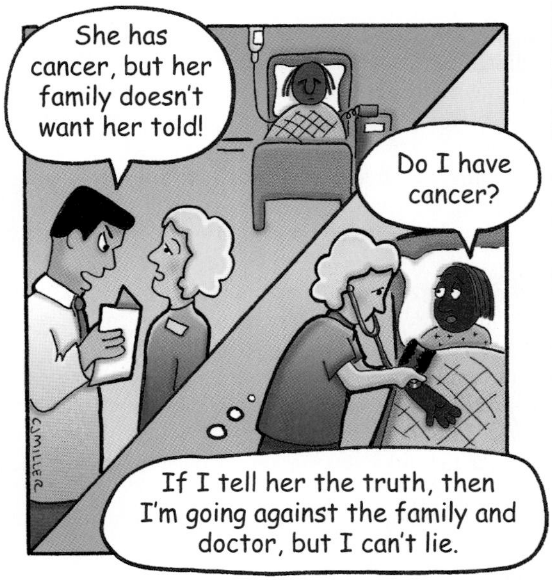
She has cancer, but her family doesn't want her told!
Do I have cancer?
If I tell her the truth, then I'm going against the family and doctor, but I can't lie.

Ethical dilemmas are not easy situations.

After completing this chapter, you should be able to:

- Define terminology commonly used in discussions about ethical issues.
- Analyze personal values that influence approaches to ethical issues and decision making.
- Discuss the moral implications of the American Nurses Association and International Council of Nurses codes of ethics.
- Discuss the role of the nurse in ethical health care issues.

Concern about ethical issues in health care has increased dramatically in the past two decades. This interest has soared for a variety of reasons, including advances in medical technology; social and legal changes involving abortion, euthanasia, patient rights, end-of-life care, and reproductive technology; and growing concern about the allocation of scarce resources, including a shortage of nurses. Nurses have begun to speak out on these issues and have focused attention on the responsibilities and the possible conflicts that they experience as a result of their unique relationship with patients and their families and their role within the health care team.

UNDERSTANDING ETHICS

Let us begin by defining commonly used terms (Box 19-1).

WHAT ARE YOUR VALUES?

Clarification of your values is suggested as a strategy to develop greater insight into yourself and what you believe to be important. Values clarification involves

BOX 19-1 Definition of Terms

Advance directive: A written statement of a person's wishes about how he or she would like health care decisions to be made if he or she ever loses the ability to make such decisions independently.

Bioethics: Ethics concerning life.

Bioethical issues: Subjects that raise concerns of right and wrong in matters involving human life (e.g., euthanasia, abortion).

Durable power of attorney for health care decisions: A document that allows a person to name someone else to make medical decisions for him or her if he or she is unable to do so. This spokesperson's authority only begins when the patient is incompetent to make those decisions.

Ethics: Rules or principles that determine which human actions are right or wrong.

Ethical dilemma: 1. A situation involving competing rules or principles that appears to have no satisfactory solution. 2. A choice between two or more equally undesirable alternatives.

Living will: A document that allows a person to state in advance that life-sustaining treatment is not to be administered if the person later is terminally ill and incompetent.

Moral or ethical principles: Fundamental values or assumptions about the way individuals should be treated and cared for. These include autonomy, beneficence, nonmaleficence, justice, fidelity, and veracity.

Moral reasoning: A process of considering and selecting approaches to resolve ethical issues.

Moral uncertainty: A situation that exists when the individual is unsure which moral principles or values apply in a given situation.

Values: Beliefs that are considered very important and frequently influence an individual's behavior.

a three-step process: choosing, prizing, and acting upon your value choices in real-life situations (Steele, 1983). Opportunities to make choices and improve your decision making are included in the following pages. As you consider your values, you will, I hope, gain more understanding about the underlying motives that influence them. It is not intended as a "right" or "wrong" activity, rather, it is a discovery about the "what" and "why" of your actions. Do not be surprised if your peers or family hold different views on some topics. And remember: the values that are "correct" or "right" for you may not always be the "right" values for others. Your values may also change over time as you face different life experiences.

Evaluate the critical-thinking questions, write down your responses to them, and consider the possible reason or reasons for your choices. The critical-thinking exercise (Critical Thinking Box 19-1), Listing Values, is suggested as a means of clarifying your values. Discuss your answers with peers and decide how comfortable you are in discussing and defending your values, especially if they differ from the values of your peers. Critical Thinking Box 19-2 involves reproductive issues and has been included here because of the proliferation of reproductive technology, including genetics, and the ongoing moral and political debate regarding abortion.

CRITICAL THINKING BOX 19-1

LISTING VALUES

List 10 values that guide your daily interactions.

Choose a partner (if available).

1. Discuss with a partner each of the values you listed and how they guide your interactions.
2. Compare your list of values with your partner's, and discuss similarities and differences in the two lists.
3. Prioritize your list, and discuss why you feel some are more important than others.

From Steele S, Harmon V: *Values clarification in nursing,* ed 2, East Norwalk, Conn, 1983, Appleton-Century-Crofits, p 90; with permission.

CRITICAL THINKING BOX 19-2

REPRODUCTIVE EXERCISE

Identify your degree of agreement or disagreement with the statements by placing the number that most closely indicates your value next to each statement.

1 = Strongly Disagree
2 = Disagree
3 = Ambivalent
4 = Agree
5 = Strongly Agree

________ 1. Contraception is a responsibility of all women.
________ 2. Some types of contraception are more valuable than other types.
________ 3. Abortion as a form of contraception is completely unacceptable.
________ 4. Abortion decisions are the responsibility of the pregnant woman and her physician.
________ 5. The birth of a "test tube baby" is a valuable medical advance.
________ 6. Genetic screening should be done frequently.
________ 7. Genetic counseling should provide information so that clients can make informed choices about future reproductive decisions.
________ 8. Amniocentesis should be required as part of prenatal care.
________ 9. Genetic engineering should be advanced and promoted by federal funding.
________ 10. Artificial insemination should be available to anyone who seeks it.
________ 11. Sperm used in artificial insemination should come from all strata of society as do blood transfusions.
________ 12. Fetal surgery should be done even when it places another fetus at risk (i.e., a twin).
________ 13. Surrogate mothers play an important role in the future of families.
________ 14. Fetuses who survive experimentation should be raised by society.
________ 15. Women should be encouraged to participate in fetal research by carrying fetuses to desired dates and then giving the fetus to the scientist for research.
________ 16. Contraception is reserved for women of legal age.
________ 17. Adolescents should require a parent's signature for abortion.

Continued

CRITICAL THINKING BOX 19-2

REPRODUCTIVE EXERCISE—cont'd

_______ 18. Information about genetically transmitted diseases should be provided to all pregnant women.

_______ 19. Women at high risk for genetically transmitted diseases should be encouraged to have amniocentesis.

_______ 20. Infants born with severe defects should be allowed to die through a natural course.

From Steele S, Harmon V: *Values clarification in nursing,* ed 2, East Norwalk, Conn, 1983, Appleton-Century-Crofts, p 169; with permission.

MORAL/ETHICAL PRINCIPLES

What Is the Best Decision, and How Will I Know? Despite different ideas regarding which moral or ethical principle is most important, ethicists agree that there are common principles or rules that should be taken into consideration when an ethical situation is being examined. As you read through each principle, consider instances in which you have acted on the principles or perhaps felt some conflict in trying to determine what was the best action to take (Figure 19-1).

Autonomy: A Patient's Right to Self-Determination Without Outside Control. Autonomy implies the freedom to make choices and decisions about one's own care without interference, even if those decisions are not in agreement with those of the health care team. This principle assumes rational thinking on the part of the individual and may be challenged when the individual infringes upon the rights of others.

Consider this:

What if a patient wants to do something that will cause harm to himself or herself? Under what circumstances can the health care team intervene?

Beneficence: Duty to Actively Do Good for Patients. For example, deciding what nursing interventions should be provided for patients who are dying when some of those interventions may cause pain. In the course of prolonging life, harm sometimes occurs.

Consider this:

Who decides what is good? Patient, family, nurse, or physician? How do you define good?

Nonmaleficence: Duty to Prevent or Avoid Doing Harm, Whether Intentional or Unintentional. Is it harmful to accept an assignment to "float" to an unfamiliar area that requires the administration of unfamiliar medications?

Consider this:

Is it acceptable to refuse an assignment? When does an assignment become unsafe?

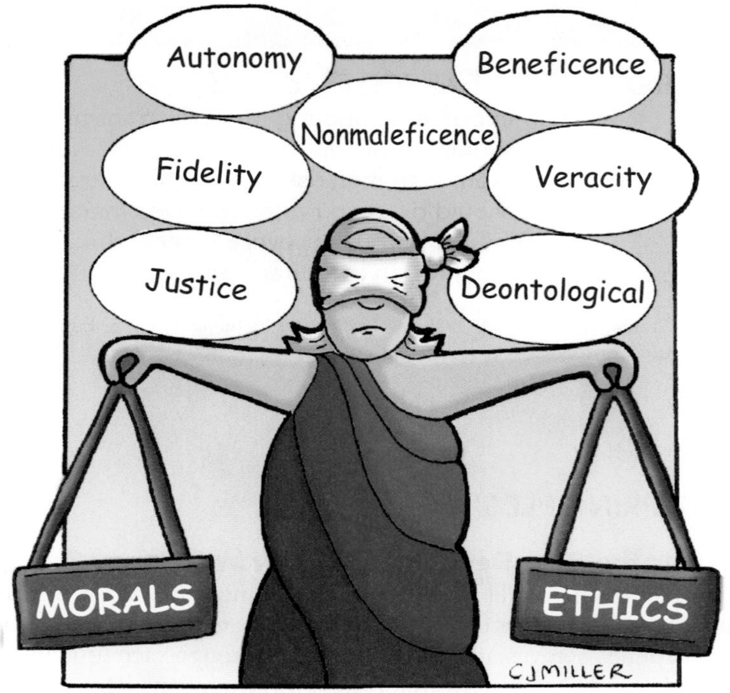

FIGURE 19-1
Moral/ethical principles.

Fidelity: The Duty to Be Faithful to Commitments. Fidelity involves keeping information confidential and maintaining privacy and trust (e.g., maintaining patient confidentiality regarding a positive HIV test or "blowing the whistle" about unscrupulous billing practices).

Consider this:

To whom do we owe our fidelity? Patient, family, physician, institution, or profession? Who has the right to access patient medical records? When should we "blow the whistle" about unsafe staffing patterns?

Justice: The Duty to Treat All Patients Fairly, Without Regard to Age, Socioeconomic Status, or Other Variables. This principle involves the allocation of scarce and expensive health care resources. Should uninsured pregnant patients have access to epidural anesthesia for childbirth, or is this a luxury reserved for those who have insurance or who pay out of pocket?

Consider this:

What is fair, and who decides? Why are some patients labeled very important persons? Should they receive a different level of care? Why or why not? What kind of access to health care should illegal immigrants receive: preventive or just more costly emergency room care?

Veracity: The Duty to Tell the Truth. The principle of veracity may become an issue when a patient who suspects that her diagnosis is cancer asks you "Nurse, do I have cancer?" Her family has requested that she not be told the truth because their culture believes bad news takes away all hope for the patient.

Consider this:

Is lying to a patient ever justified? If a patient finds out that you have lied to them, will they have any reason to trust you?

Each of the aforementioned principles sounds so right, yet the "consider this" questions indicate that putting them into practice is sometimes easier said than done. Reality does not always offer textbook situations that allow flawless application of ethical principles. As Oscar Wilde, an Irish playwright, once said, "The truth is rarely pure, and never simple." You will encounter clinical situations that challenge the way in which you apply an ethical principle or that cause two or more principles to be in conflict, creating moral uncertainty, which is often referred to as an ethical dilemma.

Which Principle or Rule Is Most Important? Current thinking on the part of ethicists favors autonomy and nonmaleficence as preeminent because they emphasize respect for the person and the avoidance of harm. However, there is no universal agreement, and many individuals rely on spiritual beliefs as the cornerstone to ethical decision making.

Another useful approach to decision making is to consider the relative benefits and burdens of an ethical decision for the patient. Clients may choose a different approach than the care team if they are capable of rational decision making. If they are not capable of autonomous decision making, substituted judgment (decision making) by their designated family is then used. Problems frequently arise when family members disagree regarding a treatment choice or quality of life issues, as evidenced by the recent Terry Schiavo case in Florida (2003), when the husband's wishes to discontinue life support for his wife were granted after a prolonged court case.

Traditional and contemporary models of ethical reasoning offer worldviews from which ethical principles, spiritual values, and the concepts of benefits and burdens can be derived, interpreted, and comparatively emphasized. Nevertheless, they are not without their critics, including nurses, who feel that abstract ideas about right and wrong are not helpful or "enough" at the bedside.

In recent years, nursing ethicists have advanced a new approach to ethical issues emphasizing an ethic of caring as the moral foundation of nursing. Nurses have been encouraged to consider all ethical issues from the central issue of caring. Because caring implies concern for preserving humanity and dignity and promoting well-being, the awareness of rules and principles alone does not adequately address the ethical issues that nurses confront, such as suffering or powerlessness. Research regarding the application of caring to ethical issues is under way, but a practical model for applying this ethic of caring to clinical situations does not yet exist. Currently, the most care-centered approach to ethical dilemmas is to consider the relative "benefits versus burdens" that any proposed solution offers to the patient.

So How Do I Make an Ethical Decision? There are a number of approaches to ethical decision making. Here is a brief overview of the three most commonly applied models of ethical reasoning. The first two types are considered normative because they have clearly defined parameters or norms to influence decision making. The third type is a combination of the other two models.

Deontological. Derived from Judeo-Christian origins, the deontological normative approach is duty-focused and centered on rules from which all action is derived. The rules represent beliefs about intrinsic good that are moral absolutes revealed by God. This approach reasons that all persons are worthy of respect and thus should be treated the same.

All life is worthy of respect.

As a result of the rules and duties that the deontological approach outlines, the individual may feel that he has clear direction about how to act in all situations. Right or wrong is determined on the basis of one's duty or obligation to act, not on the consequences of one's actions. Therefore, abortion and euthanasia are never acceptable actions because they violate the duty to respect the sanctity of all life, and lying is never acceptable because it violates the duty to tell the truth. The emphasis on absolute rules with this approach is sometimes seen as rigid and inflexible, but its strength is in its unbending approach to many issues, emphasizing intent of actions.

Teleological. Derived from humanistic origins, the teleological approach is outcome-focused and places emphasis on results. Good is defined in utilitarian terms: That which is useful is good. Human reason is the basis for authority in all situations, not absolutes from God. Morality is established by majority rule, and the results of actions determine the rules. Because results become the intrinsic good, the individual's actions are always based on the probable outcome.

That which causes a good outcome is a good action.

Simplistically, this view is sometimes interpreted as "the end justifies the means." Abortion may be acceptable because it results in fewer unwanted babies. Euthanasia is an acceptable choice by some patients because it results in decreased suffering. Limiting hospitalization coverage after delivery is acceptable because it saves money and does not adversely affect outcome for most mothers and newborns. The rights of the individual may be sacrificed for the majority utilizing this approach.

Situational. Derived from humanistic and Judeo-Christian influences and most commonly credited to Joseph Fletcher, an Episcopalian theologian, the situational view holds that there are no prescribed rules, norms, or majority-focused results that must be followed. Each situation creates its own set of rules and principles that should be considered in that particular set of circumstances. Emphasizing the uniqueness of the situation and respect for the person in that situation, Fletcher appeals to love as the only norm. Critics of this approach argue that this can lead to a "slippery slope" of moral decline.

Decisions made in one situation cannot be generalized to another situation.

Abortion is the best choice for an unmarried 16-year-old because it gives her the opportunity to finish school and mature, but it may not be the best answer for all girls in such a situation. "Pulling the plug" on a terminally ill patient who does not want any more extraordinary care is an act of compassion. Withholding or withdrawing treatment is ethically correct from the individual patient's perspective if the burden of treatment outweighs the benefit of merely extending life. Defining "burden" has to be approached from the patient's perspective, not from others who may feel burdened by the patient's need for care. Coming from the perspective of benefit versus burden can assist patients and families to make difficult decisions on the basis of the patient's clear or intended wishes discussed over a period of time. Nurses and other health care providers need to be patient advocates, speaking out for those who are disadvantaged and cannot speak for themselves.

Table 19-1 compares the relative advantages and disadvantages of each approach. Remember that there is no perfect worldview. If there were, debate would stop, and the need for continued ethical deliberation would cease. The ethical models presented here are not intended to be all-inclusive or exhaustive in depth. Rather, they should whet your appetite for further content. Many journals and texts are devoted to the topic, and you are encouraged to see how ethicists apply these and other models to issues that affect your area of practice. Surveys of nurses indicate an ongoing interest and expressed need for ethical discussion and support in practice. Nurses increasingly serve on hospital ethics committees and are encouraged to contribute their perspective to ethical debates.

TABLE 19-1

Three Approaches to Ethical Decision Making: Comparison of Advantages and Disadvantages

Ethical Approach	Advantages	Disadvantages
Deontological	Clear direction for action. All individuals are treated the same. Does not consider possible negative consequences of action.	Perceived as rigid. Does not consider possible negative consequences of actions.
Teleological	Interest of the majority is protected. Results are evaluated for their good, and actions may be modified.	Rights of individual may be overlooked/denied. What is a good result? Who determines good? Morality may be arbitrary.
Situational	This approach mirrors the way most individuals actually approach day-to-day decision making. Merits of each situation are considered. Individual has more control/autonomy to make decision in his or her own best interest.	What is good? Who decides? Morality is possibly arbitrary. Lack of rules of generalizability limits criticism of possible abuse.

How Do I Determine Who Owns the Problem? The decision to choose a particular model of ethical reasoning is personal (see Table 19-1) and based on your own values. Familiarize yourself with various models to decrease your own moral uncertainty and gain some understanding of the values of others. The following guidelines are suggested as a means of analyzing ethical issues that will confront you in nursing practice. You will not be a pivotal decision-maker in all situations, but these guidelines can assist you in making your own mind up and help patients to voice their wishes and ask questions.

First, Determine the Facts of the Situation. Make sure you collect enough data to give yourself an accurate picture of the issue at hand. When the facts of a situation become known, you may or may not be dealing with an ethical issue.

As an intensive care unit (ICU) nurse, you believe that the wishes of patients regarding extraordinary care are being disregarded. In other words, resuscitation is performed despite expressed patient wishes to the contrary. You need to

- Determine whether discussion about extraordinary care is taking place among patients, families, and attending physicians.
- Clarify the institution's policy regarding cardiopulmonary resuscitation (CPR) and do-not-resuscitate (DNR) orders.
- Determine what input the families have had into the decisions (i.e., whether the families are aware of the patient's wishes).
- Explore the use of advance-directive documentation at your institution, and determine whether patients are familiar with the use and possible limitations of living wills.
- Share your concerns with the attending physicians to obtain their views of the situation. Discuss the situation with your clinical manager to clarify any misconceptions regarding policy and actual practice.

Second, Identify the Ethical Issues of the Situation. In the ICU scenario, if competent patients have expressed their wishes about resuscitation, this should be reflected in the chart. If a living will has been executed and is recognized as valid within your state, its presence in the chart lends considerable weight to the decision. The patient should be encouraged to discuss his or her decision with family to decrease the chances for disagreement if and when the patient can no longer "speak" for himself or herself. If immediate family members disagree with the living will, the physician may be reluctant to honor the will, at least in part because of concern regarding possible liability. If a living will is executed without prior or subsequent discussion with the attending physician, there may be reluctance to honor the will because the physician was not informed of the patient's decision. The physician may feel that the patient did not make an informed decision. However, a durable power of attorney for health care (DPAHC), combined with a living will and completed before the patient's present state of incapacitation, would stand as clear and convincing evidence of the patient's wishes, preventing such a problem. The example of extraordinary care in the ICU illustrates the existence of values and principles in conflict. When the care team, family, and patient have different views of the situation, the patient is likely to be burdened with less than the best outcome, unless differences are resolved.

Patient: Values autonomy, including the right to decide when intervention should stop.

Family: May value life at all cost and be unwilling to "let go" of the patient when a chance exists to prolong life regardless of life quality.

Physician: May feel that the patient has a fair chance to survive and that the living will was executed without being "fully informed." The duty to care/cure may outweigh the physician's belief in the exercise of patient autonomy and fidelity.

Nurse: Values patient autonomy and the need to remain faithful to the patient's wishes. Concern for the needs of the family, in addition to respect for the physician-patient relationship, may cause some conflict.

Institution: Examination of institutional policy may reveal a conflict between stated policy (e.g., honoring living wills) and actual practice (e.g., code all patients unless written physician orders indicate otherwise).

In this situation, the ethical components of this second step involve autonomy and fidelity versus beneficence.

Third, Consider Possible Courses of Action and Their Related Outcomes. Having collected data and attempted discussion on the issue with all involved parties, you are faced with the following options:

1. Advocate for the patient with physicians and the family by facilitating communication.
2. Encourage the patient and family to share feelings with each other regarding desires for care.
3. Encourage the family, patient, and attending physicians to discuss the situation more openly.

If the advocacy role does not bring about some change in behavior, consider the possible input and assistance of an interdisciplinary ethics committee (IEC). In the past decade, such committees have evolved in response to the growing number of ethical issues faced in clinical practice. Currently, more than 65% of hospitals have such a committee, and it may become an integral aspect of every institution if Medicare reimbursement is linked to the presence of an ethics resource. The IEC is typically composed of physicians, clergy, social workers, lawyers, and, increasingly, nurses. Any health team member can access the committee with the assurance of receiving at least a helpful, listening ear. If necessary, the committee will convene to review a clinical case and will offer an unbiased opinion of the situation. Committee members may be helpful in clarifying issues or offering moral support; they may also be persuasive in suggesting that involved parties (i.e., family, physician, patient, and nurse) consider a suggested course of action. The authority of an IEC is usually limited, because the majority of IECs are developed with the understanding that the advice and opinions offered are not binding to the individual. However, it can serve as a potent form of moral authority and influence if used.

Taking the initiative to express your values and principles is not necessarily easy. As a recent graduate, it may seem safer to "swallow hard," remain quiet, and invest your energies into other aspects of your role. You may risk ridicule, criticism, and disagreement when you speak out on an ethical issue, especially if your view is different or unpopular. However, you risk something far more important if you do not speak out. Silence diminishes your own autonomy as a person and as a professional. Depending on the situation, it may raise eyebrows, but it is important to make your concerns known because some values may be imposed on the patient or you in the clinical setting and those values may not be morally correct. You may not agree with these values or feel that they are in the best interest of the patient.

Fourth, After a Course of Action Has Been Taken, Evaluate the Outcome. In the ICU scenario, did improved communication occur among patients, families, and physicians? Were your efforts to advocate met with resistance or a rebuff? What could you try differently the next time? What values or principles were considered most important by the decision-makers? What kind of assistance did you receive from the IEC? What role did nursing play in this situation, and was it appropriate?

What Other Resources Are Available to Help Resolve Ethical Dilemmas? Professional resources are also available to provide direction about ethical issues and behavior. The first of these is the American Nurses Association (ANA) *Code of Ethics for Nurses* (2001) (see Box 9-1 on p. 185). The code is a statement to society that outlines the values, concerns, and goals of the profession. It should be compatible with individual nurses' personal values and goals. The code provides direction for ethical decisions and behavior by repeatedly emphasizing the obligations and responsibilities that the nurse-patient relationship entails.

The provisions of the *Code of Ethics* allude to the ethical principles mentioned earlier in this chapter and certainly imply that fidelity to the patient is foremost. A copy of the code with interpretive statements is available from the ANA. If you did not purchase a copy as a reference for school, consider buying it for your own use in practice.

Critics of the *Code of Ethics* for nurses cite its lack of legal enforceability. This is a valid criticism because the code is not a legal document like licensure laws. However, it is a moral statement of accountability and can add weight to decisions involving legal censure. Many practicing nurses claim ignorance of the *Code of Ethics* for nurses or believe that it is a document for students only. However, the *Code of Ethics* for nurses is for all nurses and was developed by nurses. Take the opportunity to become familiar with its contents. Box 19-2 lists the *International Council of Nurses Code for Nurses*.

BOX 19-2 International Council of Nurses Code for Nurses

ETHICAL CONCEPTS APPLIED TO NURSING

- The fundamental responsibility of the nurse is fourfold: to promote health, to prevent illness, to restore health, and to alleviate suffering.
- The need for nursing is universal. Inherent in nursing is respect for life, dignity, and rights of man. It is unrestricted by considerations of nationality, race, creed, color, age, sex, politics, or social status.
- Nurses render health services to the individual, the family, and the community and coordinate their services with those of related groups.

NURSES AND PEOPLE

- The nurse's prime responsibility is to those people who require nursing care.
- The nurse, in providing care, promotes an environment in which the values, customs, and spiritual beliefs of the individual are respected.
- The nurse holds in confidence personal information and uses judgment in sharing this information.

Continued

BOX 19-2 International Council of Nurses Code for Nurses—cont'd

NURSES AND PRACTICE

- The nurse carries personal responsibility for nursing practice and for maintaining competence by continual learning.
- The nurse maintains the highest standards of nursing care possible within the reality of a specific situation.
- The nurse uses judgment in relation to individual competence when accepting and delegating responsibilities.
- The nurse, when acting in a professional capacity, should at all times maintain standards of personal conduct which reflect credit upon the profession.

NURSES AND SOCIETY

- The nurse shares with other citizens the responsibility for initiating and supporting action to meet the health and social needs of the public.

NURSES AND COWORKERS

- The nurse sustains a cooperative relationship with coworkers in nursing and other fields.
- The nurse takes appropriate action to safeguard the individual when his care is endangered by a coworker or any other person.

NURSES AND THE PROFESSION

- The nurse plays the major role in determining and implementing desirable standards of nursing practice and nursing education.
- The nurse is active in developing a core of professional knowledge.
- The nurse, acting through the professional organization, participates in establishing and maintaining equitable social and economic working conditions in nursing.

From International Council of Nurses: *ICN Code for Nurses: ethical concepts applied to nursing,* Geneva, 1973, Inprimeres Populaires; with permission.

In 1973, the American Hospital Association published a *Patient's Bill of Rights.* Now revised (Box 19-3), this document reflects acknowledgment of patients' rights to participate in their health care and was developed as a response to consumer criticism of paternalistic provider care. The statements detail the patient's rights with corresponding provider responsibilities. Read over each statement and consider whether they seem reasonable. When first developed, many of the statements were considered radical. This document reflects the increasing emphasis on patient autonomy in health care and defines the limits of provider influence and control. Earlier beliefs that the hospital and physician know best (paternalism) have been challenged and modified. This document is likely to be further refined as joint responsibilities between patients and health care providers.

Consider the settings in which you have had clinical experiences and decide how well these rights have been acknowledged and supported. In your future practice keep these rights in mind. Observing them is not only the "right thing to do," it is enforceable by law.

BOX 19-3 The Patient Care Partnership: Understanding Expectations, Rights, and Responsibilities

Our goal is for you and your family to have the same care and attention we would want for our families and ourselves. The sections explain some of the basics about how you can expect to be treated during your hospital stay. They also cover what we will need from you to care for you better. If you have questions at any time, please ask them. Unasked or unanswered questions can add to the stress of being in the hospital.

WHAT TO EXPECT DURING YOUR HOSPITAL STAY

- **High quality hospital care.** Our first priority is to provide you the care you need, when you need it, with skill, compassion, and respect. Tell your caregivers if you have concerns about your care or if you have pain. You have the right to know the identity of doctors, nurses and others involved in your care.
- **A clean and safe environment.** We use special policies and procedures to avoid mistakes in your care and keep you free from abuse or neglect. If anything unexpected and significant happens during your hospital stay, you will be told what happened and any resulting changes in your care will be discussed with you.
- **Involvement in your care.** Please tell your caregivers if you need more information about treatment choices. When decision making takes place, it should include:
  - *Discussing your medical condition and information about medically appropriate treatment choices.* To make informed decisions with your doctor, you need to understand:
    —The benefits and risks of each treatment, and whether the treatment is experimental or part of a research study.
    —What you can reasonably expect from your treatment and any long-term effects it might have on your quality of life.
    —What you and your family will need to do after you leave the hospital.
    —The financial consequences of using uncovered services or out-of-network providers.
  - *Discussing your treatment plan.* When you enter the hospital, you sign a general consent to treatment. In some cases, such as surgery or experimental treatment, you may be asked to confirm in writing that you understand what is planned and agree to it.
  - *Getting information from you.* Your caregivers need complete and correct information about your health and coverage so that they can make good decisions about your care. That includes:
    —Past illnesses, surgeries, or hospital stays; past allergic reactions; any medicines or dietary supplements (e.g., vitamins, herbs) that you are taking; and any network or admission requirements under your health plan.
  - *Understanding your health care goals and values.* Make sure your doctor, your family, and your care team know your wishes.
  - *Understanding who should make decisions when you cannot.* If you have signed a health care power of attorney stating who should speak for you if you become unable to make health care decisions for yourself, or a living will or advance directive that states your wishes about end-of-life care; give copies to your doctor, your family, and your care team.
- **Protection of your privacy.** State and federal laws and hospital operating policies protect the privacy of your medical information. You will receive a Notice of Privacy Practices that describes the ways that we use, disclose and safeguard patient

Continued

BOX 19-3 The Patient Care Partnership: Understanding Expectations, Rights, and Responsibilities—cont'd

information and that explains how you can obtain a copy of information from our records about your care.

- **Preparing you and your family for when you leave the hospital.** The success of your treatment often depends on your efforts to follow medication, diet and therapy plans. You can expect us to help you identify sources of follow-up care and to let you know if our hospital has a financial interest in any referrals. You can also expect to receive information and, when possible, training about the self-care you will need when you go home.
- **Help with your bill and filing insurance claims.** Our staff will file claims for you with health care insurers or other programs, such as Medicare and Medicaid. If you have questions about your bill, contact our business office. If you need help understanding your insurance coverage or health plan, start with your insurance company or health benefits manager. If you do not have health coverage, we will try to help you and your family find financial help or make other arrangements.

This is an abridged text. Full text is available at *www.aha.org*.

Another document was developed in 1992 and revised in 1996 as a response to the rapidly growing home health care area of community nursing. The National Association for Home Care established a *Home Care Bill of Rights* for patients and families to inform them of the ethical conduct they can expect from home care agencies and their employees when they are in the home. This document is widely used and addresses the rights of the patient and provider to be treated with dignity and respect; the right of the patient to actively participate in decision making; privacy of information; financial information regarding payment procedures from insurance, Medicare, and Medicaid; quality of care; and the patient's responsibility to follow the plan of care and notify the home health nurse of changes in his or her condition. Surprising as it may seem, there are instances of nurses who have lost their license as a result of unethical behavior toward patients in their homes. These abuses include financial and sexual exploitation—major violations of professional boundaries.

Home care nurses often face difficult ethical dilemmas about the delivery of care to patients. For example, a patient will require or desire more care or visits than Medicare or private insurance will pay for. All home care agencies have policies written to guide them through the decision-making process when they can no longer receive reimbursement for a patient's care. Often it is the responsibility of the home care nurse to find another community agency that can meet the patient's needs at a cost the patient can afford.

A fifth document that you should be familiar with is the *Nuremberg Code* (Box 19-4). This code grew out of the blatant abuses perpetrated by Nazi war criminals during World War II in the name of science. Experiments were conducted by health care professionals without patient consent and resulted in horrific mutilations, disability, and death. The *Nuremberg Code* identifies the need for voluntary informed consent when medical experiments are conducted on human beings. It delineates the limits and restrictions that researchers must recognize and respect. Because of the preponderance of research in many clinical settings, nurses have a responsibility to understand the concept of

BOX 19-4 The Nuremberg Code

The great weight of the evidence before us is to the effect that certain types of medical experiments on human beings, when kept within reasonably well-defined bounds, conform to the ethics of the medical profession generally. The protagonists of the practice of human experimentation justify their views on the basis that such experiments yield results for the good of society that are unprocurable by other methods or means of study. All agree, however, that certain basic principles must be observed in order to satisfy moral, ethical, and legal concepts:

1. The voluntary consent of the human subject is absolutely essential. This means that the person involved should have legal capacity to give consent; should be so situated as to be able to exercise free power of choice, without the intervention of any element of force, fraud, deceit, duress, overreaching, or other ulterior form of constraint or coercion; and should have sufficient knowledge and comprehension of the elements of the subject matter involved as to enable him to make an understanding and enlightened decision. This latter element requires that before the acceptance of an affirmative decision by the experimental subject there should be made known to him the nature, duration, and purpose of the experiment; the method and means by which it is to be conducted; all inconveniences and hazards reasonably to be expected; and the effects upon his health or person which may possibly come from his participation in the experiment.

   The duty and responsibility for ascertaining the quality of the consent rests upon each individual who initiates, directs, or engages in the experiment. It is a personal duty and responsibility that may not be delegated to another with impunity.
2. The experiment should be such as to yield fruitful results for the good of society, unprocurable by other methods or means of study, and not random and unnecessary in nature.
3. The experiment should be so designed and based on results of animal experimentation and a knowledge of the natural history of the disease or other problem under study that the anticipated results will justify the performance of the experiment.
4. The experiment should be so conducted as to avoid all unnecessary physical and mental suffering and injury.
5. No experiment should be so conducted where there is an a priori reason to believe that death or disabling injury will occur; except, perhaps, in those experiments where the experimental physicians also serve as subjects.
6. The degree of risk to be taken should never exceed that determined by the humanitarian importance of the problem to be solved by the experiment.
7. Proper preparations should be made and adequate facilities provided to protect the experimental subject against even remote possibilities of injury, disability, or death.
8. The experiment should be conducted only by scientifically qualified persons. The highest degree of skill and care should be required through all stages of the experiments of those who conduct or engage in the experiment.

Reprinted from *Trials of war criminals before the Nuremberg Military Tribunals under Control Council Law* No. 18, vol. 2, Washington, DC, 1949, U.S. Government Printing Office, p 181.

voluntary informed consent and support the patient's rights throughout the research process. After reading this code, you should have increased awareness of the patient's right to autonomy and the health care provider's responsibility to be faithful to that right.

CONTROVERSIAL ETHICAL ISSUES CONFRONTING NURSING

Situations that raise ethical issues affect all areas of nursing practice. The following is a sampling of issues that consistently cause controversy.

Abortion. This issue has raged in the United States since the 1973 *Roe v. Wade* Supreme Court decision. The resolution of this case struck down laws against abortion but left the possibility of introducing restrictions under some conditions. Efforts toward that end continue today with mixed results for both pro-choice and pro-life factions. Increasing efforts are focused on the need for parental notification/consent.

Historical references to abortion can be found as far back as 4500 BC (Rosen, 1967). It has been practiced in many societies as a means of population control and terminating unwanted pregnancies, yet sanctions against abortion are found in both ancient biblical and legal texts. Interestingly, the ancient sanctions against abortion generally related to fines payable to the husband if the pregnant woman was harmed. This form of sanction derived from the concept of woman and fetus as male property. Greek philosophers, including Aristotle and Plato, made a distinction between an unformed fetus and a formed fetus. A fine was levied for aborting an unformed fetus, whereas the aborting of a formed fetus required "a life for a life." The number of gestational weeks that determine whether a fetus was formed was not stated, although the time of human ensoulment was understood: Aristotle believed that a male fetus was imbued with a soul at 40 days gestation (*quickening*), versus 90 days for a female (Feldman, 1968). The subject of ensoulment became part of the ongoing debate regarding the time when the developing fetus becomes human. In other words,

> When does life begin?

Judeo-Christian theologians generally came to identify the beginning of life at conception or the time of implantation. Yet, even within this tradition, the Jewish Talmud and Roman law stated that life begins at birth because the first breath represents the infusion of life. These varied views continue to the present.

Social customs and private behavior regarding abortion have frequently differed from theological teaching. The first legal sanctions against abortion in the United States began in the late nineteenth century. Before that time, first-trimester abortions were not uncommon and, in fact, were advertised, supporting the idea that abortion before quickening was acceptable.

The ethical debate about abortion today is a continuing struggle to answer the question of when life begins and to determine an answer to the following questions:

- Does the fetus have rights?
- Do the rights of the fetus (for life) take precedence over the right of the mother to control her reproductive functions?
- When is abortion morally justified?
- Should minors have the right to abortion without parental consent or awareness?

The struggle to answer these questions has polarized individuals into "pro-life" or "pro-choice" camps. Yet opinion polls on the subject have found very few people to be against abortion in all circumstances or to favor abortion as a mandatory solution for some pregnancies. Most Americans express views anywhere between these extremes, and the legal battle to maintain or restrict abortion access continues. The controversy has escalated into violence in some areas of the country, with abortion clinics and personnel subjected to attack; some abortion providers have even died. This violence has resulted in the decreased availability of abortion services in a number of areas. In recent years, some pharmacists have refused to fill prescriptions for birth control pills and the "morning after" pill, claiming that this violates their moral beliefs, an exacerbation of the pro-life/pro-choice debate.

The Roman Catholic Church has been the religious group most frequently identified with the pro-life movement, but there are other groups—religious and otherwise—that support a ban on abortion. Pro-life proponents generally condone abortion only to save the life of the mother. These antiabortion groups are criticized by pro-choice as extremists, antiwoman, and repressive.

The pro-choice movement is vocal in championing the woman's right to choose and promoting the safety of legalized abortion. They cite the tragedy of past "back-alley" abortions and compare restrictions on abortion to infringements on the civil liberties of women. Within the pro-choice movement are many individuals who favor restrictions on abortions after the first trimester and oppose the use of abortion as a means of birth control. Pro-life proponents view pro-choice supporters as antifamily extremists who do not represent the views of the majority of Americans.

How Does the Abortion Issue Affect Nursing? Nurses are involved both as individuals and professionals. Some general guidelines to consider are as follows:

- Consider what your values and beliefs are in relation to abortion and how you can best apply these values to your work and possible political action.
- If you choose to work in a setting in which abortions are performed, review statement one of the ANA's *Code of Ethics for Nurses*: "The nurse, in all professional relationships, practices with compassion and respect for the inherent dignity, worth and uniqueness of every individual, unrestricted by considerations of social or economic status, personal attributes, or the nature of the health problems" (ANA, 2001).
- This statement outlines your responsibility to care for all patients. If you do not agree with an institution's policy or procedure regarding abortion, the patient still merits your care. If that care (e.g., assisting with abortions) violates your principles, you should consider changing your job or developing an agreement with your employer regarding your job responsibilities. If you cannot provide the care that the patient requires, make arrangements for someone else to do so.

You do not have to sacrifice your own values and principles, but you are barred by the ANA code of ethics for nurses from abandoning patients or forcing your values on them. Such abandonment would also constitute legal abandonment, and you would be subject to legal action.

Some hospitals have developed conscience clauses that provide protection to the hospital and nurses against participation in abortions. Find out if your institution has such a clause.

Consider your response and possible conflict in the following situations:

You are a labor and delivery nurse working on a unit that performs second-trimester saline abortions in a nearby area. You are not a part of the staff for the abortion area, but today, because of short-staffing, you are asked to care for a 16-year-old who is undergoing the procedure.

You work in a family-planning clinic that serves low-income women. Because of escalating violence against abortion providers, the nearest abortion clinic is 100 miles away. You are restricted from giving information regarding abortion services because of federal guidelines.

A 41-year-old mother of five has expressed interest in terminating her pregnancy of 6 weeks gestation. She confides that her husband would beat her if he knew she was pregnant and contemplating abortion.

You are teaching a class on sexuality and contraception to a group of high school sophomores. Two of the girls state that they have just had abortions. In response to your information regarding available methods of contraception, one of the girls states, "I'm not interested in birth control. If I get pregnant again, I'll just get an abortion. It's a lot easier."

You have a history of infertility and work in the neonatal ICU. You are presently caring for a 24-week-old baby born to a mother who admits to taking "crack" as a means of inducing labor and "getting rid of the baby." The mother has just arrived in the unit and wants to visit the baby.

These sample scenarios are meant to illustrate the conflicts that personal values, institutional settings, and patients may create for the recent graduate. In your responses, consider how you might lobby or participate in the political process to change or support existing policies regarding abortion and access to such services.

Euthanasia. *Euthanasia* refers to "mercy killing." It is a Greek word that means "good death" and implies painless actions to end the life of individuals suffering from incurable or terminal diseases. Euthanasia has been closely tied to a "right-to-die" argument, which has gained a good deal of attention in the past decade. Euthanasia is classified as *active, passive, or voluntary. Active euthanasia* involves the administration of a lethal drug or another measure to end life and alleviate suffering. Regardless of the motivation and beliefs of the individuals involved, active euthanasia is legally wrong and can result in criminal charges of murder if carried out. In recent years, incidents of active euthanasia have become periodic news events as spouses or parents have used measures to end the suffering of their mates or children (from, for example, advanced Alzheimer's disease or persistent vegetative state). *Passive euthanasia* involves the withdrawal of extraordinary means of life support (e.g., ventilator, feeding tube). *Voluntary euthanasia* involves situations when the dying individual expresses his or her desires regarding the management and time of death to a sympathetic physician who then provides the means for the patient to obtain a lethal dose of medication.

As technology has advanced, patients are routinely kept alive today who would never have survived a few short years ago. Concerns regarding prolonging life and suffering for those individuals have resulted in a movement to have "right-to-die" statutes and living wills accepted (Figure 19-2). In those states that have such statutes and recognize living wills, termination of treatment in such cases has become easier.

Right-to-die statutes free health care personnel from possible liability for honoring a person's wishes that life not be unduly prolonged (Rudy, 1985).

Another document, the DPAHC, helps ensure that a living will is carried out. The DPAHC identifies the individual who will carry out the patient's wishes in the event that he or she is incapacitated and also informs health care providers about the specific wishes of the patient regarding life-support measures.

ADVANCE DIRECTIVE
Living Will and Health Care Proxy

Death is a part of life. It is a reality like birth, growth and aging. I am using this advance directive to convey my wishes about medical care to my doctors and other people looking after me at the end of my life. It is called an advance directive because it gives instructions in advance about what I want to happen to me in the future. It expresses my wishes about medical treatment that might keep me alive. I want this to be legally binding.

If I cannot make or communicate decisions about my medical care, those around me should rely on this document for instructions about measures that could keep me alive.

I do not want medical treatment (including feeding and water by tube) that will keep me alive if:

- I am unconscious and there is no reasonable prospect that I will ever be conscious again (even if I am not going to die soon in my medical condition), *or*
- I am near death from an illness or injury with no reasonable prospect of recovery.

I do want medicine and other care to make me more comfortable and to take care of pain and suffering. I want this even if the pain medicine makes me die sooner.

I want to give some extra instructions: *[Here list any special instructions, e.g., some people fear being kept alive after a debilitating stroke. If you have wishes about this, or any other conditions, please write them here.]*

The legal language in the box that follows is a health care proxy.
It gives another person the power to make medical decisions for me.

I (name)____________________, who lives at ____________________

____________________, phone number ____________________

to make medical decisions for me if I cannot make them myself. This person is called a health care "surrogate," "agent," "proxy," or "attorney in fact." This power of attorney shall become effective when I become incapable of making or communicating decisions about my medical care. This means that this document stays legal when and if I lose the power to speak for myself, for instance, if I am in a coma or have Alzheimer's disease.

My health care proxy has power to tell others what my advance directive means. This person also has power to make decisions for me, based either on what I would have wanted, or, if this is not known, on what he or she thinks is best for me.

If my first choice health care proxy cannot or decides not to act for me, I (name) __________

____________________, address ____________________

phone number ________________, as my second choice.

(over, please)

FIGURE 19-2
Advance directive. *(From Choice in Dying [formerly Concern for Dying/Society for the Right to Die], 200 Varick Street, New York, 10014-4810.)*

Continued

I have discussed my wishes with my health care proxy, and with my second choice if I have chosen to appoint a second person. My proxy(ies) has(have) agreed to act for me.

I have thought about this advance directive carefully. I know what it means and want to sign it. I have chosen two witnesses, neither of whom is a member of my family, nor will inherit from me when I die. My witnesses are not the same people as those I named as my health care proxies. I understand that this form should be notarized if I use the box to name (a) health care proxy(ies).

Signature ______________________________

Date ______________________________

Address ______________________________

Witness' signature ______________________________

Witness' printed name ______________________________

Address ______________________________

Witness' signature ______________________________

Witness' printed name ______________________________

Address ______________________________

Notary [to be used if proxy is appointed] ______________________________

Drafted and Distributed by Choice In Dying, Inc.—the National Council for the Right to Die. Choice In Dying is a National not-for-profit organization which works for the rights of patients at the end of life. In addition to this generic advance directive, Choice In Dying distributes advance directives that conform to each state's specific legal requirements and maintains a national Living Will Registry for completed documents.

CHOICE IN DYING INC.—
The National Council for the Right to Die
(formerly Concern for Dying/Society for the Right to Die)
200 Varick Street, New York, NY 10014 (212) 366-5540

5/92

FIGURE 19-2
Advance directive—cont'd.

A major impact on the availability of living wills and the DPAHC (which are referred to as advance medical directives) resulted from the introduction of the Patient Self-Determination Act in December 1991. Passed as part of the Consolidated Omnibus Budget Reconciliation Act (COBRA), advance directives are federally mandated for all institutions receiving Medicare or Medicaid funds. On admission, all competent adults must be offered information about advance directives. This means that all adults are told about the purpose and availability of living wills *(treatment directive)* and

DPAHCs *(appointment directive)*. They are then offered assistance with completing these documents if desired. After 10 years of having advance directive information available to patients, the impact of this document on decision making is varied. It certainly has influenced the communication that many patients have with their families, physicians, and other health care providers regarding their wishes at the timing of signing, but patients often change their minds when their health care status changes, frequently opting for the prolongation of life. A problem has surfaced regarding the timing of information to patients regarding advance directives. If patients first hear about advance directives on admission to acute-care settings, anxiety regarding their admission and the separate concept of advance directives may seriously affect informed decision making at that time. Advance directives should ideally be discussed before serious illness and at the very least in a noncrisis environment to encourage nonpressured decision making. Cultural, religious, and racial issues regarding DPAHC have also surfaced and need to be researched to determine the best approaches for a culturally diverse society. Patients and families need reassurance that declining extraordinary care does not mean the abandonment of caring and palliative care when needed. Both patients and families need to be reassured that comfort care will never stop, even when aggressive curative efforts are withdrawn.

Decisions to withdraw or withhold nutrition and hydration from patients is complex and the subject of ongoing debate by ethicists, health care personnel, and the legal system. In response to the issues of hydration and nutrition, the Ethics Committee of the ANA developed guidelines in 1988. These guidelines state that there are instances when withholding or withdrawing nutrition and hydration are morally permissible. Although intended only as a guideline, this document provides direction for nurses who face such issues. Its wording has been both praised for its clarity and criticized for possible ambiguity. The primary exception to hydration and nutrition withdrawal is when harm from these measures can be demonstrated. This document is available from the ANA.

Futile Care and Physician-Assisted Suicide. Futile care (futility) and physician-assisted suicide (PAS) are two ethical and human rights issues that have drawn a great deal of attention and debate. In a survey conducted by the ANA's Center for Ethics and Human Rights in June 1994, respondents were asked to identify 10 of the most frequently occurring ethical issues. Approximately 55% identified "end-of-life decision" as one of the top four issues, and 37% identified "providing futile care" as an important priority issue facing nursing (Scanlon, 1994).

What Is Futility? *Medical futility* refers to the use of medical intervention (beyond comfort care) without realistic hope of benefit to the patient. *Benefit* is defined as improvement of outcome. A concrete example of futility would be the continuation of ICU care for a patient in a persistent vegetative state who would, on discharge from the hospital, return to a nursing home incapable of interacting with the environment. The futility debate concerns the very nature of the definition of *benefit,* in addition to who defines it. The economic pressure to control health care costs is also causing a focus on ways to eliminate "unnecessary" intervention.

On paper, futility can be defined, but its application to diverse clinical situations remains a challenge. The debate involves multiple parties whose interests and values are not always compatible. For example, patients and families have argued both for the right to refuse care that they believe is futile and the right to receive all possible care in the face of a medical opinion of futility. This argument raises two related questions:

- Do patients or families have the right to demand and receive treatment that health care providers believe to be futile?
- Do physicians have the right to refuse treatments that they believe to be futile, despite patient or family desire to initiate or continue such treatment?

Ethics committees have struggled to agree on a working definition to provide support for clinicians and patients and families who are faced with difficult decisions regarding care. Many institutions have developed guidelines for the withdrawal of treatment (except for comfort care). These guidelines emphasize the importance of clear, ongoing communication among all health care team members and with the patient and family. Accurate, compassionate discussion is essential to convey a unified approach to the realities and limitations of possible medical care. The guidelines should never be used as a threat or to imply abandonment. They are, as their name implies, guidelines. Lack of agreement among the patient, the family, and the health care team is likely to delay or prevent withdrawal of treatment, primarily because of the fear of liability, even in cases of brain death. Supporting the patient or family decision may be difficult because of personal values and professional opinions. It is crucial to clarify where professional loyalties should lie and keep the discussion patient-centered.

Pressures to eliminate unnecessary costs also influence the futility debate. Insurers, clinicians, and health care institutions increasingly question medical expenditures that produce futile outcomes and prolong the inevitability of impending death. Insurance reimbursement is likely to further limit and deny payment for treatment judged to be of no benefit. A possible risk is that beneficial treatment may be eliminated or denied solely because of economic concern in cases having an uncertain outcome. Nurses need to keep informed on institutional guidelines regarding medical futility and communicate clearly with patients, families, and physicians regarding expected goals and likely outcomes of care. The patient's welfare—and not economic concerns—should be the primary driving force for withdrawal of treatment.

Physician-Assisted Suicide. PAS has gained national attention because of Dr. Jack Kevorkian's persistent efforts to publicize and bring legitimacy to a formerly taboo topic. Kevorkian assisted or attended in the deaths of more than 130 terminally and chronically ill patients (Hyde, 1999). His work caused the state of Michigan to pass legislation barring PAS. Proponents of PAS have managed to put the issue on the ballot in three Western states since 1991, with passage occurring in the November 1994 Oregon election. PAS was immediately challenged in the Oregon court by right-to-life advocates but finally went into effect October 27, 1997. A first-year review of the law's impact indicated that 15 people had died as a result of prescriptions for lethal medications. Reasons cited for the use of a lethal dose include concern with loss of control over autonomy. Fear of uncontrolled pain or financial pressure was not mentioned (Chin et al, 1999).

PAS has been debated for years, and opinions on both sides among physicians and the public are very strong. The American Medical Association opposes PAS because it violates the most basic ethical principle: "First, do no harm." Physicians have traditionally taken care of the living patient, and support for PAS threatens to destroy this fundamental relationship. Many individual physicians have, however, changed their minds in recent years because of their work with terminally ill patients. More than a few of these clinicians have come to believe that the only option for the relief of some patients' intractable pain and suffering is death.

Although the legalization of PAS continues to be debated in the courts, the practice goes on—generally in private without headlines. Both critics and supporters of PAS state that the secrecy goes on because of the fear of arrest for homicide. There have been some court rulings supporting the right to PAS by terminally ill patients on the basis of the Fourteenth Amendment's guarantee of personal liberty. These decisions have been assailed by the right-to-life groups as an anti-life philosophy, which dishonors the intrinsic value of life.

PAS affects nursing practice because a decision to perform PAS may involve the nurse. The term PAS implies that the physician is the active agent, but a lethal dose may be ordered by the physician for the nurse to administer. Nurses need to be aware of the legal and ethical implications of such an order. The administration of a lethal dose for the explicit purpose of ending a patient's life is an illegal act that can be prosecuted as homicide. From an ethical point of view, many would consider this the ultimate act of mercy, yet it is an illegal act. Clinicians, ethicists, the public, and the courts continue to struggle with how best to respect the life and wishes of terminally ill patients without "doing harm." Nurses need to remain aware of their nurse practice acts, and the *Code of Ethics for Nurses*, as they balance patient needs with their conscience and value systems.

Ethicists generally agree that although the prolongation of life by extraordinary means is not always indicated, clarifying the circumstances when such care may be stopped (withdrawn) or possibly never begun (withheld) frequently creates controversy, particularly when the quality of life (coma, persistent vegetative state) is likely to be questionable.

Opponents of the right-to-die movement believe that it represents the erosion of the value of human life and may encourage a movement toward the acceptance of suicide as part of a "culture of death." They caution that the lives of the weak and disabled may come to be devalued as society concentrates on the pursuit of "quality life." If passive euthanasia achieves societal acceptance, who will speak out in favor of protecting incompetent or dependent individuals who are not living society's view of a quality life? The well-publicized Schiavo controversy demonstrates the political polarization that this topic can cause (Nagourney, 2005).

Proponents of the right-to-die movement believe that it provides a more natural course of living and dying to the individual and family by avoiding the artificial prolongation of life through technology. The availability of technology to prolong life often raises the question "we can, but should we?"

Surveys of medical and nursing school curricula in the United States continue to reveal minimal content on end-of-life care issues. Schools continue to focus curricula more on the curative approach to illness and disease, neglecting to address the palliative, comfort-directed needs of individuals who require care in the last months and days of their lives. This fact, combined with the aging of our population, points out the need for improvement in the education of both current clinicians and students in health care institutions. A growing number of proactive clinicians and educators concerned with the quality of care provided to dying patients and their families have created an educational movement called *End of Life Care*. The specific program targeted for nursing is called End of Life Nursing Education Consortium Project targeting nursing faculty and nursing leadership in many specialty organizations. This consortium project has educated hundreds of nurses in the past few years, slowly influencing a change in both education and clinical practice. Studies of patients facing end-of-life issues indicate that pain and symptom management, communication with one's physician, preparation for death, and the opportunity to achieve a sense of life completion are the most consistently important issues (Steinhauser et al, 2000). It will be interesting to see the impact of these efforts on patient care over the next decade. Perhaps we will be better prepared to accept the reality that everyone does die. As nurses, we are challenged to make this last event of life a better experience for all.

Consider your response and possible conflict in the following critical-thinking situations:

A 22-year-old quadriplegic repeatedly asks you to disconnect him from the ventilator. His family rarely visits, and he believes that he has nothing to live for.

The spouse of an advanced Alzheimer's patient states that he can no longer watch his wife of 43 years suffer. "She would not have wanted to live this way." His wife is being treated for dehydration, malnutrition, and a urinary tract infection. She is confused and is frequently sedated to manage her combativeness. The use of a feeding tube is being contemplated because of her refusal to eat.

The attending physician for a patient with terminal AIDS refuses to order increasing doses of pain medication because of her concern that it may cause a repeat episode of respiratory depression. The patient's pain is unrelieved, and he begs you for medication. "Please help me. I know I'm dying."

The parents of a 29-week-old premature infant with Down syndrome and tracheoesophageal fistula request that no extraordinary care be provided. They want the baby kept warm and nurtured but refuse to sign the consent form for surgery.

For each of these scenarios, consider both what your reaction would be and the possible resources you would use to resolve the conflicts.

Use of Reproductive Technology. Depending on the source, data indicate that 10% to 20% of all couples in the United States are identified as infertile. Because of this and the legalization of abortion, the development and use of reproductive technology is a subject of considerable interest and controversy.

What Is the Ethical Consideration in Artificial Insemination? Artificial insemination (AI) involves the use of husband or donor sperm in cases of infertility or when a single woman wishes to be artificially impregnated. The ethical arguments surrounding the issue involve beliefs about the use of reproductive interventions both inside and outside of marriage. For example, the Roman Catholic Church opposes AI, involving donor sperm because it violates the intimacy of marriage.

Proponents of AI cite the ability of a woman to achieve pregnancy with a relatively simple intervention. The issue is more controversial when donor sperm is used and the woman is single. The way in which we define family and parenthood may be challenged, particularly when lesbian couples or single women are involved.

What Are the Ethical Issues Surrounding Surrogate Motherhood? The flip side to AI is surrogate motherhood. Unlike simple AI, there is no anonymity of the donor uterus. The surrogate mother is known, having been selectively chosen and contracted for the purpose of carrying a fetus for another couple to claim as their own. To date, some genetic fathers and artificially inseminated surrogate mothers have fought bitter legal and emotional wars to gain custody of the offspring.

Concern for the well-being and rights of the newborn, genetic father, and surrogate mother have been discussed at great lengths in the courts, the media, and ethical circles. Efforts have been made to remove the financial incentives for surrogate motherhood, because carrying a pregnancy for the purpose of making money has been likened to selling a human being. Contracting for the "sale" of a human being has raised disturbing issues, including the refusal of the biological mother to relinquish the child despite a "contract" (Baby M) and the birth of a grossly deformed child to a surrogate mother, resulting in the refusal of anyone to accept the child as his or her own. The latter case was most damning because the child was likened to "damaged goods," abandoned by both the buyer and seller. Reducing the meaning of a human life to the terminology of retail marketing is a damning indictment of consumerism run amuck.

What Is the Ethical Issue Regarding the Use of Fetal Tissue? Fetal tissue from elective abortions has been identified as potentially beneficial in the treatment of Parkinson's disease and other degenerative disorders because of its unique embryonic qualities. Proponents argue that it is available tissue that can be put to some beneficial use in patients who at present do not have any other hope of significant improvement or cure.

Critics who assail the use of fetal tissue for stem cell research as a further erosion of respect for the unborn were successful in spurring a federal ban on the use of fetal tissue for research in the United States during the 1980s. They believe that the limited research that has already occurred regarding fetal tissue has created the mentality that pregnancy can be used as a means of providing parts and tissues for others. This ban was removed in early 1993 after President Clinton took office and, in 2001, received narrowly defined approval by the Bush administration for genetic research. A similar line of thinking has been used regarding the use of anencephalic infants as organ donors. Does the good (beneficence) achieved from the use of fetal tissue for patient's with Parkinson's disease outweigh the harm inflicted by viewing a fetus as a source of parts?

What Are the Ethical Issues Regarding In Vitro Fertilization? This procedure involves the fertilization of a mother's ovum with the father's sperm in a glass laboratory dish followed by implantation of the embryo in the mother's uterus. Since the birth of the first successful in vitro fertilization baby in 1978, the procedure has gained popularity as a last-chance method for some infertile couples to have a child. The availability of the technique has created a new subspecialty practice in obstetrics and raised ethical issues for consideration. Opponents of the procedure argue that it is an unnatural act and removes the biologic act of procreation from the intimacy of marriage. The cost of the procedure is also a source of criticism, calling into question whether it should be covered by insurance and whether the procedure should be available to all couples, regardless of ability to pay. Many couples are now lobbying to select the sex of their baby, choosing the desired embryo for implantation and destroying the undesired embryos. If technology can be made to meet our desires for a "designer baby," does that make it a morally correct course of action?

Questions concerning informed consent for the procedure merit attention as well. Many infertility clinics offer this service but have not been upfront about their success rates or qualifications. Standardized methods of reporting this information have just recently been established. To be ethical, all such clinics should define success the same way; for example, success equals pregnancy or success equals live birth. The two definitions are very different. Information about the qualifications of the staff should be available to patients, and the subspecialty should lobby for standards of practice that are enforceable and available to the public. Possible side effects from the drugs used to induce hyperovulation and from anesthesia or surgical injury during the laparoscopy should be explained.

Should anyone who desires the procedure have access, or should the procedure be limited to those in a heterosexual marriage? Most clinics have limited their services to heterosexual couples to avoid adverse publicity, but this policy is starting to change as single and lesbian women seek out avenues of becoming biological parents.

Most importantly, to whom does the embryo belong and what are his or her rights? There have been court cases involving marital disputes regarding the custody of frozen embryos. What are the rights of the embryos in such instances? Can a parent choose to destroy the embryos over the objection of the estranged spouse, or should one parent be able to obtain custody of the embryos when his or her spouse wants them to be thawed out and destroyed? What responsibility does the staff have for maintaining parental ownership of the embryos?

How Should the Ability to Diagnose Genetic Defects Prenatally Be Used? Genetic disorders such as Tay-Sachs disease, cystic fibrosis, Huntington's chorea, and retinoblastoma can be diagnosed early in pregnancy. As this technology advances, how should it be used? Should screening remain voluntary, or, as some have suggested, should it be mandatory to detect fetal disorders that could be aborted or possibly treated? Should the results of such genetic screening be made available to insurance companies? Critics argue that this information could be used as a means of coercion for couples regarding reproductive decisions if future insurance coverage is then limited. As this technology advances, safeguards need to be applied to prevent invasion of privacy and any societal movement toward eugenics. As the human genome project allows us to become capable of knowing our genetic code and possibilities for disease, it raises the question of who should have access to that information.

Allocation of Scarce Resources. When the subject of scarce resource allocation is mentioned, justice is the core issue. What is fair and equal treatment when health care financing decisions are made? Who should make such decisions and on what basis? Critics argue that health care is not a scarce resource in this country, but that the access to such care is scarce for many. They believe that this scarcity of access could be eliminated if our priorities in governmental spending were altered. Managed care put a temporary brake on runaway costs in the 1990s, but that brake seems to have failed in the past few years. However, 44 million individuals living in the United States are without health insurance or a reasonable means of accessing anything but stopgap emergency care (see *www.nchc.org/facts/coverage.shtml*). The solution to this issue remains unclear and highly politicized. Thus far, any form of national health insurance has been soundly defeated. In the meantime, managed care of one form or another is influencing a larger and larger share of the insured population, raising related issues of restricted access to specialized care and loss of patient and physician autonomy.

Allocation also raises a number of questions. For example, do all individuals merit the same care? If your answer is an immediate "yes," would you change your mind if the patient were indigent, with no chance of paying the bill? If you still say "yes," should this same indigent patient receive a liver transplantation as readily as someone who has insurance or cash to pay for it? Should taxpayers be responsible for the medical bills for organ transplants, cardiac bypass surgery, or joint replacements for incarcerated felons? These and other questions are being asked by individuals, government, and ethicists, in addition to health care providers. Perhaps at the core of this subject is a more fundamental question: Is health care a right or a privilege that comes with the ability to pay? If access to health care is a right that should be provided to all citizens, are we as a society prepared to pay the bill? And is there a level of health care that is essential for all, beyond which financing becomes a private matter?

The type of care that is provided and supported is another aspect of the debate. For example, should health promotion and prevention be emphasized as much as or more than illness-oriented and rehabilitative care? It is widely acknowledged that each dollar spent on preventive care (e.g., prenatal care) saves three or more dollars in later intervention (e.g., neonatal ICU), yet our national and state health care expenditures (Medicare and Medicaid) are traditionally weighted in favor of an illness model for reimbursement. Managed care is an effort to control health care costs, yet it is increasingly criticized as prioritizing the financial bottom line over the quality of care.

What Are Some of the Possible Solutions Being Debated? In recent years, some individuals, including the former Colorado Governor Richard Lamm, have proposed the idea of health care rationing for the elderly, specifically as it relates to the use of expensive technology that often prolongs the last few weeks of life and suffering (Lamm, 1986). He believes that such 11th-hour expenditures are unwanted by many elderly and consume disproportionate amounts of health care resources. He has been criticized for his views but defends his ideas as an example of acknowledging the finite resources of society.

Lamm believes that other, more vulnerable groups, such as uninsured children, should be given a more equitable portion of health care services (e.g., well-baby clinics). Others argue that health care is already being rationed and that we should recognize this fact and articulate our priorities.

The state of Oregon has gone one step further, imposing guidelines on the type of care that its Medicaid funds will cover. Deciding that preventive care affects a majority of its citizens, Oregon made funding for such measures as immunizations and prenatal care a priority, whereas extraordinary care that benefits only a few individuals, such as a bone marrow transplantation, will not be covered (Rooks, 1990). This utilitarian approach, emphasizing the greatest good for the greatest number, is not without its critics, but it is an effort to provide direction for health care priorities. Oregon's plan was initially vetoed by the federal government and has undergone some revision, still emphasizing preventive care and treatment for disorders that affect a majority of citizens. Other states are now looking at the Oregon model as they plan health care reform.

Health Care Rationing. You may have already experienced situations of health care rationing or limited access. As a nurse you may, on one hand, feel powerless and frustrated when patients do not receive care because they cannot afford it or, on the other hand, feel angry because indigent patients are placing heavy burdens on both private and public facilities. Consider your values and professional responsibilities as you think through this issue. As an individual and a nurse, you need to take a stand regarding health resource allocation and support efforts to improve access, while determining in your mind what type of health care you believe to be ethically justifiable.

CONCLUSION

As medical technology advances, ethical issues and concerns will play an ever-increasing role in your nursing practice. The general public, the health care professions, religious traditions, and the legal system will all have influence in the attempts to resolve the ethical issues affecting health care in the 21st century. Keeping an open mind in these controversial dilemmas is difficult, but it is hoped you will examine your personal values and continue to make decisions that are based on the welfare of the patients.

REFERENCES

American Nurses Association (ANA): *Code of ethics for nurses*, Kansas City, Mo, 2001, ANA.

Chin AE et al: Legalized physician-assisted suicide in Oregon—the first year's experience, *N Engl J Med* 340(7):577-583, 1999.

Conner D: Assisted suicide ban in Washington struck down, *Los Angeles Times*, May 4, 1994:A, 17:1.

Feldman DM: *Marital relations, birth control and abortion in Jewish law*, New York, 1968, Schocker.

Fletcher JF: *Situation ethics*, Philadelphia, 1966, Westminster.

Holm S: The ethical case against stem cell research, *Cambridge Quarterly of Healthcare Ethics* 12, 372-383, 2003.

Hyde J: *Prosecutors drop assisted suicide charge against Kevorkian*, 1999, *http://detnews.com/1999/metro/9903/13/031301.htm.*

Lamm RD: Rationing of health care: the inevitable meets the unthinkable, *Nurs Pract* 11(5):57, 61-64, 1986.

Nagourney A: 44 million with no health insurance… and more to come, *NY Times*, Mar 23, 2005:A, 14.

New York Advance Legislative Service: Regular session, Ch 308, SB 1906, 1992.

Rooks JP: Let's admit we ration health care—then set priorities, *Am J Nurs* 90(6):38-43, 1990.

Rosen H (Ed.): *Abortion in America*, Boston, 1967, Beacon Press.

Rudy EB: The living will: are you informed?, *Focus Crit Care* 12(6):51, 1985.

Scanlon C: Ethics survey looks at nurses' experiences, *Am Nurse* 26(10):22, 1994.

Shapiro R: Legislative research bans on human cloning, *Cambridge Quarterly of Healthcare Ethics* 12, 393-400, 2003.

Steele SM: *Values clarification in nursing*, ed 2, East Norwalk, Conn, 1983, Appleton & Lange.

Steinhauser KE et al: Factors considered important at the end of life by patients, family, physicians, and other health care providers, *JAMA* 284(19): 2476-2482, 2000.

Trials of war criminals before the Nuremberg Military Tribunals under Control Council Law No. 18, vol 2, Nuremberg Code, Washington, DC, 1949, U.S. Government Printing Office.

CHAPTER 20

LEGAL ISSUES

ROBIN L. PERIN, RN, BS, JD

"The law is good, if a man use it lawfully."
—*The First Epistle of Paul the Apostle to Timothy 1:8*

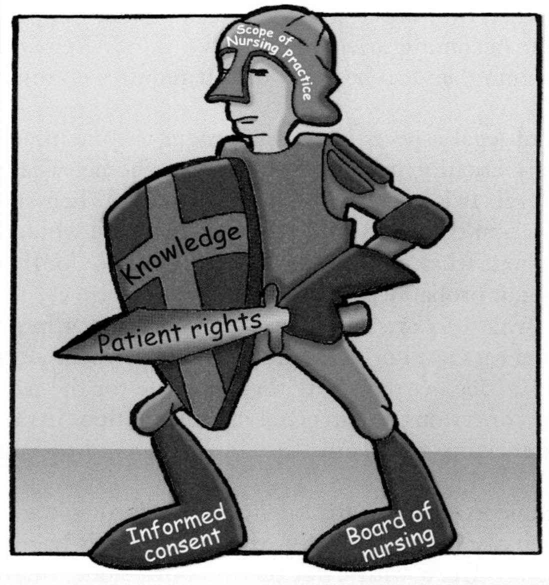

Knowledge regarding legal aspects is the best defense a nurse can have.

After completing this chapter, you should be able to:

- Discuss various sources and types of law.
- Relate the Nurse Practice Act to the governance of your profession.
- Understand the functions of a state board of nursing.
- Describe your responsibilities for obtaining and maintaining your license.
- Be able to identify the elements of nursing malpractice and how they are proved in a malpractice claim.
- Incorporate an understanding of legal risks into your nursing practice, and recognize how to minimize these.
- Identify legal issues involved in the medical record and your documentation, including the use of electronic medical records.
- Take an active role in improving the quality of health care as required by legal standards.
- Participate as a professional when dealing with nurses who are impaired or functioning dangerously in the work setting.
- Discuss the concerns surrounding at least two controversial legal issues in nursing practice.

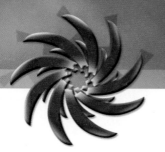

When you graduate and become a registered nurse, you will also be achieving a new status under the law. An example of this change is that after meeting certain criteria, you will have a license to practice nursing. This license sets certain standards that you must follow as a nurse in the state. Should you not live up to these standards, your state can take away your ability to practice as a nurse. Also as a professional, you may be sued. Of course, a person can always be sued if his behavior is negligent (unreasonable) and someone gets harmed. However, when you are working as a professional, the expectations for your behavior are higher than simply being a reasonable person. You are expected to perform as a reasonable nurse. If your actions are not what a reasonable nurse would do, and this causes someone to be injured, you can be sued in malpractice.

People react to these changes in legal status differently. Some nurses see the law as a big monster that is unpredictable, very frightening, and out to do them harm. They tend to act like ostriches and stick their heads in the sand whenever a legal subject is raised. If they become involved in a legal action, they are terrified and presume that terrible things will happen to them. Other nurses find the law to be quite interesting and attempt to learn all they can about how it may affect their practice. These nurses often find the law to be a very helpful tool to ensure safe practices. They also are much better able to protect themselves when they are dealing with legal issues. I hope that this chapter will be a start in your becoming a legally educated nurse. Remember, though, that the law is always changing, and to keep up with it requires continuous vigilance.

Before beginning a discussion of legal aspects in nursing, there is some practical advice that you can always use in any situation in which you wonder whether what you are doing or proposing to do is legal. It is called the "Mother Rule." When such a question about the legality of an action comes to you, ask yourself if you would feel comfortable telling your mother about what you are doing or propose to do. If your answer to this question is "no," then it probably is not legal. Why?

If you are uncomfortable with what you are doing, it may involve lying in some manner, which is involved in a claim for **fraud** or **defamation**. Perhaps you are doing something outside your scope of practice or something that is unsafe for the patient and could cause injury. These types of actions are involved in **malpractice. Invasion of privacy** and **breach of confidentiality** are claims that involve gossip or talking about patients unnecessarily.

In addition to the aforementioned, mothers are on juries. As jurors, they are instructed about laws, but they often cast their "votes" for what they think is "right" or "wrong." In every lawsuit, jurors are faced with evidence for both sides. In some respects, this forces them to simply make a human decision regarding the events. If you can feel comfortable when telling your mother (a jury) about what happened—truthfully and without hiding anything—then it is likely that you can do the same confidently with a jury. It is also likely that you will be believed and found to have acted reasonably. Simplified, that is all you need to do. Now let us address the more formal aspects of this thing called "law."

SOURCES OF LAW

WHERE DOES "THE LAW" COME FROM?

People will often tell you that you cannot do something because it is "illegal." Or, they will make a statement that the law is this or that. Some nurses, who are afraid of laws, will simply believe what they are told. Other nurses will ask, "What law?" This is an important question because there is often much misinformation regarding the law floating around institutions where nurses work.

The most common type of law affecting nurses is "**statutory law**" or "**statutes**" or "**laws**." These are the documented rules for living in your state (state laws) or the United States (federal laws) that are passed by state legislatures and by Congress. Statutes cover the rules for our relationships with each other and can be viewed as the ethics of our society written down. The section on definitions is one of the most important parts of a statute. There you can find what the authors of the statute mean when they use a certain word. Of course this is helpful because we all use words differently, but when reading laws, a more precise understanding is necessary. (Box 20-1 has a listing of definitions of common legal terms.)

BOX 20-1 Common Legal Terms

Advance directive: A document made by a competent individual to establish desired health care for the future or to give someone else the right to make health care decisions if the individual becomes incompetent; examples include living wills and medical powers of attorney.

Defamation: A civil wrong in which an individual's reputation in the community, including the professional community, has been damaged.

Defendant: The person who is being accused of wrongdoing. The person then must defend himself or herself against the charges. In a malpractice claim, the nurse or other health care provider.

Deposition: Out of court oral testimony given under oath before a court reporter. The purpose is to enable attorneys to ask and have answered questions related to a case. The deposition process may involve expert witnesses, fact witness, defendants, or plaintiffs. It may be used to impeach (find inconsistencies or untruths) testimony in trials.

Diversion program: A program for treatment and rehabilitation of substance abusers. Such programs may be used by boards of nursing for encouraging treatment but are independent of such boards.

Expert witness: A person who has specific knowledge, skills, and experience regarding a specific area and whose testimony will be allowed in court to prove the standard of care.

Good Samaritan law: Provides civil immunity to professionals who stop and render care in an emergency. Care rendered cannot be done so in a grossly negligent manner.

Continued

BOX 20-1 Common Legal Terms—cont'd

Interrogatory: A process of discovering the facts regarding a case through a set of written questions exchanged through the attorneys representing the parties involved in the case.
Jurisdiction: The court's authority to accept and decide cases. May be based on location or subject matter of the case.
Malpractice: Improper performance of professional duties; a failure to meet the standards of care that results in harm to another person.
Negligence: Failure to act as an ordinary prudent person when such failure results in harm to another.
Plaintiff: The person who files the lawsuit and is seeking damages for a perceived wrongdoing. In medical malpractice, the patient and/or the patient's family.
Reasonable care: The level of care or skill that is customarily rendered by a competent health care worker of similar education and experience in providing services to an individual in the community or state in which the person is practicing.
Standard of care: Standards based on various types of evidence as to what is reasonable and prudent behavior for a health care professional.
Statute of limitations: Laws that set time limits for when a case may be filed. Differ from state to state.
Telemedicine: Using telecommunication technology, usually interactive, to provide medical information and services.
Torts: Civil (not criminal) wrongs committed by one person against another person or property. Includes the legal principle of assault and battery.
Whistleblower: Individual "on the inside" who reports incorrect or illegal activities to an agency with authority to monitor or control those activities.
Whistleblower statute: Law that protects a whistleblower from retaliation. Usually involves specific criteria about how whistle was blown.

Nurse practice acts are examples of state statutory laws and can be easily found online, in a public library, or obtained from the state board of nursing. It would first be important to see how a "registered nurse" is defined in your state to see whether there is a clue there about what nurses can or cannot do. Usually, however, these laws are quite general and might not answer your specific question about whether registered nurses in your state can administer intravenous (IV) conscious sedation.

Hypothetical case study #1:

You are working in a hospital where a very well-known actor is admitted with a diagnosis of pneumocystic pneumonia. You know that this is usually associated with AIDS. During the patient's stay, you are asked by a physician to give an IV drug to sedate this patient while she does a procedure. The patient becomes oversedated, has a respiratory arrest, and dies. You are so upset about this that you call your best friend, who is also a nurse, to talk about the incident. You mention the actor's name and the fact that he had AIDS. Your friend says that it was "illegal" for you to be giving what he calls "IV conscious sedation," and you are in deep trouble. Where might you be able to search to determine whether this is true? What type of legal trouble might you have?

CRITICAL THINKING BOX 20-1

In hypothetical case study #1, can you identify where a constitutional law might have been broken?

The next type of law is constitutional law. This type of law refers to the rights, privileges, and responsibilities that were stated in, or have been inferred from, the U.S. Constitution, including the Bill of Rights. States may not pass laws or institute rules that conflict with constitutionally granted rights or rules because the Constitution is the highest law of our country. Freedom of speech and religion are such rights. The right to privacy is an example of a right inferred from the Constitution (Critical Thinking Box 20-1).

The third type of law to consider is a**dministrative law**. This body of law is made by administrative agencies that have been granted the authority to pass rules and regulations and render opinions, which usually explain in more detail the state statutes on a particular subject. Examples of this type of law are the rules and regulations passed by boards of nursing to control nursing practice in each state. This might well be a source for finding out specifically about nurses giving IV conscious sedation in your state. There may also be an "advisory opinion" given by the state board of nursing on this topic. Your state board of pharmacy may also have other regulations that describe their rules for administering medications and who may do this.

Another type of law is **common law**, which includes decisions made by judges in court cases or is established by rules of custom and tradition. **Case law** is composed of the decisions rendered in court cases by appeal courts. Often, nurses will hear about something happening in a court case and think that there must be a document somewhere talking about that case. This is not necessarily true, because not all cases reach the level of an appeal court, where a record of the court's opinion and reasoning is recorded. Cases are usually appealed to higher courts because there is an issue of statutory law involved. Many cases do not have such issues and are, therefore, not appealed or recorded.

Once there is a recorded court opinion, the result is the legal principle of ***stare decisis***, which means that if an issue has been decided, all other cases concerning the same issue should be decided the same way. Another word for this is **precedent**. Although you may hear of a case in which a nurse was found negligent in administering IV conscious sedation, there may not be case law on this issue to set a legal precedent in your state. Each state has its own case law. Each state's body of case law differs because it is based on the decisions of individual judges, who often do not resolve issues in the same way as judges in another state and who base their decisions on differing state statutes.

COURT ACTIONS BASED ON LEGAL PRINCIPLES

There are two major classifications of legal actions that can occur as a result of either deliberate or unintentional violations of legal rules or statutes. In the first category are **criminal actions**. These occur when you have done something that is considered harmful to society as a whole. The trials will involve a prosecuting attorney, who represents the interests of the state or the United States (the public), and a defense attorney, who represents the interests of the person accused of a crime (defendant). These actions can usually be identified by their title, which will read "*State v. [the name of the defendant]*" or "*U.S. vs. Smith [the name of the defendant]*." Examples include murder, theft, drug violations, and some violations of the Nursing Practice Acts such as misuse of narcotics. Serious crimes that can cause the perpetrator to be imprisoned are called **felonies**. Less-serious crimes resulting in fines are **misdemeanors.** The victim, if there is one, may sometimes be involved in a decision to prosecute a case, and sometimes not, and is considered only a witness in the criminal trial. Laws differ in states as to victim rights and/or if the person or the state will receive any of the money from fines. In the hypothetical case study #1, your actions would not likely result in a criminal action. Recently, however, there have been instances in which a nurse was thought to have recklessly caused a patient's death, and a case was brought in criminal court for negligent homicide. The issues involved in such criminal actions will be discussed later in this chapter.

In the second category of legal claims are **civil actions**. These actions concern private interests and rights between the individuals involved in the cases. Private attorneys handle these claims, and the remedy is usually some type of compensation that attempts to restore injured parties to their earlier positions. Examples of civil actions include malpractice, negligence, and informed consent issues. The victim (patient) or victim's family (patient's family) brings the lawsuit as the **plaintiff** against the **defendant** who may be the individual (nurse) or company (hospital) who is believed to have caused harm. In the situation presented, you might be sued for malpractice by the actor's spouse if it is felt that you acted below a standard of care and caused the actor's death.

Sometimes an event can have both criminal and civil consequences. When that happens, two trials are held with different goals. The amount of evidence required to support a guilty verdict is different for each type of trial. The criminal case requires that the evidence show that the defendant was guilty beyond a shadow of a doubt. The civil case requires only that the evidence show that the defendant was more likely guilty than not guilty. That is why you may see situations where someone such as O.J. Simpson can be found not guilty in the criminal trial, and "guilty" or negligent in the civil trial.

LEGAL CONTROL OVER NURSING PRACTICE

Having a license to practice nursing brings you into close contact with laws and government agencies. The nurse practice act is the statute governing nurses in your state. The board of nursing is the agency designated to apply the laws to individuals.

There are nurses who do not understand their responsibilities in relationship to their licensing board. Do not become one of these. State boards act under the police power granted each state from the federal government to protect the safety of its residents. Persons serving on such boards take this responsibility seriously. They expect that you will also.

Hypothetical case study #2:

After your incident with the actor, you decide to leave the state. You have to answer detailed questions on your licensure application for the new state about any previous malpractice claims.

You had heard something about a claim being filed against the hospital but had left shortly after that. Now you have received a notice from the state board of nursing of your previous residence inquiring about the incident with the actor and asking for a response within 2 weeks. The letter has taken a long time to be forwarded to you, and you have passed the deadline given to you. What should you do?

WHAT ARE THE LEGAL ASPECTS OF LICENSURE?

Receiving a license to practice nursing is a privilege, not a right. Even the successful completion of an educational program in nursing and/or passing the National Council Licensure Examination for Registered Nurses (NCLEX-RN) does not guarantee that a license will be granted. A license is granted by a state after a candidate has successfully met all the requirements in that particular state. Examples of these requirements may include high school education, successful completion of a nursing education program, application to the appropriate national and state agencies, fee payment, not being a felon (i.e., not having a criminal record), and passing the national examination for the appropriate level of licensure (NCLEX-RN or PN). Because the license is intended to guarantee public safety, the level of expertise necessary to pass the test is the minimum level needed to provide safe care. The state also continues to monitor your practice and to investigate complaints regarding this practice.

When you move to a new state, you need to make certain decisions with regard to your license. You may want to continue being licensed in the state of past residence. It is important to keep your past state board informed of your current residence so you receive important documents in a timely fashion that can affect your future ability to practice. You also need to be informed of licensure and practice requirements of a new state of residence before you begin to practice there.

Each state's practice act may be different from any other state's act. In the past, this has posed many hurdles for nurses who traveled or had practices across state lines. States have attempted to resolve these issues by developing a licensure model that will allow participating states to recognize licensure of another state. This works in the same manner as your state driver's license being recognized in other states, but your having to adhere to that state's driving laws. As of March 2005, 19 states had passed laws to accept the Nurse Licensure Compact, or the Mutual Recognition Model (National Council of State Boards of Nursing [NCSBN], 2005). You can practice in those states if your home state is part of the model.

If you travel to another state, or cross state lines in the normal course of your practice, either with a specific patient or to perform some nursing services in another state, you need to check with the board of nursing in the states in which you are performing nursing care to determine their rules about practice within their borders. An example of this would be telephone triage or telemedicine programs with patients outside of your state. You can obtain copies of a state practice act from the board of nursing or licensing agency for nurses in that state (see Appendix A for addresses of state boards of nursing).

Some practice acts regulate nursing by controlling who may use the titles "Registered Nurse" and "Licensed Practical Nurse" or "Licensed Vocational Nurse." Others regulate by controlling the scope of practice and determining the specific activities for each level of nursing—that is, who can perform what functions. In most states, the nurse practice act does the following:

1. Describes how to obtain licensure and enter practice within that state.
2. Describes how and when to renew your license.
3. Defines the educational requirements for entry into practice.
4. Provides definitions and scope of practice for each level of nursing practice.
5. Describes the process by which individual members of the board of nursing are selected and the categories of membership.
6. Identifies situations that are grounds for discipline or circumstances in which a nursing license can be revoked or suspended.
7. Identifies the process for disciplinary actions, including diversionary techniques.
8. Outlines the appeal steps if the nurse feels the disciplinary actions taken by the board of nursing are not fair or valid.

Some practice acts are very specific and detailed, others simply grant the board authority to declare the rules and regulations (administrative law) and to establish the details. To understand the scope of practice within a specific state in which you are practicing or wish to practice, you must obtain a copy of the state's nurse practice act that includes the law, rules, and regulations that the board or administrative agency has established in that state.

Because you have gone to a great deal of expense and work to obtain your nursing license, you should guard it carefully. Never ignore or take lightly any document received from your state board of nursing. Even if you think you have received a notice in error, contact the board of nursing immediately (Box 20-2).

The power of the board to discipline is the power that can have an adverse effect on the nurse's ability to practice. It is important that each nurse carefully review the power of the Board within the state of their practice. Several levels of disciplinary actions can occur based on the severity of the problem. Boards of nursing have the authority to censure, to suspend, to revoke, or to deny licensure. Each of these actions can be temporary or permanent. It would be prudent to consult an attorney who is versed in health care law if you should receive notice of any possible action against your license.

BOX 20-2 Protect Your License

- Do not let anyone else borrow it.
- Do not let anyone copy it unless you write "copy" across it. In some states it is illegal to copy your license.
- If you lose it, report it immediately and take the necessary steps to obtain a duplicate.
- Be sure that the Board of Nursing knows whenever you change your address, whether you move across the street or across the nation.
- Practice nursing according to the scope and standards of practice in your state.
- Know your state law so you will not do anything that could cause you to be disciplined by the removal of your license.
- Meet all renewal requirements on time.

Such a person can be your advocate and explain your rights and how best to deal with the state board. Seeking legal advice is an investment to protect your investment. Some institutions assist nurse employees in these instances, and some nurse insurance policies will also defend nurses in these "administrative actions."

WHAT ABOUT THE IMPAIRED NURSE?

Impaired nurses are nurses who are unable to function effectively because of some type of substance abuse (i.e., alcohol, prescription drugs, illegal drugs). More attention is currently being given to this area because of the heightened awareness of substance abuse in our society as a whole, in addition to the increasing recognition of the severity of the problem among health care workers. One of the most common reasons for state board action against nurses involves the taking of hospital medications for personal use (Brent, 2001). Boards of nursing are increasingly concerned about this issue, because it has significant impact on rendering safe, effective patient care (NCSBN, 2001). Some states will also discipline a nurse who knows about but fails to report an impaired nurse. Yet, in a recent study, it was found that only 37% of nurses who had experiences of working with an impaired colleague reported them to supervisors (Beckstead, 2002). "Helping the impaired nurse is difficult, but not impossible. The choices for action are varied. The only choice that is clearly wrong is to do nothing" (NCSBN, 2001). You are never doing a colleague a favor by not reporting impairment. A dead patient at the hands of an impaired nurse is a terrible outcome if it could have been prevented.

Do not ever assume that you or your colleagues are immune from impairment. High stress and easy access to drugs seem to contribute to this common problem for health care providers. There is a slippery slope that occurs when a nurse first takes any medication, even an aspirin, that does not belong to him or her. It is best to see that first wrong as a prelude to many future wrongs and never do it. If you do find yourself in trouble with drugs or alcohol, it is far better to voluntarily report this to your state board of nursing, rather than to be caught or to harm other persons. Most boards react favorably to the nurse who seeks assistance, rather than one who is reported by law enforcement agencies or a hospital as required by law.

Many states have taken a rehabilitative approach to this problem, rather than a punitive one, particularly to those who self-report (Brent, 2001; Nursefriendly, Inc., 2005). These states have programs set up to allow nurses to meet specific behavioral criteria, such as blood or urine testing, ordered evaluations, and attendance at rehabilitation programs, either while disciplinary action is being taken or instead of bringing formal proceedings. The primary concern is to assist the impaired nurse back to full and appropriate nursing practice. If a nurse is involved in a voluntary rehabilitation program through a contract with a state board and backslides or has additional problems, the board may bring formal action against the nurse that will negatively affect licensure for the rest of his or her life and can also involve criminal sanctions.

WHO KNOWS ABOUT THE DISCIPLINARY ACTIONS AGAINST NURSES?

When an action is taken by a state board against a nurse, states have differing methods of reporting such action to health care providers and others to protect the public. **NURSYS** is a comprehensive electronic information system that includes the collection and warehousing of nurse licensing information and disciplinary actions. Previously called NIS and ELVIS, as it underwent different stages of development, the term "NURSYS" is a derivative of "nurse" and "system." NURSYS contains data on a nurse's personal information (identity, residence), license information, education information, disciplinary action information, verification and fee tracking requests, and historical information (any changes to the aforementioned data). NURSYS is the information system that supports the mutual recognition of nurses' licenses. In 2003, NURSYS announced that it would be available to the public for nursing license verification. Nurses can also access the system to provide nursing license verification for a fee of $30.00 (NCSBN, 2003).

Another national storehouse of information is The National Practitioner Data Bank, which was part of a federal law under Medicare called The Health Care Quality Improvement Act. Although initially set up to identify physicians who had committed malpractice and/or who had licensure problems across state lines, it now extends to many licensed individuals, including nurses. Information related to malpractice payments made on behalf of a nurse and licensing actions are required to be made by professional insurance companies, federal and state agencies, and health care institutions (National Practitioner Data Bank [NPDB], 2004).

TORTS

Civil, as opposed to criminal, actions are also called torts. Remember that civil actions occur when a plaintiff files a lawsuit to receive compensation for damages he or she suffered as a result of a perceived wrong. The economic reason for filing the suit should never be forgotten. This is important to keep in mind should you or a colleague become involved in a tort action. Try not to interpret everything in terms of a personal insult and/or an intentional desire to cause you personal and professional harm. This is not a criminal action, and the terms "guilty" or "innocent" are not appropriate, nor are words such as "killed" that can sometimes be heard in the gossip mill or read in the media.

There are two categories of tort actions. Unintentional torts are those that usually involve an inadvertent, unreasonable act that causes harm to someone. We might call these acts "incidents" or "accidents." Intentional torts are those acts done deliberately by a defendant. Although sometimes occurring in the heat of a moment, they are not considered accidental in nature.

NURSING MALPRACTICE

The most common unintentional tort action brought against nurses is a malpractice claim.

According to the NPDB 2003 report, 16,339 nurses and nursing-related practitioners had a report made against them between the years 1990 to 2003. This represents claims where payment is made on behalf of a specifically named nurse and so does not touch upon the number of claims naming only a facility, yet involving nursing actions. Because malpractice can potentially affect every nurse, it is important to explore what this means.

Hypothetical case study #3:
You are a nurse working in a hospital. The physician tells you that you need to give an injection of Vistaril (hydroxine pamoate). You make sure that the order is documented in the medical record. The medication comes up from the pharmacy, and you check it against the physician's order and find it to be correct. You walk into the patient's room and use at least two patient identifiers to make sure it is the right patient. You give the injection in the patient's right upper outer quadrant of the buttocks and document this in the medical record.

The patient leaves the hospital. A year later you are told that a lawsuit has been filed against the hospital by the patient. It seems the patient is claiming that the injection you gave him caused sciatic nerve damage and his whole leg is numb (Critical Thinking Box 20-2).

LEGAL COMMENTARY

Many times nurses worry about being sued for something when, in the eyes of the law, no malpractice has occurred. Not all poor outcomes are malpractice. A nurse also may legitimately make an error in judgment. Therefore, it is important for a nurse to know the basic elements that must be proved before malpractice can occur. Then the nurse can evaluate incidents realistically.

BASIC ELEMENTS OF MALPRACTICE

What Are the Basic Elements of Malpractice?

1. You must have a duty. In other words there must be a professional nurse-patient relationship.
2. You must have breached that duty. In other words you must have fallen below the standard of care for a nurse.
3. Your breach of duty must have been a foreseeable cause of the patient's injury.
4. Damages or injury must have occurred.

These four elements need to be present in each malpractice case. The job of the patient's (plaintiff's) attorney is to prove to a jury that each element has occurred. Your attorney, on the other hand, defends you by proving that all or even just one element

CRITICAL THINKING BOX 20-2

Who may have malpractice liability in this situation and why? You? The physician? The hospital? What defenses may be available to you?

did not happen. This is not always a black and white process, which can often be frustrating and confusing. Still, it is important for the nurse to evaluate events in light of these elements and to know how they are proved in court.

Do You Have a Professional Duty? To make a claim of malpractice against a nurse, the plaintiff must establish that there is a nurse/patient relationship, or in legal terms, that you had a professional duty to a patient. A duty is implied if you are employed by and render services at a health care institution such as a hospital or nursing home. This would also be true if you work as a registered nurse for a home health agency in the home, or in a school, or in a physician's office.

In the case studies, you are working as a nurse in a hospital, and the nurse-patient relationship is implied. Therefore, the first element can easily be proved. What if you are giving medical advice in your home informally as a friend, relative, or neighbor? In this setting, it is not implied that you are acting as a nurse; and proving that you owed your friend a duty as a professional might be difficult. There is no payment, or institution, or formal contract. Therefore, although nurses are continually warned about being sued in this situation, it is unlikely that a plaintiff's attorney would easily prevail on the element of duty for such casual comments to others outside your employment.

What if you stop at an accident to assist someone who is injured? Because most states want to encourage medical professionals to help people at accidents without fear of a lawsuit, Good Samaritan Statutes have been passed. These laws give immunity from malpractice to those professionals who attempt to give assistance at the scene of an accident. In essence, you do not have any professional duty to stop, although you may feel an ethical duty to do so. If you do, know that in most—if not all—states you cannot be sued in malpractice for what you might or might not do. That is, you do not have a professional standard of care to adhere to unless you are a professional at the scene as part of your employment. All persons, of course, are expected not to leave the victim in a position that is more dangerous than when you found them.

Sometimes nurses volunteer to give nursing assistance at sports events or other activities in which it is foreseen that professional services may be needed. In thinking about this, you may see that such a situation is not quite as clear as other situations. If you are at a first aide station and/or wear a badge indicating you are a nurse, then you have an appearance that you are a professional, and people may rely on that when seeking advice or assistance. Some states give immunity to professionals under these circumstances by statute (Arizona Revised Statutes §32-1472).

> It is important to know your status under such circumstances in your state, and/or if you have immunity and/or are covered by malpractice insurance.

What Is the Professional Duty Owed? Once it is established that you owe a duty to the person, the question becomes what is that duty? How does a plaintiff's attorney establish what the duty might be? A nurse's duty owed is different than that of a physician or nursing assistant. The duty of a nurse will be to act as a reasonable nurse under the same or similar circumstances. The duty or standard of care for the physician will be to act as a reasonable physician. You can see that the two will be different. Of course, the most interesting question in any malpractice case will be how will my attorney prove that I acted as a reasonable nurse? The following will be considered when attempting to establish through evidence what the standard of care for the nurse might be.

What About the Nurse Practice Act? Perhaps the most important guideline for nurses will be the nurse practice act in the state in which you are practicing. Most acts describe in fairly general terms what a nurse may do. Prohibitions, or things that are considered unprofessional conduct, are usually more specific. A violation of such a license prohibition means that you have fallen below a standard of care set by the state for nurses. It also may mean that you risk an action against your license. If you do not know what these prohibitions are, then you are putting yourself in jeopardy. As stated previously, and applied here to the standard of care, be sure to keep up with your licensing standards.

What Is an Expert Witness? The most common way to establish the duty owed by a nurse is by the testimony of a registered nurse usually, but not always, with training and background similar to yours. This expert witness will then testify regarding what a reasonable nurse in the same or similar circumstances would be expected to do, and that you did not do it. If a plaintiff's attorney cannot find an expert nurse to testify that you did not act reasonably, then in most instances the case cannot go forward. In general, a patient cannot simply claim professional malpractice without having a professional witness to prove this.

In the same manner, if the plaintiff has an expert witness to prove you fell below the standard of care, you will need an expert witness to testify that you did not. Some nurses enjoy being expert witnesses either for the defense of a nurse, or as part of the plaintiff's claim against a nurse. Either role requires both integrity and professionalism to be effective and believed by a jury (Di Luigi, 2004).

There is a type of malpractice case in which an expert is not required. This type of claim is called *res ipsa loquitur*, or "the thing speaks for itself." This claim is very difficult to prove, because the patient must have enough evidence to show that: (1) the injury would ordinarily not occur unless someone were negligent; (2) the instrumentality causing the injury was within the exclusive control of the defendant; and (3) the incident was not owing to any voluntary action on the part of the plaintiff. If a patient can prove that all of these exist, the burden then shifts to the defendant nurse to prove that malpractice did not take place. Incidents such as operating on the wrong body part or leaving a surgical sponge in a patient fall into this category of claims.

What Are Established Policies and Procedures? Policies and procedures established by the institution in which you work are most crucial pieces of evidence for establishing a standard of care. Most good plaintiffs' attorneys will request a set of hospital policies as soon as a lawsuit is filed. For instance, in hypothetical case studies #1 and #3, a lawyer might ask for the hospital's policies on documentation and administration of medications. If you did not follow that policy, then you fell below a standard of care set by your institution.

You can see why you need to know and read the policies within your health care facility or corporation. These policies should also be a resource when you have questions about how to do certain procedures, or what your rights are in a certain situation. Policies are the laws under which you must live. It is also important for you as a professional to participate in making or changing policies so that they accurately reflect what nurses are doing in your institution. In addition, the policies set standards for giving quality and consistent patient care. If you have followed a policy, it can also be used proactively to prove that you followed the standard of care set by your institution.

What About Accreditation and Facility Licensing Standards? Most health care facilities and other health care organizations such as health maintenance organizations (HMOs) must go through a process whereby they become licensed and/or accredited. The Joint Commission for Accreditation of Healthcare Organizations (JCAHO) and the National Committee of Quality Assurance (NCQA) are two such organizations that set standards for health care organizations. These standards can often be used as evidence of the standard of care for nurses working in such facilities. For instance, the JCAHO has issued National Patient Safety Goals for 2005 that include standards to improve patient identification by requiring the use of two sources of identity not including the patient's room number (JCAHO, 2005). A state facility licensing requirement might be that the facility develop policies and procedures that govern the safe administration of drugs and that "each dose of medication administered shall be recorded in the patient's medication record and shall show the date, time, dosage, and method of administration and a method of identifying the person who administered the dose" (Arizona Administrative Code R4-23-660). Should a malpractice claim involving medications occur, the patient's attorney in Arizona will require proof that you have followed these requirements.

What About Textbooks and Journals? If you become a defendant in a lawsuit, you may be asked about texts used in the workplace such as the ***Physician's Desk Reference (PDR)***. You may also be asked whether you subscribe to a nursing journal. Articles or portions of such publications may be used as evidence of the standard of care for nurses to follow. For instance, if a nursing journal has published a recent article on correct administration of intramuscular injections, that may be used to demonstrate what you should have done. The fact that a PDR is available on a nursing unit might be used to demonstrate that a source for the correct dose of any medication and its correct administration was/is immediately available to you where you work.

What Are Professional Standards for Organizations? Professional organizations such as the American Nurses Association (ANA) or the Association of Perioperative Registered Nurses (APRN) may publish certain standards or practice guidelines. These may also be used as evidence for what a reasonable nurse should do under certain circumstances. If you are ever part of a group that sets professional standards, be sure that the standards are practical and reasonable. Knowing they can be used against nurses in malpractice claims explains why using unattainable ideals for standards, although sounding nice, can be harmful. Such standards can also be used to demonstrate that the nurse did or did not follow the standard of care.

In summary, there are many different types of evidence used by plaintiff attorneys to demonstrate an expected standard of care. The nurse needs to remember that these same documents can be used to demonstrate that you did follow the standard of care. Let us see how.

Applying the Standard of Care to the Case Study In the hypothetical case study #3, the plaintiff will have to find a nurse that will testify to the correct method of giving intramuscular injections. If you did not give the injection in such a manner, then the jury can infer that you did not act reasonably. However, if the correct method is to give the injection intramuscularly in the upper, outer, quadrant of the buttocks and you have documented that you did this, an expert's testimony will not help prove anything. Also, if you can show that you followed hospital policies in the administration of the medication, again, there will be no proof of falling below a standard of care.

What if the patient attempts to claim a case using the theory of *res ipsa loquitur*? Again, the patient's lawyer must prove that the claimed injury could not have happened unless there was negligence. As demonstrated earlier, you would be able to prove through your documentation that you were not negligent. In addition, your attorney would also be demonstrating your lack of liability through the third element of malpractice. Do you remember what that is?

Was There a Breach of Professional Duty? Not only must a plaintiff prove what the standard of care is in a given situation, the plaintiff must prove that you did not meet the standard of care. Other legal terms used regarding this needed element might be that you "fell below the standard of care" or you "breached the duty owed the patient." In other words, the plaintiff must demonstrate through the evidence listed earlier that you did not act as a reasonable and prudent nurse under the circumstances. Please remember that even if you did not act reasonably, there are other elements that must be proved to have a malpractice claim.

Did the Breach of Duty Cause the Injury? Causation is an element often overlooked by the nurse, and yet is most often hotly argued by attorneys. Did the difficult birth cause the child to have cerebral palsy or did a genetic birth defect cause the baby to have a difficult delivery? Was the injury caused by the auto accident or by the medical care? Did the patient have the physical problem before the medical care or after? Was the injury caused subsequently by the patient's lack of compliance with the treatment plan, or did the patient subsequently injure herself after the medical care was rendered?

The causation requirement must be proved by the plaintiff's attorney, and as you can imagine, this may not be easy. Certain well-documented observations will make such proof impossible.

1. Clearly document the patient's physical and mental condition upon admittance to and discharge from your health care facility or unit. Both of these observations can be used to demonstrate that either the patient had the symptom when she came and/or did not have the symptom upon leaving. Therefore, whatever happened during her stay in your unit or facility did not cause the problem.
2. After any incident, such as a patient fall, the patient's physical and mental condition must be documented. This will help demonstrate that subsequent complaints cannot be attached or caused by the incident.
3. Document clearly any actions of a patient that demonstrate noncompliance with medical directives. When a patient states or clearly demonstrates that he is not taking medications as ordered or is not following a prescribed physical therapy regimen, this can cause therapeutic failure, rather than the treatment itself. A documented "no show" at an outpatient clinic can dispel later claims that you ignored complaints and so caused the injury.
4. Document clearly when a patient complains and does not complain. If, in the case study #3, it is documented that the patient has been up and walking after the injection and has no complaints, it will be very difficult to prove that the injection caused the problem.

5. Be very careful when documenting what a patient states as opposed to what you think may have happened. If a patient states that an injection caused a problem, it is best to document clearly "Patient states, 'My leg has felt numb since I received an injection in the hospital,'" rather than document, "Hospital injection caused patient's leg to be numb." The latter documentation may inadvertently be condemning a health care provider who has done nothing wrong.
6. Document the patient's own admissions. "I knew I shouldn't have gotten out of bed so soon" can be helpful if a patient falls and then later tries to blame the nursing staff. "My wife tried to remove the stitches, but she could not get that deep one" can raise doubt regarding what caused the incision to become infected. Infection is very rarely considered to be malpractice unless it can be proved to have been caused by negligence such as not using good aseptic technique.
7. Document clearly discharge instructions. In today's managed-care environment, many acutely ill patients are sent home to care for themselves. If they and/or their families have not been given clear instructions on not only their care, but also symptoms to watch for that may need immediate medical attention, they may attempt to blame health care professionals for what occurs at home. A clear, documented discharge plan after any procedure that can have adverse outcomes is imperative, not only to prevent law suits, but for good patient care. A warning to a patient to call a specific number if adverse symptoms occur can save a life and prevent a lawsuit. Emergency departments have long understood the importance of such instructions and the age of specialized computer software programs makes them easily accessible to everyone. Even veterinarians are able to do computerized discharge planning for pets (Figure 20-1).

A patient's allergies or lack thereof is another way of preventing a malpractice claim. Neither nurses nor physicians cause patient's to have allergies. They do have a duty to not give medications to patients when previous experience has demonstrated that the medication has caused an allergic reaction. "No known allergies" can completely eliminate a claim involving an allergic reaction.

APPLYING "CAUSATION" TO THE CASE STUDY

Returning to the case example, the patient will have to prove that your injection caused the numbness in his leg. There are many intervening factors that could have caused this numbness. You do not have to prove anything because you, as a defendant, do not have the "burden of proof." The plaintiff may have a very difficult time, especially if there are no documented complaints by the patient of problems at the time of the injection or shortly thereafter.

Just remember that a patient's claim that you or another provider caused some particular injury or problem should not automatically be assumed to be true. Although you do not have to argue the point with the patient, you also do not have to agree. Injuries have many causes and many stories behind them.

- Document the facts.
- Document what you see and do.
- Your role is to render nursing services, not to judge.
- Leave the determination of fault to the courts.
- Your actions and truthful documentation will be your best defense.

SAGUARO CANYON PET CLINIC

8959 E. Tanque Verde	Invoice Nbr: 011365
Tucson, Arizona 85777	Date: February 14, 1996
520/999-9999	Doctor: Kitty Friend
Client Number: 975	Home telephone: 999-9999

Iam A. Goodguy	Animal: Lexie
1234 N. Paseo	Species: Feline
Tuscon, AZ 85777	Altered: Yes
	Breed: Manx
	Age: 1 Year
	Sex: Male

HEALTH CARE MESSAGES

February 14, 1996

Your pet has had an operation that requires special precautions and follow-up care at home under your supervision. These are covered in the instructions below. A decreased appetite for one or two days may be normal. However, if any of the following symptoms should occur, please contact our office:

(1) Loss of appetite for over two days.
(2) Refusal to drink water for over one day.
(3) Depression.
(4) Elevated or sub-normal temperature.
(5) Diarrhea.
(6) Vomiting.

It is very important, and your responsibility as the owner, to follow the instructions below to ensure a satisfactory recovery for your pet.

DIET:	Feed your pet his/her regular diet.
ACTIVITY:	Restrict activity for 10 days to inside the house or on other clean, dry, confined area. Replace litter in catbox with thin strips of shredded newspaper to protect paws.
CARE OF PAWS:	Check paws twice daily for any signs of excessive licking or separation of surgery incision sites. Keep claws clean and dry. Call us if you are unable to discourage chewing or if the paws are excessively tender or your cat is lame.
MEDICATION:	Give antibiotic medication as directed on perscription label twice daily.
POST-SURGERY:	We suggest that the declawed cat be kept indoors for its protection; although the escape mechanisms are still functional, your pet may not be able to defend itself adequately outdoors.

If you have any questions or problems, please call us at 999-9999.
Thank you.

FIGURE 20-1
Even veterinarians are able to do computerized discharge planning for pets.

Did the Patient Suffer Damages or Injury? The last element that must be proved is that your breach of duty caused injury to the patient. This last element of malpractice can also be overlooked, as the nurse becomes embroiled in the fact that a mistake has been made. For instance, in many cases of medication error, the patient is not permanently harmed, because a single dose of most medications will not cause a permanent change. This does not mean that medication errors should be taken lightly or that some medications cannot cause death with a single mistake. They can. It only means that it is very unlikely that a malpractice claim will be brought for a medication error that does not cause injury.

Damages can be viewed as the sum of money a court or jury awards as compensation for a tort action. **General damages** are those given for intangibles such as pain and suffering, disfigurement, interference with ordinary enjoyment of life, and loss of consortium (marital services) that are inherent in the injury itself (Guido, 2001). **Special damages** are the patient's out-of-pocket expenses such as medical care, lost wages, and rehabilitation costs. **Punitive damages** are those damages that seek to punish those whose conduct goes beyond normal malpractice. Claims in which this might occur are rare, but they involve issues such as changed medical records, lies being told to patients, or intentional misconduct while under the influence of alcohol or drugs. Such punitive awards can add millions of dollars to an otherwise low-damage claim. Some states have limited the amount for specific types of damages that a plaintiff can receive (Critical Thinking Box 20-3).

For a malpractice plaintiff's attorney to take a claim to trial, it may cost that person more than $100,000 and this does not count the attorney's time. Malpractice claims take much expertise and are time intensive (Larson, 2005). Because malpractice claims are brought on a contingency fee basis, the attorney will get paid only if he/she wins the claim. In this situation the damages must be greater than the costs to make the claim worthwhile. When worrying about an incident and whether or not a suit will result, it is helpful to understand what factors make claims worthwhile.

1. In the majority of claims, the most important factor involved with damages is the age of the patient. The younger the patient with a permanent injury, the longer will be the time of suffering, the costs of future medical care, the loss of wages or income, and the emotional loss to the family. Therefore, to assess damages, the first question an attorney asks is the age and status of an individual. An 83-year-old widower who has a numb leg will not have a large claim for damages. He will not lose wages. He does not have to support a family. It is likely that he has other illnesses or physical problems that might contribute to difficulty with ambulating. His life expectancy is not great. A 30-year-old single mother with three dependent children who has made her living as a waitress might well have costly damages if a numb leg hinders her ability to walk and provide for her family. However, in recent years, claims by nursing home patients have become more common because of statutes involving abuse of "vulnerable adults." These statutes can give plaintiffs triple damages and other monetary awards, including the right to "punitive damages," thus making these claims very attractive to attorneys.

CRITICAL THINKING BOX 20-3

Does your state limit the amount of damages a plantiff can receive?

2. **The nature of the injury** is also a consideration in evaluating damages. Is the injury permanent? Is it one for which a jury will have great sympathy, as when there is a huge disfiguring facial scar? Is it one that demonstrates a blatant mistake such as surgery performed on the wrong limb?
3. Does the claim involve any act of **malicious misconduct** or an **intentional cover up**? Such acts inflame juries and can cause them to award punitive damages.

Again, the principles of good documentation can make the damages of a claim not worth pursuing. It is particularly important that there is accurate evidence of damages at the time the injury occurred. Any time there is an incident involving a patient, such as a fall, an immediate and thorough examination can greatly assist in substantiating the patient's condition and thus, damages. The examination and findings need to be accurately documented. Subsequent examinations and evaluations should be completed. Documentation of the patient's complaints, or lack of complaints, at the time of an incident can prove extremely beneficial. A simple, "no complaints" or "denies pain" will refute a patient's later claim that "I was terribly injured by the fall."

Sometimes when a clear mistake has been made that falls below the standard of care and has caused an injury, your attorney will admit negligence. This is often a relief to the nurse who does not wish to try to defend a mistake and/or not tell the truth. The case is then brought solely on the amount of damages. Often the patient's perception of the injury is greatly augmented. Usually the patient will have to go through what is called an "independent medical examination" (IME) to substantiate injury.

Damages Applied to the Case Study. In the case study, numbness of a limb may be difficult to prove. Nerve conduction studies may be performed in an independent medical examination to demonstrate that the injection could not have caused the neurologic injury of which the patient complains. Numbness also does not mean lack of function and would not usually prevent any activity of daily living. Again, the age and status of the claimant would play an important role, as would your documentation of the patient's lack of complaints and ability to ambulate.

WHO MIGHT HAVE LIABILITY (RESPONSIBILITY) IN A CLAIM?

Hypothetical case study #4:

You are a nurse working on a surgical unit in a hospital. One evening you are asked to float to pediatrics. The only experience you have with children happened when you were a student. A physician asks you to give digoxin to an infant and writes an order for 2 cc. This seems like a lot of medication to you, so you ask the head nurse on the unit about the dose. The head nurse assumes you are speaking about an oral dose of the medication and states that this is normal. You give the medication by injection and shortly thereafter the child's heart stops beating and he is coded. When you attempt to use an Ambu bag, it is not on the crash cart. The child eventually recovers. Twenty-one years later, you receive notice that a young man is suing you for giving him the wrong dose of digoxin when he was an infant.

Personal Liability. There is often confusion about who can be held accountable for your actions as a nurse. You may hear things such as, "Don't worry, I'll take responsibility for this." Understand that in the eyes of the law, each individual is accountable for their own actions. There is no defense called "She made me do it." Even if you are not personally named in a lawsuit, you will be asked to give evidence regarding your involvement and will have to be able to defend your actions under oath. "I was just following orders" does not explain why you as a professional made a medication error. You are held to a professional standard of care to know about the medications you are administering, including the correct dose. In hypothetical case study #4, you may be named, and would most likely have liability.

Physician and Other Independent Practitioner Liability. For many years, physicians were seen as "The Captain of the Ship" and thus ultimately responsible for everything that happened to the patient. This doctrine is no longer true. Unfortunately, some physicians still mislead nurses by ordering them to do things and then assuring them that they will assume any risk involved. Although nurses do have a duty to follow physician's orders under most circumstances, this is never true if the nurse believes or has reason to believe that the order is unsafe for the patient, or not within the nurse's scope of practice. In hypothetical case study #1, giving an order for the nurse to give IV conscious sedation does not relieve the nurse of a duty to determine whether this is within his or her scope of practice. If not, the order must be refused. In hypothetical case study #4, if the nurse did not know the correct dose of digoxin, there was a duty to look up the correct dose. It is also true that if the physician's order is wrong, or done in a negligent manner such as in the hypothetical, it does not relieve the physician from having liability in addition to the nurse.

In instances when a nurse is hired directly by a physician to work in an office practice, the physician, as the employer, can be held vicariously liable on a theory of ***respondeat superior***. This is a Latin term meaning that the master is responsible for acts of the servant, translated in modern day to "the employer is responsible for the acts of the employee." The physician, then, rather than the nurse, may be named in the lawsuit. Remember, though, that you will still have to answer for your actions.

Another issue is what the nurse should accept as delegated or ordered by other independent health care practitioners, such as nurse practitioners (NPs), and physician assistants (PAs). States may have different rules about who can give orders to the RN.

The general rule is that the RN can accept orders from other licensed health care providers who are working within their scope of practice. To be sure about your state, contact the board of nursing. When accepting delegated duties, remember that you should only accept duties you are competent to carry out and that are within your scope of practice.

Supervisory Liability. Questions often arise regarding the nurse's responsibility for acts of those working under him or her. The standard of care for a supervisor is to act as a reasonable supervisor under the same or similar circumstances. A supervisor can be expected to ensure the following:

- The task was properly assigned to a worker competent to safely perform it.
- Adequate supervision was provided to the worker if needed.
- The nurse provided appropriate follow-up and evaluation of the delegated task.

As in hypothetical case study #3, a supervisor could be expected to more closely supervise a float nurse or a recent graduate than someone who is an experienced nurse on a pediatric unit. It is also incumbent upon a person being supervised to ask for assistance if they are faced with a problem for which they lack the necessary skills to resolve. In hypothetical case study #4, this was done, but the nurse administering the medication and the supervisor miscommunicated on the method or route of administration. Do you think this can happen?

Delegation of nursing duties to unlicensed health care workers presents supervisory nurses with some special risks. Changes in health care delivery systems and financing are resulting in some unfamiliar categories of unlicensed caregivers with a wide variety of skills and expertise. Some boards of nursing have informed their licensees that each nurse remains personally liable for any task delegated to an unlicensed worker on the theory that the delegated task is considered the nurse's responsibility, rather than within the scope of practice of the unlicensed worker. Other boards of nursing have stated that they will apply to delegation the traditional standards for supervising any health care worker as described earlier.

Certain nursing responsibilities, such as nursing diagnosis, assessment, some portions of planning, evaluation, and documentation, and teaching, should not be delegated to unlicensed staff. Contact the board of nursing in your state to better understand your responsibilities in the delegation of nursing duties.

Institutional Liability. As in the aforementioned case involving physician liability, health care institutions such as hospitals are usually sued under a theory of ***respondeat superior*** for the actions of their employees. An institution cannot really do or not do any act that can cause a lawsuit except through its employees or agents. That is why almost all health care institutions carry insurance to cover the acts and omissions of their employees. Otherwise, a corporation could go bankrupt if sued. For the most part, institutions and not individual nurses, are named defendants in a lawsuit, but again this does not relieve the nurse from having to formally answer to the court for his or her own actions or inaction. An institution's policies or lack thereof is also a common claim in a lawsuit. For instance, there can be a claim in hypothetical case study #4 that the institution should have had a policy on floating nurses to other units in the hospital, and that such persons should never be given the responsibility of taking off physician's orders. Additionally, in case study #4, there may be institutional liability through the pharmacy. If the pharmacy filled the wrong medication dose, and there are systems in place to check dosages, the pharmacist and/or technician may also be brought into the claim through the institution. There are certainly more systems in place in most hospitals to prevent medication errors than ever before. When they all fail, many persons can be involved in the liability.

Student Liability. Nursing students have responsibility for their own actions and can be liable (Guido, 2001). Again, the adage that "students practice under their instructor's license" is not true. As a student you may have an instructor supervising you closely in the early stages of your education, but at the end of your program, it is likely that you will have less supervision. Student nurses at all times will be held to the standard of an RN for the tasks they perform (Guido, 2001). It is, therefore, important that students never accept assignments beyond their preparation and that they communicate frequently with their instructors for assistance and guidance.

Instructors are responsible for reasonable and prudent clinical supervision, a standard that may be higher than other worker supervision because of the student's lack of experience.

Nurses performing as preceptors for students have the same supervisor liability they have for any other worker.

Instructors and preceptors need to remember that the level of expertise of individual students may vary, and the standard used to evaluate the student's performance usually requires more supervision than some more experienced workers may need.

WHAT DEFENSES MIGHT BE AVAILABLE IN MALPRACTICE CLAIMS?

If the plaintiff in a malpractice claim does not prove each of the elements previously discussed, the defense can ask for a dismissal of the claim by making various motions (formal requests) to the court. There are several other issues that may have an effect on the outcome of a malpractice claim.

A **statute of limitations** is a law that sets a time period after an event during which a lawsuit must be filed. States have different statutes and case law surrounding this time limit. Usually the time is measured from the time of the event or incident, last date of treatment, or from the time the event was or should have been discovered. For minors, some states allow the time to be counted from the time they reach majority (usually 18 years old), unless a suit has already been brought on their behalf by parents or others. Therefore, in hypothetical case study #4, a suit could be brought 2 or 3 years after a person turns 18 years (majority) for an injury occurring as an infant. Other states do not permit this delay. Lack of mental competence will also delay the time requirements in some states.

Failure to file the lawsuit within the statute of limitations time results in the loss of the right to sue. This can be considered a defense, because filing after the date allows the defendants to have the case dismissed. It is important to know, however, that in most states, the statute starts running when the patient knows of the injury. If there is any type of cover-up regarding an incident, the statute will not run.

Proving that the patient assumed the risk of harm, or that the patient contributed to the harm by his or her actions provides another type of defense. **Assumption of the risk** defense states that plaintiffs are partially responsible for consequences if they understood the risks involved when they proceeded with the action (Guido, 2001). An example would be a mentally competent patient who has been warned to use a call light but who insists on crawling out of the bottom of the bed and, thus, injures herself.

Contributory negligence is an older doctrine that used to be an all or nothing rule. Patients who had any part in the adverse outcome were barred from compensation. Today, most jurisdictions use a comparative negligence theory and reduce the money award by the injured party's responsibility for the ultimate harm done (Guido, 2001). One case found that a patient could be negligent and thus be at least partially responsible by (1) refusing to follow advice or instructions; (2) causing a delay in treatment or not returning for follow-up; (3) furnishing false, misleading, or incomplete information to a health care provider; or (4) causing the injury that causes a need for medical care (*Harvey v. Mid-Coast Hospital*, 1999).

WHAT EVIDENCE CAN HELP ME IN A LAWSUIT?

The Medical Record. An estimated one in four malpractice cases are decided on the basis of what is in the medical record (Sullivan, 2004). In many instances, you can become a nurse hero or in deep trouble, having to do simply with your accurate and timely documentation in the medical record. One of the most important tools for all providers in a malpractice claim is the medical record. This is the first piece of evidence asked for by the attorney for the plaintiff. The nurses' notes are often the first part of the record to be examined. Their integrity, accuracy, and completeness will make a claim defensible or indefensible. Good documentation, therefore, is one of the best defensive actions a nurse can take. By recording the care administered, the specific time it was administered, the patient's response, and the overall status of the patient's condition, the nurse can demonstrate that the standard of care was met (Figure 20-2).

Your defense attorney will use the medical record extensively and will very early in a claim make a time line of events that surrounded the incident. The most effective defense is to put on a play to a jury regarding what occurred to demonstrate all that was done for the patient. A good educational exercise is to take any patient's chart and see whether you can present a play regarding what happened to that patient during your care.

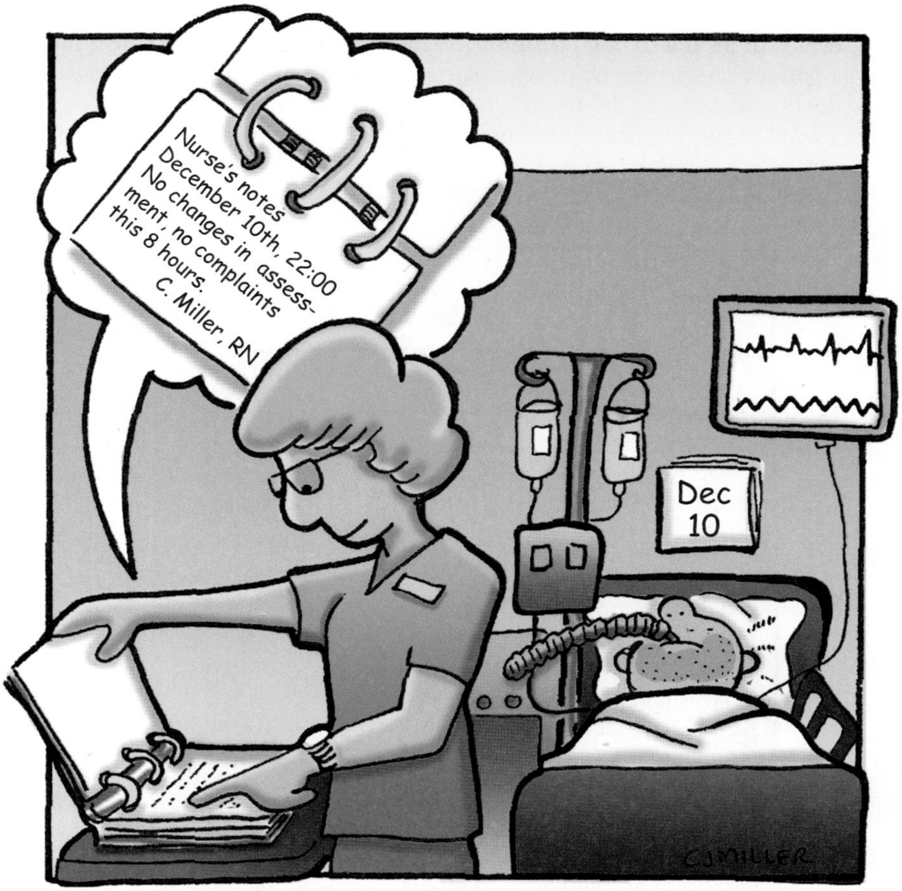
Nurse's notes
December 10th, 22:00
No changes in assess-
ment, no complaints
this 8 hours.
C. Miller, RN
Dec
10
CJ MILLER

FIGURE 20-2
It is critical that the nurse's notes reflect the current condition of the patient.

Some nurses have advocated the maintaining of personal notes regarding the circumstances of a particular incident. The rationale for this is so they can carefully review the notes; it will also assist them to more clearly recall the situation should they be required to do so. However, another consideration is that these notes are also discoverable by the other side and may be extremely dangerous. These notes are frequently written on an emotional level. In most states what you write, unless to your attorney or under a peer-review privilege, will have to be produced. Personal documentation about what others did or did not do or what you think they did wrong or should have done will always come back to haunt the nurse. Documentation regarding an incident should be thoroughly and factually done in the medical record and not in personal records or a diary (Figure 20-3).

There is an adage that "If it is not documented, it wasn't done." In reality, it is simply difficult to prove it was done if there is no documentation and the plaintiff claims it was not done. It is then a "He said, She said" type of argument. A more accurate statement might be "If it is documented, it was done." Once it is documented at the time of the event, there is a strong presumption that the documentation is accurate and whatever a patient says to the contrary is simply self-serving. That is why it is so important to document extensively, accurately, and very factually in the medical record (Box 20-3). This is especially true when there is an adverse event.

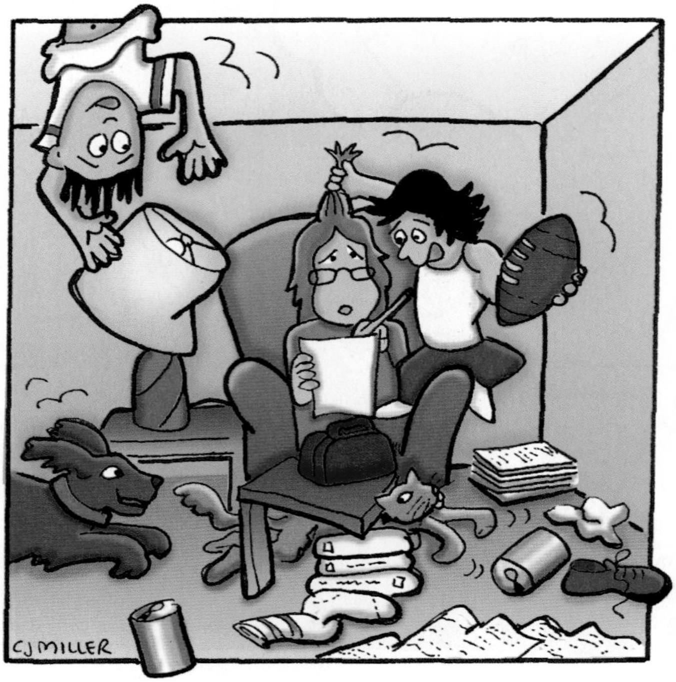

FIGURE 20-3
Charting in the home setting can be challenging.

BOX 20-3 Guidelines for Defensive Charting

- All entries should be accurate and factual.
- Make corrections appropriately and according to agency or hospital policies. Do not ever obliterate or destroy any information that is or has been in the chart.
- If there is information that should have been charted and was not, the nurse should make a "late entry," noting the time the charting actually occurred and the specific time the charting reflects. Example: 10/13/03, 10:00 late entry, charting to reflect that on 10/13/03 ...
- All identified patient problems, nursing actions taken, and patient responses should be noted. Do not describe a patient problem without including the nursing actions taken and the patient response.
- It is often as important to document why you did not do something that you would routinely do, as why you did do something. For instance, "Pt. refused to ambulate because of ... "
- Be as objective as possible in charting. Rather than charting "the patient tolerated the procedure well," chart the specific parameters checked to determine that conclusion. Example: "ambulated, tolerated well" would be more effective if charted "ambulated complete length of hall, no shortness of breath noted, pulse rate at 98, respirations at 22."
- Each page of the chart should contain the current date and time. Frequently, chart forms are stamped ahead of time. Each time you enter information on a new page, make sure it reflects the current time of charting.
- Each page of the chart should include the full name and professional designation of every person making an entry on that page.
- Follow through with who saw the patient and what measures were initiated. Particularly note when the physician visited; if you had to call a physician for a problem, record the physician's response, the nursing actions, and the patient's response. If orders were received, be sure they are signed according to policy. This is especially important if you had to make several calls to the physician.
- Make sure your notes are legible and clearly reflect the information you intended. It is a good idea to read over your nurse's notes from the previous day to see if they still make sense and accurately portray the status of the patient. If the notes do not make sense to you the next day, imagine how difficult it would be to decipher the information at a later date.
- Pertinent notes from other providers should also be reviewed. The medical record is for communication. A jury will never understand if team members are not coordinating efforts and thought.

Forms often provide a difficult problem for defense attorneys when they are not completed. A blank space on the form, or a box that is not checked when it appears that the space or box were part of needed therapy can be very detrimental to the nurse involved.

Do not have forms in the record if they are not routinely completed in a correct manner.

Many, if not most, institutions are in the process of implementing an electronic medical record (EMR). The cardinal rules of documentation still apply, but additional safeguards might have to be considered. This is especially true when some of the record is paper and some electronic. Both records then need to be accessed, coordinated, and made complete to safeguard the patient. It is believed that the EMR is more likely to promote more accurate and safe record keeping. For instance, the problem of eligible handwriting will be eliminated. Additionally certain programs have automatic safeguards to catch errors. It is therefore tempting to think that all problems will be solved (Sullivan, 2004). Of course, this is not true as long as there are humans entering information. No jury will appreciate blame being placed on a computer "glitch." This means education and problem solving to ensure safe computer documentation systems must continue as always.

HOW CAN I AVOID A MALPRACTICE CLAIM?

There are certain situations that contain a high risk for a lawsuit against nurses. These situations most often relate to patient safety, improper treatment, problems with monitoring, medication errors, and failing to follow proper procedures and policies.

Medication Errors. A recent study of 36 hospitals and nursing homes found that 20% of all medications administered involved some sort of mistake. All of these involved a violation of the classic five "rights" of medication administration—the failure to administer the **right** drug to the **right** patient, in the **right** amount, by the **right** route, and at the **right** time (Lafleur, 2004). Another study claims that 770,000 hospital patients experience an adverse drug event yearly and that almost half are preventable, such as those attributable to miscalculations, drug interactions, or drug allergies (Guido, 2001). Increased hospital costs for inpatients experiencing these errors may be $2 billion for the nation as a whole (Kohn et al, 2000). Claims involving medication errors are augmented when the nurse fails to record the medication administration properly, fails to recognize side effects or contraindications, or fails to know a patient's allergies.

JCAHO's 2004 and 2005 National Patient Safety Goals also include requirements that institutions develop bar code technology for matching patients with their medications and other treatments, as well as improve the safety of using infusion pumps (Lafleur, 2004). Particularly with the use of patient controlled anesthesia (PCA) pumps, the chance of patient harm is increased threefold (Santell, 2005). Any initiative that improves patient safety also lowers the chance of someone being sued. But, it also sets a standard on which the standard of care may rest and, therefore, becomes important for every nurse to know and follow.

The nurse's ability to listen to a patient or family member who notices that a medication is new, or recheck when anything such as color or amount seems unusual, may prevent a serious error. Many nurses feel rushed by the amount of work they are expected to accomplish and do not want to take extra time for anything. Making this check a priority will prove to be time well spent. Dealing with an error and the consequences to the patient will be longer and more painful.

Although many medication errors do not cause permanent or serious damage to patients, there are certain medications that can. New JCAHO Standards require each institution to identify high-risk medications used in the institution and to initiate safety procedures for managing these medications (JCAHO, 2004; Rich, 2004).

Medications, such as chemotherapy, should be stored separately, ordered on a special form to verify dosages, and attached to protocols that help ensure safe administration by qualified staff with specialized training.

Whenever a medication error occurs, the source of the error and the system failure should be carefully investigated. Most institutions are now attempting to ensure that punitive measures are not attached to medication errors. This is to facilitate reports to be made and systems involving the team of ordering practitioner, dispensing pharmacy, and administering nurse to have checks and balances to prevent any team member from causing harm to a patient (Kohn et al, 2000) (Box 20-4). JCAHO also requires that health care organizations have a plan for responding to adverse drug events and medication errors (e.g., send reports to the U.S. Pharmacopeia, FDA, and Institute for Safe Medication Practices) (Rich, 2004).

Provide a Safe Environment. Patient safety is being more and more recognized as a duty of health care institutions (JCAHO, 2004). Ensuring patient safety has many aspects. Nurses sometimes do not recognize the multiple roles that they must play in this area. They are responsible for knowing how equipment should work and not using it if it is not functioning correctly; removing obvious hazards such as chemicals, which might be mistaken for medications; and making the environment free of hazards such as inappropriately placed furniture or equipment, and spills on the floor. An additional preventive measure is knowing how to document correctly if an incident occurs, so that there cannot be a doubt regarding the facts of what happened and all you did to protect the patient.

BOX 20-4 Tips for Being at Your Best When Administering Medications

- Be very careful if you have been interrupted during a task. This is very common in nursing. Many accidents happen because the nurse did not remember what he or she had been doing or where he or she was in a task. Shift change is also a common time for mistakes.
- If you are fatigued, you are more likely to make mistakes. Follow all the steps thoroughly when you are tired. This is one of the reasons that double or long shifts may not be wise.
- Listen to your patients. Often they will tell you if what you are planning to do is different or unusual. Being able to take the time to do a second check may save you and your patient trouble.
- Never do a procedure you do not know how to do at the appropriate standard of performance. It is better to be embarrassed by admitting you need help or supervision than to risk hurting someone.
- Never be afraid to admit you made a mistake. Corrective action may stop or at least reduce harm.
- Keep current and up to date in your practice knowledge base. An article in a professional journal may keep the lawsuit away.
- Do not rush when you are extra busy. Set priorities on what must be done, and do it carefully.

From the Joint Commission for Accreditation of Healthcare Organizations.

Patient Falls. Patient falls represent one of the primary risks in this category and second to medication errors in numbers of untoward events (Guido, 2001). This may include falls out of bed, falls on something spilled on the floor, or falls because a nurse has not provided adequate supervision for the patient. Falls, particularly repeated falls, are a major source of both physical and psychological injury to elderly patients (Tideiksaar, 1998). They are, therefore, among the most common sources of claims against nurses.

Many people have spent much time and effort in attempts to change patient care so that falls do not occur. Proposals coming out of such efforts range from total lack of restraints (Walker, 1992), to environmental modifications (Tideliksaar, 1998), to decreasing the number of certain types of medications (Haumschild et al, 2003). It is important to keep up with the latest information in order not to be caught without defenses in a malpractice claim (see Critical Thinking Box 20-4).

If a patient falls, the nurse's first duty is to the patient. This involves the following:
Notifying a physician to assess and treat the patient.
Making sure that the patient is protected from a second fall.
Notifying the family so that they are not surprised by a patient's injury.
Documenting what occurred.

Nurses are best able to defend themselves in these cases when their institution has a policy regarding protecting vulnerable patients against falls, sometimes called a "fall protocol." These policies establish levels of risk in patients, such as age, confusion, sedation, and steps the nurse must take to protect the patient, such as side rails, soft restraints, or bed position. If the nurse follows such a protocol, it is difficult for a plaintiff to prove that the nurse fell below a standard of care. In developing such protocols, however, it is important to know the laws in your state, Federal CMS guidelines, and JCAHO standards regarding restraints. Unnecessary and unsafe restraining of patients has become the focus of public and private attention and restraint injuries can also be the basis of legal action (Medscape Medical News, 2000).

Documentation is extremely important when a patient falls. The following should be considered:

- Document factually how the fall was discovered, where the patient was found, the facts surrounding the fall. An example is to document that the patient was found beside the bed, with the side rails up, and the bed in the low position.
- Document what the patient says in regard to the fall. A statement such as "I know you told me to put on the call light, but you all seemed so busy that I didn't want

CRITICAL THINKING BOX 20-4

What fall protocols have you observed in your clinical settings? How are they the same, and how are they different?

to bother you," can be of great benefit to the nurse. "I put on the call light, but nobody came" can, of course, have the opposite effect.

- Document whom you notified, such as the physician, the family.
- Document what was done for the patient, such as an examination, radiographs, orientation to surroundings, monitoring after the incident, restraints, and assistance with further ambulation.
- Document your adherence to any policies of the hospital regarding vulnerable patients or those at risk for falls.

Equipment Failure. Today many nurses feel that they spend more time nursing equipment than the patient. This can be true. What nurses do not understand is that there is a certain standard of care connected with equipment. It must be used as directed by the manufacturer, and the nurse has a duty to know what that is and follow such directions. There is also a duty to make sure that the equipment is properly maintained and that records are kept of this maintenance. The equipment needs to be working properly and not used when a known defective condition exists. Additionally, the device must be available for use. In hypothetical case study #4, the fact that the Ambu bag was not available can be viewed as a liability for either the nurse responsible for checking crash carts, or the institution for not seeing that the carts are checked.

When there is a failure of a devise or piece of equipment and a patient is injured, the focus should of course initially be on helping the patient. After that, it is extremely important that the device (e.g., catheter, pump, instrument) be sequestered and a clear record of its handling (chain of custody) be maintained. In a lawsuit, the nurse will need to prove that equipment failure, rather than human error, caused the injury. Part of that proof will rest in the piece of equipment itself. Therefore, one of the most important aspects of the defense will be to not lose or let go of the equipment or device before it is thoroughly evaluated by a neutral party after an incident. Often the manufacturer will ask for the equipment, but their interests might be adverse to yours to prove user error rather than equipment failure. Information regarding the failure can be given, but never let the device or equipment out of the custody of the institution. In addition, the nurse should adhere to any institutional policies regarding incidents involving equipment failure.

Nurses may also have a duty to be sure their institution complies with the Safe Medical Device Act of 1990. This federal law requires that all medical device-related adverse incidents be reported to manufacturers and in the case of death, to the U.S. Food and Drug Administration (FDA), within 10 days. The purpose of this act is to protect the public from devices that may be defective (Guido, 2001).

Hypothetical case study #5:

A 67-year-old woman with chronic obstructive pulmonary disease is having increasingly difficult respirations, increased cyanosis, and increased anxiety. She tells you she just cannot breathe. You have done all the measures for which you currently have orders, without her getting relief. It is 2 AM. You call the physician. She orders Valium 10 mg intramuscularly now. Even as a recent graduate you know that Valium is contraindicated by the respiratory status. You call your supervisor, who tells you that Dr. Jones is a good physician and must know what she is doing. What should you do?

Failure to Adequately Assess, Monitor, and Obtain Assistance. Most often, the nurse should not delegate to another the responsibility of assessing and evaluating patient care and progress. If some portions of this duty are done by others (e.g., another RN, licensed practical nurse, unlicensed personnel), the nurse primarily responsible for the care of the patient must still be aware of the findings and confirm them when they indicate a change in patient condition or progress. Documentation of the changes and events surrounding the changes is critical.

Rapidly increasing numbers of cases are occurring when there is an inadequate nursing assessment, or a failure to monitor and obtain needed medical assistance for a patient whose condition is changing.

Considering the previous case study, there may also be liability for failure to challenge an inappropriate order.

These areas are uncomfortable for many experienced nurses, not just for the recent graduate. Frequently, these areas involve challenging a physician or other health care professional. They require that the nurse have current and accurate information. They also require the difficult balance between assertiveness and diplomacy.

It is not enough to identify problems. The nurse must identify the problems and contact the physician or other individuals to get appropriate care.

Of most help in situations such as hypothetical case study #5 is a policy that clearly delineates the chain of command for the institution. With a policy in place, the nurse can be clear about who must be notified about a potentially problematic order, and it can be documented appropriately. It is important that the nurse be protected from any retaliation in such instances by the institution that stands to lose if the patient's safety is not put first.

Accurate documentation of the nursing assessment and of frequent monitoring will be required to prove what you have done. Flow charts and forms can be timesaving devices in this area. Electronic communications now make such time-consuming documentation more readily available. This documentation is especially important in the critical care setting and in the obstetric suite. The attachment of accurate times to such monitoring activities will be your best defense tool in many malpractice claims.

Failure to Adequately Communicate. Perhaps the most important role of everyone on the health care team is to adequately communicate. JCAHO included improved communications in its National Patient Safety Goals for 2003. The patient's total care rests on this whether it is communication in the medical record or through verbal communication.

The most frequent claim against nurses in this area is the failure to communicate changes in the patient's condition to a professional with a need to know.

This is especially true in acute-care settings during the night hours, as in hypothetical case study #5. Communication is not always welcomed in the middle of the night and is impaired because it is not face to face, and the receiver may not be fully awake and alert. JCAHO now requires a verification "read back" of all verbal and telephone orders (not limited to medication orders) by the person taking the order and the use of a standardized set of abbreviations, acronyms, and symbols throughout the organization. Thorough documentation of the communication will protect the nurse, but it should not be done defensively or thought of as a substitute for proper care.

Communication with certain hearing- and speech-impaired patients and with ethnically and culturally diverse patients will often provide a challenge to good nursing care. The Americans with Disabilities Act is a federal statute that has requirements for institutions rendering health care to have certain translators available for key health care interactions. The failure to do so may put the institution at risk for fines, and penalties (Freydel v. New York Hospital, 2000).

Failure to Report. States have many statutes that require health care providers to report certain incidences or occurrences. If the provider fails to report as required and a person is injured, there can be **negligence per se**, and no expert testimony will be needed to prove a case. In addition, both institutional and professional licensure can be affected. It is important that nurses are aware of the reporting statutes in the state in which they are practicing. In some states, it is not only a duty, but also the law to report certain incidences. The following are examples of such statutes involving a duty to report.

- A duty to report other health care professionals whose behaviors are unprofessional and/or could cause harm to the public. This includes drug and alcohol abuse.
- A duty to report evidence of child or adult or elder abuse and neglect, including any acts of a sexual nature against vulnerable (i.e., anesthetized) patients.
- A duty to report certain communicable diseases.
- A duty to report certain deaths under suspicious circumstances including deaths during surgery.
- A duty to report certain types of injuries that are or could be caused by violence.
- A duty to report evidence of Medicare fraud.
- Emergency Medical Treatment and Labor Act (EMTALA) violations.

The nurse must know what areas must be reported, who should report, how the report should be accomplished, and to whom a report should be made. Institutional policies and Nurse Practice Acts on these topics are invaluable.

Many nurses are afraid to report their employers, other professionals, or other agencies because of the possibility of retaliatory action against them. Most mandatory reporting statutes give immunity to those who report in good faith. Some states have specific "Whistleblower Statutes" that not only protect nurses from retaliatory action but also may reward them. The content of these statutes differs from state to state, so the nurse must know whether one exists in the state of practice, and what protection is provided. A federal statute, the False Claims Act, provides protection under certain situations for reporting Medicare fraud. Additionally, federal compliance standards require that institutions maintain a mechanism to report unlawful activities such as a "hotline" where problems can be reported anonymously. In response to such reports,

CRITICAL THINKING BOX 20-5

Which states have "whistleblower" protection?

institutions must demonstrate that they responded appropriately and disciplined all individuals engaged in the illegal activities (Critical Thinking Box 20-5) (Green, 2000).

INTENTIONAL TORTS

Intentional torts are civil claims that are closely related to criminal acts in that they involve intent to do the wrong. Instead of seeking to put the bad actor in jail, however, these claims attempt to right the wrong by compensating the plaintiff. These lawsuits are less common than malpractice claims, but the following can be brought against a nurse.

Assault and battery are the legal terms that are applied to nonconsensual threat of touch (assault) or the actual touching (battery). Of course, in health care, there is a lot of touching. Permission to do this touching is usually implied when the patient seeks medical care. Sometimes, however, a patient refuses to have certain procedures done, or has certain procedures done without giving an informed consent. Also, a patient may wish to leave an institution "against medical advice" (AMA) and nurses use physical restraint or touching to keep them from leaving. All of these actions can lead to a civil claim of assault and battery.

False imprisonment means making someone wrongfully feel that he or she cannot leave a place. It is often associated with assault and battery claims. This can happen in a health care setting through the use of physical or chemical restraints, or the threat of physical or emotional harm if a patient leaves an institution. Threats such as "If you don't stay in your bed, I'll have to sedate you" constitute false imprisonment. This tort might also be telling a patient that he or she may not leave the emergency department until the bill is paid. Another example is using restraints or threatening to use them on competent patients to make them do what you want them to do against their wishes. Unless you are very clearly protecting the safety of others, you may not restrain a competent adult (Critical Thinking Box 20-6) (Guido, 2001).

Even in the psychiatric case in which someone is thought to be a danger to self or others, there are many very specific state and federal laws to follow. The tension, of course, is preventing the patient from committing suicide while also maintaining the patient's rights to liberty. This is not an easy balance, and very specific policies are needed to give legal guidance for those in the many difficult situations of emergency

CRITICAL THINKING BOX 20-6

In what situations would it be acceptable to restrain a patient?

department. and psychiatric nursing. As described elsewhere, there are also many restrictions on the appropriate use of both hard and soft restraints and elevated scrutiny on their use in long-term care facilities (Tideliksaar, 1998). Sometimes there can be a claim of elder abuse for the misuse of restraints. You must be aware of the policies in your agency and state statutory requirements.

Defamation (libel and slander) refers to causing damage to someone else's reputation. If the means of transmitting the damaging information is written, it is called **libel**; if it is oral or spoken, it is called **slander**. The damaging information must be communicated to a third person. The actions likely to result in a defamation charge are situations in which inaccurate information from the medical record is given out, such as in hypothetical case study #1 or speaking negatively about your coworkers (supervisors, doctors, other nurses).

Two defenses to defamation accusations are *truth and privilege*. If the statement is true, it is not actionable under this doctrine. However, it is often difficult to define truth, because it may be a matter of perspective. It is better to avoid that issue by not making negative statements about other people unnecessarily. An example of "privilege" would be required good faith reporting to Child Protective Services of possible child abuse or statements made during a peer review process. If statements made during these processes are made without maliciousness, state statutes often protect the reporter from any civil liability for defamation.

Recovery in defamation claims usually requires that the plaintiff submit proof of being injured, that is, loss of money or job. Some categories, such as fitness to practice one's profession, do not require such proof, as they are considered sufficiently damaging without it. Comments about the quality of a nurse's work or a physician's skills in diagnosing illness would fit in this category. You can avoid this claim by steering clear of gossip and/or writing negative documents about others in the heat of the moment and without an adequate factual basis.

INVASION OF PRIVACY AND BREACHES OF PRIVILEGE AND CONFIDENTIALITY

A good general rule in relationship to torts involving the sharing of patient information is to always ask yourself, "Do I have the patient's consent to share this information, or is it necessary to the health care services for this patient?" If the answer to either is "no," then the information should not be communicated.

The public's attention has been recently focused on privacy because of new privacy regulations under an older federal law called the Health Insurance Portability and Accountability Act of 1996 (HIPAA). These specific privacy regulations became effective in April 2003 and have an elaborate system for ensuring privacy for individually identifiable health information. Information used to render treatment, payment, or health care operations does not need the patient's specific consent for its use. This includes processes such as quality assurance activities, legal activities, risk management, billing, and utilization review. However, the rules require that the disclosure be the "minimum necessary" and a clear understanding of what information can be shared under this exception is necessary (Annas, 2003). Notice must be given to the patient of how the information will be used. All nurses working in health care must be aware of this law and how their institutions specifically comply with it.

Another aspect of HIPAA has to do with electronic information and security measures necessary to make sure that protected patient information is not accessed by those without a right or need to know. These rules came into effect in April of 2005. Each institution must have data security policies and technologies in place based on their own "risk assessment." Many institutions will now require that any health information transmitted under open networks, such as the Internet, telephones, and wireless communication networks, be encrypted (coded).

Many states have physician-patient privilege laws that protect communications between caregivers and their patients. This enables information to pass freely between physician and patient without concern that it will be shared with those who do not need to know it. This includes law enforcement. The privilege usually extends to information about a patient in the medical record or obtained in the course of providing care. Most states extend physician-patient privilege to nurses and sometimes to other health care givers as well. This privilege belongs to the patient, not the health care giver, which means that only the patient can decide to give it up.

As a professional it is important to observe **confidentiality** when talking about patients at home and at work (Figure 20-4). Nurses must be very careful to keep information about the patient or from the patient to themselves and to share it only with health care workers who must know the information to plan or give proper care. This is often difficult to do as seen in hypothetical case study #1.

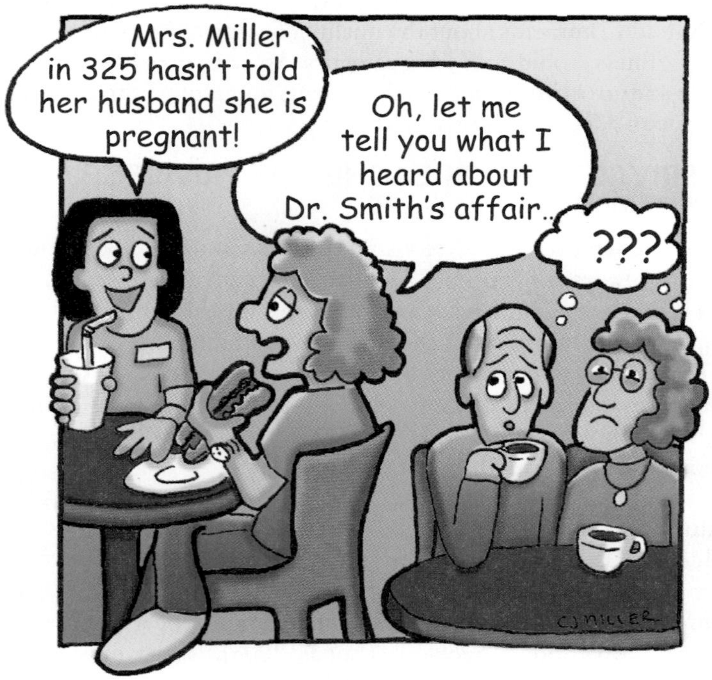
Mrs. Miller in 325 hasn't told her husband she is pregnant!
Oh, let me tell you what I heard about Dr. Smith's affair...
???
CJ MILLER

FIGURE 20-4
Maintaining confidentiality is both an ethical and a legal consideration in nursing.

Computer documentation and national clearing houses for health information present significant confidentiality issues. Such technologies offer many advantages, including easier and broader access to needed information and more legible documentation. These same advantages also present concerns because it is more difficult to ensure confidentiality. Many hospitals and agencies already have policies and procedures in place, such as access codes, limited screen time, and computers placed in locations that promote privacy. The nurse is still responsible for the protection of confidentiality when computers, faxes, e-mail, or other rapid communication techniques are used.

A similar cause of action is for **invasion of privacy**. This cause of action can apply to several behaviors, like photographing a procedure and showing it without the patient's consent, going through a patient's belongings without consent, or talking about a patient's private life publicly.

MISCELLANEOUS INTENTIONAL TORTS AND OTHER CIVIL RIGHTS CLAIMS INVOLVED WITH EMPLOYMENT

The aforementioned torts and others can be relevant to nurses in regard to their employment. These intentional torts can be brought personally against the nurse, and are not usually covered by any insurance. **Tortious Interference with Contract** is a claim that someone maliciously interfered with a person's contractual (often employment) rights. This can occur, for instance, if a nurse attempts to get another nurse fired through giving false or misleading facts to a supervisor. **Intentional Infliction of Emotional Distress** is described in its title, and can also be attached to malicious acts in the employment setting. These and certain civil rights claims such as **sexual harassment** and **discrimination** are both rights and potential liabilities for every person in the work force. Although beyond the scope of this text, policies and information regarding these issues demand further investigation by each health care employee to ensure that their rights and the rights of others are not violated.

WHAT IS A DEFENSE TO INTENTIONAL TORTS?

Informed Consent. Consent is usually a complete defense to all of the aforementioned intentional torts. You cannot have a claim for assault and battery, if the patient has given consent for the procedure. Likewise, there can be no invasion of privacy if the patient has given consent to share confidential information with someone else such as their lawyer.

There is much confusion about informed consent in that many people believe it to be a piece of paper with "informed consent" written on it. This is not true.

Informed consent in the health care setting is a process whereby a patient is informed of:

1. The nature of the proposed care, treatment, services, medications, interventions, or procedures;
2. The potential benefits, risks, or side effects, including potential problems related to recuperation;
3. The likelihood of achieving care, treatment, and service goals;
4. Reasonable alternatives and their respective risks and benefits including the alternative of refusing all interventions (JCAHO, 2004).

After being thus informed, the patient then gives consent for the procedure to be done. The piece of paper is simply evidence that the informed consent process has taken place.

The nurse's role in the consent process is often confusing. Remember that it is ultimately the responsibility of the person doing the procedure to provide the basic explanation of its risks, benefits, and alternatives. In regard to most procedures and operations, this means the physician. However, in some settings, the nurse is part of an educational process involving videos, booklets, handouts, and other aids to the patient's understanding.

As nurses perform more invasive procedures, the process of informing the patient of what is to occur is the nurse's.

For surgeries and other physician-performed procedures, nurses may be asked, "to get the consent." Be clear what this means. In essence it means to witness the patient's voluntary signature on a form that should be filled out by the person performing the procedure. That is all. However, as a witness to a signature, documentation of the patient's level of understanding, or the patient's refusal to receive information, or reluctance to have the procedure done, is critical to the witnessing role.

Consent forms must be signed when a patient is considered able or competent to make informed decisions and before the procedure is done. This means that the form must be signed before the administration of preprocedure medications, which often contain narcotics or other mind-altering drugs. The patient is the only person who may give consent if he or she is competent. Competency (also called "capacity") is defined differently from state to state and the nurse should be aware of how it is defined in his or her state of practice. Competency is presumed and therefore any claim of incompetence would have to be proved.

States differ with regard to how consent can be given if the patient is incompetent or lacks capacity to make medical decisions. Advance directives such as a medical power of attorney or a living will may give information about the patient's wishes. These documents allow individuals to prepare for possible incompetence in advance by formalizing their wishes about their further health care decisions in writing. The living will is used to allow a competent adult to direct what he or she wishes in regard to health care upon becoming incompetent. This may include that he or she does not want any unusual medical procedures or life-saving equipment used to prolong life.

Often used in conjunction with the living will is the "durable" or "medical" power of attorney. This document allows the competent adult to appoint a specific person to authorize care if he or she becomes incompetent. The durable power of attorney does not usually become effective until a person loses competency. This document may be used in conjunction with or without a living will (see Chapter 19 for more information on advance directives). Congress has passed the Patient Self-Determination Act of 1990 requiring hospitals to inform their patients of the availability of advance directives. State law defines the required wording for these documents and any other formalities necessary in their preparation. Because patients must be educated on these laws and documents, so should nurses. If not, you could be caught in violation of law at a crucial moment of life and death.

If a family challenges a living will, or medical power of attorney, a nurse will need to go through the administrative chain of command, where, it is hoped, a lawyer will be involved. A general rule is for nurses to follow the advance directives unless or until there is a court order to do otherwise. This means that families need to obtain legal services and go to court to overturn or challenge these documents. All persons, no matter what their age, should complete advance directives. The recent Terri Schiavo case is a sad demonstration of the difficulties faced by families when there are no documented advance directives, and family members differ in beliefs about what should or should not be done. Questions then arise whether acts or omissions of health care providers prolong life or prolong the dying process. Judges are certainly not the preferred ultimate decision-makers.

When a patient does not have an advance directive and is incompetent, there are also state laws that give guidance regarding who can act as a *surrogate decision-maker*. Parents must usually sign for minor children. Spouses or immediate family members may usually sign for unconscious patients. In other instances, if no one is available or designated, a court can appoint someone for the purpose of medical decisions in a very short time. Informed consent is not required if the procedure is necessary to save a life and is done during an emergency. A special consent under stricter standards applies to research studies, and often surrogates may not be able to make such decisions (Truog, 2002).

Competent patients may always decline to give consent for a procedure, even if doing so may have serious consequences for their health status. This legal standard respects the fundamental liberty interest in personal autonomy protected by American jurisprudence (Moore, 1999). In certain instances, pregnant women may not be permitted to refuse a treatment if doing so will result in serious harm to the fetus. Such a case should be referred to risk management and resolved before the procedure is done. Consent may be withdrawn at any time before the procedure. Documentation of events surrounding such incidents should be accurate and complete.

CRIMINAL ACTIONS

Nurses who violate specific criminal statutes, such as those having to do with illegal drug use, negligent homicide, and assault and battery, risk criminal prosecution. Conviction of certain types of crimes must be reported to the state board of nursing and will usually result in a review of licensure status. You must be aware of the rules in the state in which you practice.

WHAT CRIMINAL ACTS POSE A RISK TO THE NURSE?

Theft and Misappropriation of Property. Sometimes, nurses fail to adequately protect a patient's property and thus open themselves up to claims of theft. Many patients bring valuables to health care facilities or think that they do. Clear notice to the patients before admittance to leave valuables at home is helpful. A thorough and documented list of property upon admission is imperative to prevent such claims, as is the locking up of valuables. When dentures and other property have not been adequately stored or monitored, the nurse may be held responsible.

Another aspect of this problem is theft from the employer. Because of the extensive and costly nature of this problem, many employers have developed elaborate systems to try to discourage theft. With an ever-increasing focus on lowering health care costs, those related to employee theft will not be tolerated. Occasionally, nurses accidentally leave the job with tape, bandages, or other supplies in their pockets. These should be returned. Better yet, establishing a routine of checking your pockets before leaving for home will help reduce this risk. No employer's property should ever be intentionally taken by a nurse.

Nursing Practice Violations. Scope-of-practice violations that result in the death of a patient may be the result of nurses doing tasks or procedures that have not been accepted by the State Board of Nursing as within the appropriate scope for nurses, or doing actions that have been approved for advanced practice nurses only. In some states these violations and other possible violations of the Nurse Practice Act are misdemeanors, but in other states they may be felonies. In rare cases, charges of murder or negligent homicide may be filed against the nurse (Kowalski & Horner, 1998). In November 2000, the State of Hawaii convicted an individual of manslaughter in the death of a nursing home patient for permitting the progression of decubitus ulcers without seeking appropriate medical help (Di Maio & Di Maio, 2002). This fairly new trend should be of concern to all nurses as mistakes will always occur in medicine. To err is human. "Making an error that endangers the patient is terrifying; making one that kills a patient can be career-ending because of the guilt, regret, and self-blame" (Kohn, Corrigan, & Donaldson, 2000). If fear of criminal prosecution and prison are added to these personal responses, how can we believe thoughtful, caring people will continue in the profession? As Curtin (1997) asks, "What conceivable social good will be achieved by putting these nurses in jail?" (Kowalski & Horner, 1998).

Violations of the Food and Drugs Act. Participating in any activity with illegal drugs or the misappropriation or improper use of legal drugs may result in criminal action against the nurse. Conviction for a crime in this area will almost always result in action against a nurse's license. As described earlier, there is a high incidence of substance abuse in the medical profession, so nurses need to be aware of the risks and avoid them. Writing prescriptions for drugs without the authority to do so is a criminal activity. Obtaining drugs illegally for friends and/or family needs, even if they seem legitimate, will still have criminal consequences.

RISK MANAGEMENT AND QUALITY IMPROVEMENT

HOW DO I PROTECT MYSELF AND MY PATIENT FROM ALL THESE RISKS?

The safety of patients often involves many different formalized processes in institutions. One involves quality and goes by many names such as "quality assurance" (QA), "continuous quality management" (CQM), or "continuous quality improvement" (CQI). In relationship to nursing practices, *peer review* is the process of using nurses to evaluate the quality of nursing care. This means that you, as a professional nurse, will be continuously involved in evaluating the care that you and other nurses provide. In the past, this was only done through retroactive review of care using techniques such as nursing audits to evaluate care already given. The current focus is on looking for ways to do better all the time. Examples of activities that may be involved in this process include the following:

1. Evaluation of what nurses are doing for patients
2. Policy and procedure development
3. Staff preparation, competency, and skill documentation
4. Continuing education and certification
5. Employee evaluations
6. Ongoing monitoring, such as infection control and risk-management systems

JCAHO requires that peer review be driven by the following: (1) The organization's delineation of circumstances that require review; (2) The designation of who will participate in the process; (3) The time frame of the review; (4) The timely reporting of the results (JCAHO, 2004).

Risk management is a process that becomes involved when incidents or untoward events occur that may pose a financial risk or risk of lawsuit to the institution. This department, through a risk manager, will often take the first step, and that is to gather evidence surrounding the event in "anticipation of litigation." Such evidence will include interviews with those involved and physical evidence such as relevant documents. If you are being interviewed, understand that a truthful accounting is the most important aspect of this process and will best serve the institution and yourself.

Risk management will then often evaluate how to prevent a reoccurrence by changing systems that have broken down to allow an adverse occurrence. This might mean setting a new standard that can then be evaluated and ensured through a quality assurance process.

One tool used by risk management is the **incident report**. Incident reports generate many legal concerns as in most states they must be produced in a lawsuit and can be used as evidence against individuals and the institution (Guido, 2001). Therefore extreme caution should be used when completing an incident report, and only the person directly involved should objectively document the facts. Conclusions, opinions, defensiveness, and judgment or blame of others have absolutely no place in this document or process. In addition, the form should never be used for punitive reasons, as this will almost certainly increase the possibility that it will not be filled out honestly if at all (Kohn, Corrigan, & Donaldson, 2000).

Although you would not mention that you filled out an incident report in the medical record, the same objective, factual documentation of an incident should be made in the medical record by the person involved in the incident. Lack of documentation in the face of a known occurrence will always be considered a cover-up and thus will be extremely detrimental to any subsequent legal action. Never speculate about who or what caused an incident, as this may inadvertently give the plaintiff "causation" proof, which may not be true.

An example of risk management and quality assurance working together would be the following. A fire breaks out in the operating room, and a patient is burned. Immediately after this event, a risk manager might be notified through a telephone call and then later an incident report. The risk manager would come immediately to the scene and collect all items and/or equipment involved in the fire (evidence) to determine the cause of the fire. He or she would also interview those who saw the fire (witnesses) to determine facts involved. The risk manager may also take specific actions to assist the patient and/or family, in addition to giving advice to those involved regarding documentation of the event and/or communications. Sometimes financial settlements are made very early to avoid the costly process of a lawsuit. Risk management might also identify ways to prevent another occurrence, such as removal of all alcohol-based skin preparations from the operating room. This standard may then be periodically evaluated by the quality assurance department to ensure the continued safety of a patient.

Risk managers usually work very closely with insurance companies that cover institutions and their employees for all types of financial risk including malpractice and general liability. The defense and prevention of many claims starts with good risk management. Yet such efforts must also be made by every individual on the health care team who identifies a risk to patient safety and does something constructive to correct it. Several simple risk-management actions by nurses can often prevent a lawsuit. These include the following:

1. Approaching angry patients with an apology and an offer to help (Gutheil et al, 1984). Moving toward the patient who has experienced an unexpected outcome rather than away is always the best policy. Isolation and a feeling of abandonment in the face of an untoward event can only augment the feeling that a wrong was done.
2. Sharing uncertainties and bringing patient's expectations down to a realistic level during the informed consent process can also prevent claims based on disappointment that an outcome is not perfect (Gutheil et al, 1984).
3. Refusing to participate in hospital gossip, jousting in the medical record, or judging others on the medical team will contribute to an atmosphere of teamwork and compassion, rather than competition, blame, and retaliation. The latter can ultimately contribute to unsafe patient care. The inadvertant negative remark to patients and families about a physician, or the pharmacy, or laboratory or other nurses is very frequently the genesis of a lawsuit. Such remarks are often based on limited knowledge and personal bias. The fact is that you may then end up as a witness in a malpractice claim against your peers and/or other medical team members. This is seldom a desirable position for anyone.

MALPRACTICE INSURANCE

One of the more controversial topics for nurses involves the need for nurses to purchase individual malpractice insurance policies (Guido, 2001; Kelly & Joel, 1999; Murphy, 1998; Simpson, 1998). There is often misinformation about what these individual policies will do or cover, and there is little substantiation for what most authors say. Part of the problem is that lawyers, rather than insurance professionals, talk about what the policies mean. In addition, sometimes insurance companies use scare tactics to induce nurses to purchase their products. An informed nurse should at least know what questions to ask.

WHAT ABOUT INDIVIDUAL MALPRACTICE INSURANCE?

Some individual nurse policies claim that you can prevent settlement of a claim if you wish to do so (have a consent clause). However, a close reading of the policy might demonstrate that should the case then be lost at trial or settled for more than the insurance company wished to offer, they have the right to collect that difference and the cost of defense from you. Therefore, the consent you have a right to withhold has very little meaning.

The fact that registered nursing insurance costs have not changed much since introduced on the market, although all other malpractice insurance costs have risen drastically, is an indication of its lack of use. For instance, you can buy an individual nursing malpractice policy for $ $19.00 for employed nurses (because employed nurses already have coverage that is primary) or $59.00 for $1 million per claim and $5 million per year coverage (Medmal4Nurses.com, 2005). Whereas a policy for physicians ranges from $40,000 to $200,000, and for extended-practice nurses functioning in a physician's office, it is approximately $1200 (Physicians Mutual Insurance Company, 2004). This also is an indication of how often the registered nursing insurance policy is actually used.

WHAT IS INSTITUTIONAL COVERAGE?

Almost all health care corporations or institutions carry very large insurance policies that specifically cover acts or omissions of their employed nurses. This includes both when the institution only is named under the previously described ***respondeat superior*** doctrine, or when an individual nurse employee is named. Most individual personal nursing malpractice policies are secondary to this policy. This means they cannot be used in any manner if the institutional policy is used to cover the claim. It is not correct to assume that you can have your personal attorney present to represent your personal interests in addition to the institutional attorney. Even if you could, having two attorneys will often divide the defense and augment the claim.

A representation that the institutional attorney will only look out for the institution's interests and not yours is questionable in that attorneys ethically must represent both your interests and the institution's. In addition, the institution's interests are rarely, if ever, adverse to yours. Both of you wish to settle claims that have liability and defend claims when there is no liability.

The claim that an institution will insure you, but then turn around and sue you is belied by the fact that one cannot find statistics to verify this common claim. Institutions spend millions of dollars on insurance to specifically cover the acts of nurses. In addition, if institutions sued the nurses working for them, they would not keep nurses. Recently, one case was cited in the literature as demonstrating that an institution sued its nurse (*St. Anthony's Hospital v. Whitfield*, 1997), but a reading of that case as reported does not disclose the reasons for the claim (Murphy, 1998).

It is true that if an employee commits a criminal act that by its nature is outside the scope of their employment, such as forced sexual intimacies with a patient, an institution may not defend the employee, nor cover costs. In this regard, however, criminal acts are not insurable under laws in most states and therefore are not covered by any policy (Simpson, 1998).

WHAT SHOULD I ASK ABOUT INSTITUTIONAL COVERAGE?

There are certain things that a prudent nurse concerned about coverage should do. All nurses should request and have a right to a document, which gives them the following information regarding their employer's insurance coverage for them:

1. The name of the institution's insurance carrier, the limits of the policy, and the rating of the insurance company (Best Rating A+++ is the highest).
2. Whether they are covered for all acts occurring within the scope of their employment and during the time they are employed.

3. The acts for which they do not have coverage.
4. If the hospital will cover them if they need to appear before the State Board of Nursing in relationship to a malpractice claim. If not, an individual insurance policy that clearly does may be valuable.
5. If the nurse is an independent practitioner and/or in an extended practice role, he or she should be absolutely certain how they are covered by their institutional employers.
6. If a nurse does utilization review for an insurance company that is involved in an employee benefit plan, there may be individual exposure (Murphy, 1998).
7. If the nurse is working in a physician's office that has limited coverage.
8. If the nurse is self-employed, then of course individually purchased coverage is essential.

You may obtain individual policies from all companies selling insurance to nurses. If you are concerned about your institutional coverage, obtain such policies and determine whether they truly offer more or additional coverage. As stated earlier, the cost is very low, and although the protection may also be limited, some nurses feel more secure owning these policies.

WHAT HAPPENS WHEN I GO TO COURT?

Sometimes, despite all your efforts, you find yourself in litigation as a defendant. Know that very few claims go to trial. Therefore, you do not need to picture yourself in a setting from "Law and Order" with a prosecutor tearing you apart. Ninety-five percent of personal injury lawsuits are either dismissed or settled out of court, usually after an investigatory process called "discovery" (Fish et al, 1990). This involves written questions about situations surrounding a case called **interrogatories,** and a recorded oral questioning process called a **deposition**.

Depositions are oral statements given under oath and are extremely important in any malpractice claim. They are used to evaluate the merits of the case, the credibility of the witnesses, and the strength of the defendants. Cases are won or lost in this process. Therefore, with the help of your attorney, you must be very prepared. If you have not been offered the chance to meet with your attorney well before your deposition, request the time to do so. This is your right and an ethical obligation of the attorney. Being prepared ahead of time can have a significant effect on your performance under stress. Many attorneys will role-play situations with you so you will get the feel of the process. There are also good books, videos, and other aids that should be considered. Ask your attorney, or check with your hospital Risk Management Department, in addition to the public library and websites.

Depositions occur in a less formal setting than the courtroom. Attorneys for both sides will be present, but this is not the time to tell your story. The attorney questioning you will be either the attorney for the plaintiff or for the other defendants whose interests may be adversarial to yours. Your attorney can object to certain questions, but on the whole you will have to answer them anyway because in the deposition there is no judge to rule on the objections.

Remember, in a deposition you are there to answer questions in a truthful manner, but not to teach or inform.

The following are tips for how a nurse should act in a deposition.

1. You need to look and act like a professional. That means that you must be prepared. Know the case; and review your documented record ahead of time.
2. Be clear, accurate, and very concise. It is often said that if you say more than seven words, it is too much. If you do not know an answer, say so—do not guess.
3. Never give opinions unless asked for them. Stick to the facts!
4. Speak slowly and in a well-modulated tone of voice. Do not allow yourself to be rattled by the opposing attorney.
5. If you do not remember a question or do not understand it, ask for it to be repeated or clarified. Many attorneys use long, multi-part questions to confuse you. Do not get caught in this trap.
6. If you have made a statement and later realize it is not correct, do not be afraid to say so, rather than to skirt issues or contradict yourself.
7. Do not allow yourself to be goaded into an angry or emotional response. You can always ask for a break during a deposition to collect yourself and your thoughts.
8. Avoid the use of "always" and "never" and vague comments like "maybe," "I think," or "possibly."
9. Do not answer more than is asked for by the question. This helps maintain focus and clarity. The attorney desires to catch you in contradictory statements. The shorter your statements, the less likely that is to happen.

A lawsuit is a very disconcerting and disheartening process to everyone involved. Your ability to realize this and not feel alone in the process is extremely important. Often institutions mandate that persons involved in litigation receive counseling to help them resolve the anger and depression that almost everyone feels at some point. Be sure to use resources available to you including your lawyer. Your risk management team also is often a good resource and can usually answer questions or help resolve problems you might be having in relationship to the case. Remember that the old adage of "this too will pass" is true.

CONTROVERSIAL LEGAL ISSUES AFFECTING NURSING

Because developments and advances in medical and nursing care occur constantly, there are many areas of practice that do not have firm rules to follow when making decisions. Changes in health care delivery and society's values have sparked controversy about a variety of issues.

HEALTH CARE COSTS AND PAYMENT ISSUES

One example is third-party reimbursement, or the right of an individual nurse, usually a nurse practitioner, to be paid directly by insurance companies for care given. Medicare has passed rules that allow nurse practitioners to bill independently under their own provider number. This is a very important step in the field of independent practice for nurses, as many health care insurers follow the lead of Medicare in billing issues.

In relationship to the right to bill, all nurses need to understand billing and reimbursement rules so that they cannot be accused of participating in fraudulent billing schemes. For instance, although a bill can be generated for certain follow-up care performed by nurses in the outpatient clinic as services rendered "incident to" what the physician does, there are strict requirements of physician involvement that nurses must understand. Nurse practitioners need to be careful that their services are not also being illegally billed for by physicians with whom they collaborate.

The seven most frequent areas where nurses can inadvertently become involved in fraud and abuse claims are the following:

1. Questionable accuracy and monitoring of physician visit coding
2. Improper use of diagnosis codes
3. Failure to provide patient care or providing patient care that is sloppy
4. Anesthesia services
5. Unneeded critical or acute care services
6. Billing for physician assistant services
7. Improper billing of nursing or physician services (Nelson & Sanders, 2004)

To avoid these areas, it is important to know about and understand your institution's compliance plan and to report suspected abuses through the required "hot line" or directly to nursing administration (Green, 2000).

From another perspective, the high cost of health care is also driving the proliferation of health care workers with less training and education than nurses, who can be hired for less money. Often these unlicensed workers have no laws circumscribing their practice and are doing tasks that have traditionally been done by RNs or LPNs, such as administering medications and giving injections. This is an important issue for nurses, especially when asked to supervise such workers and/or compete for positions in the health care market.

Controversial legislative changes have been made in an attempt to address some of these problems. In response to concerns of whether or not increased acuity of patients, increased caregiver workload, and declining levels of training among patient-care personnel have threatened the quality of patient care, California passed Assembly Bill 394. This bill set a minimum nurse-patient ratio in acute care general, special, and psychiatric hospitals (Lang et al, 2004). A year after it went into effect, nurses were battling Governor Arnold Schwarzenegger to keep what they fought so hard to obtain, and that is a ratio of RN to patient of 6 to 1 in 2004 and 5 to 1 in 2005. The controversy seems to stem from the difficulty of maintaining ratios "at-all-times" and in finding enough nurses to fill the ratios.

Related topics involve practice models and case management. Practice models involve attempts by institutions to answer what types and ratios of health care providers should constitute a patient-care team (Batcheller et al, 2004). Case management looks at how patient care teams can best derive better outcomes and continuity for patients while effectively managing the variable costs of care delivery. Decisions on these matters by institutions become policies and thus the "laws" under which you must deliver patient care.

Your knowledge of the issues, participation in the processes, and support for legislation and policies that are favorable for your profession and for patient care will be important when your state and/or institution decides such issues. Professional behavior includes concern with and participation in the direction health care, and particularly nursing care, will take in the future.

HEALTH CARE DELIVERY ISSUES

Changes made in the types of systems used to deliver health care and in the techniques used by the systems have created many concerns for nurses. Hospitals and other expensive acute-care settings are giving way to outpatient clinics and same-day surgery centers. This means that people are being sent home while still acutely ill to take care of themselves or relatives without the benefit of hospital nursing services. This makes the nurse's role in discharge planning and patient education an extremely important one to prevent deterioration of certain health or surgical conditions in the home. In addition, it means that home health care nurses are routinely organizing care that used to be only rendered in hospitals. For example, respirators in the home are not unusual. With this change, however, come more independent responsibilities for nurses. Responsibility can translate into liability.

Telephone nursing triage and telemedical nursing care present new and unusual legal concerns because of the difficulties of providing accurate long-distance care and the independent nature of these tasks. Although these nurses bring nursing care to many areas that have not had access to this care in the past, selecting appropriately prepared individuals to provide the care and educating them to function effectively when they cannot see the patient are challenging tasks.

HMOs and other forms of prepaid health care have helped reduce the rapidly growing costs of health care through a process called **utilization review**. Nurses hired to do this review are often asked to make judgments regarding whether or not a patient should be discharged. Early discharge of patients and limits on insurance reimbursements for certain allowable medications, equipment, and external services have sometimes caused ethical and legal problems for health care professionals (Deloughery, 1998).

Past laws protecting the HMOs from malpractice claims when patients were harmed because of flawed utilization review practices are now being challenged. There is a growing public concern that managed-care organizations are making large profits while patients covered under their programs are not receiving adequate care. Both Congress and state legislatures are attempting to pass statutes to curb this practice (Kongstvedt, 2001).

The many changes occurring in the workplace often create levels of confusion and frustration, which make it more difficult to focus on the quality of the care being given on a day-to-day basis. These issues are examples of how legal issues interweave with all the other events in your professional life. Nurses must remain involved in these matters to stay aware of how their legal responsibilities are influenced by them.

ISSUES ABOUT LIFE-AND-DEATH DECISIONS

Controversial ethical issues surrounding life and death also, of course, present controversial legal issues. Scientific research and new technologies can blur the line between life and death. As a nurse, you can often find yourself in the center of such controversies, so you need to be very aware of what your state's laws are on at least the following subjects.

Abortions. Where can abortions be performed? Who can perform them? When can an abortion be performed? Under what conditions? Under what if any conditions can teenagers obtain an abortion without parental consent?

Fetal Rights. If a fetus is born alive, what rights does it have? What rights do the parents have? What rights do health care workers have? What are the laws surrounding fetal death and/or the cessation of life-preserving treatments?

Human Experimentation or Research. What can be done legally with the products of conception? What types of consent are necessary to enroll a patient in research studies? What types of boards and oversight must be involved to approve and monitor human research studies?

Patient Rights. What rights do patients have in your state in relationship to medical records, medical information, giving consent, participating in their care, suing providers, dictating issues surrounding their death, donating organs, being protected from abuse, receiving emergency treatment, being protected from the practice of unlicensed providers, transplantation of organs, accessibility of the disabled to health care, privacy, and confidentiality?

CONCLUSION

As time goes on, laws will be changing and new areas will arise that nursing will have to address. Continuing education, critical thinking, and an open mind will help you to learn about and deal with the legal issues that will touch your professional life daily. Get involved whenever possible with safety, quality, and risk-management processes in your institutions. Be someone who has an educated opinion about conflicts inherent in medicine and nursing. Take the opportunity to visit the hearings conducted by your state's board of nursing and by the state legislature. By becoming involved with the legal and disciplinary process, you will be much more aware of how you can protect yourself and your patients and influence the direction of health care issues. By concluding this chapter, it is hoped that you also feel more confident when faced with "the law."

REFERENCES

American Society for Healthcare Risk Management: *Perspective on disclosure of unanticipated outcome information*, Chicago, 2001, ASHRM.

Annas GJ: HIPAA regulations—a new era of medical-record privacy?, *N Engl J Med* 348(15): 1486-1490, 2003.

Beckstead J: Modeling attitudinal antecedents of nurses' decisions to report impaired colleagues, *J Nurs Res* 24(5):537-551, 2002.

Bolin JN, Clark LS: Avoiding charges of fraud and abuse, *JONA* 34(12): 546-550, 2004.

Brent N: *Nurses and the law*, ed 2, New York, 2001, Saunders.

Curtin LL: When negligence becomes homicide, *Nurs Manage* 28(7):7-8, 1997.

Deloughery G: *Issues and trends in nursing*, St Louis, 1998, Mosby.

Di Luigi K: What it takes to be an expert witness, *RN* 67(2): 65-66, 2004.

Di Maio VJ, Di Maio TG: Homicide by decubitus ulcers, *Am J Forensic Med Pathol* 23(1):1-4, 2002.

Fish RM, Ehrhardt ME, Fish B: *Malpractice: managing your defense*, Montvale, NJ, 1990, Medical Economics Books.

Freydel v. New York Hospital, No. 97 Civ 7926 (SHS), Jan 4, 2000.

Goedert J: It's time to 'address' the final security rule, *Health Data Management* 11(4), 2003.

Green E: Creating an effective corporate compliance program, *Drug Benefit Trends* 12:37-38, 2000.

Guido GW: *Legal and ethical issues in nursing*, Upper Saddle River, NJ, 2001, Prentice Hall.

Gutheil TG: On apologizing to patients, *Risk Management Foundation of the Harvard Medical Institutions* 6:3-4, 51, 1987.

Gutheil TG, Bursztajn H, Brodsky A: Malpractice prevention through the sharing of uncertainty.

Informed consent and the therapeutic alliance, *N Engl J Med* 311(1):49-51, 1984.

Harvey v. Mid-Coast Hospital, 36 F. Supp. 2d 32, D. Maine, 1999.

Haumschild M, Karfonta T, Haumschild M, et al: Clinical and economic outcomes of a fall-focused pharmaceutical intervention program, *Am J Health-Syst Phar* 60(10), 2003.

Joint Commission on the Accreditation of Healthcare Organizations: *National patient safety goals*, Oakbrook Terrace, Ill, 2005, JCAHO.

Joint Commission on the Accreditation of Healthcare Organizations: *Comprehensive accreditation manual for hospitals: the official handbook*, Oakbrook Terrace, Ill, 2004, JCAHO.

Kelly LY, Joel JA: *Dimensions of professional nursing*, New York, 1999, McGraw-Hill.

Kohn LT, Corrigan JM, Donaldson MS: *To err is human: building a safer health system*, Washington, DC, 2000, National Academy Press.

Kongstvedt PR: *Essentials of managed health care*, ed 4, Rockville, Md, 2001, Aspen.

Kowalski K, Horner MD: A legal nightmare. Denver nurses indicted, *MCN Am J Maternal Child Nurs* 23(3):125-129, 1998.

Lafleur K: Tackling med errors with technology, *RN* 27(5):29-31, 2004.

Lang TA, Hodge M, Olson V, et al: Nurse-patient ratios: a systematic review on the effects of nurse staffing on patient, nurse employee and hospital outcomes, *JONA* 34(7/8):326-327, 2004.

Larson A: Medical malpractice law and litigation (1998 to 2005), Law Offices of Aaron Larson.

Medmal4Nurses.com, 2005.

Medscape Medical News: *Joint Commission releases revised restraints standards for behavioral Healthcare*, 2000.

Moore R: A guide to the assessment and care of the patient whose medical decision-making capacity is in question, *Medscape Gen Med* 1(3), 1999.

Murphy EK: Individual malpractice insurance decisions revisited, *AORN J* 67(6):1234-1236, 1998.

National Council of State Boards of Nursing (NCSBN): *2005 Nurse Licensure Compact, www.ncsbn.org/nlc/rnlpvncompact_mutual_recognition_state.asp.*

National Council of State Boards of Nursing (NCSBN): *NCSBN introduces online public access to NURSYS*, letter, February 12, 2003.

National Council of State Boards of Nursing: *Chemical dependency handbook for nurse managers—a guide for managing chemically dependent employees*, Chicago, 2001, NCSBN.

National Practitioner Data Bank (NPDB): *2004 Annual report*, 2004, U.S. Department of Health and Human Services.

Nelson R: Staffing in California one year later, *AJN* 105(2):25-26, 2005.

Nursefriendly, Inc.: Nursing & healthcare directories on: The nursefriendly chemical dependence, substance abuse impaired nurses, New Jersey, 1997–2005.

Physicians Mutual Insurance Company, Scottsdale, Ariz, 2005, *http://phoenix.jobing.com/jobfair_company.asp?i=3888.*

Rich D: New JCAHO Medication management standards for 2004, *Am J Health-Syst Pharm* 61(13):1349-1358, 2004.

St. Anthony's Hospital v. Whitfield, 946 SW2d 174 (Tex App 1997).

Simpson KR: Should nurses purchase their own professional liability insurance?, *Am J Maternal Child Nurs* 23(3), 1998.

Sullivan GH: Does your charting measure up?, *RN* 17(3): 2004.

Tideliksaar R: *Falls in older patients: prevention and management*, Baltimore, 1998, Health Profession Press.

Truog R: *Inadequacies in use of informed consent may limit potential for research in intensive care*, 15th Annual Congress of European Society of Intensive Care Medicine, Sept 19-Oct 2, 2002, Barcelona, Spain.

Walker RS: *Falls and serious injuries before, during and after a nursing home became restraint free*, thesis, Tuscon, Ariz, 1992, University of Arizona.

Yocum CJ, Haack MR: *Interim report: a comparison of two regulatory approaches to the management of chemically impaired nurses*, Chicago, 1996, NCSBN.

UNIT VI

Contemporary Nursing Practice

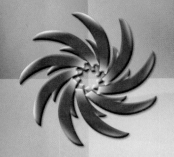

CHAPTER 21

Cultural and Spiritual Awareness

VALERIE S. ESCHITI, RN, MSN, CHTP, AHN-BC

It gives me a deep comforting sense that "things seen are temporal and things unseen are eternal."

—Helen Keller

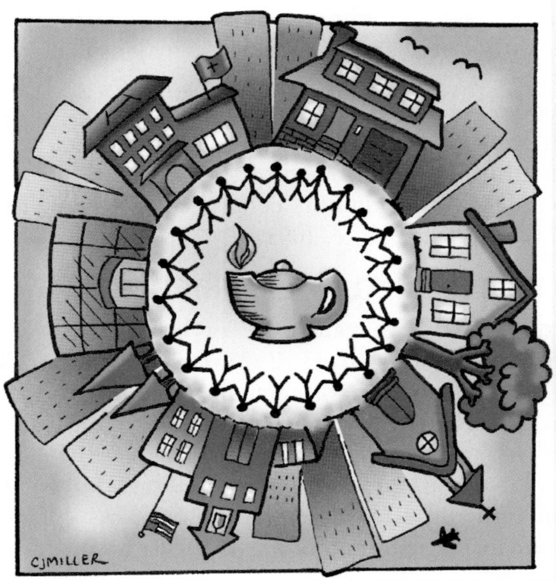

Nursing is a vital part of community health.

After completing this chapter, you should be able to:

- Define cultural competence.
- List practice issues related to cultural competence.
- Identify challenges in defining spirituality.
- Determine cultural and spiritual beliefs of clients in the health care setting.
- Assess spiritual needs of patients in the health care setting.

CULTURE AND SPIRITUALITY

WHAT IS MEANT BY CULTURAL COMPETENCE?

In a global society that is becoming increasingly diverse, cultural competence is necessary for excellence in nursing care. The American Nurses Association (ANA) indicates the necessity of the nurse being sensitive to individual needs in the *Code of Ethics*: "The need for health care is universal, transcending all individual differences. The nurse establishes relationships and delivers nursing services with respect for human needs and values, and without prejudice. An individual's lifestyle, values system, and religious beliefs should be considered in planning health care with and for each patient" (ANA, 2001). But what exactly is cultural competence? It is defined as "developing an awareness of one's own existence, sensations, thoughts, and environment without letting it have an undue influence on those from other backgrounds; demonstrating knowledge and understanding of the client's culture; accepting and respecting cultural differences; adapting care to be congruent with the client's culture" (Purnell & Paulanka, 2003).

The culturally competent nurse has enhanced ability to provide quality care, which fosters better patient understanding of the plan of care.

"'Inattention to cultural competence in patient care leads, at best, to sub-optimal patient outcomes and, at worst, to active harm,' says Carla Serlin, PhD, RN, director of ANA's Ethnic/Racial Minority Fellowship Programs. 'When we fail to address issues of difference such as language, ethnicity and race, our patients will have lower levels of compliance with care instructions and longer hospital stays.'" (Stewart, no date)

Campinha-Bacote created a model of cultural competence called "The Process of Cultural Competence in the Delivery of Healthcare Services." This model defines cultural competence as "the process in which the healthcare professional continually strives to achieve the ability and availability to work within the cultural context of a client—individual, family, or community" (Campinha-Bacote, 2003).

WHAT PRACTICE ISSUES ARE RELATED TO CULTURAL COMPETENCE?

Barriers to Cultural Competence. Two categories of barriers to cultural competence exist: provider barriers and systems barriers (Mazanec & Tyler, 2003). Provider barriers are those such as a nurse may have, including lack of information about a culture. The mnemonic CULTURE, developed by Zerwekh and Claborn (2006), can be helpful for nurses in assessing and improving their level of cultural competence (Box 21-1). In addition, nurses need to use effective cultural interviewing questions, which are best if semi-structured and open-ended. Spector (2000) has identified nine suggestions for enhancing communication when gathering cultural data (Box 21-2).

BOX 21-1 CULTURE: A Nursing Approach

C **C**onsider your own cultural biases and how this affects your nursing care.
U **U**nderstand the need to recognize cultural implications in planning and implementing nursing care.
L **L**earn how to utilize cultural assessment tools.
T **T**reat clients with dignity and respect.
U **U**se sensitivity in providing culturally competent care.
R **R**ecognize opportunities to provide specific culturally based nursing care.
E **E**valuate your own previous encounters with clients from other cultures and backgrounds.

BOX 21-2 Nine Suggestions for Gathering Cultural Data

- Determine the level of fluency in English and arrange for an interpreter if needed.
- Ask how the client prefers to be addressed.
- Allow the client to choose seating for comfortable personal space and eye contact.
- Avoid body language that may be offensive or misunderstood.
- Speak directly to the client, whether an interpreter is present or not.
- Choose a speech rate and style that promotes understanding and demonstrates respect for the client.
- Avoid slang, technical jargon, and complex sentences.
- Use open-ended questions or questions phrased in several ways to obtain information.
- Determine the client's reading ability before using written materials in the teaching process.

From Spector RE: *Cultural diversity in health and illness,* ed 5. Upper Saddle River, NJ, 2000, Prentice-Hall Health, as cited in Ignatavicius, D, Workman, L: *Medical-surgical nursing: critical thinking for collaborative care.* St. Louis, 2006, Elsevier.

Systems barriers are those that exist in an agency, because the agency's structure and policies are not designed to support cultural diversity (Mazanec & Tyler, 2003). For instance, an American Indian family may wish to spend the night in the intensive care unit room with a critically ill family member. However, the room does not have a cot on which to sleep, and the waiting room is not large enough to accommodate all the family and extended family members who are present to support the patient. The community in which the hospital is located has a large American Indian population. The nurse, as an advocate for patients and their families, can intervene through activities such as joining a hospital committee focused on hospital redesign. The nurse can point out the need for space for family members to stay the night near their loved ones. In this way, the nurse supports the needs of the cultural diversity in her community.

Health and Health Care Disparities. One of the goals of *Healthy People 2010* is to eliminate health disparities. Health disparities are inequalities in disease morbidity and mortality in segments of the population. These disparities may be due to differences in race or ethnicity. They are believed to be the result of the interaction among genetic variations, environmental factors, and health behaviors. For instance, the infant death rate among blacks is more than double that of whites. American Indians and Alaska Natives have an infant death rate almost double that for whites. Their rate of diabetes is more than twice that for whites. Hispanics are almost twice as likely to die from diabetes as are non-Hispanic whites. New cases of hepatitis and tuberculosis also are higher in Asians and Pacific Islanders than in whites (Healthy People 2010, 2000).

Healthy People 2010 goals:
1. Increase quality and years of healthy life.
2. Eliminate health disparities.

Inequalities in income and education are at the root of many health disparities. In general, those populations who have the worst health status are those that have the highest poverty rates and the least education. Low income and education levels are associated with differences in rates of illness and death, including heart disease, diabetes, obesity, and low birth weight. Higher incomes allow better access to medical care, enable people to afford better housing and live in safer neighborhoods, and increase the opportunity to engage in health-promoting behaviors (Healthy People 2010, 2000).

"Disparities in health care are defined as racial or ethnic differences in the quality of health care that are **not** due to access-related factors or clinical needs, preferences and appropriateness of intervention" (Smedley, Stith, & Nelson, 2002, p. 4). Some of the causes of health care disparities include provider variables and patient variables. Provider variables are provider/patient relationships, lack of minority providers, as well as provider bias and discrimination. Patient variables are mistrust of the health care system and refusal of treatment (Baldwin, 2003).

The solutions to challenges of health and health care disparities are complex, and still being discovered (Critical Thinking Box 21-1). Some solutions are increasing diversity of health care providers, ensuring that all people have access to affordable, basic health care; promoting wellness and a healthy lifestyle; strengthening

CRITICAL THINKING BOX 21-1

Can you think of ways to decrease health and health care disparities in your community? What projects could you do as a nursing student to make a positive impact? Could you devise a project as part of a class assignment or a Student Nurses Association activity?

provider/patient relationships; increasing cultural competency of health care providers; and conducting research to determine why certain diseases impact minorities so greatly, and to discover effective intervention strategies (Baldwin, 2003).

WHAT IS THE MEANING OF SPIRITUALITY?

One of the challenges for the nurse in providing spiritual care to patients is that there is not yet a clear definition of spirituality (MacLaren, 2004). Many people confuse religion with spirituality, when in fact, they can be separate entities. McSherry (2000) presents several components of spirituality with relevance to nursing, which is a helpful framework for understanding the concept (Box 21-3). At times, a spiritual advisor or chaplain may be called upon for a patient's or family's spiritual needs. But there are times these spiritual needs may be met most appropriately by the nurse (Van Dover & Bacon, 2001).

A definition of spiritual nursing care is "an intuitive, interpersonal, altruistic, and integrative expression that is contingent upon the nurse's awareness of the transcendent dimension of life but that reflects the patient's reality" (Sawatzky & Pesut, 2005). Spiritual Distress is an approved nursing diagnosis (Carpenito-Moyet, 2004). Examples of spiritual nursing interventions include: prayer, presence, scripture reading, peaceful environment, meditation, music, pastoral care, inspiring hope, active listening, validation of patients' thoughts and feelings, values clarification, sensitive responses to patient beliefs, and developing a trusting relationship (Callister et al, 2004).

BOX 21-3 Components of Spirituality

- Spirituality is a universal concept relevant to all individuals
- The uniqueness of the individual is paramount
- Formal religious affiliation is not a prerequisite for spirituality
- An individual may become more spiritually aware during a time of need

From McSherry W: *Making sense of spirituality in nursing practice: an integrative approach,* Edinburgh, 2000, Churchill Livingstone, p 27.

CULTURAL AND SPIRITUAL ASSESSMENT

WHAT ARE CULTURAL AND SPIRITUAL BELIEFS ABOUT ILLNESS AND CURES?

Patients will have different responses to illness based on their cultural and spiritual beliefs. It is vital for the nurse to be aware of the variety of responses that may be encountered (Table 21-1).

TABLE 21-1

Cultural and Spiritual Beliefs Affecting Nursing Care

ASIAN/PACIFIC ISLANDER
Extended family has large influence on client.
Older family members are honored and respected, and their authority is unquestioned.
Oldest male is decision-maker and spokesman.
Strong emphasis on avoiding conflict and direct confrontation.
Respect authority and do not disagree with health care recommendations—but, they may not follow recommendations.
CHINESE
Chinese clients will not discuss symptoms of mental illness or depression because they believe this behavior reflects on family; therefore, it may produce shame and guilt. As a result, there may be psychosomatic symptoms.
Use herbalists, spiritual healers, and physicians for care.
JAPANESE
Believe physical contact with blood, skin diseases, and corpses will cause illness.
They also believe improper care of the body, including poor diet and lack of sleep, cause illness.
They believe in healers, herbalists, and physicians for healing, and energy can be restored with acupuncture and acupressure. Their high regard for the status of physicians decreases the likelihood that they will question their care.
They use group decision making for health concerns.
Disability is a source of family shame. Mental illness is taboo.
Pain is not expressed as it is considered a virtue to bear pain.
Addiction is a strong taboo.
HINDU AND MUSLIM
Indians and Pakistanis do not acknowledge a diagnosis of severe emotional illness or mental retardation because it reduces the chance of other family members getting married.
Medical beliefs are a blend of modern and traditional practice.
VIETNAMESE
Vietnamese are slow to trust authority figures due to their refugee experiences. They accept mental health counseling and interventions particularly when they have established trust with the health care worker.
Very patriarchal society.
Although home remedies are tried first, they are compliant with Western health care treatment, once sought.

Continued

TABLE 21-1

Cultural and Spiritual Beliefs Affecting Nursing Care—cont'd

HISPANIC/LATINO

Older family members are consulted on issues involving health and illness.

Patriarchal family—men make decisions for family.

Illness is viewed as God's will or divine punishment resulting from sinful behavior.

Prefer to use home remedies and consult folk healers known as curanderos or curanderas rather than traditional Western health care providers.

Many believe in the hot and cold theory of disease, although they may differ about what constitutes hot or cold.

AFRICAN-AMERICAN

Family and church oriented.

Extensive family bonds.

Key family member is consulted for important health-related decisions.

Illness is a punishment from God for wrongdoing, or is due to voodoo, spirits, or demons.

Illness is prevented through good diet, herbs, rest, cleanliness, and laxatives to clean the system.

Wear copper and silver bracelets to prevent illness.

Some distrust health care providers, especially due to an under representation of African-American health care providers.

AMERICAN INDIAN

Oriented to the present.

Value cooperation, family, and spiritual beliefs.

Strong ties to family and tribe.

Believe state of health exists when client lives in total harmony with nature.

Illness is viewed as an imbalance between the person and natural or supernatural forces.

May use medicine man or medicine woman instead of or in conjunction with seeking Western health care.

Illness is prevented through rituals and prayer.

Some mistrust health care providers, due to historical conflicts in the United States, lack of culturally competent care, and underrepresentation of American Indians as health care providers.

Adapted from Smith SF, Duell DJ, Martin BC: *Clinical nursing skills: basic to advanced skills*, ed 6. Upper Saddle River, NJ, 2004, Pearson-Prentice Hall, p 111.

The nurse needs to be careful, however, not to stereotype a patient based on his or her cultural or spiritual background.

People of many cultures may use complementary, alternative, or integrative modalities that can affect their health status (Box 21-4). Because the public is increasingly using integrative therapies in the United States (Eisenberg et al, 1998), it is vital that the nurse have a basic understanding of various therapies, as well as their benefits and risks. For instance, a diabetic Chinese patient may be ingesting ginger. Ginger may decrease blood glucose levels (*Nursing2004*, 2004). It is possible that ginger ingestion by the patient could influence the dosage of an oral antidiabetic agent needed by the patient (Figure 21-1).

BOX 21-4 Definitions of Terms

Complementary therapies: those that are used in conjunction with mainstream treatments.
Alternative therapies: those that are used instead of mainstream medical therapies.
Integrative therapies: those for which there is some scientific basis for usage.

From National Center for Complementary and Alternative Medicine: *What is complementary and alternative medicine?*, 2002, *http://nccam.nih.gov/health/whatiscam/*.

The American Holistic Nurses Association (AHNA) says, "Holistic nursing embraces all nursing which has as its goal the enhancement of healing the whole person from birth to death" (AHNA, 2004). Vital components of a holistic nursing assessment are identification of cultural and spiritual practices and needs.

The Joint Commission on the Accreditation of Healthcare Organizations (JCAHO) acknowledges a patient's right to care that respects their cultural and spiritual values.

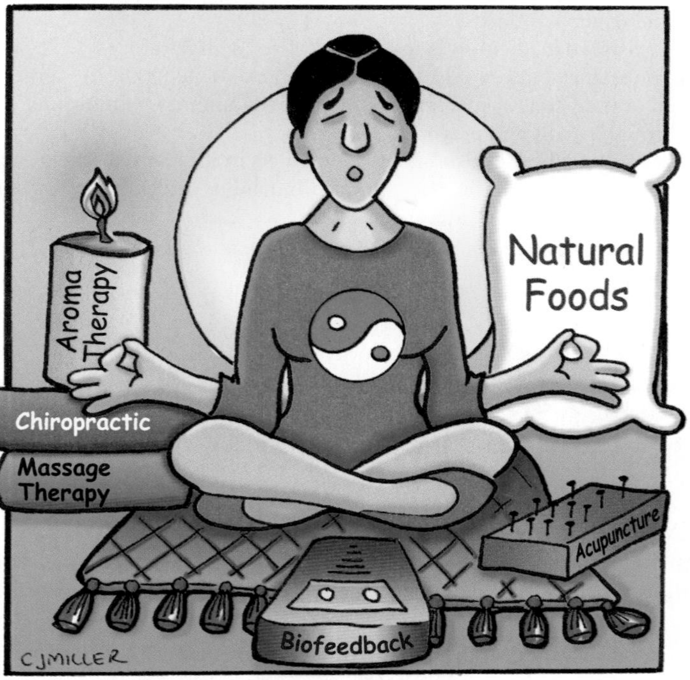

FIGURE 21-1
Complementary health care therapy is on the rise.

CRITICAL THINKING BOX 21-2

How much knowledge do you have regarding various integrative therapies, such as acupuncture, healing touch, reiki, herbal medicine, and aromatherapy? Use the additional readings and Internet resources listed at the end of the chapter to enhance your knowledge base. Identify possible referral sources for integrative therapies in your community. You never know when a patient may ask you for information and/or referral regarding integrative therapies.

"JCAHO recommends that health care organizations (1) acknowledge patients' rights to spiritual care and (2) provide for these needs through pastoral care and a diversity of services that may be offered by certified, ordained, or lay individuals" (LaPierre, 2003, p. 219). It is imperative that the nurse performs a spiritual assessment; to assess the patient's individual needs (Critical Thinking Box 21-2 and Figure 21-2).

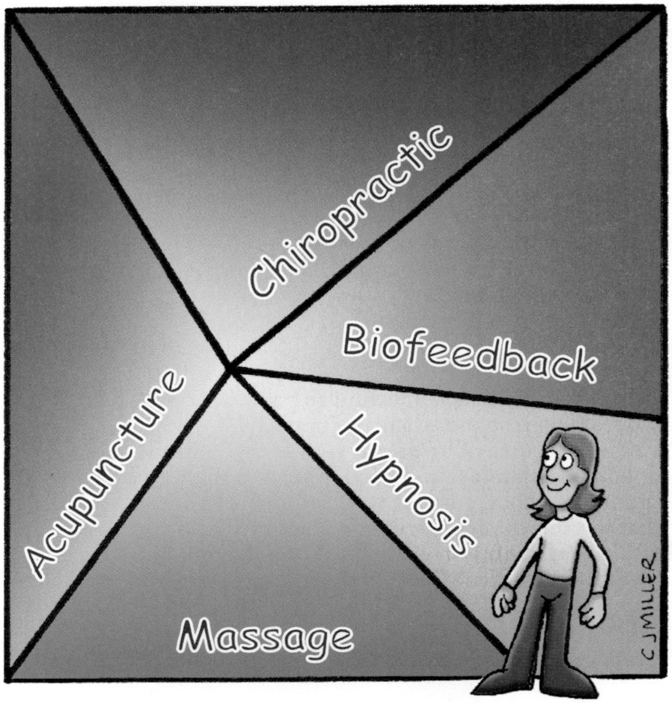

FIGURE 21-2
The five most reported integrative therapies.

HOW DO YOU ASSESS SPIRITUAL NEED?

Specific spiritual assessment tools can be used as guides by the nurse to determine the spiritual needs of her patients. Aspects of these tools may also be integrated into an agency assessment document. Box 21-5 lists dimensions of spirituality with corresponding assessment questions. These questions can assist the nurse in determining needs that exist in any of the seven spiritual dimensions.

BOX 21-5 Dimensions of Spirituality with Corresponding Assessment Questions

SPIRIT-ENHANCING PRACTICES OR RITUALS

How do you express your spirituality (or philosophy of life)?
What spiritual or religious practices or activities are important to you?
How has being sick affected your spiritual practices?
How does being sick have an impact on your praying (or meditation, scripture reading, fasting, receiving sacraments, service attendance, etc.)?
How and for what do you pray?
What spiritual or religious books or symbols are helpful to you?
What effect do you expect your illness to have on your spiritual practices or beliefs?
What kinds of readings, artwork, or music are inspirational for you?
How do Holy Scriptures (e.g., Koran, Bible) help you in daily life?
How can I as a nurse help you with your spiritual practice?
How do your religious practices help you to grow spiritually?

EXPERIENCE OF GOD OR TRANSCENDENCE

Is religion important to you? Why or why not?
Does God/Higher Power/Ultimate Other/The Transcendence, etc. seem personal to you?
Do you feel close now?
How does God or a deity function in your personal life?
How is God working in your life?
How would you describe your god and what you worship?
What is your picture of God?
What do you feel you mean to God?
Are there any barriers between you and God? Is there anything you think God could not forgive you?
How do you make sense of feeling angry with God?
How does God respond when you pray?
Do you feel a source of love from God or any spiritual being? Where is God in all this?
What kind of relationship do you have with the leader of your spiritual community (e.g., priest, rabbi, guru)?
In what ways does your spiritual community help you when times are bad?
What kinds of confusion or doubt do you have about your religious beliefs?
Are you having difficulty carrying out your religious duties?

SENSE OF MEANING

What gives most meaning to your life? What is the most important thing in your life?
When you are sick, do you have feelings that you are being punished or that it is God's will for you to be sick?

Continued

BOX 21-5 Dimensions of Spirituality with Corresponding Assessment Questions—cont'd

What are your thoughts about or explanations for suffering? Are these beliefs helpful?
What do you see as the cosmic/God's plan or purpose for your life?
Have you been able to answer any of the "why" questions that often accompany illness?
What, if any, have been the good outcomes from having this difficult time in life?
What, if anything, motivates you to get well?

GIVING AND RECEIVING LOVE, OR CONNECTEDNESS TO SELF (DEGREE OF SELF-AWARENESS) AND OTHERS
What do you do to show love for yourself?
What are some of the most loving things that people have done for you?
What are the loving things that you do for others?
How do others help you now? How easy is it to accept their help?
For what do you hope? How do you experience hope?
How have you experienced forgiveness during your life/illness? (Forgiveness toward self, toward or from others and God)

SOURCES OF HOPE AND STRENGTH
What helps you to cope now?
What (or who) is your source of hope? Of strength? How do they help?
To whom do you turn when you need help? Are they available?
What helps you most when you feel afraid or need special help?
How can I help you maintain your spiritual strength during this illness?
To what degree do you trust your future to God?
What brings you joy and peace in your life?
What do you believe in?
What do you do to make yourself feel alive and full of spirit?

LINKAGE BETWEEN SPIRITUALITY AND HEALTH
How does your spirituality affect your experience of being sick?
How has your current situation/illness influenced your faith?
How has being sick affected your sense of who you are (or how has being sick affected you spiritually)?
What has bothered you most about being sick (or in what is happening to you now)?
What do you do to heal your spirit?
Has being sick (or your current situation) made any difference in your feelings about God or your faith experience (or in what you believe)?
Is there anything especially frightening or meaningful to you now?
Do you ever wish for more faith to help you with your illness?
Has being ill ever made you feel angry, guilty, bitter, or resentful?
How involved in a spiritual/religious community/organization (e.g., church, temple, covenant group) are you? (As a visitor? Member? Leader?)

From Taylor EJ: *Spiritual care: nursing theory, research, and practice,* Upper Saddle River, NJ, 2002, Pearson-Prentice Hall, pp 121-124.

CONCLUSION

As you enter the world of nursing, you are going to come into contact with patients from various cultures, and they are going to have many different spiritual beliefs. As nurses, we must be able to address these issues as they relate to health care. Nurses need to become more "culturally competent" to better understand the health care needs of our vast, multicultural patient population. It will not be enough to recognize and accept these cultural implications; we must plan nursing and health care that will achieve the most positive patient results. With the melting pot of cultures in the patient population, nurses must begin to implement a more holistic approach to providing health care. The place to begin is with each individual nurse, who must begin with an assessment of his or her own value system and become more culturally competent.

In clinical settings, spiritual assessment tools can help the nurse gain a deeper understanding of the patient from a holistic perspective (Box 21-6). However, these

BOX 21-6 Spiritual Assessment Tool

To facilitate the healing process in clients/patients, families, significant others, and yourself, use the following reflective questions to assist in assessing, evaluating, and increasing awareness of the spiritual process in yourself and others.

MEANING AND PURPOSE

These questions assess a person's ability to seek meaning and fulfillment in life, manifest hope, and accept ambiguity and uncertainty.

- What gives your life meaning?
- Do you have a sense of purpose in life?
- Does your illness interfere with your life goals?
- Why do you want to get well?
- How hopeful are you about obtaining a better degree of health?
- Do you feel that you have a responsibility in maintaining your health?
- Will you be able to make changes in your life to maintain your health?
- Are you motivated to get well?
- What is the most important or powerful thing in your life?

INNER STRENGTHS

These questions assess a person's ability to manifest joy and recognize strengths, choices, goals, and faith.

- What brings you joy and peace in your life?
- What can you do to feel alive and full of spirit?
- What traits do you like about yourself?
- What are your personal strengths?
- What choices are available to enhance your healing?
- What life goals have you set for yourself?
- Do you think that stress in any way caused your illness?
- How aware were you of your body before you became sick?
- What do you believe in?
- Is faith important in your life?
- How has your illness influenced your faith?
- Does faith play a role in regaining your health?

Continued

BOX 21-6 Spiritual Assessment Tool—cont'd

INTERCONNECTIONS

These questions assess a person's positive self-concept, self-esteem, and sense of self; sense of belonging in the world with others; capacity to pursue personal interests; and ability to demonstrate love of self and self-forgiveness.

- How do you feel about yourself right now?
- How do you feel when you have a true sense of yourself?
- Do you pursue things of personal interest?
- What do you do to show love for yourself?
- Can you forgive yourself?
- What do you do to heal your spirit?

  These questions assess a person's ability to connect in life-giving ways with family, friends, and social groups and to engage in the forgiveness of others.
- Who are the significant people in your life?
- Do you have friends or family in town who are available to help you?
- Who are the people to whom you are closest?
- Do you belong to any groups?
- Can you ask people for help when you need it?
- Can you share your feelings with others?
- What are some of the most loving things that others have done for you?
- What are the loving things that you do for others?
- Are you able to forgive others?

These questions assess a person's capacity for finding meaning in worship or religious activities and a connectedness with a divinity or universe.

- Is worship important to you?
- What do you consider the most significant act of worship in your life?
- Do you participate in any religious activities?
- Do you believe in God or a higher power?
- Do you think that prayer is powerful?
- Have you ever tried to empty your mind of all thoughts to see what the experience might be like?
- Do you use relaxation or imagery skills?
- Do you meditate?
- Do you pray?
- What is your prayer?
- How are your prayers answered?
- Do you have a sense of belonging in this world?

  These questions assess a person's ability to experience a sense of connection with all life and nature, an awareness of the effects of the environment on life and well-being, and a capacity or concern for the health of the environment.
- Do you ever feel at some level a connection with the world or universe?
- How does your environment have an impact on your state of well-being?
- What are your environmental stressors at work and at home?
- Do you incorporate strategies to reduce your environmental stressors?
- Do you have any concerns for the state of your immediate environment?
- Are you involved with environmental issues such as recycling environmental resources at home, work, or in your community?
- Are you concerned about the survival of the planet?

From Dossey BM, Keegan L, Guzzetta CE: *Holistic nursing: a handbook for practice*, Sudbury, Mass, 2000, Jones & Bartlett, pp 106-107.

CRITICAL THINKING BOX 21-3

If your patient requested for you to pray with him, would you feel comfortable? If not, what other resources could you call upon to meet the spiritual needs of this patient?

tools are merely guides, not multipurpose checklists that can be completed all at once during an initial assessment period. "Rather than considering completion of an instrument to be an end point, these guides are most effective when the questions are used as openings or referent points for discussing spirituality with patients. As we reflect with patients and explore the deeper sense of their responses, we come to better know and understand them in their wholeness. We can adapt the different ways of approaching spirituality assessment to fit the specific situation and person" (Burkhardt & Nagai-Jacobsen, 2002) (Critical Thinking Box 21-3).

REFERENCES

American Holistic Nurses Association (AHNA): *What is holistic nursing?*, 2004, *www.ahna.org/about/whatis.html.*

American Nurses Association: *Code of ethics for nurses with interpretive statements*, Kansas City, Mo, 2001, ANA, *www.nursingworld.org/ethics/code/ethicscode-150.htm.*

Baldwin DM: *Disparities in health care: focusing efforts to eliminate unequal burdens.* Washington, DC, 2003, American Nurses Association, *http://nursingworld.org/mods/mod560/cebrdnfull.htm.*

Burkhardt MA, Nagai-Jacobsen MG: *Spirituality: living our connectedness*, Albany, NY, 2002, Delmar.

Callister LC, Bond AE, Matsurmura G, et al: Threading spirituality through nursing education, *Hol Nurs Practice*, 18(3):160-166, 2004.

Campinha-Bacote J: *The process of cultural competence in the delivery of healthcare services: a culturally competent model of care*, Cincinnati, 2003, Transcultural C.A.R.E. Associates, *www.transculturalcare.net/Cultural_Competence_Model.htm.*

Dossey BM, Keegan L, Guzzetta CE: *Holistic nursing: a handbook for practice*, ed 3, Sudbury, Mass, 2000, Jones & Bartlett.

Eisenberg DM, Davis RB, Ettner SL, et al: Trends in alternative medicine use in the United States: 1990-1997, *JAMA*, 280(18):1569-1575, 1998.

Healthy People 2000: what are its goals?, Washington, DC, U.S. Department of Health and Human Services, *www.healthypeople.gov/About/goals.htm.*

Healthy People 2010: understanding and improving health, Washington, DC, 2000, U.S. Department of Health and Human Services, *www.healthypeople.gov/Document/html/uih/uih_2.htm#goals.*

LaPierre LL: JCAHO safeguards spiritual care, *Holistic Nurs Pract* 17(4):219, 2003.

MacLaren J: A kaleidescope of understandings: spiritual nursing in a multi-faith society, *J Adv Nurs*, 45(5):457-462, 2004.

Mazanec P, Tyler MK: Cultural considerations in end-of-life care: how ethnicity, age, and spirituality affect decisions when death is imminent, *Am J Nurs* 103(3):50-58, 2003.

McSherry W: *Making sense of spirituality in nursing practice: an integrative approach.* Edinburgh, 2000, Churchill Livingstone.

National Center for Complementary and Alternative Medicine: What is complementary and alternative medicine?, 2002, *http://nccam.nih.gov/health/whatiscam/.*

Nursing 2004 herbal medicine handbook, ed 2, Philadelphia, 2004, Lippincott Williams & Wilkins.

Purnell LD, Paulanka BJ: *Transcultural healthcare: a culturally competent approach*, ed 2, Philadelphia, 2003, F.A. Davis.

Sawatzky R, Pesut B: Attributes of spiritual care in nursing practice, *J Holistic Nurs* 23(1):19-33, 2005.

Smedley BD, Stith AY, Nelson AR: *Unequal treatment: confronting racial and ethnic disparities in health care*, Institute of Medicine report, Washington, DC, 2002, National Academy Press.

Smith SF, Duell DJ, Martin BC: *Clinical nursing skills: basic to advanced skills*, ed 6. Upper Saddle River, NJ, 2004, Pearson-Prentice Hall, p 111.

Stewart M: *Nurses need to strengthen cultural competency for next century to ensure quality patient care*, Washington, DC, no date, NursingWorld, *http://nursingworld.org/tan/98janfeb/cultcomp.htm.*

Taylor EJ: *Spiritual care: nursing theory, research, and practice*. Upper Saddle River, NJ, 2002, Pearson-Prentice Hall.

Van Dover LJ, Bacon JM: Spiritual care in nursing practice: a close-up view. *Nurs Forum* 6(3):18-30: 2001.

Zerwekh J, Claborn J: *CULTURE: a mnemonic for assessing and improving cultural competence*. Ingram, TX, 2006, Nursing Education Consultant, Inc.

CHAPTER 22

Quality Patient Care

TESS M. PAPE, PhD, RN, CNOR

"A pessimist sees the difficulty in every opportunity; an optimist sees the opportunity in every difficulty."

—Sir Winston Churchill

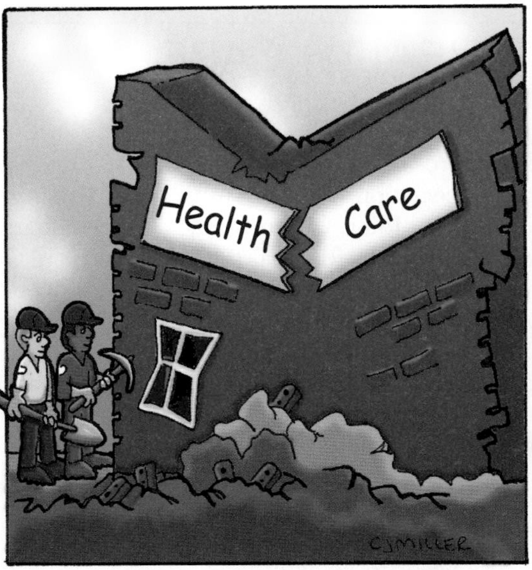

By working together in our quality circles we can fix our broken health care system.

After completing this chapter, you should be able to:

- Describe the history and evolution of quality in health care.
- Discuss the use of key indicators to measure performance.
- Describe your role in quality and performance improvement.
- Identify tools and processes for continuous quality improvement.
- Identify the role of regulatory standards and agencies.
- Incorporate successful process improvement strategies.
- Consider the value and requirements of quality credentialing.

You may wonder why nurses need to know about quality issues to provide patient care. All nurses know to give high quality care, right? Of course they do, at least in an ideal world—but soon many new graduates find out that not all nurses care about truly doing the right thing for the patient and the health care environment. That is why we have quality improvement departments within health care settings. Someone must monitor quality care compliance.

Have you ever wondered why on a hot summer day, you notice the best parking place is determined by shade instead of distance? This is because the value placed on the issue is determined by the person doing the valuing. It also depends on the situation. For example, a person may park under the shade tree on a hot summer day, but park in the sun on a cold day. If the space is far from the building, the temperature of the day will play a role. So, too, is quality in health care settings.

Issues that are on the forefront of news will take precedence over those that are routine or commonplace. Recently, medical errors have become of primary concern. Illegible handwriting as a contributing factor to errors has led to regulations about what medical abbreviations are appropriate (Institute of Medicine [IOM], 2000).

In the 1980s, the hot topic of HIV and hepatitis caused great concern over the use of gloves to prevent transmission of infection. Because of the introduction of foreign supplies of latex gloves, more latex allergies surfaced. In the 1990s, more emphasis was placed on using needleless systems, and legislation was passed to prevent more needlestick injuries. Each decade seems to have critical topics that need to be addressed with quality initiatives. This does not mean that other issues are not just as important, but it simply shows how history and events shape the quality paradigm.

STANDARDS OF QUALITY HEALTH CARE MANAGEMENT

Several agencies have established standards that guide quality in health care. Some of these include the American Nurses Association (ANA) Standards of Nursing Care, accrediting group standards such as the Joint Commission on Accreditation of Healthcare Organizations (JCAHO). The Agency for Healthcare Research and Quality (AHRQ) established clinical practice treatment guidelines. These guidelines are designed to improve patient outcomes and reduce costs. Each health care facility also sets its own standards of practice.

The JCAHO publishes a sentinel event alert monthly. A *sentinel event* is an unexpected occurrence involving death or loss of limb or function. Such events are called "sentinel" because they sound a warning of the need for immediate investigation and response (Figure 22-1).

WHAT IS ROOT CAUSE ANALYSIS?

When errors occur, the primary cause needs to be determined so that a solution can be found. *Root cause analysis* (RCA) is a process designed for use in investigating and categorizing the root causes of events that occur. In the health care setting, there are many factors that can affect the cause of errors. Rather than to place blame on any one

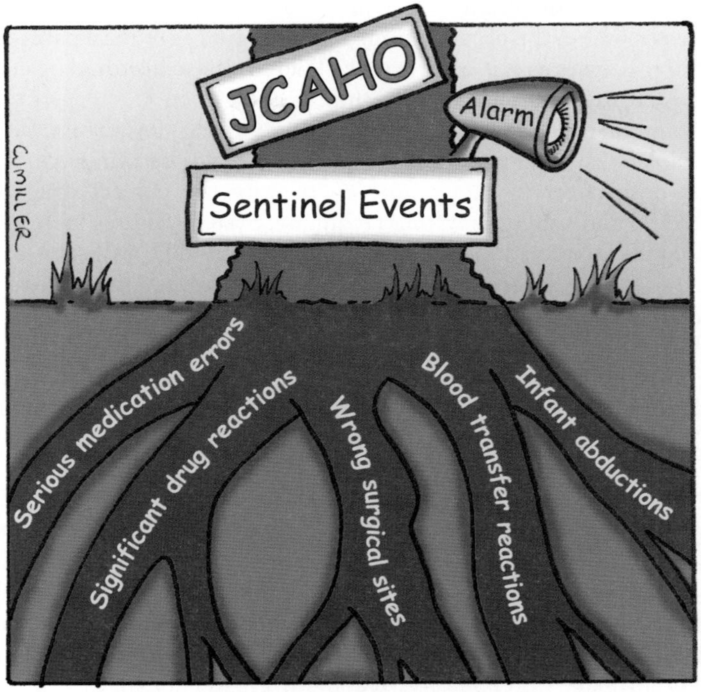

FIGURE 22-1
Root causes of sentinel events.

person or thing, RCA, when conducted appropriately, can identify all factors leading up to the error. Often an RCA is conducted by a hospital's risk management department, and the results are presented to the *quality improvement* (QI) department for follow-up action. The role of the QI department is to become proactive at finding ways of preventing similar incidences from occurring.

Imagine an occurrence during which a nurse administers the wrong dose of a medication instead of the correct dose. The typical investigation would probably conclude that the nurse was at fault. However, if the analysis stops here, the reasons for the mistake may not be fully understood. Therefore, we may never discover what to do to prevent it from occurring again.

In the case of the nurse who gave the wrong medication dose, we are likely to make recommendations such as punishing the nurse, re-educating the nurse, and reminding all other nurses to be alert when giving the same medication. But, this does little to resolve the real problem. That is because medication administration involves a complex set of steps in achieving the desired goal of getting the correct medication to the patient in a timely manner. A multitude of contributing factors often lead to medication errors as nurses encounter problems within the system, work-design problems, or human and environmental factors.

The environment and behavior are as much a part of the system as they are the processes within the organization. Technology is as much a part of system components within processes as it is of structure. Therefore, each should be considered when evaluating a cause and effect relationship.

Common causes of medication errors are: wrong-dose errors; lack of drug knowledge; rule violations; slips; memory lapses; inadequate monitoring; misuse of infusion pumps; faulty-dose checking and failure to identify the correct drug; medication-stocking problems; and using the wrong technique. System failures included lack of easy access to drug information, look-alike packaging, sound-alike drug names, transcription errors, lack of patient information, poor communication, distractions, interruptions, and excess workloads.

Therefore, a root cause factor chart should be generated to find the real origin of the error. Figure 22-2 depicts a simplified version of the root cause analysis performed in the example. As the investigation proceeded, it became evident that the nurse was not entirely at fault because of a look-alike vial.

WHAT IS FMEA?

Failure mode and effects analysis (FMEA) is a proactive quality method that is often used to identify and remedy weak points in the early phase of obtaining products and/or processes. The process is highly structured and quite time consuming for the team tasked with its completion; however, the benefits are important for preventing errors. The JCAHO currently requires at least one hospital FMEA be conducted annually.

The primary differences in RCA and FMEA are that the first is reactive and the second is proactive. However, FMEAs should not be done on everything that could possibly go wrong. Instead they are usually conducted when a new piece of equipment is obtained, or when implementing a high-risk process. For example, if the hospital is planning to implement a physician order-entry program, a FMEA would be useful to pinpoint problem areas before they occur. Other times, an FMEA choice may be based on an error that occurred in the latest news of the press. For example, when there was a case of mistaken identity with a patient undergoing cardiac catheterization, many hospitals performed FMEAs to prevent such an incident from occurring at their facility.

HISTORY AND EVOLUTION OF QUALITY IN HEALTH CARE

The advent of quality in health care became important when hospitals found the need to look outside their own expertise for error prevention strategies. The year is not as important as the fact that health care found a need to borrow from other industries that were successful at managing risk. However, manufacturing industries began focusing on error prevention in the early 1920s. The evolution of improved quality techniques in health care was not adopted until the 1960s and is still evolving.

Historically, the focus of quality improvement was in controlling processes by inspection so that errors were prevented. Later, the emphasis changed from inspection to proactive approaches to error prevention. Included with prevention are monitoring processes to keep errors under control.

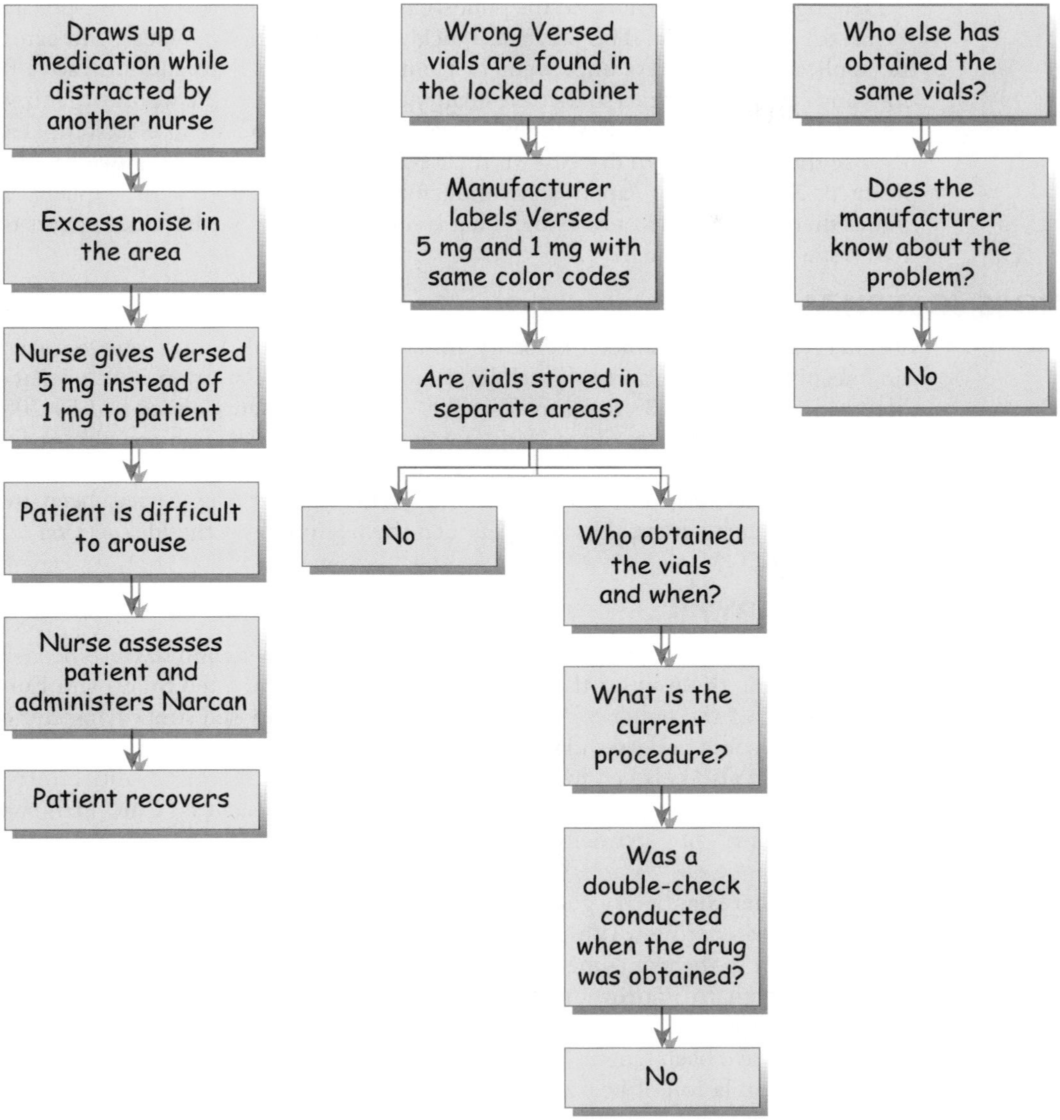

FIGURE 22-2
Root cause factor chart.

WHO IS EDWARD DEMING?

Edward Deming is often considered the father of quality improvement. Yet, quality concepts have developed and improved over several decades. What once began simply as a method for discovering how to prevent defects has evolved into highly skilled methods for tracking and improving quality today.

Deming's teachings embraced the philosophy that quality is everyone's responsibility within the organization. The Japanese quickly adopted Deming's ideas, and extended the application of process improvement from manufacturing to administrative functions and service industries so that the quality concept affected the whole organization. Japanese companies started taking over product markets on small electronic devices because they were able to drive down their costs, while improving the quality of their products. Subsequently, American manufacturers began to use the same quality techniques that the Japanese were using. That is one reason why we have better cars today than just a few decades ago.

WHO IS JOSEPH M. JURAN?

Another valuable forefather of quality initiatives is Joseph Juran, who emphasized the meaning of the Pareto principle. Remember the Pareto principle that was discussed in Chapter 13? It means that 80% of the problems are caused by 20% of sources, people, or things. Therefore, if you can fix the 20%, you can almost fix the entire system. From his entry job as a factory troubleshooter, he developed a career as a writer, educator, and consultant. Juran's major contribution has been in the field quality management. His work marked the beginning of the idea of *total quality management* (TQM).

WHO IS PHILLIP CROSBY?

Phillip Crosby published 14 books about quality management and has also been credited with paving the way for the quality revolution in the United States and Europe. He is considered the father of *"zero defects."* He often proposed simplifying things so that everyone could understand it. (Now, where was he in your Nursing Fundamentals textbooks?) He also believed in the importance of communicating quality efforts and their results to the entire organization. Subsequently, ideas such as "lean" manufacturing, "just-in-time" product delivery, and *"Six Sigma"* methods have crossed over into health care.

Recently, there has been a genuine paradigm shift in quality improvement strategies within health care settings. What once was considered only work for the QI Department is now brought to the front-line workers, who can best impact the outcomes. An ongoing commitment to improvement strategies supports an atmosphere of teamwork. The focus is on the process, rather than blaming the people doing the work according to what they have been taught (Figure 22-3).

Still, the regulation of health care is conducted at the national level by regulatory governmental bodies. These governmental agencies are responsible for approving many of the licenses for educational institutions that educate personnel. Institutional accreditation is also conducted by these government agencies.

The JCAHO is the primary agency used for hospital accreditation. The mere mention of JCAHO can strike fear in the minds of nurses and hospital administrators. This is because hospitals must meet certain quality standards to pass the JCAHO inspections. Total quality management and related approaches are sometimes referred to as total quality improvement, world-class quality, continuous quality improvement, total service quality, and total quality leadership.

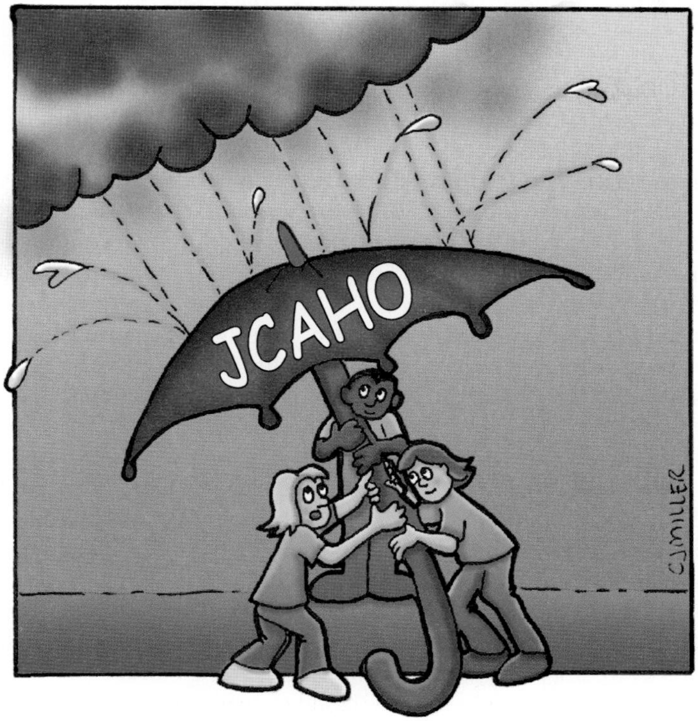

FIGURE 22-3
Error prevention is everyone's responsibility.

In the 1990s, the JCAHO first began to mandate the use of *continuous quality improvement* (CQI) and promoted that organizations adopt a model to carry out process improvement activities. The JCAHO also endorses the use of *plan-do-study-act* cycle (PDSA) as one tool for process improvement.

Some hospital QI departments have combined newer strategies with PDSA, including *define-measure-analyze-improve-control* (DMAIC) and *rapid cycle tests* (RCTs) of change, which further incorporate a team focus. These are components of Six Sigma methodology, and more discussion of these methods will come later.

JCAHO has also mandated specific quality outcome measures for all hospitals. Some of these include outcome measures for patients admitted with a diagnosis of acute myocardial infarction, congestive heart failure, community-acquired pneumonia, surgical-infection prophylaxis, pregnancy-related conditions, and deep vein thrombosis. Outcome or core measures are those that the public consumer considers important for choosing one hospital over another. However, discussion of techniques for measuring these institutional outcomes is beyond the scope of this text. Instead, we focus on general CQI outcomes for nursing units.

JUST WHAT IS THE JCAHO?

The JCAHO is the prime accrediting body for health care institutions that are Medicare and Medicaid funded. This means that nearly all hospitals must be JCAHO-accredited in order to stay in business.

In the past, the JCAHO standards have directly addressed patient safety in many areas. Beginning on July 1, 2001, additions to the standards required hospitals to develop a systematic approach to error reduction and design patient care processes with safety in mind. For CQI initiatives, JCAHO recommends using such things as flow charts, Pareto charts, run charts or line graphs, control charts, and histograms to depict data. Once the data have been collected; these tools help visualize results of performance improvement and can readily be completed and understood by most nurses. This is not an exhaustive list of tools; other valuable tools are discussed later.

WHAT ARE PATIENT SAFETY GOALS?

A primary driving force for CQI activities is the JCAHO National Patient Safety Goals (NPSG). In 2001, the JCAHO began instituting annual patient safety goals intended to improve quality of health care. The goals for 2006, which include some of the goals from 2005, are summarized in Table 22-1.

The first NPSGs were approved by the Joint Commission's Board of Commissioners in July 2002. The Joint Commission established these goals to help accredited organizations address specific areas of concern regarding patient safety. Each goal includes no more than two succinct, evidence-based or expert-based recommendations. Each year, the goals and associated recommendations are re-evaluated; some may continue while

TABLE 22-1

JCAHO 2005 Hospital National Patient Safety Goals Summarized

Goal 1: Improve the accuracy of patient identification	Use at least two patient identifiers (neither to be the patient's room number) whenever administering medications or blood products; taking blood samples **and other specimens for clinical testing, or providing any other treatments or procedures.**
Goal 2: Improve the effectiveness of communication among caregivers	For verbal or telephone orders or for telephonic reporting of critical test results, verify the complete order or test result by having the person receiving the order or test result "read-back" the complete order or test result. Standardize a list of abbreviations, acronyms, and symbols that are not to be used throughout the organization. Measure, assess and, if appropriate, take action to improve the timeliness of reporting, and the timeliness of receipt by the responsible licensed caregiver, of critical test results and values. **Implement a standardized approach to "hand off" communications, including an opportunity to ask and respond to questions.**

Continued

TABLE 22-1

JCAHO 2005 Hospital National Patient Safety Goals Summarized—cont'd

Goal 3: Improve the safety of using medications	Remove concentrated electrolytes (including, but not limited to, potassium chloride, potassium phosphate, sodium chloride >0.9%) from patient care units. Standardize and limit the number of drug concentrations available in the organization. Identify and, at a minimum, annually review a list of look-alike/sound-alike drugs used in the organization, and take action to prevent errors involving the interchange of these drugs. **Label all medications, medication containers (e.g., syringes, medicine cups, basins), or other solutions on and off the sterile field in perioperative and other procedural settings.**
Goal 4: Improve the safety of using infusion pumps	Ensure free-flow protection on all general-use and PCA (patient controlled analgesia) intravenous infusion pumps used in the organization.
Goal 5: Eliminate wrong-site, wrong-patient, wrong-procedure surgery	Create and use a preoperative verification process, such as a checklist, to confirm that appropriate documents (e.g., medical records, imaging studies) are available. Implement a process to mark the surgical site and involve the patient in the marking process. [Disease-Specific Care]
Goal 6: Improve the effectiveness of clinical alarm systems	Implement regular preventive maintenance and testing of alarm systems. Assure that alarms are activated with appropriate settings and are sufficiently audible with respect to distances and competing noise within the unit.
Goal 7: Reduce the risk of health care-associated infections—hand hygiene, report infections that are sentinel events	Comply with current Centers for Disease Control and Prevention (CDC) hand hygiene guidelines. Manage as sentinel events all identified cases of unanticipated death or major permanent loss of function associated with a health care-associated infection.
Goal 8: Accurately and completely reconcile medications across the continuum of care	**Develop a process for obtaining and documenting a complete list of the patient's current medications upon the patient's admission to the organization and with the involvement of the patient. A complete list of the patient's medications is communicated to the next provider of service when it refers or transfers a patient to another setting, service, practitioner, or level of care within or outside the organization.**
Goal 9: Reduce the risk of patient harm resulting from falls	**Assess and periodically reassess each patient's risk for falling, including the potential risk associated with the patient's medication regimen, and take action to address any identified risks.**
Goal 10: Reduce the risk of influenza and pneumococcal disease in institutionalized older adults	**Develop and implement a protocol for administration and documentation of the flu vaccine. Develop and implement a protocol for administration and documentation of the pneumococcus vaccine.** [Assisted Living, Disease-Specific Care, Long Term Care]. **Develop and implement a protocol to identify new cases of influenza and to manage an outbreak.**

Continued

TABLE 22-1

JCAHO 2005 Hospital National Patient Safety Goals Summarized—cont'd

Goal 11: Reduce the risk of surgical fires	**Educate staff, including operating licensed independent practitioners and anesthesia providers, on how to control heat sources and manage fuels, and establish guidelines to minimize oxygen concentration under drapes.** [Ambulatory, Office-Based Surgery]
Goal 12: Implementation of applicable NPSF and associated requirements at practitioner sites	Inform and encourage components and practitioner sites to implement the applicable National Patient Safety Goals and associated requirements. [Networks]
Goal 13: Encourage the active involvement of patients and families in the patient's care as a patient safety strategy	**Define and communicate the means for patients to report concerns about safety and encourage them to do so.**
Goal 14: Prevent health care-associated pressure ulcers	Assess and periodically reassess each patient's risk for developing a pressure ulcer (decubitus ulcer) and take action to address any identified risks. [Long-Term Care]

Note: New goals and requirements are indicated in **bold.**
From Joint Commission on Accreditation of Healthcare Organizations (JCAHO): *Hospitals' national patient safety goals*, 2005, *www.jcaho.org/accredited+organizations/hospitals/npsg/05_npsg_hap.htm.*

others will be replaced because of emerging new priorities. New goals and recommendations are announced in July and become effective on January 1 of the following year (JCAHO, 2004a).

MONITORING QUALITY OF HEALTH CARE

It is important for nurses to know how to design and conduct simple projects within their group to improve processes on their nursing units. Nurses need to know the basics of collecting and analyzing data and what to do with the results, and they must be able to carry out simple performance improvement projects.

WHAT IS QUALITY ASSURANCE?

Quality assurance (QA) is a term often used synonymously with QI. The term may refer to the process or activities that are used to monitor, evaluate, and control services providing some measure of quality to consumers. It often includes reports that must be generated to track progress. Incidence reports are sometimes referred to as QA reports or variance reports. These help guide the hospital risk management department and QI department to make system improvements (Box 22-1).

BOX 22-1 Common Quality Terms

Audit: a formal periodic check on quality measures to verify correctness of actions.

DMAIC (define, measure, analyze, improve, control): a Six Sigma process for improving existing processes that fall below institutional goals or national norms.

Outcome or core measures: measures that the public consumer considers important for choosing one hospital over another.

Quality indicators: data that indicate whether high-quality care is being maintained. An item of concern that has come about due to a nursing practice problem (i.e., Foley catheter securing).

Quality assurance: activities that are used to monitor, evaluate, and control services providing some measure of quality to consumers.

Key indicators: selected data based on JCAHO mandates or on specific problem areas that may reveal the need for more extensive data collection or remedial action to resolve an identified problem (i.e., fall rates, medication error rates).

Key performance indicators (KPI): reflect the things that the team wants to change. Typical KPIs are time, costs, distance, numbers of incidents, or items.

Metric: a measurement for the rate of compliance or noncompliance with an indicator.

Monitor: similar to auditing; checking or verifying that an established practice has been retained.

Operational definitions: a statement detailing the thing or event using specific identifiable and measurable wording with written inclusion and exclusion criteria.

Pareto principle: 80% of the problems are caused by 20% of sources, people, or things. If you can fix the 20%, you can fix the system.

Patient safety goals: goals established by the JCAHO that highlight problematic areas in health care and describe evidence and expert-based solutions to these problems. Goals are derived primarily from informal recommendations made in the Joint Commission's safety newsletter, Sentinel Event Alert.

Plan-do-study-act (PDSA): contained within an RCT for planning, doing, studying, and carrying out actions intended to drive and maintain change.

Performance improvement: a plan and documentation method that demonstrates what procedures will be and have been implemented for changes in the quality of services based on previous data collection.

Total quality management (TQM): a management style where the goal is producing quality services for the customer and where the customer defines what quality means.

Rapid cycle tests (RCT) of change: a strategy for process improvement as a part of DMAIC where changes are made and implemented in very short time frames.

Six Sigma: a measurement standard in product variation that began in the 1920s when Walter Shewhart showed that three sigma from the mean is the point where a process requires correction. No fewer than 3.4 errors per million opportunities.

Stakeholders: key people who will be affected by change, and can either influence or derail the improvement.

HOW DO WE MONITOR QUALITY?

As stated earlier, someone must monitor quality care compliance. The QI department is typically the department that receives data, analyzes trends, and recommends actions to facilitate improvement in the organization. However, there should also be a CQI Council as a primary decision-making nursing team, and *quality circles* (QC) who function along service lines that collaborate to improve care for a group of patient types.

Examples of service lines include surgical units, medical units, neurologic units, rehabilitation units, and outpatient units. These teams audit indicators each month to determine whether quality care issues are being missed.

Each service line sets out an annual quality plan for the next year, based on recent problem areas or hot topics. Because it is impossible to track everything that nurses consider important to quality care, QCs use various methods to prioritize or target their reviews. They establish unit-specific *quality indicators* for tracking using measurable questions that provide data for trending improvement.

WHAT IS AN INDICATOR AND A METRIC?

A *quality indicator* is an item of concern that has come about due to a nursing practice problem. For example, a QC team may have identified a problem with Foley catheters being secured properly. Perhaps several patients had Foley catheters that were inadvertently pulled out. After some investigation, the problem was identified as having to do with not properly securing the catheters. Thus, the team will monitor a metric or measurement for the rate of Foley catheters that are secured properly.

A unit-based QI nurse is usually assigned the responsibility to audit charts or verify a procedure by direct observation to determine compliance. The results are compiled and sent to the QI department. This is done until noncompliance reaches pre-established criteria, such as <5% and/or compliance is 95%. The indicator may have been selected due to a risk issue. For example, there may have been a patient who suffered an injury due to a catheter not being taped correctly. The critical thinking exercise (Critical Thinking Box 22-1) can help you discover another example of how important chart auditing can be.

Metric descriptors are the indicator measures, called *rates of noncompliance* or *compliance*, that identify the issue more specifically. Some examples of metrics are in Table 22-2. Metrics and key indicators are developed after careful consideration, and data collection about how things really are, and not simply based on hearsay. The results are analyzed on a monthly or quarterly basis by the QI department, tracked, and trended with graphic displays and written committee reports. Based on the results, over time process improvement strategies may need to be changed, and more education instituted. The QI department produces reports to major hospital committees, the Chief Nursing Officer, and other Councils. Such reports are usually reviewed at each JCAHO visit.

WHAT ARE KEY INDICATORS?

JCAHO mandates that certain key indicators continue organization-wide to monitor such areas as advance directives, autopsy rates, AMAs and elopement rates, blood-product utilization rates, blood-transfusion reaction rates, code blue rates, conscious-sedation complication rates, fall rates, medication-error rates, mortality rates, pain-management

CRITICAL THINKING BOX 22-1

An audit review committee composed of the Quality Coordinator, 3 nurses, 2 case managers, a physical therapist, and a pharmacist, was charged with the task of reviewing the care of the patients having a total hip replacement. The patients' care did not seem to conform to the expected length of stay (LOS) as established by Medicare DRG reimbursement charts. As they reviewed the chart and discussed the care of all 20 patients, they noted that Mr. Garcia had been ready for discharge at 10:00 AM on Tuesday, but the case manager for that nursing unit was not able to place him in a rehabilitation unit until 48 hours later. Many of the other 19 charts depicted this same scenario. As a result, the hospital was not reimbursed for the entire LOS at a loss of approximately $4000 per incident.

1. Who is responsible for the error?
2. What do you think should be done in this situation?
3. What steps can be taken (if any) to prevent the situation in the future?

TABLE 22-2

Indicator and Metric Descriptors

Indicator	Metric Descriptor
Admission documentation	Metric 1—Rate of learning needs not documented within 24 hours of admission. Metric 2—Rate of skin assessment (Braden scale) not documented within 24 hours of admission. Metric 3—Rate of spiritual needs not documented within 24 hours of admission.
Foley securing	Metric 1—Rate of Foley catheters not secured in place according to the procedure described in Perry and Potter.
IV tube labeling	Metric 1—Rate of continuous flow IV tubing that has not been labeled with the date and time it is due to be changed. Metric 2—Rate of intermittent flow tubing (IVPB) has not been labeled with the date and time it is due to be changed.
Skin care	Metric 1—Rate of high-risk patients, as defined by the Braden scale (<17), who have pressure ulcers within 2 to 4 days of admission. Metric 2—Rate of those patients with pressure ulcers that are: Stage 1 Stage 2 Stage 3 Stage 4 Eschar
TORAV/VORAV Verbal or telephone orders	Metric 1—Rate of telephoned physician's orders that did not contain read back verification by using "TORAV" *(telephone order read back and verified)* documentation with signature of person taking the order on the first 2 charts of each odd numbered day. Metric 2—Rate of verbal physician's orders that did not contain read back verification by using "VORAV" *(verbal order read back and verified)* documentation with signature of person taking the order on the first 2 charts of each odd numbered day.

effectiveness, restraint use, and surgical-site infection rates. Simply put, these are tracked routinely, and remain a part of the JCAHO accreditation standards. Key indicators are selected based on JCAHO mandates or on problem areas that must be monitored on an ongoing basis. These may reveal the need for more extensive data collection or remedial action to resolve an identified problem. Regardless of whether there is improvement, JCAHO key indicators must be tracked. However, some changes to the indicator questions asked may be made when improvement is found.

WHAT IS PERFORMANCE IMPROVEMENT?

Performance improvement (PI) includes a plan and documentation method that demonstrates what procedures will be and have been implemented for changes in the quality of services based on previous data collection. PI is similar to the nursing process (assess, diagnose, plan, implement, and evaluate). Often QI nurses are called on to conduct small data collection processes and provide reports. Critical Thinking Box 22-2 provides a sample scenario for you to try out these skills.

The hospital system and services rendered are assessed regularly for problems. A diagnosis of sorts is made that demonstrates where the Pareto principle or 80% of the problems are. Planning involves fixing the 20% of sources, people, or things that contributed to the problem. Implementation occurs as specific strategies are put into place to resolve the errors. Evaluation takes place as data is collected over a period of time that demonstrates compliance or noncompliance with the issue.

WHAT ARE THE BARRIERS TO QUALITY IMPROVEMENT?

One of the primary barriers to implementing effective QI programs is cost. The cost of providing high-quality services within the health care organization has increased greatly over the past few decades, primarily due to decreased payments and the increased costs of doing business. Health care organizations continue to look for ways to cut expenses by reducing the high cost of supplies, or by reducing staff. However, with the continuing shortage of qualified registered nurses, reducing labor costs is

CRITICAL THINKING BOX 22-2

METRICS AND INDICATORS

Your nursing unit has experienced a lack of labeling of the IV tubing as to when it needs to be changed. You are the QI (quality improvement) nurse who must collect data for a process improvement project. The nurse manager has asked you to determine baseline data for a month and report to her what your findings are.

1. How would you go about doing this?
2. What would be your indicators?
3. What would be the metrics?
4. Pretend you have some results after a month. How will you report the information to the manager?

neither advisable nor acceptable, considering the errors that can occur as a result. However, improving quality can serve to offset many of the factors associated with initial expenses. Liability risks are reduced as quality initiatives begin to establish prevention strategies. Soon, the organization begins to reap the rewards of "fire prevention" rather than "fire fighting."

The United States Pharmacopeia has a great deal of information on medication-error rates related to patient deaths. Once the organization realizes that the cost of a lawsuit for each medication-error related death or disability far outweighs the cost of nurses, then quality becomes critical.

Other barriers to QI are tradition, and failure to recognize that changes are needed. Hospital administrators often oppose change of any kind, because they value tradition, have an authoritative management style, and do not value innovators.

Nurses are often unaware or unwilling to change practice from the way they have always done things. Many practicing nurses remain resistant to change because it seems threatening, requires effort, retraining, and restructuring old work habits.

However, having new knowledge provides the confidence nurses need in justifying decisions to patients, physicians, and other nurses. Providing high-quality care is in itself a magnet for more nurses to join the organization. It is critical to become informed providers, recognizing that there is always uncertainty in decision-making. However, answers can be found using a system for developing new, quality knowledge.

QUALITY IMPROVEMENT METHODS

There are several flavors of quality improvement, but primarily include the values of the institution. Top management must be committed to CQI or it will not work. They must empower nurses and other employees to help plan and carry out the needed strategies for change. Data must be collected systematically and not sporadically. Blaming previous personnel does nothing to improve things. The work involves examining systems issues with a proactive approach rather than always being reactive. Working groups or QCs must have a sense of collaboration and appreciation for the value each one brings to the table. They must be committed to being a part of the solution, and not a part of the problem.

Some problems we typically encounter in hospitals are delays in room assignments, medication delivery, treatments or other care, and internal system delays (e.g., dietary, linen). All of these time delays ultimately cost us more.

Efficient people may not even realize these time traps are occurring because they are so accustomed to developing "work-arounds" to eliminate them. And, other people simply ignore the time traps, and instead just put in their 8 or 12 hours and go home, hoping perhaps tomorrow will be better.

Everyone wins when nurses become involved in being a part of those who are willing to make things work well. Thus, it is critical to be knowledgeable about current CQI methods.

TOOLS AND PROCESSES FOR CONTINUOUS QUALITY IMPROVEMENT

Tools are any organizational or analytical technique that assists in understanding a problem. Quality tools are more specific, because they include tools applied to solving organizational or unit-specific problems. The discussion is not all inclusive of tools that can be used for CQI, but provides an overview of more recent tools used (Figure 22-4).

WHAT IS SIX SIGMA?

Six Sigma methodologies are the newest wave of change initiatives for CQI. As with any new wave before it (root cause analysis, FMEA, or pain as the fifth vital sign), the JCAHO will most likely be inclined toward recommending Six Sigma methods in the future for accreditation purposes. Specific CQI employees will need Six Sigma education to understand and utilize the information to benefit the institution.

Six Sigma as a measurement standard in product variation began in the 1920s when Walter Shewhart showed that three sigma from the mean is the point where a process requires correction. Walter Shewhart was one of Edward Deming's teachers, and is responsible for the PDSA cycle of process improvement. Many measurement standards (zero defects, lean manufacturing, etc.) later came on the scene, but credit for coining

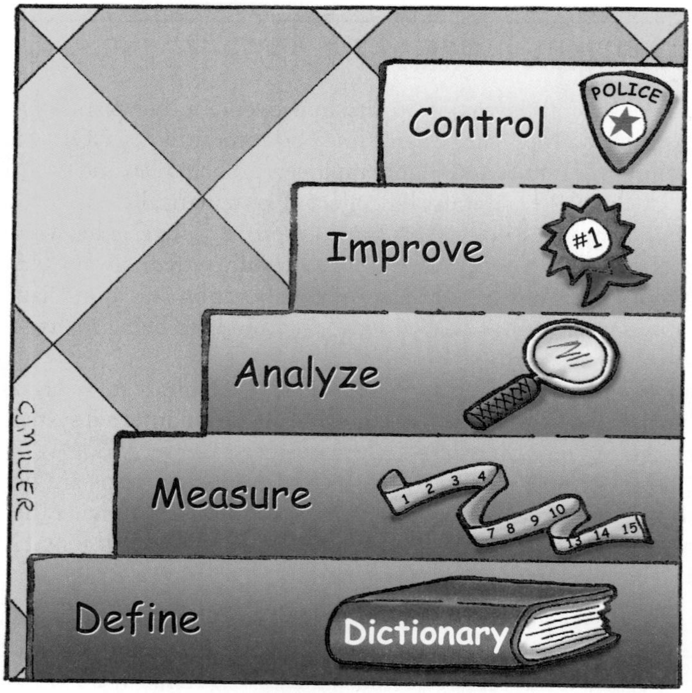

FIGURE 22-4
Stair steps to quality health care.

the term "Six Sigma" goes to a Bill Smith of Motorola. Bill Smith is considered the father of Six Sigma, which is a federally registered trademark of Motorola. Six Sigma (SS) is a methodology that uses analytical tools to improve the efficiency and capability of business processes. The primary goal of SS is to increase profits by improving standard operating procedures, reducing errors, and decreasing misuse of the system.

SS methodology is based on strategies that focus on CQI and variation reduction through the application of DMAIC. The Six Sigma DMAIC process (define, measure, analyze, improve, control) is primarily for improving existing processes that fall below institutional goals or national norms. DMAIC can save companies thousands of dollars per project, and teams can complete four to six projects per year.

DMAIC is a process with the potential to lead to Six Sigma or having near "zero" defects. Six Sigma means having no more than 3.4 defects per million opportunities or 99.99966% accuracy. The idea is to focus on the voice of customer (VOC), whether internal or external, and attempt reduce risks associated with high volume, high risk, problem-prone areas of practice.

From the time of inception of DMAIC, the executive team must be supportive and must be trained in rapid cycle tests (RCT) of change. They must create financial and human resources, and allow sufficient time for project teams to work, and then proceed to be supportive of the efforts put forth. The entire organization must be behind the effort and be enthused about change. If the organizational culture is too resistant to change, it will be difficult. Often a cultural change is needed before the process will be successful.

Data driven means real results are measured using numbers (calculations) to support ideas for change. The bottom line is that we know that we are not perfect, but we can strive to perform up to this 99.99966% goal.

So, if you take a million blood pressure readings, there should be no fewer than 3.4 that were incorrect.

Another important point is that processes function most effectively if kept within a certain range, which reduces system errors significantly. The main idea is to control peaks and valleys in performance (those things that are way off target).

The DMAIC process (Table 22-3) provides more reliability and validity than other QI models, and has become a national trend in QI strategies. Many companies will only do business with those who are using DMAIC.

TABLE 22-3

DMAIC

DMAIC IS PRONOUNCED DUH-MAY-ICK AND INCLUDES:

DEFINE	Define the issue, possible causes, and goals.
MEASURE	Measure the existing system with metrics.
ANALYZE	Analyze the gap between existing and goal.
IMPROVE	Improve the system with creative strategies.
CONTROL	Control and sustain the improvement.

HOW DO WE USE DMAIC?

The DMAIC flow diagram (Figure 22-5) provides an overview of the DMAIC process. The framework depicts the flow from the starting point of Define through Control to the next project. However, depending on the project, the steps may not always follow the path directed by the arrows. Teams may need to change direction at times.

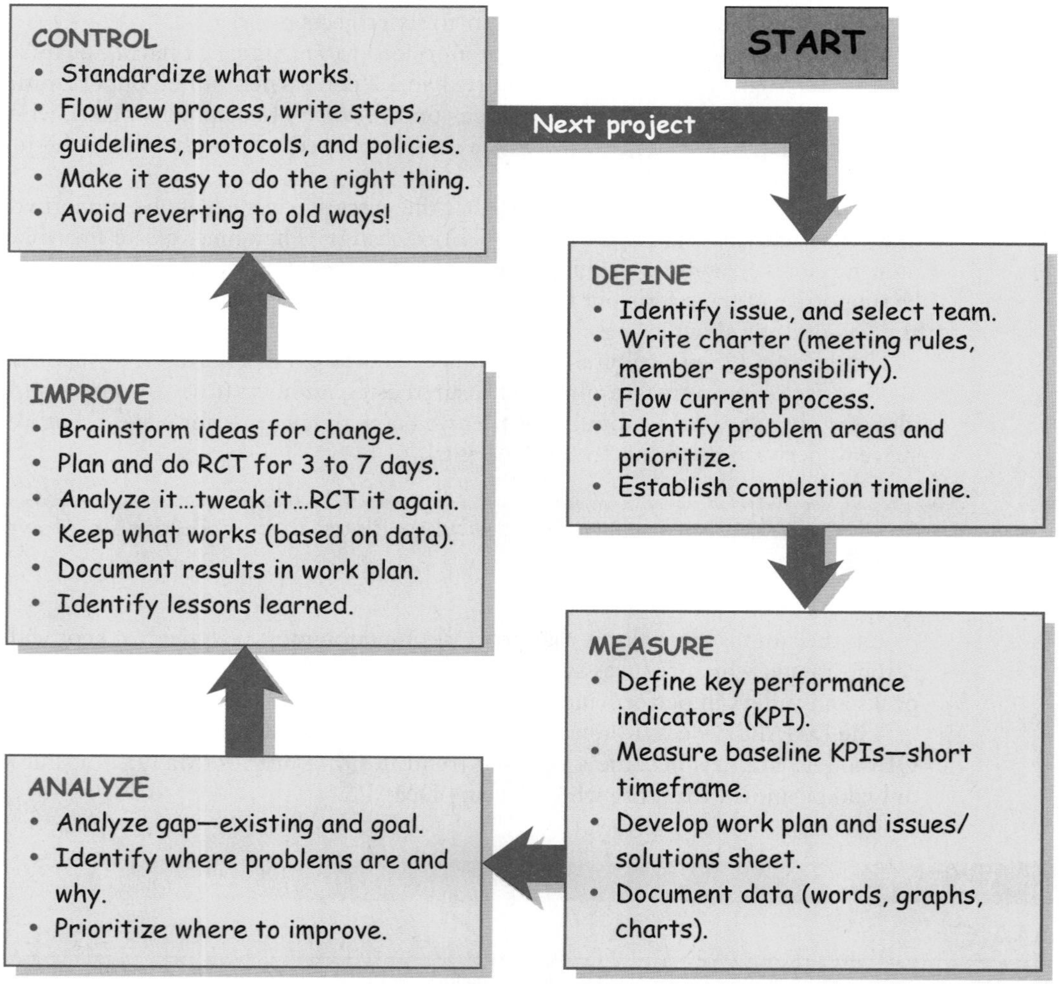

FIGURE 22-5

This flow diagram provides an overview of the define-measure-analyze-improve-control (DMAIC) process used at University Health System (UHS). The framework depicts the flow from the starting point of Define through Control to the next project. However, depending on the project, it may not always follow the path directed by the arrows. Teams may need to change direction at times.

Sometimes the process may need to stop at the measure phase and go back to the design phase to develop formats for measuring. For example, the team may want to do some brainstorming or conduct RCTs to develop the best data collection form before moving on.

The Six Sigma engine (Figure 22-6) uses the parts of DMAIC to (1) improve processes, (2) design or re-design processes and to (3) manage processes. The most powerful difference between Six Sigma's DMAIC and other improvement methods is the rigorous discipline of finding and keeping solutions to problems. Now we see that the Plan–Do–Study–Act (PDSA) cycle also fits well with DMAIC.

PDSA is used to plan and conduct RCTs of change. However, there is no "one size fits all" for organizations using DMAIC to move toward Six Sigma. Nevertheless, the organization needs to standardize the DMAIC process somewhat so that everyone will understand their roles and functions during each step.

As indicated, the PDSA cycle is contained with the RCT. Thus each project will be done slightly differently. The main things are to keep on track with the goal in mind, and use real data not guesswork or gossip to direct decisions.

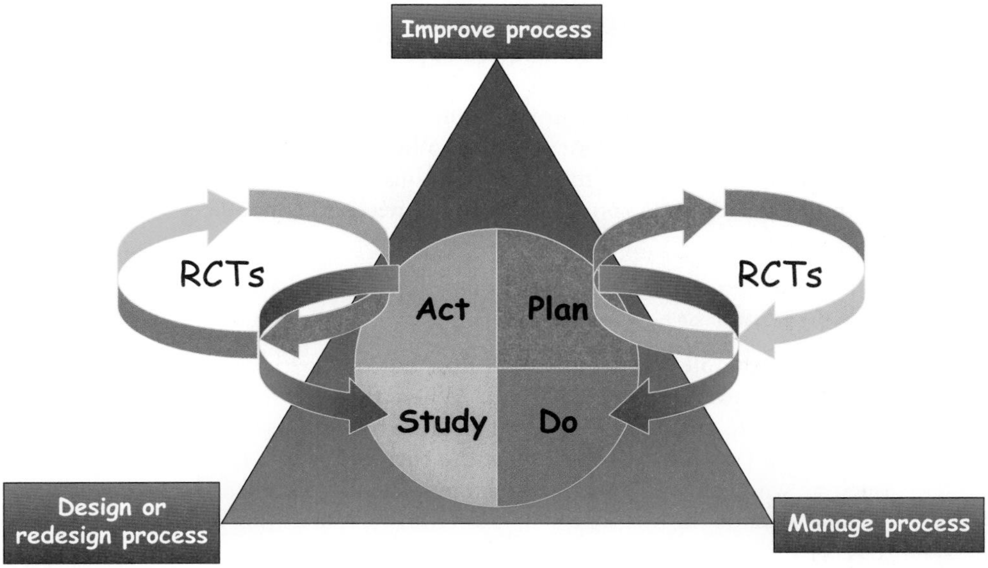

FIGURE 22-6

The Six Sigma engine uses the parts of DMAIC to (1) improve processes, (2) design or redesign processes and to (3) manage processes. The most powerful difference between Six Sigma's DMAIC and other improvement methods is the rigorous discipline of finding and keeping solutions to problems. The plan-do-study-act (PDSA) cycle also fits well with DMAIC (define-measure-analyze-improve-control). PDSA is used to plan and conduct rapid cycle tests (RCTs) of change. There is no "one size fits all" for organizations using DMAIC to move toward Six Sigma. However, we still need to standardize our DMAIC process at UHS so that everyone will be on the "same page" when it comes to teamwork. This will help everyone understand roles and functions during each step. As indicated, the PDSA cycle is contained with the RCT of change.

THE DEFINE PHASE

In the define phase, a charter is developed as a written document of the work the team will accomplish. Identify the business case, goal, team leaders, membership, team responsibilities or roles. Include as team members only those who want to be a part of the solution, and not a part of the problem. This is no place for "whiners" or complainers. Set team rules (attendance, absence, how decisions are made). During meetings, ask that only one conversation go on at a time (no sidebars). Determine who will be key people needed to hold a meeting. Determine what the constraints or limits on resources might be.

Assign responsibility for each aspect of a problem and resolution. Allow brainstorming during meetings, which may cause some delays in meeting goals, but is a valuable part of the process. During meetings, identify who the stakeholders are, how they will be affected.

Stakeholders are key people who will be affected by change, and can either influence or derail the improvement. Consider how to sell ideas to them. Also, identify support resources. Who will fund or support any changes recommended?

Next, write the problem statement and goal statement. Determine the cost of doing nothing different (fire fighting) versus the cost of improving. These costs can be in dollar amounts or lost time, injury, errors, or dissatisfaction, for example. Set the goal in terms of how much saving is planned. 10%? 25%? By what date?

Problem statement—The number of patients waiting to be seen by an MD in the emergency department (ED) is excessive, and patients are dissatisfied. Controls are needed so that there are a limited number of minutes between bed placement and MD arrival to bedside. Patients need to be cared for efficiently so that they can get through the system in a timely manner, thus making room for more patients who are waiting in the waiting room. The hospital needs to contain costs and improve patient satisfaction.

Example: Goal Statement = there will be a 25% decrease in amount of time patients must wait in the ED after being placed in a bed.

In the example, the team would flow out or diagram the processes (Figure 22-7) that take place with the problem. When flow diagramming, use large sheets of paper or write on an erase board. If an erase board is used, someone should take notes and record the flow on paper. Flow the current "as is" process. Ask lots of questions, such as why things happen at each step. Identify problem areas for improvements. Think "outside the box" and slay "sacred cows!" Be willing to be innovative and objective in thinking of possible solutions. The letters in the boxes represent the usual process. The blue letters represent things that altered the process, and indicate a need for change. There are inputs, processes, and outputs in a typical flow diagram.

At the start of each team meeting, review the agenda or plan for the meeting. Ask for any additions needed, then review the ground rules, and the progress made to date. At the end of the meeting, review lessons learned, and set assignments for the next meeting.

Develop the workplan (Table 22-4). This is done with an Excel spreadsheet used for tracking plans. The issues/solutions sheet, also done with an Excel spreadsheet, keeps the team focused and is used to track brainstorming. The issues/solutions

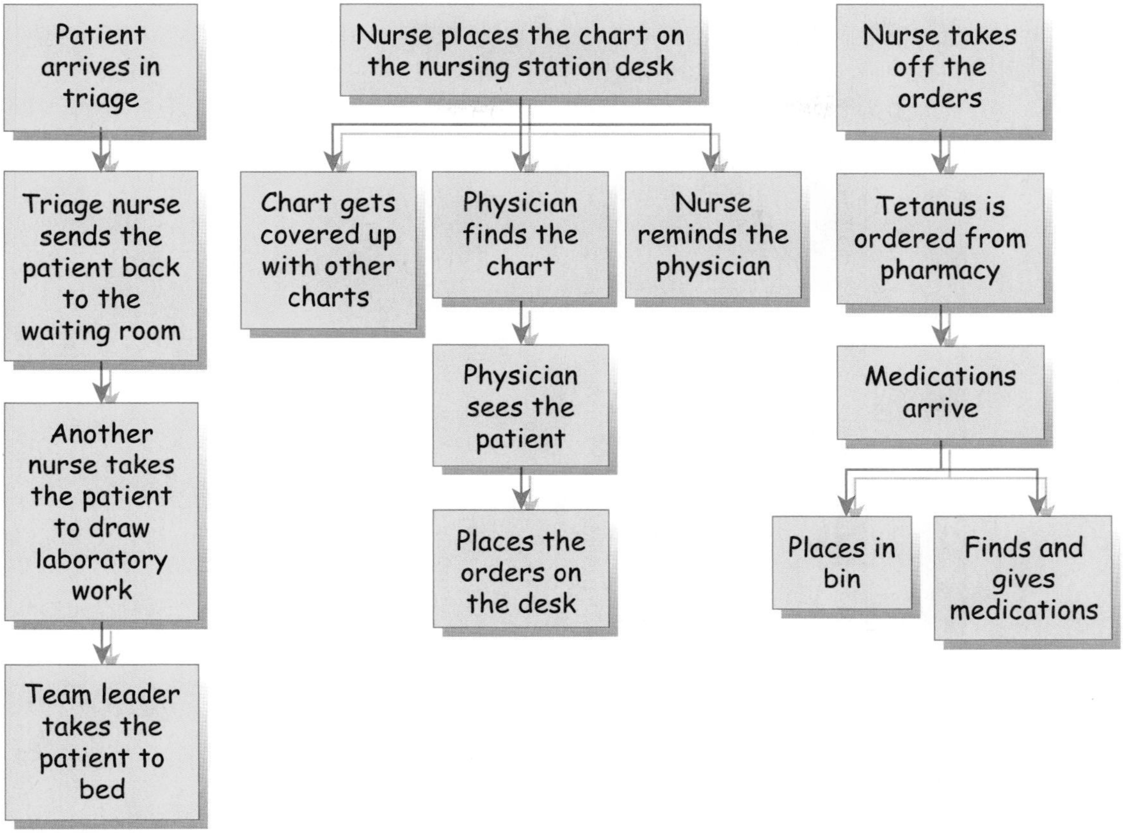

FIGURE 22-7
This is a process flow example. There are inputs, processes, and outputs in a typical flow diagram.

sheet (Table 22-5) and the workplan keep the team progressing and on track. Figure 22-8 provides another flow process example with a medication delivery process diagrammed step-by-step as a group.

THE MEASURE PHASE

Everyone within the team needs to agree on what is to be measured. These are called *key performance indicators* (KPI). KPIs should reflect the things that the team wants to change. Typical KPIs are time, costs, distance, numbers of incidents, or items. It is best to use whole numbers (with decimals), and measurable facts. Never use what someone thinks is a problem. Measure the problem first. It is also important to identify who will be responsible for data collection, retrieval, and analysis. If the team fails to document everything, things will fall apart quickly.

TABLE 22-4

Emergency Center Rapid Cycle Testing System

RCT #	Date	RCT Initiative	Urgent Matters Workplan	Responsible Persons	Data Collection Process	Summary Results	KPI Most Affected	% Improved
1	????	MD Awareness: Time in Bed	Use a special table called the "deck" to place the charts for the MDs. The RN Team Leader will be tasked with placing the time the patient was placed in a bed on the triage note to make the MD aware. In addition, post weekly "Bed to Provider" time in a graphic format at the chart pick-up station.	Team Leader (TL) and/or Patient Care Coordinator (PCC or Charge Nurse)	We collected pre-RCT data via First Net (Bed tracking software) for June 1-3 on 278 patients and compared it to RCT data for June 4-6 on 268 patients (for time from bed placement to evaluation). The tow times were 121 minutes vs. 110 minutes. (Trisha)	This RCT is considered successful and will be implemented immediately. The initial process or change occurred slowly because some of the nurses failed to put the time on the note as directed. Nurses that receive ambulance patients place their note on "deck" and did not place the time initially.	Bed Placement to MD Exam	10%

2	????	Chart on Deck	Implement chart placement on bedside table with log book. Record time chart is placed on "deck" and when chart is picked up.	PA, MD	Manual tracking: pre RCT: Mon, Tues, Wed; post RCT: Thurs, Fri, Sat. Data revealed an average turnaround time for MD to receive charts of 2.5 hours.	RCT was successful. The MD saw the patient after charts placed on deck at an average of 60 minutes instead of 2.5 hours for a 40% improvement.	Bed Placement to MD Exam	40%
3	6/16/04	"Deck" Officer	Creation of a "deck" officer concept to inhance the MD awareness initiative. A PA is assigned to monitor the "deck" and assign patients to housestaff and other MD/PAs if the patient's chart is not picked up within 15 minutes of bed placement. In addition, this individual is also seeing patients.	Medical Director, PAs	First Net (tracking system): pre RCT days without deck officer. RCT data: Days with Deck Officer by secretary June 24-26 Pre RCT = 61 minutes, RCT July 6-8; 26 minutes	RCT overall was successful. Barriers include not always having the extra PA to act as deck officer. On days that the deck officer was utilized, most patients were seen in under 30 minutes.	Bed Placement to MD Exam	42%

TABLE 22-5

Brainstorming Results: Hospital Solutions Issues Sheet

Date	Persons	Issue	Detail	Proposed Solution	Responsible
6/1/06	MDs	MD to see patient	Average time from patient arrival to bed placement is 3 hours. Delays in time for MDs to see patients still remains problematic. A new RCT is being developed for this.	When patients are placed in a bed, a copy of the triage note is placed on the "deck." "Deck" is a term used for the location of charts on patients pending MD evaluation. The MD cannot determine how long the patient has been in a bed based on a chart that only has a triage time.	TL, charge nurse
6/3/06	EC staff nurses	Chart on deck	Some of the nurses failed to put the time on the note as directed. Nurses that receive ambulance patients place their note on "deck" and did not place the time initially. The Team Leader (TL) or Patient Care Coordinator (PCC) had to go back and remind them for a couple of days.	The TL or PCC had to go back and remind them for a couple of days. Most patients brought from waiting area by TL or PCC were done correctly.	TL, charge nurse
6/6/06	EC staff	Chart on deck	Still having problems getting charts in hands of MDs so they will see patients quicker.	Discussion centered around the possibility of assigning an MD or PA to be the deck officer to more closely monitor the charts. This could potentially free up more inpatient beds on CPC, Gen Med, and Hartman units.	MD, PA
7/10/06	EC	EC patient flow	Arrival to bed for admitted patients is an average of 235 minutes.	Focus on having TL aggressively look for possible EC discharges and move patients to the dismissal area.	TL, charge nurse

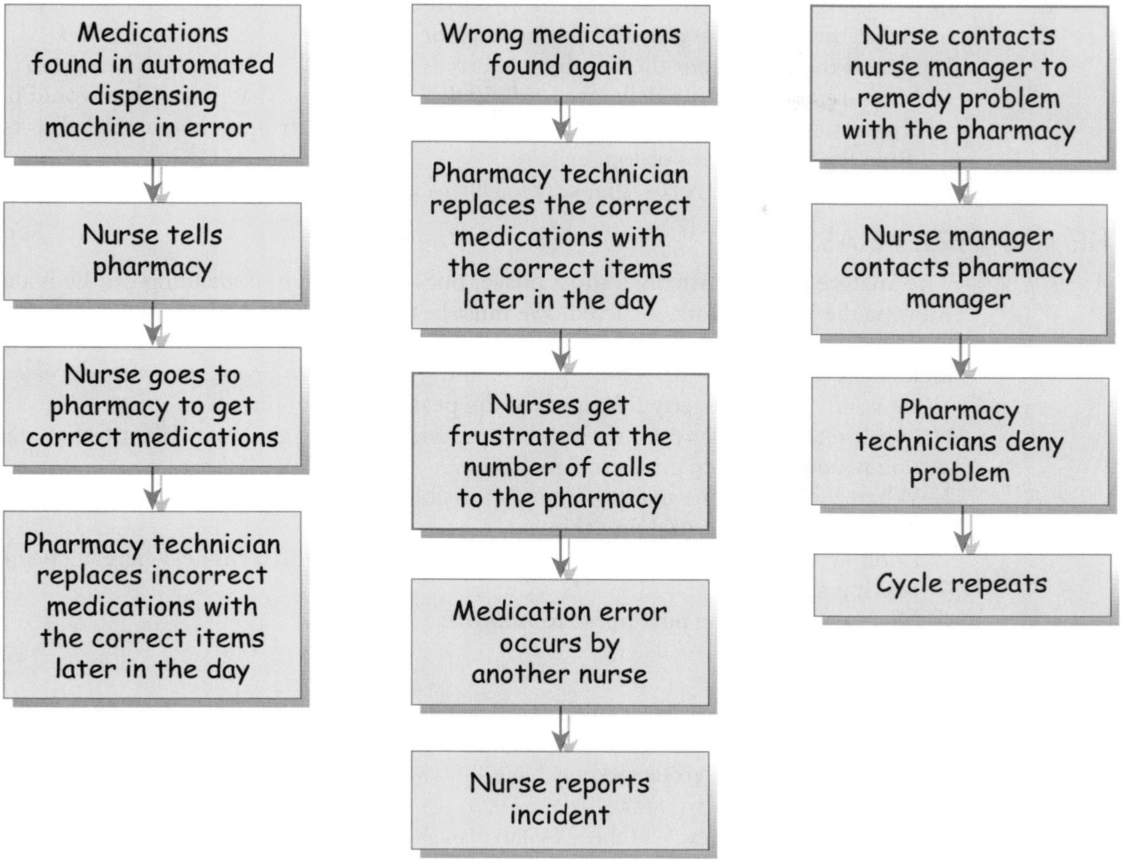

FIGURE 22-8
This is a process flow example. There are inputs, processes, and outputs in a typical flow diagram.

Identify what specifically will be measured to determine improvements and what will not be measured. Operational definitions detail the thing or event using specific wording with written inclusion and exclusion criteria. This helps get everyone in agreement on what is identifiable and measurable.

For example: KPI #1 = the number of near-miss medication incidences on the nursing unit due to wrong medications found in the automated dispensing machine. We are including only those kept in the automated dispensing machine, and excluding any kept in other areas.

Begin by measuring baseline numbers. That is, start with what exists currently before any changes are made. In other words, do not meddle with things until you know how bad the problem is. Otherwise, you will not see any true changes when you do RCTs. Baseline measures can be retrospective if data have already been collected, or you can go forward for a couple of weeks to find out what the real data show. Find out what the actual losses are in time, errors, or dollars.

1. Get all the facts about the numbers of errors first. Record them in the workplan.
2. Measure and track the issue over a defined period of time based on what would be a realistic timeframe to obtain a sample of what is occurring. This may need to be done for 2 to 4 weeks or longer.
3. Document data in words, graphs, pie charts, and bar charts.

THE ANALYZE PHASE

The analyze phase is usually a short phase, but can be longer depending on the issue. Analyze the baseline data collected. We must be objective in identifying where the real problems exist. These may be indicated by peaks in the graphs related to the number of incidences over that 2- to 4-week period, and may relate to problems with processes. What could be the underlying causes of the peaks in the graph?

1. Identify the *gaps* between the current performance and the goal. Identify how far you need to come to get to the goal.
2. When looking at the data to identify possible sources of variation, avoid blaming people or past ways of doing things.
3. Look at the current process flow diagram again, and determine where to begin making a change.
4. Move quickly to the next phase to improve.

THE IMPROVE PHASE

The improve phase is a good place to determine whether measures reflect the true problems. The problem statement and goal statement may need to be revised based on the findings. The data collected may have shown that no real problem exists or that the problem involves other issues.

Now use the PDSA cycle (Table 22-6) to plan and implement some RCTs. The idea is to think up creative ways to improve the system. Brainstorm ideas for the RCTs that you might try based on a problem process step within the flow diagram and the baseline metrics.

Brainstorming is when all team members spontaneously contribute and gather ideas without excluding any idea given. It is usually performed rapidly with all ideas considered and recorded. Be clear about what the target is, and play off of each others' suggestions.

The group may consider using a fair voting method or writing out RCT ideas. Otherwise, whoever talks the loudest gets heard. Sometimes some great ideas come from those quiet people.

1. Ask yourself: Can a step in the process be eliminated? Simplifying steps and deleting steps in a process can often eliminate big defects.
2. Could you try a new method?
3. Next, conduct the RCT using the PDSA cycle (see Table 22-6) for 3 to 7 days. Include staff education before starting the RCT so that everyone understands what is expected.
4. Conduct the RCT, and study the results. Document everything in the workplan.
5. Analyze the data with percentage calculations for improvements over baseline for last week.
6. Document all brainstorming sessions in the issues/solutions sheet.

Use data to determine whether there were improvements or a lack of improvement. What percentage of improvement was there this week compared to last week, and

TABLE 22-6

The PDSA Cycle Within the RCT

PLAN	1. State the goal of RCT cycle. Make predictions about what will be expected to happen. Who will be responsible, at what time, and place? When will it occur? Where will it take place first? 2. What are we trying to accomplish? 3. How will we know the change is an improvement? Roughly, how far do we expect to come (percentage, minutes)? Use only data that are reflective of the KPIs. For example, you would not measure time elements if you are looking at distance. 4. What change can we feasibly make that will result in improvement? Be realistic about what can be changed. 5. How long should it take? How many days should you run the RCT to see a result. Keep it as short as possible. Use the workplan and issues/solutions sheet to document, track, and analyze the data during and after RCTs. The workplan is very important to project successes in keeping track of each RCT and results.
DO	First, carry out the RCT on one or two nursing units for 3 to 7 days. If it needs tweaking, make a small change and RCT again for 3 to 7 days or longer, depending on the issue. Then move to another nursing unit.
STUDY	Compare the resulting data to your predictions, to baseline, and contrast it to previous time frames. For example: What was the improvement in time compared with last week?
ACT	Act on what was discovered after the initial RCT. What are the new changes the team can make based on results? What might be next cycle? Go on to do another RCT to improve the process further.

compared to the baseline measure? How many minutes difference is there? Make decisions based on fact not assumptions. Small improvements still mean improvement and help determine whether you are on the right track or not.

Small changes may need to be made in the process ... so tweak it ... and test it again with a change in the RCT over 3 to 7 days. Compare percentages, again to baseline or previous week, and determine whether there was any improvement.

Market the solutions to the people whose cooperation is needed. If front-line people have been involved at the outset, this part is easier. Prepare for possible objections to the implementation of the change, and plan to prevent them.

THE CONTROL PHASE

Now you are ready to establish controls to keep things going in the right direction. Controlling and sustaining the improvement is not easy and requires the development, documentation, and implementation of an ongoing monitoring plan.

1. Standardize the steps in the new process, and detail new flow diagrams. Write standard operating procedures, protocols, steps, guidelines, or policies so that it will be easier for people to do the right thing and harder for them to do the wrong thing.
2. Educate everyone about the new practice. Distribute the information in a systematic manner so that everyone in the organization has an equal chance of being informed.
3. Educate new employees in correct procedures and be an example for them to follow. Keep people informed.

4. Prevent reversion back to old ways or breaks in the "critical links" in the process by developing a process to monitor that changes have stuck and gains are sustained. Keep the process on the new course, and maintain the new practices you worked so hard to develop. Backsliding can occur easily as people tend to return to old habits. Change is difficult for some people who are used to tradition or who have been absent from the job for a time.
5. Continue to measure KPIs on a routine basis to see if solutions are still working. If slipping occurs, reinforce the new change or do more RCTs.

Box 22-2 provides a simplified example of DMAIC used successfully in one emergency center. Many of the important details have been left out for space. However, the basic process can be seen. Now see what you can do with the DMAIC process on a small scale using the scenario in Critical Thinking Box 22-3.

Practice improves results with time, and it can be a lot of fun.

BOX 22-2 Example of DMAIC in the Emergency Center

Problem statement: Emergency department patients are not seen by an MD in a timely manner.

DEFINE

The team *Defined* the cause of the problem as having to do with where the charts are placed.
Goal—Get the charts to the MDs sooner.
Business case – Cost of doing nothing different = Unhappy patients, possible patient complications, lack of bed space, and bottlenecks.

MEASURE

Key performance indicator (KPI) #1 = time between patient bed placement and being seen by MD.
The team *Measured* the actual average baseline data (KPI #1) over a period of 2 weeks. Baseline = 90 minutes (±15 min).
Target = patients should be seen within 30 minutes of bed placement (a 50% improvement) within a month.

ANALYZE

The team *Analyzed* the gap between existing situation and goal of 30 minutes (gap is 60 min). The gap also depended on which MD was on duty.
Can something be done about which MD was on duty? Not really.
The team brainstormed for other ideas. Can something be done about where charts are placed? Yes.

IMPROVE

The team *Improved* by doing RCTs
KPI #1 = time of patient bed placement to seen by MD

Continued

BOX 22-2 Example of DMAIC in the Emergency Center—cont'd

RCT #1: For the next 5 days, the team members involved placed charts in a separate bin and measured KPI #1.
Result = the MD saw patients on time 34% of the time. So they tweaked the plan and did more RCTs.
RCT #2: For the next 5 days they placed charts on separate bedside table (the deck) and set up a log book of times charts were placed and picked up.
Still measured KPI #1 = time of patient bed placement to seen by MD, and added another KPI.
KPI #2 = time between charts placed on deck and picked up off of deck.
Result = MD saw patients on time 20% of the time.
The team again brainstormed, tweaked the plan and did more RCTs.
Next 5 days, one MD was assigned as deck officer to oversee the process.
Result = MD saw patients on time 99% of the time within 30 minutes.

CONTROL

The team *Controlled* and sustained the improvement by establishing a standard practice.
They wrote a protocol and announced the new practice:
Always have charts placed on deck and assign a deck officer to monitor timeliness of chart retrieval.
The Department Director will monitor effectiveness of protocol, and watch for slippage into old ways.

CRITICAL THINKING BOX 22-3

A retrospective review of several charts revealed that documentation for 40% of PRN medications was lacking a prior assessment of pain. About 50% of the charts did not have documentation that the pain was evaluated within 30 to 45 minutes after the PRN medication was given. You have been asked to lead a team to resolve the problems that occurred mostly on your nursing unit.

1. What standard of practice has been violated?
2. How would you go about conducting your problem resolution using the DMAIC model approach for process improvement?
3. Who would you include on your team?
4. Who will develop the workplan and issues solutions sheet?
5. When will meetings be held? What are the ground rules?
6. What is the business case?
7. What are the goals and targets?
8. What are the KPIs?
9. What RCT can be done?
10. Imagine that you have some excellent RCT results, what will you do to control the improvement?

HEALTH CARE PROVIDER CREDENTIALING FOR QUALITY IMPROVEMENT

Some larger health care organizations require that an individual obtain a certification in health care quality within a certain period of time of the hire date. Persons can become a *Certified Professional in Healthcare Quality* (CPHQ) after taking a certification test to determine one's knowledge of quality management, quality improvement, case/care/disease/utilization management, and risk management at all employment levels and in all health care settings.

Although a minimum education requirement is no longer required, those who test should have worked in quality management for a minimum of 2 years, and review testing requirements prior to investing money into taking the examination. Approximately 75% of those who apply to test actually achieve certification.

CONCLUSION

Accountability is critical in nursing. We have to provide quality care that is cost-effective and meets the health needs of our clients. We do not have the luxury of giving a client all the time we would like to or the possible equipment and supplies that might be needed. Nurses must be accountable to both the quality of care and the economics of providing that care. An effective quality assurance program is a vehicle to provide accountability; if nursing does not provide its own accountability, someone else will do it for us.

Change is inevitable!
He who fails to invent change is at the mercy of those who will!

REFERENCES

Institute of Medicine (IOM): *To err is human: building a safer health system*, Kohn L, Corrigan J, Donaldson M (Eds.), Washington, DC, 2000, National Academy Press.

Joint Commission on Accreditation of Healthcare Organizations (JCAHO): *2004 Hospitals' national patient safety goals*, 2004a, *www.jcaho.org/accredited+organizations/hospitals/npsg/04_npsg.htm.*

Joint Commission on Accreditation of Healthcare Organizations (JCAHO): *2005 Hospitals' national patient safety goals*, 2004b, *www.jcaho.org/accredited+organizations/hospitals/npsg/05_npsg_hap.htm.*

CHAPTER 23

Nursing Informatics

JAN MCCLELLAN, RN, BC, MSN
JOANN ZERWEKH, EdD, RN, APRN, BC

Technology…the knack of so arranging the world that we don't have to experience it.
—*Max Frisch*

When computers (people) are networked, their power multiplies geometrically. Not only can people share all that information inside their machines but they can reach out and instantly tap the power of other machines (people), essentially making the entire network their computer.
—*Scott McNeely*

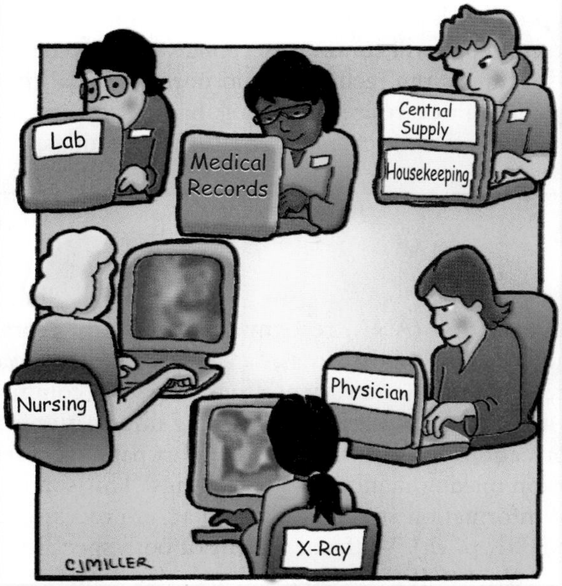

Nursing informatics—a specialty practice of nursing.

After completing this chapter, you should be able to:

- Define nursing informatics.
- Discuss the necessity of using recognized taxonomies and nursing nomenclature in nursing documentation.
- Discuss trends associated with the computerized electronic record, e-health, PDAs.
- Describe what a nurse specializing in nursing informatics might do.
- Review the steps in evaluating a website.
- Discuss future trends in nursing informatics.

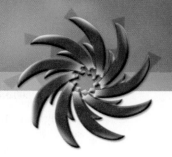

Computer automation is pervasive today. Everywhere we turn this technology is in evidence. The neighborhood grocery store has automated scanners and checkout lines. Your bank has automated tellers, check scanners, wire transfers, and online services. The local library has automated catalogs, interlibrary lending, and books online. From our homes, we can access the world through the Internet using the World Wide Web (www), researching any question, sending e-mail, and purchasing just about anything through our personal computers. A litany of computerized marvels could fill volumes.

The explosion of new technology during the past 30 years that makes all this possible is truly phenomenal. What is even more incredible, and perhaps a bit frightening, is that this seems to be just the beginning. The time is coming, in the not too distant future, when the thoughts, communications, creations, manuscripts, learning material, and financial assets of the civilized world will exist primarily in electronic form. If the lights went out, civilization as we know it will cease to exist.

Health care is not immune. Some of the most complex automated systems and certainly some of the most complex requirements for these systems can be found in the health care environment. Systems to serve the diverse needs of the health care industry from the administration and financial departments to the nursing divisions need to be implemented and integrated across the continuum of care of modern health care organizations. As a result, the demand for health care professionals who are knowledgeable in the application of this technology is growing rapidly.

Even with technology all around us, we as users do not always feel comfortable with it. Technology is sometimes confusing, intimidating, and in large part because it changes so rapidly, downright bewildering. In spite of these issues, there are some relative constants that make the field less confusing and easier to manage. One of the biggest challenges we face is how to properly harness and apply the available technology. The good news is that while the technology will continue to change and become more robust, the techniques employed to apply the technology do not. The goal of this chapter is to explore how nursing and health care are embracing, harnessing, and using this technology to increase the quality of patient care in all health care settings.

NURSING INFORMATICS

WHAT IS NURSING INFORMATICS?

In 1994, the American Nurses Association (ANA) recognized the field of Nursing Informatics. The ANA has defined nursing *informatics* as, "a specialty that integrates nursing science, computer science, and information science to manage and communicate data, information, and knowledge in nursing practice. Nursing informatics facilitates the integration of data, information, and knowledge to support patients, nurses, and other providers in their decision making in all roles and settings. This support is accomplished through the use of information structures, information processes, and information technology." (ANA, 2001, p. vii). With the advent of both specialty and integrated clinical information systems (CIS), the longitudinal electronic medical record (EMR) has become the ultimate goal of health care organizations. The EMR will reflect a record of the patient's health care throughout his/her life. Although this realization of 100% integration of all patient data in one longitudinal electronic record is becoming more available, few organizations have actually reached this goal. There are still outstanding issues of what to do with outside information that comes into your facility, old systems not able to interface with new, corrupt data from old systems, and not enough manpower to enter all the data from old charts. Although solutions are being developed to solve some of these problems, it will take time to reach the ultimate goal.

Information is power. The extensive clinical background of the nurse informaticist (NI) is invaluable to the success of the implementation of these online, computer applications. Nurses have a unique understanding of workflow, the hospital and clinical environment, and specific procedures that are necessary for effective health care information infrastructure. Moreover, the NI is critical to the translation of standard information into practical models that can be applied to improve the health care work environment (Delany, 2004).

So, what does this mean? What does a nurse specializing in NI do on a daily basis? How does one become an expert in this unique field of nursing?

THE CERTIFICATION PROCESS

In 1994, the American Nursing Credentialing Center (ANCC) *(www.nursingworld.org/ancc)* provided a method for nurses to become certified in this specialty. Their focus is to improve patient care with health care automation that encourages caregivers and physicians to make more accurate and timely decisions. Box 23-1 lists the eligibility

BOX 23-1 Qualification Criteria for Nursing Informatics Specialist Certification Examination

- Hold a baccalaureate or higher degree in nursing or a baccalaureate degree in a relevant field. Relevant areas include: science (e.g., biology, anatomy, physiology), professional disciplines (e.g., engineering, computer science, psychology, physical therapy), or academic liberal arts (e.g., mathematics, English, philosophy, history);
- Hold a current active registered nurse license in the United States or its territories;
- Have practiced as a licensed registered nurse for a minimum of 2 years;
- Have a minimum of 2000 hours in the field of informatics nursing within the past 3 years; or have completed at least 12 semester hours of academic credits in a graduate program in informatics nursing in informatics courses (e.g., computer programming, information science, systems analysis and design, management of information systems) and have practiced a minimum of 1000 hours in informatics nursing within the past 3 years; or have completed a graduate program in nursing informatics that includes at least 200 hours of clinical practicum.
- Have had 30 continuing education contact hours applicable to the specialty area within the past 3 years (American Nursing Credentialing Center, 2003).

From American Nursing Credentialing Center: *Informatics nurse certification exam,* 2003, *www.nursingworld.org/ancc/certification/cert/certs/informatics.html.*

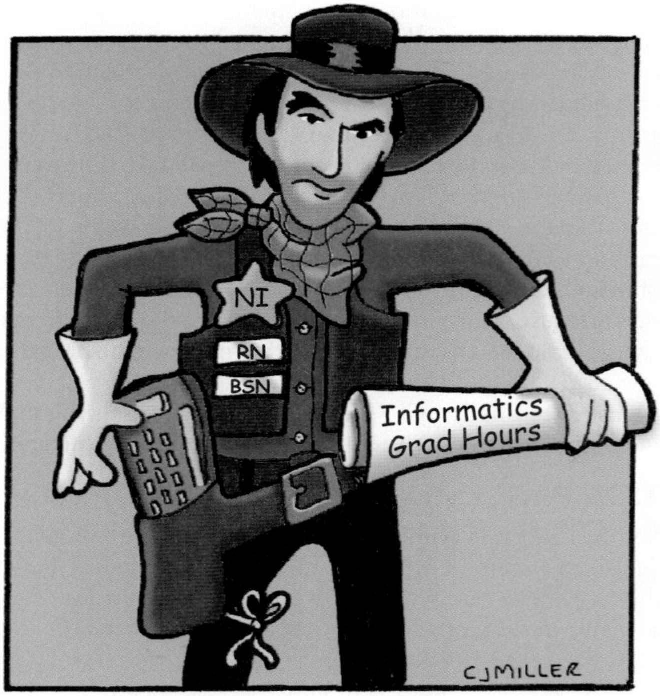

FIGURE 23-1
The new nurse entrepreneur in the competitive field of nurse informatics.

requirements for taking the ANCC nursing informatics certification examination. The following is a brief overview of the content and knowledge needed to work in nursing informatics (Figure 23-1).

SYSTEM LIFE CYCLE

This content area that the NI needs to understand includes system planning, system analysis, system design, system implementation and testing, and system evaluation, maintenance, and support. The mastery of several project management tools is necessary. Knowledge of basic system tools might include:

- A word-documenting tool
- A project management tool
- An e-mail/communication tool
- A slide presentation tool

The nursing informatics nurse can be involved in the evaluation of current systems as well as being instrumental in bringing the needs of both the clinical and technical sides of the health care organization to the attention of administration and the vendor

CRITICAL THINKING BOX 23-1

What experience have you had with management tools, such as e-mail and slide presentations?

for the "system" chosen. Having an understanding of systems theory will serve as the basis for decision making and project management (Critical Thinking Box 23-1).

Once a new system has been built, every existing system and the new system must be tested to ensure that all data elements are processed correctly and that the outputs end up at the correct place. It is standard practice to do three levels of testing new software (Saba & McCormick, 2001). These are:

- Unit testing—The actual programmers conduct this as the code is programmed.
- Alpha testing—This is the first testing of new software. It occurs within the development organization.
- Beta testing—This is the testing and running of the new software at the actual patient site.

You may have heard the term beta testing with regard to NCLEX (National Council Licensure Examination) developing a new generation of test items. It is very much the same process, checking software/test questions before implementing them as part of the test plan.

The NI could be involved in all onsite testing and evaluation. After a new software package is purchased, it is critical to integrate and test the software throughout all departments within the organization. After the new software has been thoroughly tested, it will be an ongoing process to provide adequate training for the people who will be the end users of the software. Developing meaningful testing scenarios is very important and certainly falls within their expertise, as they know the workflow of the clinician.

HUMAN FACTORS

The NI must consider human factors when assisting with purchasing and implementing a health care information system. *Ergonomics* and software and user interface are important considerations.

Many of today's jobs are performed at a computer work area, often in a "shared" area. This is the case in a hospital setting, where nurses, physicians, and ancillary caregivers use the nursing station 24 hours a day. There could be dozens of workers using the same computer almost constantly. Change, variation, and adjustment to fit an individual worker are basic to the well being of each worker. Workstations should accommodate users of many different heights, weights, and individual needs. Computer vendors must keep in mind that the average age of a nurse is creeping toward the mid-40s, and letter size and font as well as proper lighting and the avoidance of shadows are vitally important to aid in viewing computer screens.

The successful ergonomic design of an office workstation depends on several interrelated parts. The task, the posture, and the work activities all interact. The three activities alone can be difficult to deal with, but these activities also must interact positively with existing furniture, equipment, and the environment. The combination makes the picture more complicated. Important parts of the workstation are the chair, the desk, and the placement of the computer (CPU), keyboard, and monitor.

The chair should be padded appropriately, easily adjustable, and include strong lumbar supports. Usually wheels allow easy movement and armrests may or may not be used, as they sometimes cause more problems than support.

The desk must be wide and deep enough to accommodate the computer's footprint, keyboard, and mouse, with ample space around the machine to write, use the phone conveniently, and perform all other desktop activities. Keep the area clear of clutter and crowding.

The placement of the computer, keyboard, and mouse should be unique to every worker, but because this is highly unlikely, the monitor height should be approximately the 18 to 22 inches above the desk surface, causing most users to view the screen with slightly lowered eyes. The keyboard should be placed directly in front of the user and the mouse on the user's dominant-hand side of the machine. Some nursing stations designate some machines as "left handed" mouse machines so that the mouse will not need to be switched numerous times during a shift. Be sure to use a mouse pad to ensure traction, lessening the frustration and continual long movements of the mouse (Critical Thinking Box 23-2).

Poor workplace design is often the major source for cumulative trauma disorders (CTDs). CTDs have been associated with users who work for long periods of time at poorly constructed or poorly arranged workstations.

Ergonomic design of work tasks can reduce or remove some of the risks. Other solutions may include:

- Information and training to workers about body positions that eliminate the opportunity for repetitive stress injuries to occur
- Frequent switching between standing and sitting positions, reducing net stress on any specific muscle or skeletal group
- Routine stretching of the shoulders, neck, arms, hands, and fingers has proven successful

NIs may be called upon to assist in the design and layout of a work area when installing a new system. Teaching and education of work area stretches as well as

CRITICAL THINKING BOX 23-2

What is your workplace environment like? Have ergonomics been considered? How could you make it better?

CRITICAL THINKING BOX 23-3

What has been your experience and exposure to the use of computer technology in the hospital? Your school? At home? Think of ways to become more familiar with the use of computer technology.
Even with technology all around us, we do not always feel comfortable with it.

policies and procedures may fall to their area of expertise. It is necessary to understand the ergonomic principles to ensure the health of the staff working in this environment.

INFORMATION TECHNOLOGY

The NI must have a basic knowledge of how a computer works. It is important for the NI to converse with the technology staff on an intellectual level regarding hardware, software, communications, data representation, and security. As an NI gains experience with system implementation, training, testing, presenting, and facilitating knowledge in all these areas are important (Critical Thinking Box 23-3).

INFORMATION MANAGEMENT AND KNOWLEDGE GENERATION

In the past, the process of designing a database has been left to the information systems professionals. Why is it important for an NI to understand information and database management? When reviewing the basic elements of an electronic medical record, it is important to be knowledgeable of all the places and formats in which the data are stored. An understanding of database management is needed for this (Figure 23-2).

The NI should have an understanding of two types of databases:

- Operational databases—These are used wherever there is a need to collect, maintain, and modify data. This database stores dynamic data, which could change frequently. *Examples are inventory databases, order maintenance databases, and patient-tracking databases.*
- Analytical databases—These are used to track historical and time-dependent data. These data would unlikely be modified. *Examples would be chemical test databases and survey databases.*

PROFESSIONAL PRACTICE, TRENDS, AND ISSUES

WHAT ARE REGULATORY AND ACCREDITATION REQUIREMENTS?

Although there are many regulatory and governmental agencies instituting health care policy, the Joint Commission on Accreditation of Healthcare Organizations (JCAHO) and Health Insurance Portability and Accountability Act (HIPAA) are two to take notice of. The NI must have a clear understanding of these regulations to be able to guide the organization within these boundaries. To stay abreast of new regulations being signed into law and changes to existing regulations is constant effort.

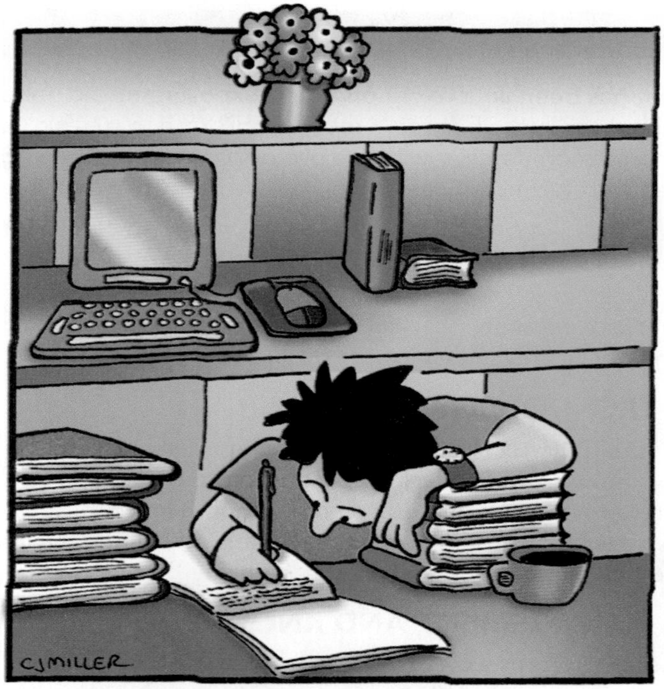

FIGURE 23-2
Even with technology all around us, we do not always feel comfortable with it.

HIPAA. In 1996, the HIPAA was developed. These standards were developed to ensure that health care organizations collect the right data in a common format so that the data can be shared (Simpson, 2001). The major areas of impact from this regulatory legislation are in these areas:

- Health Information Privacy Law
- Data Security Standards
- Electronic Transactions Standards

Although some of the sections continue to be negotiated, and final outcomes are yet to be determined, the privacy standards have been approved. Among many requirements, health care entities must adopt written privacy policies and procedures that define how they intend to abide by the highly complex regulations and protect individually identifiable health information. Each health care organization must ensure that all staff members who have access to patient information have an understanding of the consequences of noncompliance (Gale Group, 2001).

In 1998, it was purposed that all health plans, health plan providers, and health care clearinghouses that maintain or transmit health information electronically be required to establish and maintain responsible and appropriate safeguards to ensure the integrity and confidentiality of the information. Although this seems very logical, it is a very

CRITICAL THINKING BOX 23-4

How has your clinical facility made changes to accommodate the Health Insurance Portability and Accountability Act (HIPAA) requirements?

difficult and time-consuming task when using pre-existing automated systems that did not previously have these requirements (Critical Thinking Box 23-4).

JCAHO

The JCAHO wrote the Information Management (IM) Standards in the mid-1990s. The 10 standards outline the need for information management regulation (Clark, 2004). These standards are available at the JCAHO website at *www.jcaho.org*.

The JCAHO sends out a team of experts for a review of every health care organization that wishes to be JCAHO certified. This team inspects and reviews a variety of areas within each organization. The NI may be called upon to lead the effort for preparing the IM standards for the JCAHO visit and for maintaining ongoing compliance (Critical Thinking Box 23-5).

ETHICS

Privacy and Confidentiality. Every health care organization has a responsibility to itself, to its patients and to the community at large to have good control of its information systems. Because the internal workings of health care rely on accurate and timely data and information, personal data about employees and patients must be kept safe and confidential. A corporate security plan is important to an organization.

Maintaining confidentiality implies a trust of the individuals who handle that data and information. These health care workers ensure the privacy of this information and use it only for the purpose for which it was disclosed.

Security policies must be explicit and well defined. Confidentiality agreements should be reviewed and signed upon hire and yearly there after. Breeches of security, confidentiality, or privacy should be dealt with quickly, and the offender should be charged accordingly. Every lapse should be treated openly and made an example for others to note. The NI may be involved in this process and the writing of the policies and procedures. As this is outlined in both JCAHO and HIPAA standards, the NI must be aware of the importance of these topics to the health care organization.

CRITICAL THINKING BOX 23-5

Have you had the opportunity to be in clinical during a Joint Commission on Accreditation of Healthcare Organizations (JCAHO) visit? If so, what did you observe? How was the staff prepared for the visit?

MODELS AND THEORIES

Nomenclature, Classification, and Taxonomy. Nursing nomenclatures offer a recognized, systematic classification and consistent method of describing nursing practice. Nomenclatures act as descriptors or labels; classifications are group or class entities; and taxonomy is the study of the classifications.

In 1995, the ANA approved the establishment of the Nursing Information and Data Set Evaluation Center (NIDSEC^{SM}) to review, evaluate against defined criteria, and recognize information systems from developers and manufacturers who support documentation of nursing care within automated nursing information systems (NIS) or within computer-based patient record systems (CPR). They recognized the following 13 nursing practice classification systems (ANA, 2003).

- North American Nursing Diagnosis Association Approved List of Diagnostic Labels (NANDA)
- Nursing Interventions Classification System (NIC)
- Nursing Outcomes Classification System (NOC)
- Nursing Management Minimum Data Set (NMMDS)
- Clinical Care Classification (CCC) [formerly Home Health Care Classification (HHCC)]
- Omaha System
- Patient Care Data Set (PCDS)
- Perioperative Nursing Dataset (PNDS)
- SNOMED CT
- Nursing Minimum Data Set (NMDS)
- International Classification for Nursing (ICNP®)
- ABC codes
- Logical Observation Identifier Names & Codes (LOINC®)

If the unique nomenclature of these classification systems is used consistently, gathered data elements can be captured, stored, and manipulated accurately in the electronic medical record. Without a common language, data cannot be aggregated into useful language (Simpson, 2000). The need for consistency causes problems for software vendors as they attempt to produce unique and robust software packages, but need to use the recognized labels and groupings of nursing practice elements. So what happens?

Currently, each software vendor uses a unique, patented naming convention for their specific functionality and then must "explain and define" these names and labels in their literature or presentations by relating them back to recognized nursing practice or data elements. This causes confusion to the user community.

The ANA Committee for Nursing Practice Information Infrastructure requires that classifications or languages meet certain criteria, including:

- The language provides a clinical useful terminology and rationale for development
- The language consists of clear and unambiguous terms
- The developer provides evidence of reliability, validity, and utility
- The language includes a unique identifier for each item

Each of these classifications or languages has made a unique contribution to knowledge development in nursing. Learning about and working with standardized

CRITICAL THINKING BOX 23-6

What has been your experience or exposure to these different practice classification systems? What does your clinical agency use?

nursing languages will ensure nursing contributions are an integral part of any electronic medical record. Understanding those contributions through research and teaching will help to further define the scope of nursing practice. Standardized classifications or language, teaching, clinical practice, and research must be interrelated as nursing moves forward (Critical Thinking Box 23-6).

Theories. From the inception of Nursing Informatics, during the 1990s, *general systems theory* has served as a conceptual framework. Systems theory consists of six elements:

- Interdependent parts—elements of the system that interact for processing
- Input—any outside element or factor that is brought into the system
- Process—the activity within the system
- Output—any product that is produced from the processing activity
- Control—rules or procedures within the system
- Feedback—reusing output from the system as input back into the system for validation or correction

This theory organizes interdependent parts working together to produce a product that none used alone could produce. Nursing Informatics uses this theoretical foundation for analysis and design, implementation and support, and testing and evaluation of automated systems. It is used, as a basis for decision making, education curriculum needs, and foundation for system and project management.

Change is always occurring, sometimes it is planned and sometimes it happens quite unexpectedly. The effects of change range from positive to negative, from minor to major, from predictable to unpredictable. Our health care organizations are in constant change. With the advent of computers and new technology, nurses and caregivers are being invited to use this technology. An understanding of the *theory of change* offers a foundation and approach to assist nurses and caregivers in the inevitable change that will occur with the implementation of a clinical information system. Review Kurt Lewin's change theory in Chapter 10.

It is common for NIs to be called upon to answer some of these questions. They act as role models for nursing and caregiver users, as they themselves have moved from a clinical background to being very comfortable in a technical environment.

CLINICAL INFORMATION SYSTEMS

Every day nurses encounter technology, and this technology is changing the ways that health care is delivered in the hospital, physician's office, or the patient's home. CISs have replaced pencil and paper charting. Even Florence Nightingale expressed a desire for medical records that were standardized, organized, and legible.

> "In attempting to arrive at the truth, I have applied everywhere for information, but in scarcely an instance have I been able to obtain hospital records fit for any comparison." (Florence Nightingale Museum website).

An Institute of Medicine (IOM) (2001) report, *Crossing the Quality Chasm: A New Health System for the 21st Century*, identified the development and application of CISs as essential for health care to be able to leverage state-of-the-art technology to deliver the highest-quality, lowest-cost patient care.

WHAT IS A CLINICAL INFORMATION SYSTEM (CIS)?

According to Sittig and colleagues (2002), "A clinical information system is a collection of various information technology applications that provides a centralized repository of information related to patient care across distributed locations. This repository represents the patient's history of illnesses and interactions with providers by encoding knowledge capable of helping clinicians decide about the patient's condition, treatment options, and wellness activities. The repository also encodes the status of decisions, actions underway for those decisions, and relevant information that can help in performing those actions. The database could also hold other information about the patient, including genetic, environmental, and social contexts." Essentially, the CIS utilizes the computer to provide and store information and data about a patient from departments that are patient-focused or departmental-focused.

WHAT IS THE COMPUTERIZED PATIENT RECORD (CPR)?

There are many names used for the computerized patient record (CPR; no, this is not resuscitation of your computer) that basically refer to the same thing—the EMR, the electronic patient record (EPR), and the electronic health record (EHR). It is important to note that the CPR is not the CIS. It is a discrete part of the CIS.

In its simplest form, a CPR resides in a software program that offers the health care provider an instrument with which to obtain clinical information (e.g., history; physical examination findings; laboratory, radiographic, and other data) and the ability to transcribe data into a computer database repository by typing or using a mouse, a stylus pen, or voice activation information. With electronic or computer data entry, the need for a paper-based record can be eliminated. Many software products offer not only a CPR component but an "interface" that is "bundled" into practice management programs (e.g., billing, paperless registration, appointment scheduling, electronic querying/searchable databases). Figures 23-3 and 23-4 illustrate screen shots from a patient's CPR.

For practical purposes, CPR can be classified into three groups depending on where the patient record data are stored: (1) office-based or conventional (hospital) system, (2) Web-based system, and (3) handheld or wireless system. The leading proprietary software system CPRs are universally Windows products but may differ according to the language in which they are written (e.g., Java, Visual Basic). Advantages of the CPR are listed in Box 23-2.

As mentioned in the IOM (2003) report, a listing of essential features of the CPR (Box 23-3) must be addressed for our outdated health care system model to take

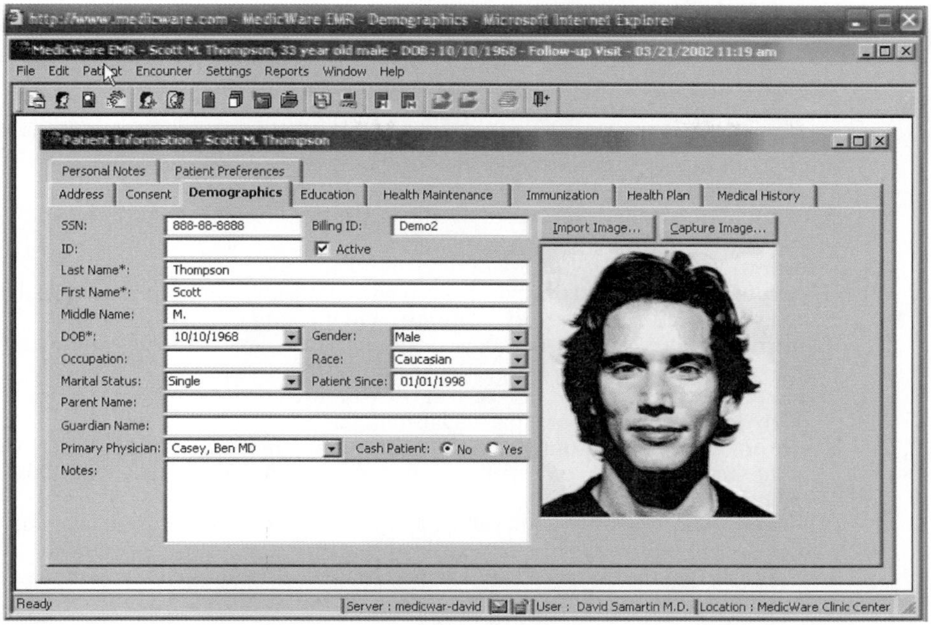

FIGURE 23-3
Client information screen. *(Courtesy of Medicware, Irwindale, Calif.)*

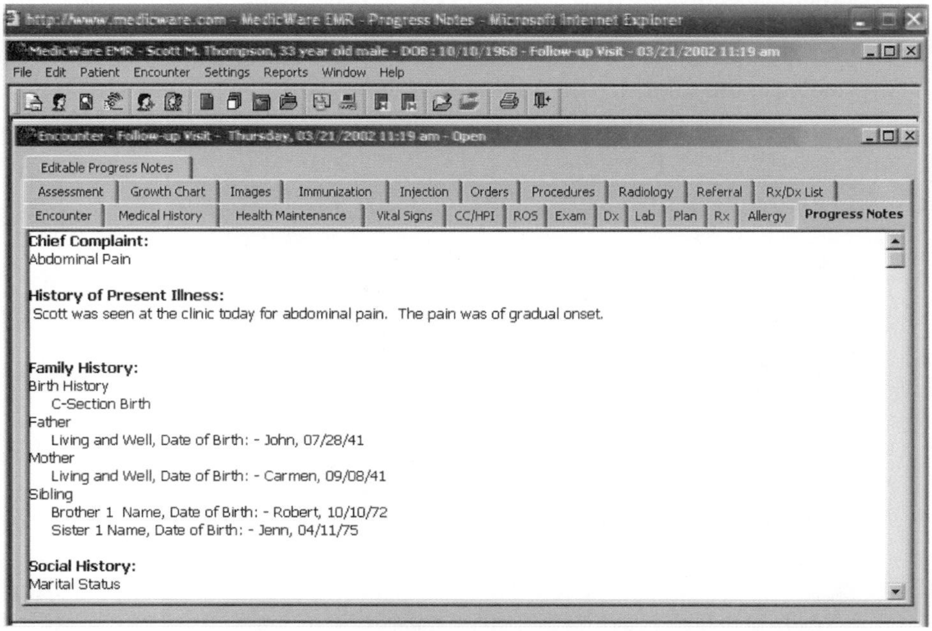

FIGURE 23-4
Client encounter screen. *(Courtesy of Medicware, Irwindale, Calif.)*

BOX 23-2 Advantages of Computer-Based Medical Records

Simultaneous, remote access to patient data from many locations
Legibility of record—no handwriting
Safer data—backup and disaster recovery system, so less prone to data loss
Patient data confidentiality—authorized use can be restricted and monitored automatically
Flexible data layout—can recall data in any order (chronically or in reverse chronological order)
Integration with other information resources
Incorporation of electronic data—can automatically capture physiologic data from bedside monitors, laboratory analyzers, and imaging devices
Continuous data processing—check and filter the data for errors, summarize and interpret data, and issue alerts and/or reminders
Assisted search—can search free-text or structured data to find a specific data value or to determine whether a particular item has ever been recorded
Greater range of data output modalities—data can be presented to users via computer-generated voice, two-way pagers, e-mail, and personal data assistants (PDA), for example.
Tailored paper output—data can be printed using a variety of fonts, colors, and sizes to help focus the clinician's attention on the most important data, as well as include images to see a more complete "picture" of the patient's condition.
Always up to date

advantage of the potential benefits of the "e-revolution." With the general public using the Internet everyday and an estimated 100 million Americans going to the Internet to obtain information, including health information, to make decisions, it is imperative to recognize the influence the Internet can have on making changes to improve patient self-management, patient satisfaction, and health outcomes (Dunn, 2003).

BOX 23-3 Eight Core Functions of the Electronic Health Record

A committee of the Institute of Medicine of the National Academies has identified a set of eight core care delivery functions that electronic health records (EHR) systems should be capable of performing to promote greater safety, quality, and efficiency in health care delivery.
The eight core functions are
- Health information and data
- Result management
- Order management
- Decision support
- Electronic communication and connectivity
- Patient support
- Administrative processes and reporting
- Reporting and population health

From Institute of Medicine (IOM): *Key capabilities of an electronic health record system*, 2003, Data Standards for Patient Safety, *www.iom.edu/report.asp?id=14391*.

WHAT IS e-HEALTH?

The all-encompassing term *e-health* is replacing the older term *telehealth* and according to Mea (2001), "e-health presents itself as a common name for all such technological fields," such as medical informatics and telemedicine and represents virtually everything related to computers and medicine. Although most "e-words" come from the commerce or business sector, the term is generally understood, despite its lack of precise definition, because of the dynamic environment that it is a part of the Internet. E-health has come to characterize not only a technical development but also a state-of-mind, a way of thinking that focuses on improvement of health care via information and communication technology.

Eysenbach (2001) feels that it stands not only for "electronic" but implies a lot of other "*e*s," which he feels represent what e-health is all about (Box 23-4), and he adds that it should also be **e**asy to use, **e**ntertaining, **e**xciting, and most of all **e**xist (Critical Thinking Box 23-7)!

BOX 23-4 The 10 *es* in "e-health"

1. **Efficiency**—leading to decreasing costs by avoiding duplicate or unnecessary diagnostic or therapeutic interventions, through enhanced communication possibilities between health care establishments, and through patient involvement.
2. **Enhancing quality of care**—by allowing comparisons between different providers, involving consumers as additional power for quality assurance, and directing patient streams to the best quality providers.
3. **Evidence based**—intervention effectiveness and efficiency should not be assumed but proven by rigorous scientific evaluation.
4. **Empowerment** of consumers and patients—by making the knowledge bases of medicine and personal electronic records accessible to consumers over the Internet, e-health opens new avenues for patient-centered medicine and enables evidence-based patient choice.
5. **Encouragement** of a new relationship between the patient and health professional, toward a true partnership, where decisions are made in a shared manner.
6. **Education** of physicians and health care providers through online sources (continuing education) and consumers (health education, tailored preventive information for consumers)
7. **Enabling** information exchange and communication in a standardized way between health care establishments.
8. **Extending** the scope of health care beyond its conventional boundaries.
9. **Ethics**—e-health involves new forms of patient-physician interaction and poses new challenges and threats to ethical issues such as online professional practice, informed consent, privacy and equity issues.
10. **Equity**—to make health care more equitable is one of the promises of e-health, but at the same time there is a considerable threat that e-health may deepen the gap between the "haves" and "have-nots," deepening the "digital divide."

Adapted from Eysenbach G: What is e-health?, *J Med Internet Res* 3(2), 2000, *www.jmir.org/2001/2/e20/*.

CRITICAL THINKING BOX 23-7

The Pew Internet and American Life Project (Pew) reported in 2003 that 80% of Americans with Internet access have used the Web to get health or medical information. How have you (or your family) used the Internet for your own health or medical care?

TRENDS

When the first edition of this textbook came out more than 10 years ago, the section on "computer technology" was new and innovative. It was the cutting edge of technology that sent many nurse educators, students, and practicing nurses scrambling to make sense of how the computer might affect them. The explosion of knowledge and technology have visibly changed our mind-set on the use of computer technology to the extent that computer literacy is a requirement in nursing education. Faced with devices, equipment, computer sensors, electronic patient records (CPR), "smart" body parts, and so on, that involve technological skills affects the way that nursing is practiced and delivered. As Dunn (2003) so cleverly states, "time to byte the bullet… the e-health train has not only left the station but is rapidly moving down the track carrying tens of millions of e-patients and many possibilities for transforming patient self-management, improving health outcomes, and enhancing [health provider] patient relationships." Although there are numerous trend areas, using the Internet to communicate and to provide patient self-care, evaluating Internet resources, and use of personal digital assistants (PDAs) come to the forefront.

USING THE INTERNET: THE NEXT GENERATION OF HEALTH CARE DELIVERY

Undoubtably, the Internet has transformed our ability to locate health information and to connect via e-mail or web bulletin boards with other individuals who have similar interests. The federal government recognizes the importance of having access and quality information and has established a series of goals in the *Healthy People 2010* action plan. According to Dunn (2003), Internet-based patient self-care is the "next generation of health care delivery." Health information on the Internet can dramatically improve the patients' abilities to manage their own health care conveniently. Not all of the Web-based information is accurate, which raises concerns about the quality of information individuals are using, and the impact this information has on the overall health of an individual.

Internet users must still proceed with caution when seeking health care information online, as there is a plethora of incomplete and inaccurate information that can be dangerous.

As nurses, we need to better understand how consumers find health information on the Internet, how to evaluate the quality of information retrieved, and how to help our patients to critically evaluate and manage information (Greenberg et al, 2004).

A 2001 study by RAND for the California Healthcare Foundation showed that information on health websites is often incomplete or out of date and is very commercialized. This might be of little concern if consumers routinely consulted health care professionals about the information. However, the Pew Internet and American Life Project (Pew) found that 69% of consumers did not discuss the information they found with a doctor or nurse, and considering that most health information on the Internet is written in a style that is above the 9th grade reading level, many individuals come away from the source of information confused, especially the underserved populations who need the information the most.

As tools and security functions are refined and advanced, components of the CPR that are being implemented or are being considered via the Internet include the following:

- Remote access to CPR from a health care provider's home or office
- Access to multiple clinical information systems in lieu of purchasing stand-alone electronic records systems
- Creation of a virtual CPR by bringing together information from multiple systems in a way that appears seamless to the end user
- Use of application service providers to provide access to the CPR
- Direct patient access to the official version of the patient's CPR

Imagine having access to your complete CPR no matter where you are in the world and being able to download portions of it to a CD-ROM or removable drive (flash or thumb drive) for whatever you need to have as documentation.

A study by Ross and colleagues (2004) describes how a patient-accessible online medical record affects patient care for patients with chronic diseases, such as congestive heart failure, and clinic operations using SPPARO (System Providing Access to Records Online) software that consisted of a Web-based electronic medical record (CPR), an educational guide, and a messaging system enable electronic communication among patient and staff. A noted trend of improved satisfaction with doctor-patient communication was found among patients, as well as how well patients felt their problems were understood, and how well doctors explained information. In interviews, the physicians and nursing staff did not feel that providing SPPARO to their patients resulted in a perceptible change in their workload.

e-MAIL

Everyone is familiar with e-mail. Your instructor may require you to complete assignments and submit your work via e-mail attachment instead of submitting a hard copy. You send e-mail to family and friends on a daily basis. Although more than 100 million Americans now use the Internet (and many access health information) and use e-mail daily, few doctors communicate with their patients through e-mail (Patt et al, 2003). Considering the popularity of e-mail and despite its potential for rapid, asynchronous, documentable communication to improve both the quality and efficiency of health services delivery, the use of e-mail communication has not been widely adopted by many physicians.

In Patt's (2003) study, physicians reported improved communication via e-mail with patients who have chronic diseases that require frequent, small changes in their treatment plans. In addition, physicians noted several other benefits including continuity of communication with patients, especially patients who travel, ability to respond to non-urgent issues on their own time, avoidance of phone tag with patients, and improved efficiency. Drug-refill requests and educational information, including links to reputable Internet sources, were also cited as examples of effective use of e-mail with patients. Physicians anticipated problems with e-mail communication, such as reimbursement problems, technical problems of failing servers or lost e-mails, and medicolegal consequences of e-mail used for urgent issues, but had not frequently experienced them, as reported in the study. With standards and guidelines for e-mail developed by the American Medical Informatics Association (1998), technically minded, electronically equipped, health care consumers will continue to accelerate the demand for e-mail access to their health care providers (Englebardt & Nelson, 2002).

PERSONAL DIGITAL ASSISTANTS (PDAs)

The PDA or personal digital assistant is a computer or information system that is located where the data is collected, which allows bedside data collection and charting. This conserves time and reduces steps to and from the nurses' station. Wilcox and La Tella (2001) report that PDAs offer easier information transmission between workers that provides for greater continuity of care. The major limitation of the PDA is the small screen size, drop/down lists for data to be displayed, and the limited storage capacity. The advantages are portability and information at your fingertips.

WHAT CAN A PDA DO TO HELP ME?

PDAs are no longer simply an appointment book and organizer. PDA applications can monitor blood glucose levels, blood pressure, diet, and activity, along with checking for drug interactions, calculating dosages, analyzing lab results, scheduling procedures, ordering prescriptions, and automating other clinical tasks, which reduces the probability of errors and increases patient safety (Abrahamsen, 2003). New PDA applications and programs are being developed at an astonishing rate. In addition, in educational settings, the PDA can be used to "beam" assignments, reading selections, and other information among students and faculty. Reference materials are readily available and some types of PDAs can connect to the Internet and provide access to *MEDLINE* and other knowledge sources in a wireless setting (Fontelo et al, 2003) (Critical Thinking Box 23-8).

CRITICAL THINKING BOX 23-8

Do you have a PDA? If so, how do you use it? If not, do you anticipate purchasing one in the near future? Do you find nurses in the hospital or clinic setting using PDAs on a regular basis? What programs do they or you use?

EVALUATING INTERNET RESOURCES

WHAT DO I NEED TO KNOW TO EVALUATE AN INTERNET RESOURCE?

McGonigle (2002) suggests a five-step plan to evaluate websites (Box 23-5).

Remember that *anybody* can publish *anything* on the Web. Make sure you critically appraise the source of the information.

BOX 23-5 How to Evaluate Websites

STEP 1: AUTHORITY
Who is/are the author(s)? Describe each author's authority or expertise. Are professional qualifications listed? How can you contact the author(s)? Who is the site's sponsor? Is the site copyright protected?

STEP 2: TIMELINESS AND CONTINUITY
When were the site materials created? When did it become active on the World Wide Web? When was it last updated/revised? Are the links up-to-date? Are the links functional? When were data gathered? What version/edition is it?

STEP 3: PURPOSE
Who is the targeted audience? What is the purpose? Are the goals/aims/objectives clearly stated?

STEP 4: CONTENT: ACCURACY AND OBJECTIVITY
Does the information provided meet the purpose? Who is accountable for accuracy? Are the cited sources verifiable? What is the value of the content of this site related to your topical needs? How complete and accurate are the content information and links? Is the site biased? Does it contain advertisements?

STEP 5: STRUCTURE AND ACCESS
Does the site load quickly? Do multimedia, graphics, and art used on the page serve a purpose or are they just decorative or fun? Is there an element of creativity? Is there appropriate interactivity? Is the navigation intuitive? Are there icons? Is this a secured site?

From McGonigle D: How to evaluate websites, *OJIN* 6(2), 2002, *http://eaa-knowledge.com/ojni/ni/602/web_site_evaluation.htm.*

It is important to encourage patients to focus their Internet searching endeavors to well known and reputable sites. For example, the U.S. Surgeon General's Family History Initiative is a great place to start with promoting attention on the importance of a well-documented family health history. In addition to the Office of the Surgeon General, other U.S. Department of Health and Human Services (USDHHS) agencies involved in this project include the National Human Genome Research Institute (NHGRI), the Centers for Disease Control and Prevention (CDC), the Agency for Healthcare Research and Quality (AHRQ), and the Health Resources and Services Administration (HRSA). A downloadable, free tool entitled, "My Family Health Portrait," is available at *www.hhs.gov/familyhistory/download.html.* The tool will help patients organize their family trees and help them identify common diseases that may run in their families. After completing the required information, the tool will create and print out a graphic representation of the patient's family generations and the health disorders that may have moved from one generation to the next. This is a powerful tool for predicting illnesses (USDHHS, 2004), and can be brought by the patient to their next health care provider's appointment.

The CARS Checklist. Acronymns are always helpful for remembering important key features. The CARS Checklist (Credibility, Accuracy, Reasonableness, Support) developed by Harris (1997) is designed for helping to evaluate a website. Although few sources will meet the majority of the criteria, the checklist will help in separating the high-quality information from the poor-quality information.

- ✓ **C**redibility—an authoritative source, a source that supplies some good evidence that allows trust.
- ✓ **A**ccuracy—a source that is correct today (not yesterday); a source that gives the whole truth.
- ✓ **R**easonableness—a source that engages the subject thoughtfully and reasonably, concerned with the truth.
- ✓ **S**upport—a source that provides convincing evidence for the claims made, a source you can triangulate (find at least two other sources that support it).

Harris (1997) notes that you need to have a little "**café**" advice to live with the information that you obtained from your Internet search.

Challenge the information and demand accountability.

Adapt and require more credibility and evidence for stronger claims—it is okay to be skeptical of the information.

File new information in your mind rather than immediately believing or disbelieving it.

Evaluate and re-evaluate regularly. Recognize the dynamic, fluid nature of information.

CONCLUSION

Nursing informatics is a specialty grounded in the present while planning for the future. NIs face many challenges in their daily activities, as they are in a position to wear many hats and bear many responsibilities. Change is the only constant. The challenge will be for the NI to assume a leadership role, while the nurse educator and practicing nurse prepare to embrace the generalized applications of working within a computerized environment, such as the clinical information system. No longer will it be sufficient to be able to turn on a computer and complete a simple task. A nurse will need to be able to use technology and access information, as well as evaluate the content of the information to provide to the patient population.

Nursing informatics is a very exciting and rewarding nursing specialty that will continue to expand and grow well into the future.

REFERENCES

Abrahamsen C: Patient safety: take the informatics challenge, *Nurs Manage* 34(4):48-51, 2003.

American Nurses Association (ANA): *ANA scope and standards of nursing informatics practice*, Washington, DC, 2001, ANA.

American Nurses Association (ANA): *Nursing Information and Data Set Evaluation Center (NIDSEC™)*. 2003, *www.nursingworld.org/nidsec/.*

American Nursing Credentialing Center: *Informatics nurse certification exam*, 2003, *www.nursingworld.org/ancc/certification/cert/certs/informatics.html.*

Clark J: *Information management: the compliance guide to JCAHO standards*, ed 4, 2004, HCPro, Inc.

Davis N, LaCour M: *Introduction to health information technology*, Philadelphia, 2002, Saunders.

Delany C: NICTF activities: Response to the President's Information Technology Advisory Committee, *CIN: Computers, Informatics, Nursing* 22(5):299, 302-305, 2004.

Englebardt SP, Nelson R: *Health care informatics: an interdisciplinary approach*, St. Louis, 2002, Mosby.

Eysenbach G: What is e-health? *J Med Internet Res*, 3(2):2001, *www.jmir.org/2001/2/e20/.*

Fontelo P, Ackerman M, Kim G, Locatis C: The PDA as a portal to knowledge sources in a wireless setting, *Telemedicine Journal and e-Health* 9:141-147, 2003.

Gale Group: HIPAA privacy rule takes effect, *Healthcare Financial Management* 55(6):9, 2001.

Greenberg L, D'Andrea G, Lorence D: Setting the public agenda for online health search: a white paper and action agenda, *J Med Internet Res* 6(2), 2004, *www.jmir.org/2004/2/e18/.*

Harris R: *Evaluating Internet research sources*, 1997, *www.virtualsalt.com/evalu8it.htm.*

Institute of Medicine (IOM): Committee on Quality of Health Care in America. *Crossing the quality chasm: a new health system for the 21st century*, Washington, DC, 2001, National Academy Press.

Institute of Medicine (IOM): *Key capabilities of an electronic health record system*, 2003, Data Standards for Patient Safety, *www.iom.edu/report.asp?id=14391.*

McGonigle D: How to evaluate web sites, *OJIN 2002*, 6(2), *http://eaa-knowledge.com/ojni/ni/602/web_site_evaluation.htm.*

Mea VD: What is e-health (2): the death of telemedicine?, *J Med Internet Res*, 3(2), 2001. Retrieved *www.jmir.org/2001/2/e22/.*

Patt MR, Houston TK, Jenckes MW, et al: Doctors who are using e-mail with their patients: a qualitative exploration. *J Med Internet Res*, 5(2), 2003, *http://www.jmir.org/2003/2/e9/.*

RAND Corporation: *Proceed with caution: a report on the quality of health information on the Internet*, San Francisco, Calif, June 2001, Rand Corporation, sponsored by the California Health Care Foundation, *www.chcf.org/documents/consumer/ProceedWithCautionCompleteStudy.pdf.*

Ross SE, Moore LA, Earnest MA, et al: Providing a Web-based online medical record with electronic communication capabilities to patients with congestive heart failure: randomized trial, *J Med Internet Res*, 6(2), 2004, *www.jmir.org/2004/2/e12/.*

Saba VK, McCormick KA: *Essentials of computers for nurses: informatics for the new millennium*, ed 3, New York, 2001, McGraw-Hill.

Simpson R: A systems view of information technology, *Nursing Administration Quarterly* 24(4):80, 2000.

Simpson R: Size up the big three, *Nurs Manage* 32(3):12, 2001.

Sittig DF: Advantages of computer-based medical records, *The Informatics Review*, 1999, *www.informatics-review.com/thoughts/advantages.html.*

Sittig DF, Hazlehurst BL, Palen T, et al: A clinical information system research landscape, *The Permanente Journal*, Spring 2002, *http://xnet.kp.org/permanentejournal/spring02/landscape.html#.*

U.S. Department of Health and Human Services: *U.S. Surgeon General's family history initiative*, December 29, 2004, *www.hhs.gov/familyhistory/.*

Wilcox RA, La Tella RR: The personal digital assistant: a new medical instrument for the exchange of clinical information at the point of care, *Medical Journal Aust* 174:659-662, 2001.

CHAPTER 24

Using Nursing Research in Practice

ELA-JOY LEHRMAN, MS, MAED, PhD, RN, CNM

Knowledge can be used deliberately for the guidance of practice decisions and the development of theoretical explanations, as well as researchable questions.

—Ada Sue Hinshaw

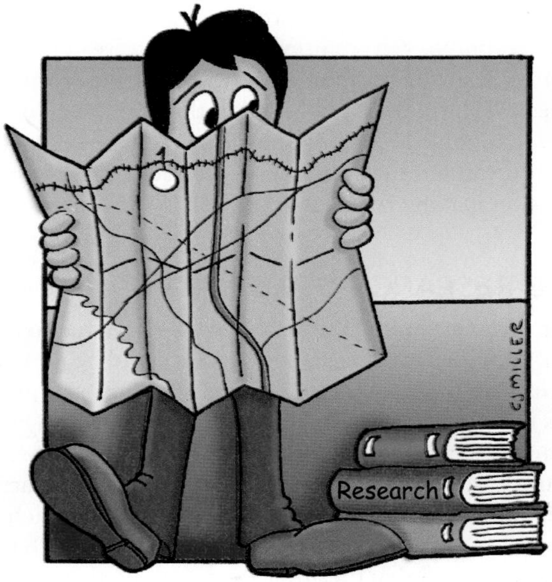

Nursing research is the road map to professional practice.

After completing this chapter, you should be able to:

- Identify the steps in the process of research utilization.
- Discuss the difference between conducting research and research utilization.
- Identify resources for evidence-based nursing practice.
- Identify the characteristics of your practice context.
- Describe the function of the National Institute of Nursing Research.

THE NEED FOR NURSING PRACTICE BASED ON RESEARCH

During the past century, there was a continuing increase in the costs associated with the delivery and receipt of health care in the United States. At the same time, there was more and more scrutiny of how health care dollars are spent. A major determinant of which heath care treatments receive funding from health care insurance is now based on documentation of favorable patient outcomes. In addition, patients want to know that the dollars they spend on health care will help them to get well and feel better—they want to purchase something that works for them. As providers of today's health care, nurses must be able to demonstrate that the nursing care they provide is cost effective and improves the health of patients.

Although in the past nursing care was largely based on traditional knowledge, given the current health care environment, today's nurses must base their practice on nursing care that has been documented as being beneficial to patients. Such practice is based on sound scientific research in which nursing care has been able to demonstrate cost-effective, predictable, and measurable practice outcomes. In this chapter, two methods of incorporating nursing research findings into nursing practice are discussed—*Nursing Research Utilization* and *Evidence-based Practice*.

WHAT IS NURSING RESEARCH UTILIZATION?

The classic research utilization project report indicates that research utilization is the process of systematically integrating the findings of completed nursing research studies into clinical nursing practice (Horsley et al, 1983). In the process of research utilization, the emphasis is on using existing data (findings) from previous nursing research studies to modify a current nursing practice. A major component of the process is reviewing completed nursing research studies that have been published in the literature. In contrast, conducting new research involves the collection of new data to answer a specific clinical practice question. Nursing research utilization is a step-by-step process incorporating critical thinking and decision making to ensure that a change in practice has a sound basis in nursing science.

WHAT ARE THE STEPS FOR NURSING RESEARCH UTILIZATION?

Step 1: Preutilization. The first step in the application of nursing research to nursing practice is the recognition that some aspect of nursing practice could be done in a more efficient, a more beneficial, or simply a different way. This begins an exploratory phase in which nursing colleagues in the practice setting are consulted regarding their opinions about the need to find a new approach for some aspect of nursing practice. An early question should be: "Is the current practice research-based?" When current practice is research-based, the next question should be "Is the research on which the practice is based outdated?" (e.g., the specific details of taking temperatures with mercury thermometers became outdated when digital thermometers were used exclusively in practice).

Consensus building constitutes a second phase of step 1 that is used to identify the specific practice to be changed. The incorporation of the principles of change theory will increase the possibility of success. (See Chapter 10 for information about the challenges of change.) In any practice setting in which there are several nurses, a change will be more acceptable if those affected by the change are included in the decisions related to the change. This consensus is crucial for the successful application of research findings.

The third and final phase of step 1 delineates the aspect of nursing practice that will be changed into a concise statement of the *practice problem*. This statement will answer the question "In our current nursing practice, what do we want to change, improve, or make more efficient?" The narrower and more specific the statement of the practice problem, the easier your task will be in step 2.

Step 2: Assessing. The second step in research utilization is the identification of and critical evaluation of published research that is related to the practice problem you have identified (Figure 24-1). Nursing literature is searched to identify those studies that deal with your practice problem. Although some studies may have explored the

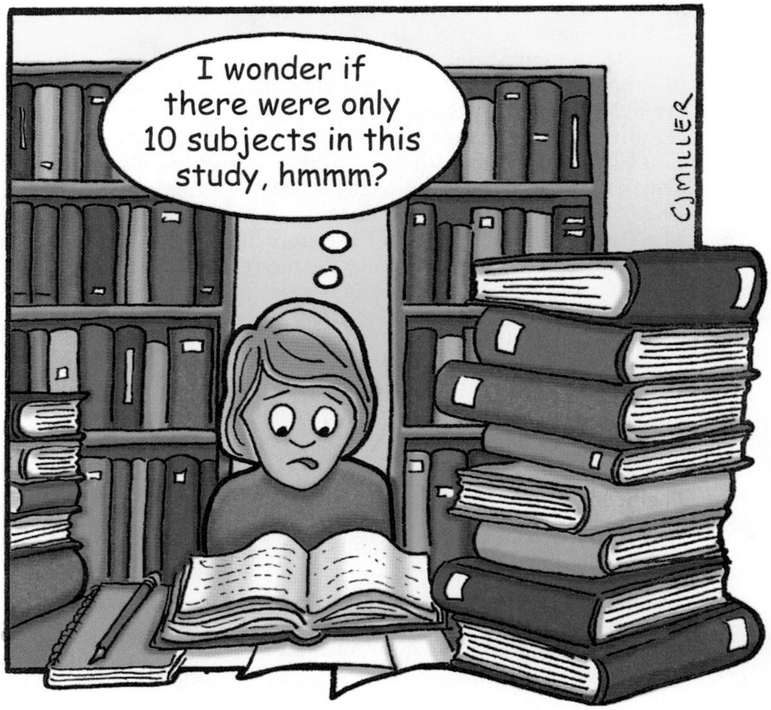
I wonder if there were only 10 subjects in this study, hmmm?
CJMILLER

FIGURE 24-1
Nine out of ten nurses recommend . . .

exact practice problem that you are examining, it is likely that most research will have approached the problem from a different point of view. Your task will be to analyze and to critically evaluate the research reports to determine which findings are adaptable to your practice problem and context. Organizing and summarizing the adaptable findings into an outline format will provide you with your primary working document for the remainder of the use plan (Box 24-1). Box 24-2 contains suggestions on reading a nursing research article.

The advent of the Internet and online searches has made a thorough search of the current literature easier. However, the volume of materials now available also increases the complexity of a review of literature. For example, the keywords used in a search

BOX 24-1 Analyzing a Research Article for Potential Use of Findings in Nursing Practice

1a. The Purpose of the study is:
1b. The importance of this study to nursing practice is:
2. The Research Question/Hypothesis is:
(If the question/hypothesis is not stated, it could be):
3a. The Independent Variable(s) is/are:
3b. The Dependent Variable(s) is/are:
(If there are no independent and dependent variables, the Research Variable(s) is/are):
3c. Definition(s) of the variable(s) of interest to me is/are:
4. The Conceptual Model/Theoretical Framework linked with this study is:
5a. The content areas in the Review of Related Literature are:
5b. The review does/does not evaluate both supporting and nonsupporting studies:
6a. The Research Design used for the study is:
6b. The design is/is not appropriate for the research question:
6c. The control(s) used in this study is/are:
6d. The Study Setting is:
7a. The Target Population is:
7b. The Sampling Method is:
7c. The Sampling Method is/is not appropriate for the design:
7d. The criteria for participants are:
7e. The sample included _______ participants
7f. The sample is/is not representative of the population:
8a. The Study Instrument(s) is/are:
8b. Instrument validity and reliability information are presented and are of adequate levels for confidence in using the results:
9a. The Data Collection Method(s) is/are:
9b. The data collection method(s) is/are—is not/are not appropriate for this study:
10. Steps were taken to protect the Rights of Human Subjects:
11a. The Data Analysis Procedure(s) is/are:
11b. The data analysis method(s) is/are appropriate for the level of data collected and the research question/hypothesis:
11c. The research question/hypothesis is/is not supported:
12. The author(s) major Conclusions and/or Implications for Nursing Practice are:

BOX 24-2 How to Read a Nursing Research Article

A research article should answer the following:

What:	Is the content of the article related to my question? Read the problem statement, purpose, research question, and results/findings.
Why:	Why was the research done? Read the problem statement, or the review of literature.
When:	When was the study done? Is it classic, current, or outdated? Do more recent findings provide a better answer? Read the date of publication.
How:	What research method was used? Read the method and design sections.
Who:	Who were the subjects, what was the sample? Read the method section.
Where:	In what setting was the research done? Read the method section.
So What:	Are the findings helpful to me and my problem? Read the findings and discussion.
Do Not:	Do not automatically accept what you read; critically evaluate the content. You can only evaluate what is written and reported; do not assume anything about what is not written.

What to Do When: When the statistical procedures are beyond your level of understanding:

- Read the results section, being alert for specific phrases that will tell you the answer to the research question. For example, "the hypothesis was not supported."
- Look at the tables; tables should be understandable without the narrative.
- Assume that the appropriate statistical analysis was done correctly and that the researcher has interpreted the results correctly.
- Have someone who understands the statistics read the article and get his or her opinion or get a consultant.

can either return no articles or hundreds of articles. When conducting an electronic search, a valuable technique is to begin searching within the most recent year, and then move back 1 year at a time until an adequate research base is identified.

There are times, however, when an electronic search is not adequate. Keep in mind that many of the classic research studies were published before electronic formats were widely used and may not be available online. Also, there may be valuable studies that are available in hard copy only. Because of these limitations of electronic sources, you may need to make a trip to the stacks in the library. Box 24-3 contains hints on conducting a search in the library.

Step 3: Planning. Planning for research utilization is accomplished in three phases. The first phase involves determining the new approach, or *innovation*, that will be used on the basis of the findings from the review of the literature. Previous research findings will be used to design the innovation in the context of your practice setting (e.g., intensive care unit, ambulatory care, home care). The expected *practice outcomes* should also be determined on the basis of the literature and may need to be adjusted according to the characteristics of your particular practice.

BOX 24-3 Hints for Conducting a Literature Search in the Library

1. Do some narrowing before you go to the library. Think about some key terms or alternate terms for your problem. Be prepared to narrow or expand your search, depending on what you find.
2. Plan to spend time in the library, but do not waste valuable time. Ask the library personnel to help you get started.
3. Begin by identifying the major professional nursing journals that publish nursing research, and start your literature review with those. If your problem is in a specialty area, review specialty journals.
4. If you find one article related to your problem, look at that author's reference list for other articles and journals.
5. Look at the table of contents in the journal where you found one related article.
6. Look at the section of books or journals in the library stacks that are about your problem.
7. Know the limitations of the library where you do your search; use interlibrary loan as needed.

Phase two of planning is the establishment of a systematic method for implementing the new approach. A *specific plan* should be established and followed so that the new approach is applied appropriately. Policies and procedures for implementation may need to be written. This phase may include staff training for the new approach.

The third phase of planning involves establishing a *method for evaluating* the practice outcomes, or effects, of the new approach. The outcomes are usually some specific improvements in patient care. Ideally, your evaluation will indicate both the quality and the quantity of the change in the outcome.

Step 4: Implementing. This step involves the implementation or application of the new approach, along with the collection of the evaluation data. By following the specific plan that you established in step 3, the new approach will be introduced into practice. It is important that you begin collecting your evaluation data at the same time so that you can clearly determine the effect of the new approach.

Step 5: Evaluating. Step 5 involves the evaluation of the implementation to determine whether the new approach improved practice outcomes. Whether you will continue using the new approach in the practice setting may also be determined on the basis of new technology, economic considerations, or changes in staffing. If there is no change in outcomes, you may want to return to the previous practice. The evaluation phase may lead to another research utilization project; for example, if the practice problem is significant and the practice outcomes were not improved, another new approach may be tried.

RESEARCH UTILIZATION: WHAT IS IT NOT?

Research utilization does *not* entail simply taking the findings of a single research study and using those findings in nursing practice. Research studies are replicated to rule out chance findings and to validate previous studies. Similar studies with different populations are conducted to determine the applicability of findings to different groups of people. For these reasons, research utilization encompasses the findings of many studies to develop the new approach that will be put into practice.

Data are collected in the process of research utilization. However, research utilization is not the collection of data to answer a research question, as is the case when conducting research. The data collected in research utilization are needed for evaluation to determine whether there is some advantage to the new approach in the practice setting.

Research utilization should not be confused with a review of nursing practice. Practice review involves a quality-control/risk-management process to evaluate the appropriate use of resources related to a specific treatment. As with research utilization, practice review use does not entail the use of nursing research findings during the process of evaluation.

When you review the nursing research literature for research utilization, as mentioned previously, there is no assurance that you will find studies that are directly applicable to your practice situation. Your specific question may not have been the topic of previous research studies. In this case, you may have to either adapt the findings from the literature or conduct your own research.

A COMPARISON OF PROCESS: RESEARCH UTILIZATION COMPARED WITH NURSING RESEARCH AND THE CONDUCT OF RESEARCH

HOW IS THE USE OF RESEARCH IN PRACTICE DIFFERENT FROM CONDUCTING RESEARCH?

As illustrated in Table 24-1, the major steps involved in both conducting and utilizing research are the same. Both are problem-solving processes involving critical thinking. For example, a clinical practice problem may provide the impetus to conduct and use research. However, there are differences. Conducting research taps into the "ways of knowing," whereas using research taps into the "ways of doing."

When we conduct research, whether in the clinical setting or the laboratory, the primary activity undertaken is the systematic collection of new data. Following specific steps called the protocol, we gather information that will answer a specific research question. For many nursing studies, the *research question* arises from a situation in nursing practice that needs an answer.

The *utilization of research* involves the systematic process of integrating the findings of completed nursing research studies into clinical nursing practice.

Research utilization also entails reviewing research that has already been completed to develop a new approach to nursing practice. All three processes, research utilization, nursing research, and the nursing process, have the same five major steps. However, the specific tasks for each process are different.

TABLE 24-1

Comparison of Processes: An Overview of the Nursing Process, Conducting Research, and Research Utilization

Nursing Process	Conducting Research	Research Utilization
Preprocess	Preplanning	Peruse
Establish a nurse-patient relationship	Identify the need for a research study	Identify a practice problem that needs a new approach
	Determine feasibility	Obtain consensus
	Scan the literature	
Assessing	Assessing	Assessing
Gather data	Identify the problem	Identify and critically evaluate published research related to your practice problem
	State research purpose	Identify the findings that are adaptable to your problem and your context
	Begin to formulate the research question	
	Review the literature	
Planning	Planning	Planning
Diagnose	Identify and define the variables	Determine the new approach and the desired outcomes
Set goals	Select a conceptual or theoretical model	Establish a systematic method for implementing the new approach
Prioritize	Select research design	Establish a method for evaluating the outcomes of the new approach
Determine nursing interventions	Finalize research question	
	Plan data analysis	
Formulate care plan	Write research proposal	
	Negotiate a site for data collection	
	Complete human subjects review	
Implementing	Implementing	Implementing
Initiate the plan	Prepare questionnaires	Begin using the new approach
	Train data collectors	Collect data about the outcomes of the new approach
	Obtain subject sample	
	Collect the data	
	Prepare data for analysis	
Evaluating	Evaluating	Evaluation of the implementation
Determine the patient response	Analyze the data	Determine whether the practice change improved patient outcomes
	Organize the data	Decide whether to continue using the new approach
	Answer the research question	
	Interpret the results	
	Report the findings	
	Plan next project	

WHAT IS THE RELATIONSHIP BETWEEN NURSING THEORY AND RESEARCH UTILIZATION?

Nursing theory used as the theoretical framework of a research study is essential for the continued development of nursing theories; research findings will support theory or will suggest the modification of theory. In contrast, when a specific nursing theory is used as the framework for nursing practice, the focus is on the intervention.

The intervention that is designed in the planning phase of research utilization must be consistent with the theory. For example, if Orem's theory of self-care requisites is used for nursing practice, a successful intervention would be one that emphasizes self-care rather than care received from others. There is a close relationship between nursing research and research utilization because of the focus of both on nursing practice.

DEFINING YOUR PRACTICE CONTEXT

Your practice context will determine to what degree you can apply the findings from nursing research to your practice problem. A *practice context* entails a blending of all those factors and systems that contribute to the delivery of nursing care. This blend includes the health, social, and ethnic characteristics of the patient population served; the type of practice setting; the economic constraints of the setting; the type of health care–delivery system; the existing policies and procedures; the staffing pattern; and the administrative structure. Each factor or system can be either enabling or inhibiting, but it is the practice context as a whole that is evaluated to determine the applicability of nursing research findings.

WHAT ARE THE HEALTH, SOCIAL, AND ETHNIC CHARACTERISTICS OF THE PATIENT POPULATION BEING SERVED?

To begin defining your practice context, you will need to identify any characteristics that are specific to the group of people who will be receiving nursing care. Is there some particular health characteristic that should be considered? For example, if you teach prenatal classes, the health characteristic will be pregnancy. Are there some particular social and ethnic characteristics that need consideration? If your prenatal classes are for pregnant teenagers who are single, then social characteristics need special consideration. Be as thorough and as specific as possible in identifying these characteristics.

WHAT ARE THE HEALTH CARE DELIVERY CHARACTERISTICS OF YOUR SETTING?

As you continue to define your practice context, specify the type of practice setting, the economic constraints of the setting, the type of health care delivery system, the existing policies and procedures, the staffing patterns, and the administrative structures. In other words, include all the characteristics of the care setting that will either contribute to or inhibit the process of applying research findings. If your practice setting is a hospital where there is a limit to the length of stay for a particular surgery, then a new approach that would increase that length of stay would not be an appropriate one for implementation. Furthermore, when implementing a new approach in practice, care must be taken to preserve or improve the current health-care delivery standards.

WHAT ARE THE MOTIVATORS AND BARRIERS FOR INCORPORATING NURSING RESEARCH INTO YOUR PRACTICE?

Identify your bridges (motivators) and roadblocks (barriers) in the practice setting (Critical Thinking Box 24-1). The more individuals in the practice setting from whom you can attain consensus on the new approach to practice; the easier it will be to implement. Those who understand the need for making a change in practice will be more likely

CRITICAL THINKING BOX 24-1

Think about...
What are the barriers that might inhibit your use of research findings?
How would you go about minimizing the barriers?

to support the change. (See Chapter 10 for information on change theory.) Those who feel that they had a part in the decision-making surrounding the new approach are also more likely to promote it. In both instances, these colleagues become motivators for the implementation of innovation and change.

As with any change process that involves a group of people, it is very likely that a small number of individuals in the practice setting will be very resistant to the new approach. Those who are resistant may present barriers that prevent the full implementation of the new process. They may complain about lack of time to learn the new approach, for example, in an effort to avoid being a part of what they do not support. These colleagues, as well as budgetary and personnel constraints, are examples of barriers.

In addition, the research literature may present barriers to implementing a new approach. For example, if there are only a few research studies reported in the nursing literature that are related to your practice problem, then the lack of replication of the findings may prevent you from developing a research-based approach for your particular practice problem. Another barrier is the time lag from the completion of a research project until the project report is published. This time lag, which may be a few years, may make the research findings obsolete. For example, research related to glass oral thermometers would be obsolete if your practice setting uses electronic ear thermometers.

WHAT IS EVIDENCE-BASED PRACTICE?

Evidence-based practice is similar to research utilization in that it is *a systematic method of applying research findings to nursing practice*. However, evidence-based practice incorporates many additional sources of data that may contribute to improved nursing care. Driever (2002) has developed the following working definition of evidence-based practice:

> Evidence on which nursing practice is based is derived from the synthesis of knowledge from research; data analyzed from the medical record; quality improvement and risk data; infection control data; international, national, and local standards; pathophysiology; cost-effectiveness analysis; benchmarking data; patient preferences; and clinical expertise. Evidence-based nursing practice involves the explicit and judicious decision making about health care delivery for individual or groups of patients based on the consensus of the most relevant and supported evidence derived from theory-derived research and data-based information to respond to consumers' preferences and societal expectations. (Driever, 2002, p. 593)

Evidence-based practice goes beyond nursing research in considering other sources of documentation that may improve nursing care. Research published by other disciplines is included (for example, medical research and social research), as well as nonresearch data that may contribute to practice (for example, financial data and clinical experts).

This is prudent at a time in history when the complexity of health problems is increasing, and at a time when the discovery of new data is more rapid than ever before.

Although there are sources of completed evidence reports readily available (for example, see the website at *www.ahrq.gov/clinic.epc.epcseries.htm*), not all aspects of practice have been evaluated to date. Therefore, the decision to implement an evidence-based practice that does not have a formal report requires a dedicated commitment on the parts of all those involved. The steps in applying evidence-based practice include definition of the problem; identifying, reviewing, and evaluating the data applicable to the problem; designing a practice change based on the data; and implementing the change in nursing practice.

Step 1: Define the problem. Because the focus remains on nursing practice, identification of the *practice problem* is identical to the first step of research utilization.

Step 2: Identify, review, and evaluate the data applicable to the problem. Like research utilization, the major source of data to be reviewed is *current nursing research, followed by current research from other disciplines.* Scientific research findings form the base with all other data building on this base. The specific nursing practice that will be changed, in addition to the practice context, will determine the types of data included for review.

Step 3: Design a practice change based on the data. Prepare a *written plan* for the new nursing practice. The plan needs to be consistent with your practice context to be effective, and it may experience motivators and barriers to the change. The plan will also require the consensus of those who will implement the plan in order for maximum benefit.

Step 4: Implement the change in nursing practice. Move the new plan into nursing practice on a *defined schedule*. Staff in-services may be required for those involved to fully understand the change. Monitor the implementation process.

THE NATIONAL INSTITUTE OF NURSING RESEARCH

WHAT IS ITS FUNCTION?

The National Institute of Nursing Research (NINR) is a branch of the National Institutes of Health (NIH), which is under the jurisdiction of the U.S. Department of Health and Human Services. Each institute within the NIH focuses on a specific area of health care research; the NINR is a major source of federal funding for nursing research. The NINR also supports education in research methods, research career development, and excellence in nursing science.

Another function of the NINR is establishing a National Nursing Research Agenda. The agenda is composed of priority topics for nursing research. These topics may be related to a national health need, or they may be in an area that requires research for the development of nursing science. Nurses incorporate topics from the agenda in research grant proposals that will be submitted to the NINR. For more information online, visit the NINR website at *http://ninr.nih.gov/ninr/*.

THE AGENCY FOR HEALTH CARE RESEARCH AND QUALITY

WHAT IS ITS FUNCTION?

As part of the Omnibus Budget Reconciliation Act of 1989, the Agency for Health Care Policy and Research (later renamed the Agency for Healthcare Research and Quality [AHRQ]) was established to enhance the quality and effectiveness of health care services. The AHRQ conducts and supports general health services research; develops clinical practice guidelines; and disseminates research findings and guidelines to health care providers, policymakers, and the public. One arm of the AHRQ supports the Evidence-based Practice Centers Program, which develops reports about interventions that are based on published scientific studies related to health care. For more information about AHRQ, visit their website at *http://www.ahrq.gov/*.

CONCLUSION

During the past few years, nursing research has been very important in establishing a platform for the development and utilization of evidence-based practice. Whether you are a new graduate or an experienced nurse, there are ample opportunities for you to apply research in your area of clinical practice. When areas of practice need to be changed, it is important to have valid information and data to support the need for change. Check out your hospital resources, establish networking and colleague support, and initiate a mini-research of your own.

REFERENCES

Driever MJ: Are evidenced-based practice and best practice the same?, *Western J Nurs Res* 24(5):591-597, 2002.

Horsley JA, et al: (1983). *Using research to improve nursing practice: a guide*, New York, 1983, Grune & Stratton.

CHAPTER 25

Workplace Issues

SUSAN AHRENS, RN, PhD, CS

Fear is the father of courage and the mother of safety.

—*Henry H. Tweedy*

The safety of the people is the supreme law. (Salus populi suprema lex.)

—*Cicero (106–143 BC)*

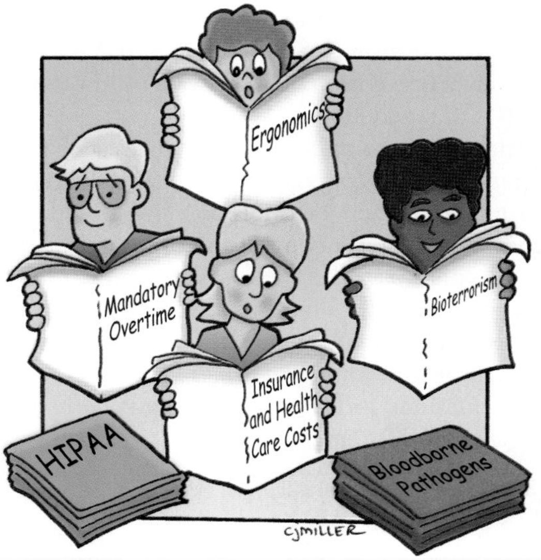

Workplace issues.

After completing this chapter, you should be able to:

- Determine your risk of encountering a workplace issue that can impact your health.
- Understand ergonomics and ways to safeguard your musculoskeletal system.
- Know the variety of diseases that are likely to be involved in a bioterrorism attack and what to look for.
- Discuss the importance of personal protective devices and how to use them.
- Understand the risk for violence at work and how to reduce your risk.
- Identify useful Internet sites to keep up to date with potential workplace issues (e.g., OSHA, CDC, ANA).

A hospital, nursing home, clinic, or physician's office can be hazardous to your future health and well-being. *This is especially true if you are not informed.* Many nurses are aware of the risk of exposure to infection, but are not aware of other hazards that exist in health care organizations. In addition to exposure to infection, being in a health care organization can expose a nurse to injury, toxic chemicals, bioterrorism, and violence. How well a health care organization plans and protects health care workers from occupational hazards is a measure of how safe you will be and what risks you may encounter as you work. This chapter addresses workplace issues that could potentially affect your health and what you need to do to avoid injury, occupational exposure, and illness.

QUESTIONS TO ASK WHEN STARTING A NEW POSITION

Is the hospital latex-free? If not, what latex will I be exposed to?

What ergonomic devices exist to protect me from harm? Will I be lifting, pulling, tugging, and using a computer?

Does the organization have an antiviolence program? How are bullying behavior and other hostile work situations being addressed by the organization?

Is the organization needleless? If not, what is my exposure risk?

What is the organization's policy for exposure to infectious agents? Does it include testing, medication, counseling, and follow-up?

What is the organizational plan for recognizing and dealing with bioterrorism?

What personal protective equipment is available to me? Is it adequate to protect against blood, bacterial, and toxic exposure?

What is the organization tuberculosis (TB) prevention plan? Does the plan adhere to Occupational Safety and Health Administration (OSHA) regulations?

Does the organization have an influenza prevention plan? Does it follow the Center for Disease Control and Prevention (CDC) guidelines?

Is there a plan for handling potentially toxic or infectious substances such as blood, chemoprophylaxis, and suction canisters? What is my potential exposure? Will I receive training in correct handling? Will annual refreshers be offered?

Who is the designated safety officer? Where is a copy of the organizational safety plan and emergency situation's response plan?

Where will I park? Is it well-lit? Is it patrolled? What is my risk?

What is the workmen's compensation program? Would I be able to return to work in a light-duty capacity if I am injured? For how long?

Does the organization provide vaccinations for infections I might be exposed to such as influenza, chicken pox, and hepatitis B?

ERGONOMIC HAZARDS FOR HEALTH CARE WORKERS

According to the American Nurses Association (ANA), ergonomic hazards have become a major safety concern among health care workers (ANA, 2004), and nurses are considered to be in a profession that puts them at risk for serious musculoskeletal injuries. The most common injuries tend to be back and shoulder injuries. Unfortunately, these types of injuries are the most debilitating of all injuries. Imagine if you cannot raise your arms or reach for things without severe pain. Or... what would happen if every step you took resulted in pain in your back and down your leg and sitting or lying down does not relieve your distress? These problems can be yours if you do not take the risk seriously.

So, what is your risk? That is somewhat unclear, as studies investigating work-related injuries in nursing are sporadic. However, it has been reported that more than 50% of nurses complain of chronic back pain. In addition, nurses in one study reported transferring to a different unit, position, or employment due to a back injury, and many of those who had remained in their position say they had considered leaving nursing all together because of back pain (Owen, 1989). More than one third of nurses have had back injuries severe enough that they were required to take a leave from work (Owen, 2000). In other words, out of every 10 nurses, four of them at one time or another will have a back injury severe enough that they need to take a leave from work. Back-related injuries reduce the already short supply of nurses, and because there are fewer nurses, the risk for back-related and other musculoskeletal injuries increases.

The reason these injuries are so common in nursing is the nature of the work that nurses do. Patient-handling tasks are repetitive and are usually done manually with very little mechanical support. Lifting, transferring, repositioning, and reaching are the actions that are associated with injuries. Often the configuration of the patient's room and the placement of furniture, monitors, blood pressure cuffs, thermometers, and other hanging devices contributes to injury as it requires nurses to reach and stretch in nonergonomic positions to perform tasks.

Until recently, it was believed that good body mechanics with proper lifting techniques could prevent back and shoulder injuries. However, according to the ANA (2004), the idea that there is a safe way to manually lift or turn a physically dependent patient is no longer valid. *Teaching nurses to use proper body mechanics to lift and turn patients does not result in fewer injuries* (ANA, 2004). These studies were not useful for nursing because the studies of body mechanics used were those of lifting static objects and this does not reflect the environment in which most nurses work. Many of the situations in which nurses are injured involve sudden, quick changes in position and human beings rather than static boxes; therefore, proper body mechanics do not work, as the nurse cannot adjust in a way that protects the back. Therefore, the current recommendations by the ANA include the use of assistive patient-handling devices for lifting, transferring, and turning patients (Box 25-1).

It is important that nurses take good care of their backs, even when they are young, flexible, and strong, because aging contributes to the risk for career-ending injury. Repetitive stress on the structures of the spine, shoulders, and hips can cause small, repeated damage that could manifest in serious, debilitating injury. The ANA has sponsored a program, "Handle with Care" to raise awareness, promote the use of ergonomic equipment and assistive devices, and encourage health care organizations to invest in a safe patient-handling program. In addition, in reducing work-related injuries to nurses, safe patient-handling programs can reduce some of the hidden costs of health care organizations and improve patient care (ANA, 2004).

BOX 25-1 Safe Patient-Handling Legislation

In the May 2005 session of the Texas legislature, a "Safe Patient Handling" bill was passed. Through the combined efforts of the Texas Hospital Association, the Texas Health Care Association, and the Texas Nurses Association, this is the first legislation in the nation to address the problems nurses encounter by manually lifting and moving patients. For the past 30 years, nurses have been on the Occupational Safety and Health Administration (OSHA) top 10 list of work-related injuries. The majority of these injuries were musculoskeletal injuries related to patient transfer and movement. The bill encourages the availability and utilization of ergonomic equipment and other assistive devices to protect the practicing nurse against back injuries, as well as other musculoskeletal injuries.

What can the nurse do to reduce the risk for a serious back injury? First of all, be aware of the potential risk by assessing each patient's dependency needs and abilities when deciding what assistive devices to use. Do not ever try to move, lift, or turn a dependent person without an appropriate assistive device or help. Next, know what assistive devices are available to you, and learn how to properly use them. If your organization does not have devices readily available, become an advocate for a safe patient-handling program. Finally, keep yourself fit and do not ever "tough it out" when you suffer an injury. Make sure you report your injury and follow the advice of your health care provider so your body can properly heal. For more information on ways to promote safe patient handling and prevent work-related injuries see the following websites: *www.patientsafetycenter.com* and *www.nursingworld.org/handlewithcare.*

BIOTERRORISM

Even before the terrorist attacks of September 11, 2001, the *Association for Professionals in Infection Control and Epidemiology* (APIC) had warned of the threat of bioterrorism to Americans. Most biological attacks will be covert, meaning that there will be no warning and no "big bang." Therefore, it is important that you know and understand what bioterrorism is and how to identify a potential event because health care workers in hospitals and clinics may have the first opportunity to recognize a covert event. Being an alert nurse can save lives, including your own. According to APIC, everyone in health care needs to be alert to signs of an unusual outbreak or pattern of illness.

As a nurse, you will be at the forefront of observing for these signs and can initiate procedures that limit the effect of an attack and help identify victims. It was the quick recognition and response of nurses in the recent severe acute respiratory syndrome (SARS) endemic that was credited with the limited impact of this disease in the United States, and many lives were saved as a result. Nurses aware of the SARS outbreak quickly recognized an individual at risk for SARS, and instituted respiratory precautions. It is believed that a much greater exposure to the health care workers would have resulted in a much larger death toll in the United States. Health care workers in Canada and other countries were the largest victim pool.

What would you do if you suspected an unusual outbreak of disease among your patient population? All health care facilities are encouraged to have a monitoring plan to identify unusual patterns of illness in their community. In most organizations, the infection control specialist does this monitoring. In the hospital, the Infection Control Nurse is responsible for hospital surveillance and is a reminder of how critical the Department of Health Epidemiologist-Infection Control Nurse relationship is for successful passive and active surveillance to be carried out. In the community setting, the local epidemiologist does the monitoring. In addition, because bioterrorist attacks can cause rapid progression to illness and the potential for the rapid spread of disease, all health care providers need to know and be able to recognize the signs and symptoms of high-risk agents. Would you be able to recognize anthrax poisoning or a small pox outbreak?

As a health care provider, you need to be able to recognize epidemiologic principles that are typical of an endemic disease (remember: most bioterrorist agents will not be endemic to an area, save for a few geographical locations [i.e., anthrax in Texas, plague in Colorado]) that should raise concern such as:

- A rapidly increasing disease incidence in a normally healthy population.
- A sharp rise and fall of incidence in a short period.
- An unusual increase in the number of people seeking care for a similar symptom presentation, especially with fever.
- An unusual pattern of an illness (e.g., influenza symptoms in June).
- People who stay indoors with filtered air are not as affected as those who are outdoors.
- Clusters of people from one geographically distinct area
- Large numbers of rapidly fatal cases
- Any person presenting with a disease that is uncommon and is high risk for bioterrorism potential *(www.bt.cdc.gov/)*.
- A sudden or steep rise in animal/livestock fatalities (often as indicator of zoonoses)

You should be familiar with your organization's response plan if bioterrorism is suspected. You should know where to find the numbers of internal contacts (infection control, epidemiologist, and your administrator-on-call) and what external contacts can be helpful (local health department, state health department, FBI office). The CDC Emergency Response Office is (770) 488-7100. State health departments and the FBI contact offices for each state are located at their respective websites. Many nurses will never need to know these numbers, but given the current climate, this is information that can save lives. The National Response Plan (NRP), which aligns federal coordination structures, capabilities, and resources into a unified, local and community response management, is identified in Figure 25-1.

Given the need to respond rapidly to a bioterrorism-related outbreak, you need to be able to recognize the major syndromes associated with high-risk agents. Anthrax, botulism, plague, and smallpox are considered the four top agents for potential bioterrorism because plague and smallpox can be spread (person-to-person) and botulism and anthrax can be disseminated to a population via airborne release (they are not spread person-to-person). See Table 25-1 for a listing of etiology, syndrome, transmission, isolation, and prevention. A great website to learn about bioterrorism agents is found at *www.bioterrorism.uab.edu/*.

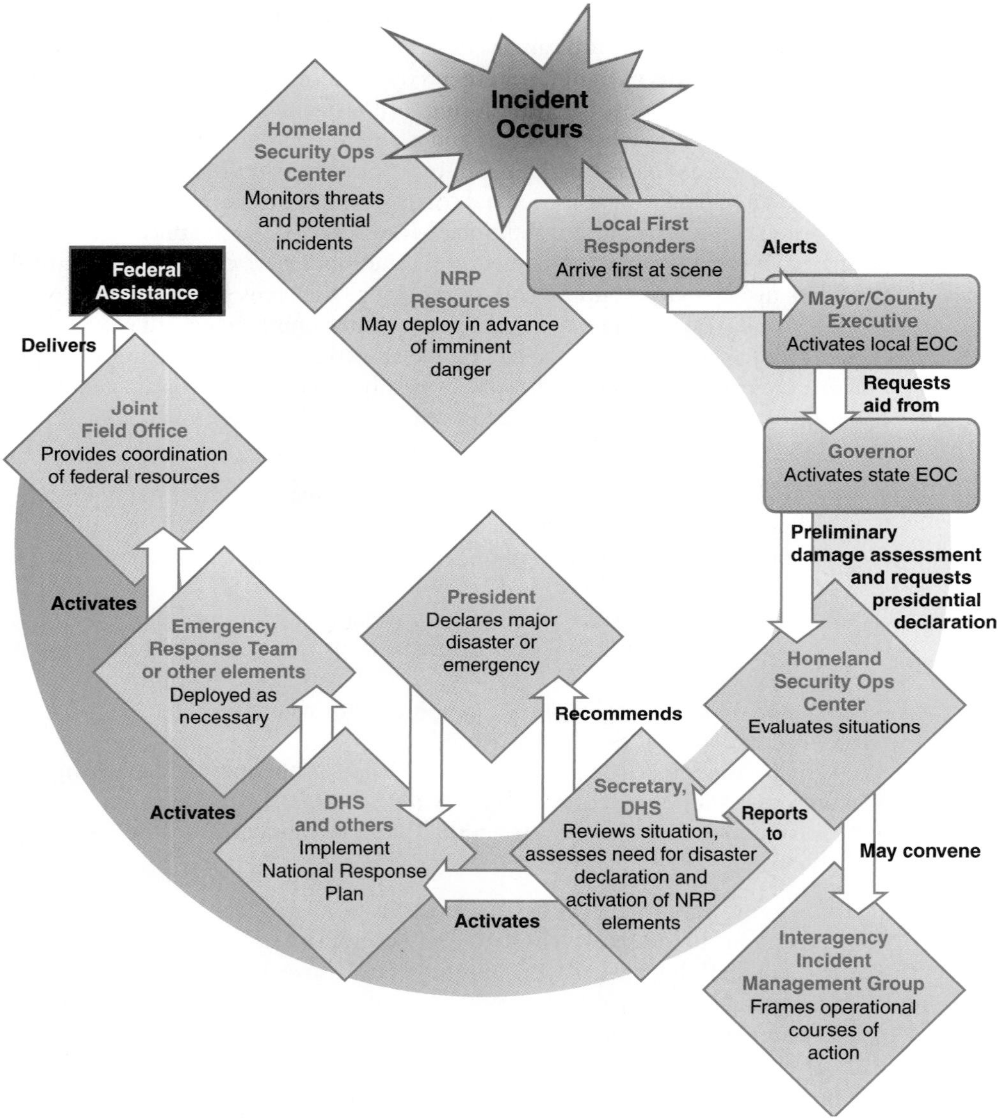

FIGURE 25-1
Overview of federal response to a community incident or threat. (*From the Department of Homeland Security:* National response plan, *December 2004*, www.dhs.gov/interweb/assetlibrary/NRPbaseplan.pdf.)

In addition to biological agents in a terrorist attack, a nuclear attack or an attack using chemical products is a risk in health care. Again, the biggest problem is that attacks can be covert and result in a few targeted victims or a mass casualty similar to the sarin gas attack in Japan. In particular, emergency room nurses need to know and understand the signs and symptoms of a chemical release and promptly respond to

TABLE 25-1

Bioterrorism Agents

Agent	Etiology	Signs and Symptoms	Transmission	Isolation/Prevention
Anthrax	*B. anthracis*	*Pulmonary:* Flu-like Respiratory failure Hemodynamic collapse Usually fatal *Cutaneous:* Local skin—head, forearms, hands Localized itching followed by a papular lesion that turns vesicular and ***develops a black eschar in 2-6 days*** Responds well to antibiotics *Gastrointestinal:* Abdominal pain, nausea, vomiting, fever Bloody diarrhea, emesis Usually fatal	Anthrax is a durable spore that lives in the soil Inhalation of the spore, contact with the spore, and the ingestion of contaminated food	There is a vaccine available. (This vaccine is not traditionally given to health care workers.) Standard isolation precautions; however, once the patient is sick, there is no person-person transmission.
Botulism	*Clostridium botulinum*-produces a neurotoxin	Responsive, no fever Drooping eyelids, weakened jaw clench, difficulty swallowing or speaking Blurred vision and double vision ***Arm paralysis followed by respiratory and leg paralysis*** Respiratory depression	Ingestion of toxin-contaminated food; the toxin can be made into an aerosol and inhaled (manmade)	There is a vaccine available. Pentavalent vaccine only works for the toxin that the person was vaccinated for (i.e., A vaccine only protects against type A). Supportive care only. No isolation precautions implemented.
Plague	*Yersina pestis*	Fever, cough, chest pain ***Bloody sputum*** Sputum can be thick and very purulent or watery with gram-negative rods Bronchopneumonia	In a bioterrorist event, most likely to be aerosolized	There is no proven vaccine for the pneumonic plague, which is the most likely version in a bioterrorist event. Droplet isolation precautions.
Smallpox	*Variola virus*	Prodrome of fever, myalagia ***Vesicles on the distal limbs (hands, feet) as compared to truncated vesicles with chicken pox***		Vaccine created in late 1700s. Routine vaccination ceased with eradication of smallpox in 1979. Droplet precautions recommended, especially if pocks develop inside the buccal cavity.

deal with the victims. In the case of a nuclear attack, nurses need to be prepared to deal with these special victims. Hospitals in most states are required to have a plan to deal with biological, chemical, or nuclear terrorist attacks. Every nurse should be prepared to take action if such an event occurs. In addition, you need to understand how to protect yourself from harm when dealing with these situations (Figure 25-2).

Understanding personal protective equipment and standard precautions is important. If you are working on a general nursing unit, you will most likely be adequately protected with masks, face shields, goggles, gowns, and gloves. You should always follow standard precautions when caring for patients. Your hospital or clinic will have additional guidelines to follow if a patient is suspected or diagnosed with communicable illnesses such as influenza, chicken pox, and methicillin-resistant *Staphylococcus aureus*. Carefully following your organization's infection control policy is considered adequate for most situations.

Nurses in the emergency department may need additional personal protective equipment for potential exposure to patients with nuclear contamination, chemical toxins, and biological threats. Yearly training on the proper methods of decontamination and use of personal protective equipment such as respirators is essential to make sure that emergency room nurses know how to prevent self-contamination.

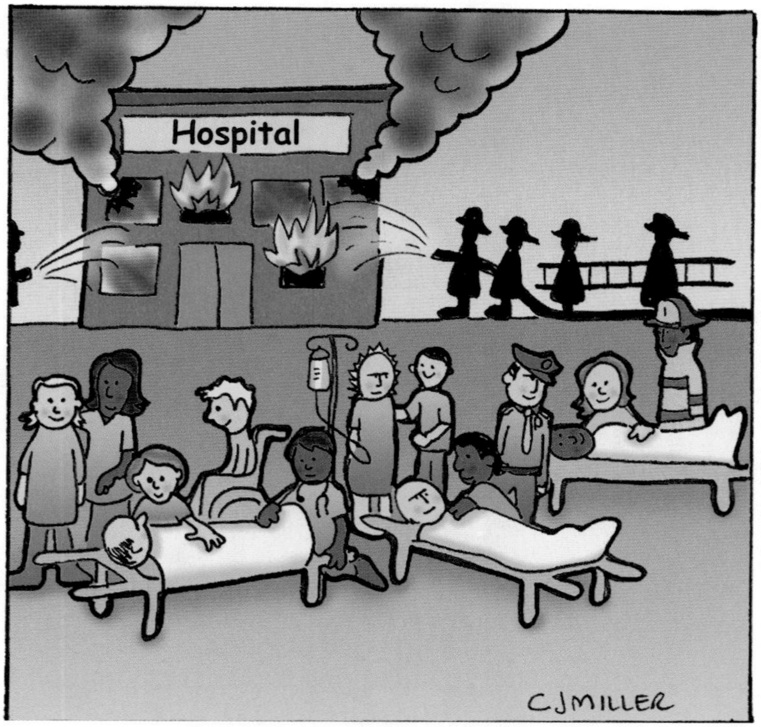

FIGURE 25-2
We are prepared.

Lastly, you need to pay attention to the threat level for terrorist attacks and know what to look for. Hospitals and other health care organizations are believed to be a likely target for attack. The current threat level and possible event can be found at the Homeland Security website at *www.whitehouse.gov/homeland/*. This website has other interesting information about what is happening to keep our world free of harm and ways each citizen can contribute.

WORKPLACE VIOLENCE: A GROWING CONCERN IN HEALTH CARE

Witnessing the aftermath of a violent attack on a nurse colleague is a powerful realization that the potential for being harmed by another person at work is very real. As a nurse, you are at risk for harm from coworkers, patients, and families. No matter what the occupation, workplace violence is a growing risk and the second leading cause of occupational death in the United States (Henry, 2002). The nature of health care workers' jobs puts them at risk for workplace violence, which can result in injury or death (Henry, 2002).

Studies on nurses and workplace violence show that 80% or more nurses have experienced some sort of violence in their career. Workplace violence is defined as violent acts, including physical assaults and threats of assault, directed at individuals at work or on duty. Violence is the intentional use of physical force that has a high likelihood or results in injury or death (Henry, 2002). This can include verbal abuse, threats, unwanted sexual advances, physical assault, and murder.

Nurses often fail to report acts of violence because of lack of understanding or a belief that "nothing will be done" (Henry, 2002). This has the risk of escalating the situation until physical harm occurs. Many times nurses have never encountered a hostile person before and do not understand how to recognize and de-escalate the situation.

Recently, a nurse in a large urban hospital was working with a young man who had been hospitalized with chest pain. He had denied any drug use; however, he habitually used cocaine and also consumed large amounts of alcohol on a regular basis. Once the physician discharged him, the patient grew increasingly agitated, as he wanted to leave the facility to resume his drug behaviors.

The nurse had been working on the unit less than a year after graduation and did not recognize the patient's increasing agitation. He used the call light to repeatedly summon the nurse to the room to find out when he could leave. When she entered the room in response to his fifth call and told him it would be another 30 minutes before she could complete the paper work for his discharge, he attacked her. Before she was able to summon help, she was assaulted. The nurse recovered physically, but was not able to return to her chosen profession due to posttraumatic stress syndrome. A huge emotional toll was also seen with the rest of the nursing staff who were fearful of another event happening.

In response to this attack and other events that had happened in local industry, the hospital leadership developed a crisis intervention program. This program taught nursing staff how to recognize signs of escalating anger that could result in an attack and strategies to de-escalate the situation. Nurses were also taught how to protect themselves during an attack. Knowing how to protect themselves and how to recognize an escalating situation helped this nursing staff believe they could deal with future situations that put them at risk for harm.

Additionally, the hospital instituted a "code white"' program. A code white stood for a potentially violent situation, which anyone could call if *any* person became loud or abusive, made threats, or started throwing objects. A code white ensured that resources were available to help de-escalate the situation and that no nurse would be alone with someone who was "acting out." Trained volunteers and other staff from the hospital, including security, will respond to a code white, which is paged overhead. It was stressed to the nursing staff that any time they felt unsafe, a code white should be called. A code white could be called by using the phone system or by pushing a strategically placed alarm button. After instituting the program, there were no further incidents in which nurses were harmed.

So what do you need to do when you start your first job? First of all, be familiar with your organization's policies regarding workplace violence. Next, take a crisis intervention course to become familiar with the signs of escalating violence such as pacing, using foul language, cursing, raised fist, threats. Learn strategies to de-escalate anger. Lastly, do not ever try to handle a potentially violent person on your own. Use whatever procedures your organization has to defuse situations; for example, call security and/or call a "code white" (Figure 25-3).

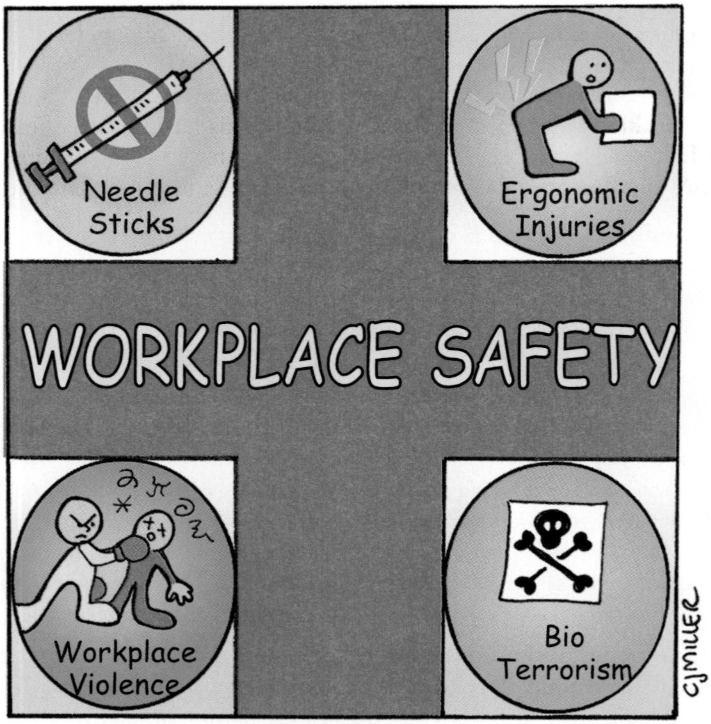

FIGURE 25-3
Workplace safety is important.

MISCELLANEOUS WORKPLACE ISSUES

In addition to the workplace issues already identified, latex allergy, SARS, HIV, tuberculosis exposure, and needlestick injuries are issues that can impact your health if you are not aware of how to prevent exposure and injury (Box 25-2). OSHA has established guidelines that organizations must follow to protect workers. The Needlestick Safety and Prevention Act (P.L. 106-430), which became law on November 6, 2000, provides important protections for health care workers regarding needlestick injuries. Advocating for workplace safety, the ANA was very instrumental in having this piece of federal legislation passed. This act amends the Blood-Borne Pathogen Standard (OSHA administered) to require the use of safer devices to protect from sharps injuries. It also requires that employers solicit the input of nonmanagerial employees who are responsible for direct patient care regarding the identification, evaluation, and selection of effective engineering and work-practice controls (Figure 25-4).

In addition, the bill requires employers to maintain a sharps injury log to document, at a minimum, the type and brand of device involved in each incident; the department or work area in which the exposure occurred; and an explanation of how the incident happened. The information would be recorded and maintained in a way that would protect the confidentiality of injured employees. The log would serve as an important source of data to help determine the relative effectiveness and safety of currently used devices and to guide the development of future products. You need to be familiar with these guidelines and any guidelines that have been established by local or state health departments. In some states, the guidelines established by health departments is more strict than those established by OSHA.

BOX 25-2 Facts About Needlestick Injuries

- Health care workers suffer between 600,000 and one million injuries from conventional needles and sharps annually. These exposures can lead to hepatitis B, hepatitis C, and HIV.
- At least 1000 health care workers are estimated to contract serious infections annually from needlestick and sharps injuries.
- Registered nurses working at the bedside sustain an overwhelming majority of these exposures.
- Needlestick injuries are preventable. More than 80% of needlestick injuries could be prevented with the use of safer needle devices.
- More than 20 other infections can be transmitted through needlesticks, including tuberculosis, syphilis, malaria, and herpes.
- According to the American Hospital Association, one case of serious infection by blood-borne pathogens can soon add up to $1 million or more in expenditures for testing follow-up, lost time, and disability payments.
- The cost of follow-up for a high-risk exposure is almost $3000 per needlestick injury even when no infection occurs.
- Safe needle devices cost only 28 cents more than standard devices.

Adapted from American Nurses Association (ANA): *Needlestick injury fact sheet,* 2005, *www.nursingworld.org/readroom/fsneedle.htm.*

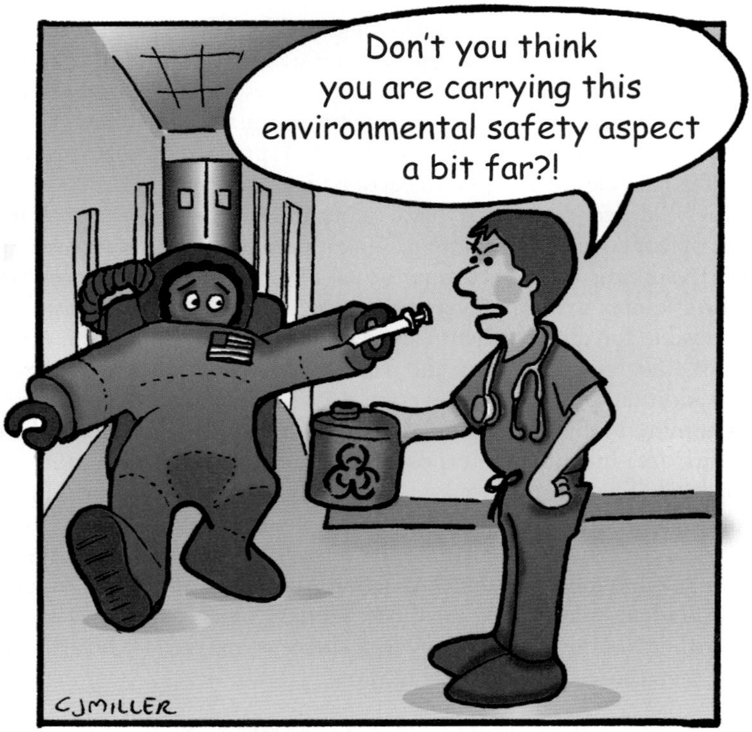
Don't you think
you are carrying this
environmental safety aspect
a bit far?!
CJMILLER

FIGURE 25-4
Nurses must be aware of potential threats to their health.

DEALING WITH STAFFING SHORTAGES

The shortage of experienced nurses has created many challenges and changes in the health care environments in which we work. Many of these changes are just beginning. We will see many more in the years to come as nurses become scarcer and the need for nursing grows. Hospitals and other health care organizations are beginning to realize that nurses have many options for employment, and often the best place to work is where they will go. As a nurse, you need to understand these issues, how to find the best place to work, and how to cope with situations like high nurse-to-patient ratios and mandatory overtime.

An organization (hospital, clinic, nursing home) that provides an environment that is conducive to good nursing care is the best place to be. It does not need to be the newest, sparkling, technologically advanced hospital in a large city. For instance:

One of the most spectacular places to practice nursing may be a modest nurse-managed clinic that meets the needs of indigent people in a rural county. The salaries may not be the best, and the clinic will always need something, but the environment is great in that it allows nurses to care for patients and make a difference in the lives of the people they serve.

Finding a good place to work can be difficult. For many years, health care organizations have ignored the needs of nursing (Duclos-Miller, 2002). To attract nurses, many health care organizations have used incentives rather than making substantial changes to the environment for nursing (workloads, autonomy). Unfortunately, the lure of higher salaries, benefits, sign-on bonuses, and tuition repayment programs can be appealing for new nurses, as education is costly and the demands are great for our financial resources. Nurse recruiters are trained to "sell" their organization as a place to work in order to fill positions. As a new nurse looking for a position, it may be challenging to find the best fit for you. Fortunately, there are research-based criteria that can help you determine if an organization provides a good environment for nursing.

In the early 1980s, the American Academy of Nursing (AAN) commissioned a study to determine what characteristics of hospitals attracted nurses. It was interesting to learn that things such as nursing autonomy, low nurse-patient ratios, and collaborative relationships with physicians were some of those reasons. From this work, magnet hospitals were identified that embodied these essential characteristics that promoted nursing. Today, in our current nursing shortage, hospitals are actively seeking "magnet" status as a marker for nurses to know that it is a good place to work. In addition, magnet hospitals are known to have better patient outcomes. The American Nurses Credentialing Center (ANCC) is responsible for judging whether hospitals achieve this status. A magnet status hospital would be a good place to work for most nurses (Critical Thinking Box 25-1).

In today's world, no matter where you work, you may need to cope with a situation in which the number of patients under your care and their needs for nursing may be greater than what you are able to provide. What should you do?

First of all, it is important to understand the chain of command for your organization. In other words, to whom should you report your concerns and what are your next steps if you are not satisfied with the response you receive. Next, remain calm and use your great assessment skills to determine exactly what your situation is. Here are some things to consider:

- How many patients do you have? What is going on with them? What nursing tasks do you need to accomplish? What are your priorities (safety issues) and those tasks that are "nice to do"?
- What are your resources? Do you have someone to delegate tasks? What family support do you have (for example, to keep an eye on a confused patient).
- Are you aware of a nurse colleague who might be able to come and help who perhaps was not considered by those who worked on staffing?

CRITICAL THINKING BOX 25-1

To find out more about the characteristics of magnet status, the website is *www.nursingworld.org/ancc/magnet/*. Determine whether your clinical practice site has magnet status.

- Is there any other way to deliver care? For example, working together as a team to take care of patients is not ideal, but it can be more efficient to function in this way for a shift, rather than not meet your patient needs.
- What are your hospital policies for high census or high patient load situations?

Gather your facts and present your concerns to the next person in authority, a charge nurse, or supervisor. Do not threaten to leave or make rash statements; just present your facts. Ask for whatever assistance is available. Tell this person what your concerns are and what you are or are not going to be able to accomplish in your shift due to the high patient load.

Document Your Concerns. If the support you receive is not appropriate, then you need to calmly tell your charge nurse or supervisor that you are going to report your concerns to the next person in charge. Again, do not threaten. If the situation is continuous rather than intermittent, use the notes you have documented to figure out the pattern of what is happening.

Remember that difficult situations tend to be in the forefront of your mind, while reality might be different. This is human nature.

Consider the following example.

A group of nurses told their nurse manager that they were always getting patients from surgery who did not meet criteria to be discharged from the recovery room. The examples that they gave were very disturbing to the new manager, so she asked them to keep a log of patients who were unstable when they reached the unit. In the next month, instead of a large number of patients coming back from the recovery room unstable, they found two. In both situations, the patient became hypotensive and required a significant amount of care to stabilize his/her condition. What the staff and the manager realized after looking at the data was that those two situations were so stressful that they "forgot" the 50 patients who came back without a problem. This is why documentation of events is so important.

If your notes tell you that poor staffing is more often than not and you are not able to get your patient care done, then you need to work with your manager to find out the reasons. Is your unit understaffed for the needs of your patients? Does your unit have many vacancies? Does your unit have a lot of sick calls? Are assignments being done correctly? Are nurses doing frequent "nonnursing" functions such as phlebotomy, running errands, or transcribing orders? Does your unit need someone to help with nonessential nursing duties such as bathing or feeding patients? Many organizations involve staff nurses in helping to solve these problems. Volunteer to work with a group to make changes. If your organization or unit is not willing to work with you to make the workload easier, then you may need to consider a job change.

Mandatory overtime is another way that hospitals deal with poor staffing. Mandatory overtime creates a loss of control for the nurse over the ability to schedule nonwork activities, including essential family functions. Mandatory overtime may also put safe patient care at risk because of nurse fatigue and subsequent loss of the ability to concentrate and make good decisions. Although many other professional groups have worked to decrease the incidence of mandatory overtime, when fatigue can jeopardize the public's safety, 67% of nurses report that they worked some sort of mandatory or unplanned overtime per month (Bosek, 2001). Mandating overtime is a major concern of our professional associations.

Although it is our professional duty to ensure that our services are continued for our patients until transferred to another nurse, our duty to ensure that patients receive safe treatment may be in conflict if mandatory overtime results in a nurse who is fatigued and may make a serious mistake. According to Duclos-Miller (2002), we all need to recognize that by accepting a nursing position, we have made a commitment to the institution to provide nursing care at specified intervals. Once we accept responsibility for a patient assignment, we have that responsibility until either our services are no longer needed or we transfer the responsibility to someone else. Does this mean we need to work beyond our capacity?

In many states there is legislation prohibiting mandatory overtime. Is your state one of them? You can go to the ANA website to find out if your state has mandatory overtime legislation.

Legislation that is opposed to mandatory overtime is a priority of the ANA. Legislating overtime of nurses may not be the only answer. Health care organizations must be able to provide care to their patients, and legislation will not be sufficient to alleviate the workloads imposed if there are not enough nurses to take care of patients.

In addition to the previous discussion related to developing a good work environment for nursing, creative solutions can be developed by management and nursing staff to deal with shortages without resorting to mandatory overtime. Some ideas might be,

- Develop an on-call system that provides one or two extra nurses per shift
- Develop policies that limit mandatory overtime and ensure rotation among all staff
- Provide incentives to encourage part-time nursing staff to pick up extra time
- Develop creative shifts for high-activity, high-volume times
- Develop processes to identify shortages with enough time to arrange coverage
- Reward nurses who do put forth extra effort for the organization. For example, one hospital provides a bonus of $100 for every 100 hours of on-call that an individual signs up to come in if needed. Another example might be a creative shift (11 AM–2 PM) to staff for admissions and transfers and reduce the workload for the rest of the staff.

What should you do if you are mandated to stay over your scheduled shift due to a staffing shortage? First, you should be familiar with your organization policies regarding mandatory overtime before this happens. If the policy is unacceptable to your life circumstances, you probably should not be working in the facility. If you find yourself in a situation in which you believe you are too fatigued to stay over your shift, you need to follow the chain of command in asking for assistance with your situation. Again, you need to assess your situation and provide the charge nurse, supervisor, or manager with the facts of your situation. You need to document your concerns and follow-up as needed after the event. If you believe your organization policy regarding mandatory overtime can be improved or eliminated, work with your manager and others to change it.

CONCLUSION

As you stand at the door, your new license in hand, the greatest human adventure awaits you. Nursing is one of the hardest and most awesome professions that exist. As a nurse, you have the opportunity to be part of and witness the most intimate moments of the lives of individuals and families. You have the ability to change people and be changed forever. However grand the profession, it is not without risk, and workplace issues exist that require your vigilance. Make sure that you wash your hands often, stay current about workplace issues, wear protective equipment, ask for what you need to be safe, take care of your back, and most of all, work hard, but not too much!

REFERENCES

American Nurses Association (ANA): *Handle with care*, 2004, *www.nursingworld.org/handlewithcare*.

Bosek M: Mandatory overtime: professional duty, harm, and justice, *JONA's Healthcare Law, Ethics, and Regulation* 3:99-102, 2001.

Department of Homeland Security: *National response plan*, December 2004, *www.dhs.gov/interweb/assetlibrary/NRPbaseplan.pdf*.

Duclos-Miller P: Mandatory overtime: is it really necessary?, *Connecticut Nursing News*, March-May 2002.

Henry J: Violence prevention in healthcare organizations within a total quality management framework, *J Nurs Admin* 32:479-486, 2002.

Martin F: TNA and nursing enjoy successful legislative session, *Texas Nursing* 79(5), 2005.

Owen BD: The magnitude of low-back problem in nursing. *Western J Nurs Res* 11:234-242, 1989.

Owen BD: Preventing injuries using an ergonomic approach, *AORN J* 72:1031-1036, 2000.

APPENDIX A

Boards of Nursing

Alabama Board of Nursing
770 Washington Avenue
RSA Plaza, Suite 250
Montgomery, AL 36130-3900
Phone: (334) 242-4060
Fax: (334) 242-4360
Contact Person: N. Genell Lee, MSN, JD, RN, Executive Officer
Website: www.abn.state.al.us/

Alaska Board of Nursing
550 West Seventh Avenue, Suite 1500
Anchorage, Alaska 99501-3567
Phone: (907) 269-8161
Fax: (907) 269-8196
Contact Person: Dorothy Fulton, MA, RN, Executive Director
Website: www.dced.state.ak.us/occ/pnur.htm

American Samoa Health Services
Regulatory Board
LBJ Tropical Medical Center
Pago Pago, AS 96799
Phone: (684) 633-1222
Fax: (684) 633-1869
Contact Person: Etenauga Lutu, RN, Executive Secretary

Arizona State Board of Nursing
1651 E. Morten Avenue, Suite 210
Phoenix, AZ 85020
Phone: (602) 889-5150
Fax: (602) 889-5155
Contact Person: Joey Ridenour, MN, RN, Executive Director
Website: www.azboardofnursing.org/

Arkansas State Board of Nursing
University Tower Building
1123 S. University, Suite 800
Little Rock, AR 72204-1619
Phone: (501) 686-2700
Fax: (501) 686-2714
Contact Person: Faith Fields, MSN, RN, Executive Director
Website: www.state.ar.us/nurse

California Board of Registered Nursing
400 R St., Suite 4030
Sacramento, CA 95814-6239
Phone: (916) 322-3350
Fax: (916) 327-4402
Contact Person: Ruth Ann Terry, MPH, RN, Executive Officer
Website: www.rn.ca.gov/

California Board of Vocational Nurse and Psychiatric Technicians
2535 Capitol Oaks Drive, Suite 205
Sacramento, CA 95833
Phone: (916) 263-7800
Fax: (916) 263-7859
Contact Person: Teresa Bello-Jones, JD, MSN, RN, Executive Officer
Website: www.bvnpt.ca.gov/

Colorado Board of Nursing
1560 Broadway, Suite 880
Denver, CO 80202
Phone: (303) 894-2430
Fax: (303) 894-2821
Contact Person: Nancy L. Smith, PhD, RN, BC, FAANP, Program Director & Education Consultant
Website: www.dora.state.co.us/nursing/

Connecticut Board of Examiners for Nursing
Department of Public Health
410 Capitol Avenue, MS# 13PHO
PO Box 340308
Hartford, CT 06134-0328
Phone: (860) 509-7624
Fax: (860) 509-7553
Contact Person: Jan Wojick , Board Liaison
Nancy L. Bafundo, BSN, MS, RN, Board President
Website: www.state.ct.us/dph/

Delaware Board of Nursing
861 Silver Lake Boulevard
Cannon Building, Suite 203
Dover, DE 19904
Phone: (302) 739-4522
Fax: (302) 739-2711
Contact Person: Iva Boardman, MSN, RN, Executive Director
Website: www.professionallicensing.state.de.us/boards/nursing/index.shtml

District of Columbia Board of Nursing
Department of Health
717 14th Street, NW, Suite 600
Washington, DC 20005
Phone: (202) 724-4900
Fax: (202) 727-8241
Contact Person: Karen Scipio-Skinner MSN, RN, Executive Director
www.dchealth.dc.gov/

Florida Board of Nursing
Mailing address:
4052 Bald Cypress Way, BIN C02
Tallahassee, FL 32399-3252
Physical address:
4042 Bald Cypress Way
Room 120
Tallahassee, FL 32399
Phone: (850) 245-4125
Fax: (850) 245-4172
Contact Person: Dan Coble, RN, PhD, Executive Director
Website: www.doh.state.fl.us/mqa/

Georgia State Board of Licensed Practical Nurses
237 Coliseum Drive
Macon, GA 31217-3858
Phone: (478) 207-1640
Fax: (478) 207-1633
Contact Person: Jacqueline Hightower, JD, Executive Director
Website: www.sos.state.ga.us/plb/lpn

Georgia Board of Nursing
237 Coliseum Drive
Macon, GA 31217-3858
Phone: (478) 207-1640
Fax: (478) 207-1660
Contact Person: Sylvia Bond, RN MSN, MBA, Executive Director
Website: www.sos.state.ga.us/plb/rn

Guam Board of Nurse Examiners
Regular mailing address:
PO Box 2816
Hagatna, Guam 96932
Street address (for FedEx & UPS):
651 Legacy Square Commercial Complex,
South Route 10
Suite 9
Mangilao, Guam 96913
Phone: (671) 735-7406 or (671) 725-7411
Fax: (671) 735-7413
Contact Person: Lillian Perez-Posadas, Interim Executive Officer

Hawaii Board of Nursing
King Kalakaua Building
335 Merchant Street, 3rd Floor
Honolulu, HI 96813
Phone: (808) 586-3000
Fax: (808) 586-2689
Contact Person: Kathleen Yokouchi, MBA, BBA, BA, Executive Officer
Website: www.hawaii.gov/dcca/areas/pvl/boards/nursing

Idaho Board of Nursing
280 N. 8th Street, Suite 210
PO Box 83720
Boise, ID 83720
Phone: (208) 334-3110
Fax: (208) 334-3262
Contact Person: Sandra Evans, MA.Ed, RN, Executive Director
Website: www2.state.id.us/ibn

Illinois Department of Professional Regulation
James R. Thompson Center
100 West Randolph, Suite 9-300
Chicago, IL 60601
Phone: (312) 814-2715
Fax: (312) 814-3145
Contact Person: Maryann Alexander, PhD, RN, Nursing Act Coordinator
Website: www.dpr.state.il.us/

Illinois Department of Professional Regulation
320 W. Washington Street
3rd Floor
Springfield, IL 62786
Phone: (217) 782-8556
Fax: (217) 782-7645

Indiana State Board of Nursing
Health Professions Bureau
402 W. Washington Street, Room W066
Indianapolis, IN 46204
Phone: (317) 234-2043
Fax: (317) 233-4236
Contact Person: Tonja Thompson, Director of Nursing
Website: www.state.in.us/hpb/boards/isbn/

Iowa Board of Nursing
RiverPoint Business Park
400 SW 8th Street
Suite B
Des Moines, IA 50309-4685
Phone: (515) 281-3255
Fax: (515) 281-4825
Contact Person: Lorinda Inman, MSN, RN, Executive Director
Website: www.state.ia.us/government/nursing/

Kansas State Board of Nursing
Landon State Office Building
900 SW Jackson, Suite 1051
Topeka, KS 66612
Phone: (785) 296-4929
Fax: (785) 296-3929
Contact Person: Mary Blubaugh, MSN, RN, Executive Administrator
Website: www.ksbn.org/

Kentucky Board of Nursing
312 Whittington Parkway, Suite 300
Louisville, KY 40222
Phone: (502) 429-3300
Fax: (502) 429-3311
Contact Person: Sue Derouen, RN, BSN, Interim Executive Director
Website: www.kbn.ky.gov/

Louisiana State Board of Nursing
3510 N. Causeway Boulevard, Suite 601
Metairie, LA 70002
Phone: (504) 838-5332
Fax: (504) 838-5349
Contact Person: Barbara Morvant, MN, RN, Executive Director
Website: www.lsbn.state.la.us/

Louisiana State Board of Practical Nurse Examiners
3421 N. Causeway Boulevard, Suite 505
Metairie, LA 70002
Phone: (504) 838-5791
Fax: (504) 838-5279
Contact Person: Claire Glaviano, BSN, MN, RN, Executive Director
Website: www.lsbpne.com/

Maine State Board of Nursing
158 State House Station
Augusta, ME 04333
Phone: (207) 287-1133
Fax: (207) 287-1149
Contact Person: Myra Broadway, JD, MS, RN, Executive Director
Website: www.maine.gov/boardofnursing/

Maryland Board of Nursing
4140 Patterson Avenue
Baltimore, MD 21215
Phone: (410) 585-1900
Fax: (410) 358-3530
Contact Person: Donna Dorsey, MS, RN, Executive Director
Website: www.mbon.org/

Massachusetts Board of Registration in Nursing
Commonwealth of Massachusetts
239 Causeway Street, Second Floor
Boston, MA 02114
Phone: (617) 973-0800 or (800) 414-0168
Fax: (617) 973-0984
Contact Person: Rula Faris Harb, MS, RN, Executive Director
Website: www.state.ma.us/reg/boards/rn/

Michigan/DCH/Bureau of Health Professions
Ottawa Towers North
611 W. Ottawa, 1st Floor
Lansing, MI 48933
Phone: (517) 335-0918
Fax: (517) 373-2179
Contact Person: Diane Lewis, MBA, BA, Policy Manager for Licensing Division
Website: www.michigan.gov/healthlicense

Minnesota Board of Nursing
2829 University Avenue SE
Minneapolis, MN 55414
Phone: (612) 617-2270
Fax: (612) 617-2190
Contact Person: Shirley Brekken, MS, RN, Executive Director
Website: www.nursingboard.state.mn.us/

Mississippi Board of Nursing
1935 Lakeland Drive, Suite B
Jackson, MS 39216-5014
Phone: (601) 987-4188
Fax: (601) 364-2352
Contact Person: Delia Owens, RN, JD, Executive Director
Website: www.msbn.state.ms.us/

Missouri State Board of Nursing
3605 Missouri Boulevard
PO Box 656
Jefferson City, MO 65102-0656
Phone: (573) 751-0681
Fax: (573) 751-0075
Contact Person: Lori Scheidt, BS, Executive Director
Website: http://pr.mo.gov/nursing.asp

Montana State Board of Nursing
301 South Park
PO Box 200513
Helena, MT 59620-0513
Phone: (406) 841-2340
Fax: (406) 841-2305
Contact Person: Sandra Dickenson, Executive Director
Website: www.discoveringmontana.com/dli/bsd/license/bsd_boards/nur_board/board_page.htm

Nebraska Department of Health and Human Services Regulation and Licensure
Nursing and Nursing Support
301 Centennial Mall South
Lincoln, NE 68509-4986
Phone: (402) 471-4376
Fax: (402) 471-1066
Contact Person: Charlene Kelly, PhD, RN, Executive Director
Website: www.hhs.state.ne.us/crl/nursing/nursingindex.htm

Nevada State Board of Nursing
5011 Meadowood Mall, #201
Reno, NV 89502-6547
Phone: (775) 688-2620
Fax: (775) 688-2628
Contact Person: Debra Scott, MS, RN, Executive Director
Website: www.nursingboard.state.nv.us/

New Hampshire Board of Nursing
21 South Fruit Street, Suite 16
Concord, NH 03301-2341
Phone: (603) 271-2323
Fax: (603) 271-6605
Contact Person: Margaret Walker, MBA, BSN, RN, Executive Director
Website: www.state.nh.us/nursing/

New Jersey Board of Nursing
PO Box 45010
124 Halsey Street, 6th Floor
Newark, NJ 07101
Phone: (973) 504-6586
Fax: (973) 648-3481
Contact Person: George Hebert, Executive Director
Website: www.state.nj.us/lps/ca/medical.htm

New Mexico Board of Nursing
6301 Indian School Road NE, Suite 710
Albuquerque, NM 87110
Phone: (505) 841-8340
Fax: (505) 841-8347
Contact Person: Allison Kozeliski, RN, Executive Director
Website: www.state.nm.us/clients/nursing

New York State Board of Nursing
Education Building
89 Washington Avenue
2nd Floor West Wing
Albany, NY 12234
Phone: (518) 474-3817, ext. 280
Fax: (518) 474-3706
Contact Person: Barbara Zittel, PhD, RN, Executive Secretary
Website: www.nysed.gov/prof/nurse.htm

North Carolina Board of Nursing
3724 National Drive, Suite 201
Raleigh, NC 27602
Phone: (919) 782-3211
Fax: (919) 781-9461
Contact Person: Polly Johnson, MSN, RN, Executive Director
Website: www.ncbon.com/

North Dakota Board of Nursing
919 South 7th Street, Suite 504
Bismarck, ND 58504
Phone: (701) 328-9777
Fax: (701) 328-9785
Contact Person: Constance Kalanek, PhD, RN, Executive Director
Website: www.ndbon.org/

Northern Mariana Islands: Commonwealth Board of Nurse Examiners
PO Box 501458
Saipan, MP 96950
Phone: (670) 664-4812
Fax: (670) 664-4813
Contact Person: Rosa M. Tuleda, Associate Director of Public Health & Nursing

Ohio Board of Nursing
17 South High Street, Suite 400
Columbus, OH 43215-3413
Phone: (614) 466-3947
Fax: (614) 466-0388
Contact Person: John Brion, RN, MS, Executive Director
Website: www.nursing.ohio.gov/

Oklahoma Board of Nursing
2915 N. Classen Boulevard, Suite 524
Oklahoma City, OK 73106
Phone: (405) 962-1800
Fax: (405) 962-1821
Contact Person: Kimberly Glazier, M.Ed., RN, Executive Director
Website: www.youroklahoma.com/nursing

Oregon State Board of Nursing
800 NE Oregon Street, Box 25, Suite 465
Portland, OR 97232
Phone: (971) 673-0685
Fax: (971) 673-0684
Contact Person: Joan Bouchard, MN, RN, Executive Director
Website: www.osbn.state.or.us/

Pennsylvania State Board of Nursing
PO Box 2649
Harrisburg, PA 17105-2649
Phone: (717) 783-7142
Fax: (717) 783-0822
Contact Person: Laurette D. Kaiser, RN, MSN, Executive Secretary/Section Chief
Website: www.dos.state.pa.us/bpoa/cwp/view.asp?a=1104&q=432869

Puerto Rico: Commonwealth of Puerto Rico Board of Nurse Examiners
800 Roberto H. Todd Avenue
Room 202, Stop 18
Santurce, PR 00908
Phone: (787) 725-7506
Fax: (787) 725-7903
Contact Person: Roberto Figueroa, RN, MSN, Executive Director of the Office of Regulations and
Certifications of Health Care Professions

Rhode Island Board of Nurse Registration and Nursing Education
105 Cannon Building
Three Capitol Hill
Providence, RI 02908
Phone: (401) 222-5700
Fax: (401) 222-3352
Contact Person: Jean Marie Rocha, MPH, RN, Executive Officer
Website: www.health.ri.gov/

South Carolina State Board of Nursing
110 Centerview Drive, Suite 202
Columbia, SC 29210
Phone: (803) 896-4550
Fax: (803) 896-4525
Contact Person: Martha Bursinger, RN, MSN, Executive Director
Website: www.llr.state.sc.us/pol/nursing

South Dakota Board of Nursing
4305 South Louise Avenue, Suite 201
Sioux Falls, SD 57106-3115
Phone: (605) 362-2760
Fax: (605) 362-2768
Contact Person: Gloria Damgaard, RN, MS, Executive Secretary
Website: www.state.sd.us/doh/nursing/

Tennessee State Board of Nursing
425 Fifth Avenue North
1st Floor, Cordell Hull Building
Nashville, TN 37247
Phone: (615) 532-5166
Fax: (615) 741-7899
Contact Person: Elizabeth Lund, MSN, RN, Executive Director
Website: www.tennessee.gov/health

Texas Board of Nurse Examiners
333 Guadalupe, Suite 3-460
Austin, TX 78701
Phone: (512) 305-7400
Fax: (512) 305-7401
Contact Person: Katherine Thomas, MN, RN, Executive Director
Website: www.bne.state.tx.us/

Utah State Board of Nursing
Heber M. Wells Building, 4th Floor
160 East 300 South
Salt Lake City, UT 84111
Phone: (801) 530-6628
Fax: (801) 530-6511
Contact Person: Laura Poe, MS, RN, Executive Administrator
Website: www.commerce.state.ut.us/

Vermont State Board of Nursing
81 River Street
Heritage Building
Montpelier, VT 05609-1106
Phone: (802) 828-2396
Fax: (802) 828-2484
Contact Person: Anita Ristau, MS, RN, Executive Director
Website: www.vtprofessionals.org/opr1/nurses/

Virgin Islands Board of Nurse Licensure
Veterans Drive Station
St. Thomas, VI 00803
Phone: (340) 776-7397
Fax: (340) 777-4003
Contact Person: Winifred Garfield, CRNA, RN, Executive Secretary

Virginia Board of Nursing
6603 West Broad Street
5th Floor
Richmond, VA 23230-1712
Phone: (804) 662-9909
Fax: (804) 662-9512
Contact Person: Jay Douglas, RN, MSM, CSAC, Executive Director
Website: www.dhp.virginia.gov/

Washington State Nursing Care Quality Assurance Commission
Department of Health
HPQA #6
310 Israel Road SE
Tumwater, WA 98501-7864
Phone: (360) 236-4700
Fax: (360) 236-4738
Contact Person: Paula Meyer, MSN, RN, Executive Director
Website: https://fortress.wa.gov/doh/hpqa1/hps6/Nursing/default.htm

West Virginia State Board of Examiners for Licensed Practical Nurses
101 Dee Drive
Charleston, WV 25311
Phone: (304) 558-3572
Fax: (304) 558-4367
Contact Person: Lanette Anderson, RN, BSN, JD, Executive Director
Website: www.lpnboard.state.wv.us/

West Virginia Board of Examiners for Registered Professional Nurses
101 Dee Drive
Charleston, WV 25311
Phone: (304) 558-3596
Fax: (304) 558-3666
Contact Person: Laura Rhodes, MSN, RN, Executive Director
Website: http://www.wvrnboard.com/

Wisconsin Department of Regulation and Licensing
1400 East Washington Avenue, RM 173
Madison, WI 53708
Phone: (608) 266-0145
Fax: (608) 261-7083
Contact Person: Kimberly Nania, PhD, MA, BS, Director, Bureau of Health Service Professions
Website: www.drl.state.wi.us/

Wyoming State Board of Nursing
2020 Carey Avenue, Suite 110
Cheyenne, WY 82002
Phone: (307) 777-7601
Fax: (307) 777-3519
Contact Person: Cheryl Lynn Koski, MN, RN, CS, Executive Director
Website: http://nursing.state.wy.us/

APPENDIX B

National Nursing Organizations

Academy of Medical-Surgical Nurses
E. Holly Avenue, Box 56
Pitman, NJ 08071-0056
Phone: 856-256-2323
Fax: 856-589-7463
E-mail: amsn@ajj.com
Website: http://amsn.inurse.com

Air & Surface Transport Nurses Association
7995 East Prentice Avenue, Suite 100
Greenwood Village, CO 80111
Phone: 800-897-NFNA (6362)
Fax: 303-770-1614
E-mail: executive-director@astna.org
Website: http://www.astna.org

American Academy of Ambulatory Care Nursing
E. Holly Avenue, Box 56
Pitman, NJ 08071-0056
Phone: 856.256.2350
Fax: 856-589-7463
E-mail: aaacn@ajj.com
Website: http://www.aaacn.org/cgi-bin/WebObjects/AAACNMain

American Academy of Nurse Practitioners
PO Box 12846
Austin, TX 78711
Phone: 512-442-4262
Fax: 512-442-6469
E-mail: admin@aanp.org
Website: http://www.aanp.org

American Academy of Nursing
555 East Wells Street, Suite 1100
Milwaukee, WI 53202-3823
Phone: 414-287-0289
Fax: 414-276-3349
E-mail: info@aannet.org
Website: http://www.aannet.org/

American Assembly for Men in Nursing
c/o NYSNA
11 Cornell Road
Latham, NY 12110-1499
Phone: 518-782-9400, ext. 346
E-mail: aamn@aamn.org
Website: http://www.aamn.org

American Association for the History of Nursing, Inc.
PO Box 175
Lanoka Harbor, NJ 08734
Phone: 609-693-7250
Fax: 609-693-1037
E-mail: aahn@aahn.org
Website: http://www.aahn.org

American Association of Colleges of Nursing
1 Dupont Circle NW, Suite 530
Washington, DC 20036
Phone: 202-463-6930
Fax: 202-785-8320
E-mail: webmaster@aacn.nche.edu
Website: http://www.aacn.nche.edu

American Association of Critical Care Nurses
101 Columbia
Aliso Viejo, CA 92656-1491
Phone: 800-899-2226
Fax: 949-362-2020
E-mail: info@aacn.org
Website: http://www.aacn.org

American Association of Diabetes Educators
100 W. Monroe Street, 4th Floor
Chicago, IL 60603-1901
Phone: 312-424-2426
Fax: 312-424-2427
E-mail: aade@aadenet.org
Website: http://www.aadenet.org

American Association of Legal Nurse Consultants
401 N. Michigan Avenue
Chicago, IL 60611
Toll free: 877/402-2562
Fax: 312-673-6655
E-mail: info@aalnc.org
Website: http://www.aalnc.org

The American Association of Managed Care Nurses, Inc.
4435 Waterfront Drive, Suite 101
Glen Allen, VA 23060
Telephone: 804-747-9698
Fax : 804-747-5316
E-mail: info@aamcn.org
Website: http://www.aacmcn.org

American Association of Neuroscience Nurses
4700 W. Lake Avenue
Glenview, IL 60025-1485
Phone: 888-557-2266
Fax: 847-375-6333
E-mail: aann@aann.org
Website: http://www.aann.org

American Association of Nurse Anesthetists
222 S. Prospect Avenue
Park Ridge, IL 60068-4001
Phone: 847-692-7050
Fax: 847-692-6968
E-mail: info@aana.com
Website: http://www.aana.com

The American Association of Nurse Attorneys
PO Box 515
Columbus, OH 43216-0515
Toll Free: 877-538-2262
Fax: (614) 221-2335
Website: http://www.taana.org

American Association of Occupational Health Nurses, Inc.
2920 Brandywine Road, Suite 100
Atlanta, GA 30341
Phone: 770-455-7757
Fax: 770-455-7271
E-mail: aaohn@aaohn.org
Website: http://www.aaohn.org

American Association of Office Nurses
52 Park Avenue, Suite B4
Park Ridge, New Jersey 07656
Phone: 201-391-2600 or 800-457-7504
E-mail: aaonmail@aaon.org
Website: http://www.aaon.org

American Association of Spinal Cord Injury Nurses
75-20 Astoria Boulevard
Jackson Heights, NY 11370
Phone: 718-803-3782
Fax: 718-803-0414
E-mail: info@epva.org
Website: http://www.aascin.org

American College of Nurse Practitioners
1111 19th Street NW, Suite 404
Washington, DC 20036
Phone: 202-659-2190
Fax: 202-659-2191
Email: acnp@acnpweb.org
Website: http://www.nurse.org/acnp

American Holistic Nurses Association
PO Box 2130
Flagstaff, AZ 86003-2130
Phone: 800-278-2462
Fax: 520-526-2752
E-mail: ahna-flag@flaglink.com
Website: http://www.ahna.org

American Nephrology Nurses' Association
E. Holly Avenue, Box 56
Pitman, NJ 08071-0056
Phone: 888-600-2662
Fax: 856-589-7463
E-mail: anna@ajj.com
Website: http://www.annanurse.org

American Nurses Association
8515 Georgia Avenue, Suite 400
Silver Spring, MD 20910
Phone: 800-274-4ANA (4262)
Website: http://www.nusringworld.org

American Nursing Informatics Association
PMB 105
10808 Foothill Boulevard, Suite 160
Rancho Cucamonga, CA 91730
Website: http://www.ania.org/

American Organization of Nurse Executives
1 N. Franklin
Chicago, IL 60606
Phone: 312-422-2800
Fax: 312-422-4503
E-mail: aone@aha.org
Website: http://www.aone.org

American Psychiatric Nurses Association
1555 Wilson Boulevard, Suite 602
Arlington, VA 22209
Phone: 703-243-2443
Fax: 703-243-3390
E-mail: info@apna.org
Website: http://www.apna.org

American Radiological Nurses Association
7794 Grow Drive
Pensacola, FL 32514
Phone: 866-486-ARNA (2762); 850-474-7292
Fax: 850-484-8762
E-mail: arna@puetzamc.com
Website: http://www.arna.net

American Society of Ophthalmic Registered Nurses
PO Box 193030
San Francisco, CA 94119-3030
phone: 415-561-8513
fax: 415-561-8531
e-mail: asorn@aao.org

American Society of PeriAnesthesia Nurses
10 Melrose Avenue, Suite 110
Cherry Hill, NJ 08003-3696
Phone: 877-737-9696
Fax: 856-616-9601
E-mail: aspan@aspan.org
Website: http://www.aspan.org

American Society of Plastic Surgical Nurses
3220 Pointe Parkway, Suite 500
Atlanta, GA 30092
Phone: 678-966-3065
info@aspsn.org
Website: http://www.asprsn.org

Association of Camp Nurses
8630 Thorsonveien NE
Bemidji, MN 56601
Phone: 218-586-2633
E-mail: acn@campnurse.org

Association of Nurses in AIDS Care
3538 Ridgewood Road
Akron, OH 44333
Phone: 800-260-6780
Fax: 330-670-0109
Website: http://www.anacnet.org

Association of Pediatric Oncology Nurses
4700 W. Lake Avenue
Glenview, IL 60025
Phone: 847-375-4724
Fax: 847-375-6324
E-mail: info@apon.org
Website: http://www.apon.org

Association of Perioperative Registered Nurses
2170 S. Parker Road, Suite 300
Denver, CO 80231-5711
Phone: 800-755-2676 or 303-755-6300
Website: http://www.aorn.org

Association of Rehabilitation Nurses
4700 W. Lake Avenue
Glenview, IL 60025-1485
Phone: 800-229-7530
Fax: 847-375-4777
E-mail: info@rehabnurse.org
Website: http://www.rehabnurse.org

Association of Women's Health, Obstetric and Neonatal Nurses
2000 L Street NW, Suite 740
Washington, DC 20036
Phone: 800-673-8499
Fax: 202-728-0575
Website: http://www.awhonn.org

Dermatology Nurses Association
East Holly Avenue, Box 56
Pitman, NJ 08071-0056
Phone: 800-454-4362
E-mail: DNA@ajj.com
Website: http://www.dnanurse.org

The Development Disabilities Nursing Association
1733 H Street, Suite 330
PMB 1214
Blaine, WA 98230
Phone: 800-888-6733
Fax: 360-332-2280
e-mail: ddnahq@aol.com
Website: http://ddna.bluestep.net/

Emergency Nurses Association
915 Lee Street
Des Plaines, IL 60016-6569
Phone: 800-243-8362
E-mail: enainfo@ena.org
Website: http://www.ena.org

Endocrine Nurses Society
4350 E. West Highway, Suite 500
Bethesda, MD 20814-4410
Phone: 301-941-0249
Fax: 301-941-0259
E-mail: staff@endo-nurses.org
Website: http://www.endo-nurses.org

Home Healthcare Nurses Association
228 Seventh Street SE
Washington, DC 20003
Phone: 800-558-4462
Fax: 202-547-3540
E-mail: hhna_info@nahc.org
Website: http://www.nahc.org/hhna

Hospice and Palliative Nurses Association
One Penn Center West, Suite 229
Pittsburgh, PA 15276-0100
Phone: 412-787-9301
Fax: 412-787-9305
Website: http://www.hpna.org

Infusion Nurses Society
220 Norwood Park South
Norwood, MA 02062
Phone: 781-440-9408
Fax: 781-440-9409
Website: http://www.ins1.org

International Association of Forensic Nurses
East Holly Avenue, Box 56,
Pitman, NJ 08071-0056
Phone: 856-256-2425
Fax: 856-589-7463
Email: iafn@ajj.com
Website: http://www.forensicnurse.org/

International Council of Nurses
3, Place Jean Marteau
1201 Geneva
Switzerland
Telephone 41-22-908-01-00
Fax 41-22-908-01-01
E-mail: icn@icn.ch
Website: webmaster@icn.ch

International Nurses Society on Addictions
PO Box 10752
Raleigh, MC 27605
Phone: 919-821-1292
Fax: 919-833-5743
Website: http://www.intnsa.org

International Transplant Nurses Society
1739 E. Carson Street, Box 351
Pittsburgh, PA 15203-1700
Phone: 412-488-0249
Fax: 412-431-5911
E-mail: itns@msn.com
Website: http://www.itns.org

National Association of Clinical Nurse Specialists
2090 Linglestown Road, Suite 107
Harrisburg, PA 17110
Phone: 717-234-6799
Fax: 717-234-6798
E-mail: info@nacns.org
Website: http://www.nacns.org

National Association of Hispanic Nurses
1501 16th Street NW
Washington, DC 20036
Phone: 202-387-2477
Fax: 202-483-7183
E-mail: info@thehispanicnurses.org
Website: http://www.thehispanicnurses.org/

National Association of Neonatal Nurses
4700 W. Lake Avenue
Glenview, IL 60025-1485
Phone: 800-451-3795
Fax: 888-477-6266
E-mail: info@nann.org
Website: http://www.nann.org

National Association of Orthopaedic Nurses
East Holly Avenue, Box 56
Pitman, NJ 08071-0056
Phone: 856-256-2310
Fax: 856-589-7463
E-mail: naon@mail.ajj.com
Website: http://naon.inurse.com

National Association of Pediatric Nurse Associates & Practitioners, Inc.
20 Brace Road, Suite 200
Cherry Hill, NJ 08034-2634
Phone: 856-857-9700
Fax: 856- 857-1600
E-mail: info@napnap.org
Website: http://www.napnap.org

National Association of School Nurses
PO Box 1300
Scarborough, ME 04070-1300
Phone: 207-883-2117 or 877-627-6476
Fax: 207-883-2683
E-mail: nasn@nasn.org
Website: http://www.nasn.org

National Association of Vascular Access Networks
11417 S. 700 East, PMB 205
Draper, UT 84020
Phone: 888-576-2826
Fax: 801-576-1824
E-mail: info@navannet.org
Website: http://www.navannet.org

National Black Nurses Association, Inc.
8630 Fenton Street, Suite 330
Silver Spring, MD 20910-3803
Phone: 301-589-3200
Fax: 301-589-3223
E-mail: NBNA@erols.com
Website: http://www.nbna.org

National Council of State Boards of Nursing, Inc.
111 East Wacker Drive, Suite 2900
Chicago, IL 60601
Phone: 312-525-3600
Fax: 312-279-1032
Toll-free service for testing: 866-293-9600
E-mail: info@ncsbn.org
Website: http://www.ncsbn.org

National Federation of Licensed Practical Nurses, Inc.
605 Poole Drive
Garner, NC 27529
Phone: 919-779-0046
Fax: 919-779-5642
Website: http://www.nflpn.org

National Gerontological Nursing Association
7794 Grow Drive
Pensacola, FL 32514
Phone: 850-473-1174
Fax: 850-484-8762
E-mail: ngna@puetzamc.com
Website: http://www.ngna.org

National League for Nursing
61 Broadway, 33rd Floor
New York, NY 10006
Phone: 800-669-1656
Fax: 212-812-0393
E-mail: nlnweb@nln.org
Website: http://www.nln.org

National Nursing Staff Development Organization
7794 Grow Drive
Pensacola, FL 32514
Phone: 800-489-1995
Fax: 850-484-8762
E-mail: e-mail@nnsdo.org
Website: http://www.nnsdo.org

National Organization for Associate Degree Nursing
7794 Grow Drive
Pensacola, FL 32514
Phone: 877-96NOADN (966-6236)
Fax: 850-484-8762
E-mail: noadn@puetzamc.com
Website: http://www.noadn.org

National Student Nurses' Association
45 Main Street, Suite 606
New York, NY 11201
Phone: 718-210-0705
Fax: 718-210-0710
E-mail: nsna@nsna.org
Website: http://www.nsna.org

Nurses Christian Fellowship
PO Box 7895
Madison, WI 53707-7895
Phone: 608-274-4823, ext. 402
E-mail: ncf@ivcf.org
Website: http://www.ncf-jcn.org

Oncology Nursing Society
125 Enterprise Drive
Pittsburgh, PA 15275
Phone: 866-257-4ONS (4667) or 412-859-6100
Fax: 877-369-5497 or 412-859-6162
E-mail: customer.service@ons.org
Website: http://www.ons.org

Sigma Theta Tau International Honor Society of Nursing
550 W. North Street
Indianapolis, IN 46202
Phone: 317-634-8171
Fax: 317-634-8188
E-mail: stti@stti.iupui.edu
Website: http://www.nursingsociety.org

Society of Gastroenterology Nurses and Associates
401 North Michigan Avenue
Chicago, IL 60611-4267
P: 800-245-7462 in Illinois: 312-321-5165
Fax: 312-527-6658
Website: http://www.sgna.org/

Society of Otorhinolaryngology and Head-Neck Nurses, Inc.
116 Canal Street
New Smyrna Beach, FL 32168
Tel : 386-428-1695
Fax : 386-423-7566
E-mail: sohnnet@aol.com
Website: http://www.sohnnurse.com

Society of Pediatric Nurses
7794 Grow Drive
Pensacola, FL 32514
Phone: 850-494-9467 or 800-723-2902
Fax: 850-484-8762
Email: spn@puetzamc.com
Website: http://www.pedsnurses.org

Society of Trauma Nurses
1926 Waukegan Road, Suite 1
Glenview, IL 60025
Phone: (847) 657-6745
FAX (847) 657-6819
Email: info@TraumaNurseSoc.org
Website: http://www.traumanursesoc.org/

Society of Urologic Nurses and Associates
E. Holly Avenue, Box 56
Pitman, NJ 08071-0056
Phone: 888-827-7862
Fax: 856-589-7463
E-mail: suna@ajj.com
Website: http://www.suna.org

Society for Vascular Nursing
7794 Grow Drive
Pensacola, FL 32414
Phone: 888-536-4786
Fax: 850-484-8762
E-mail: svn@puetzamc.com
Website: http://www.svnnet.org

Transcultural Nursing Society
36600 Schoolcraft Road
Livonia, MI 48150-1173
Phone: 888-432-5470
Fax: 732-432-5463
E-mail: barnes@smtp.munet.edu
Website: http://www.tcns.org

Wound, Ostomy and Continence Nurses Society
1550 S. Coast Highway, #201
Laguna Beach, CA 92651
Phone: 888-224-9626
Fax: 949-376-3456
E-mail: maria@wocn.org
Website: http://www.wocn.org

APPENDIX C

American Nurses Association Constituent Member Associations

All office hours listed are local times. Indiana and Arizona do not observe Daylight Savings Time.

Alabama State Nurses' Association (ASNA)
Janet Donoghue, BS, RN, President (10/06)
Joseph Decker II, Executive Director
360 North Hull Street
Montgomery, Alabama 36104-3658
(334) 262-8321
Fax: (334) 262-8578
E-mail: ed.asna@mindspring.com
www.alabamanurses.org
Office Hours: 8:00 AM to 4:00 PM Central Time

Alaska Nurses Association (AaNA)
Rebecca Bolling, BSN, RN, President (10/05)
Camille Soleil, JD, Executive Director
3701 East Tudor Road, Suite 208
Anchorage, Alaska 99507-1069
(907) 274-0827
Fax: (907) 272-0292
E-mail: csoleil@aknurse.org
www.aknurse.org
Office Hours: 8:00 AM to 4:30 PM Alaska Time

Arizona Nurses Association (AzNA)
Kathy Player, EdD, RN, President (10/05)
Patricia Rehn, MS, RN, CNA, Executive Director
1850 E. Southern Avenue, Suite #1
Tempe, Arizona 85282
(480) 831-0404
Fax: (480) 839-4780
E-mail: info@aznurse.org or patt@aznurse.org
www.aznurse.org
Office Hours: 8:30 AM to 4:30 PM Mountain Time

Arkansas Nurses Association (ArNA)
Cheryl Schmidt, PhD, RN, President (10/05)
Jan Hoskins, MSN, RN, Chief Staff Officer
1401 W. Capitol Avenue, Suite 155
Little Rock, Arkansas 72201
(501) 244-2363
Fax: (501) 244-9903
E-mail: arna@arna.org or janhoskins@sbcglobal.net
www.arna.org
Office Hours: 8:00 AM to 4:30 PM Central Time

ANA\California (ANA\C)
Louise Timmer, EdD, RN, President (04/06)
Tricia Hunter, RN, Executive Administrator
1121 L Street, Suite 409
Sacramento, California 95814
(916) 447-0225
Fax: (916) 442-4394
E-mail: ANA\C@anacalifornia.org
www.anacalifornia.org
Office Hours: 9:00 AM to 5:00 PM Pacific Time

Colorado Nurses Association (CNA)
Eve Hoygaard, MS, RN-C, WHNP, President (6/07)
Paula Stearns, MSN, RN, Executive Director
1221 South Clarkson Street, Suite 205
Denver, Colorado 80210
(303) 757-7483
Fax: (303) 757-8833
E-mail:cna@nurses-co.org or pstearnsrn@aol.com
www.nurses-co.org
Office Hours: 8:30 AM to 4:30 PM Mountain Time

Connecticut Nurses Association (CNA)
Doris (Dee) Lippman, PhD, RN, President (10/05)
Polly T. Barey, MS, RN, Executive Director
Meritech Business Park
377 Research Parkway, Suite 2D
Meriden, Connecticut 06450
(203) 238-1207
Fax: (203) 238-3437
E-mail: polly@ctnurses.org
www.ctnurses.org/
Office Hours: 9:00 AM to 5:00 PM Eastern Time

Delaware Nurses Association (DNA)
Patricia A. Winston, MS, RN, CHE, President (10/06)
Sarah J. Carmody, Executive Director
2644 Capitol Trail, Suite 330
Newark, Delaware 19711
(302) 368-2333 or (800) 381-0939
Fax: (302) 366-1775
E-mail: sarah@denurses.org
www.denurses.org
Office Hours: 9:00 AM to 4:00 PM Eastern Time

District of Columbia Nurses Association, Inc. (DCNA)
Joan J. Greaves, RN, President (1/07)
Herman Brown, Executive Director
5100 Wisconsin Avenue NW, Suite 306
Washington, DC, 20016
(202) 244-2705
Fax: (202) 362-8285
E-mail: hbrown@dcna.org
www.dcna.org
Office Hours: 9:00 AM to 5:00 PM Eastern Time

Federal Nurses Association (FedNA)
COL John S. Murray, USAF, President
Contact: Pamela C. Hagan, MSN, RN
8515 Georgia Avenue, Suite 400
Silver Spring, Maryland 20910
(301) 628-5059
Fax: (301) 628-5006
E-mail: FedNA@ana.org
www.nursingworld.org/FedNA
Office Hours: 9:00 AM to 4:30 PM Eastern Time

Florida Nurses Association (FNA)
Mary Tittle, PhD, ARNP, President (09/05)
Paula Massey, MN, RN, Executive Director
PO Box 536985
Orlando, Florida 32853-6985
(407) 896-3261
Fax: (407) 896-9042
E-mail: info@floridanurse.org or pmassey@floridanurse.org
www.floridanurse.org
Office Hours: 8:30 AM to 4:30 PM Eastern Time

Georgia Nurses Association (GNA)
Linda Easterly, MS, BSN, RN, COHN-S, President (10/06)
Deborah Hackman, Chief Executive Officer
3032 Briarcliff Road NE
Atlanta, Georgia 30329-2655
(404) 325-5536
Fax: (404) 325-0407
E-mail: ceo@georgianurses.org
www.georgianurses.org/
Office Hours: 8:00 AM to 4:30 PM Eastern Time

Guam Nurses Association (GNA)
Leonora Urbano, MSN, RN, President (12/05)
Glynis S. Almonte, BSN, RN, Executive Director
PO Box CG
Hagatna, Guam 96932
Telephone/Fax: (671) 477-6877
E-mail: guamnurs@ite.net
Office Hours: 11:00 AM to 1:00 PM Pacific Time

Hawaii Nurses Association (HNA)
Luanne Long, RN, President (5/07)
Aggie Pigao Cadiz, BSN, RN, Executive Director
677 Ala Moana Boulevard, Suite 301
Honolulu, Hawaii 96813
(808) 531-1628
Fax: (808) 524-2760
E-mail: aggie@hinurses.org
www.hawaiinurses.org
Office Hours: 8:00 AM to 4:30 PM Hawaiian Time

Idaho Nurses Association (INA)
Marni Allen, MS, RN, RNP-BC, President (10/06)
Judy Murray, PhD, RN, Executive Director
2471 Bank Drive, Suite 111
Boise, Idaho 83705
(208) 345-0500
Fax: (208) 345-1163
E-mail: idahonursesassn@hotmail.com
www.nursingworld.org/snas/id
Office Hours: 9:00 AM to 5:30 PM Mountain Time

Illinois Nurses Association (INA)
Kathleen Perry, PhD, RN, President (10/05)
Tom Renkes, Executive Director
105 West Adams Street, Suite 2101
Chicago, Illinois 60603
(312) 419-2900, ext. 229
Fax: (312) 419-2920
E-mail: trenkes@illinoisnurses.com
www.illinoisnurses.com
Office Hours: 9:00 AM to 5:00 PM Central Time

Indiana State Nurses Association (ISNA)
Joyce D. Darnell, MA, BSN, President (10/05)
Ernest C. Klein, Jr., RN, CAE, Executive Director
2915 North High School Road
Indianapolis, Indiana 46224
(317) 299-4575
Fax: (317) 297-3525
E-mail: klein@indiananurses.org or
ISNA@indiananurses.org
www.indiananurses.org
Office Hours: 8:30 AM to 4:30 PM Eastern Time

Iowa Nurses Association (INA)
Karol Joenks, BSN, RNc, President (10/05)
Linda Goeldner, MA, MA, CHE, CAE, Executive
Director
1501 42nd Street, Suite 471
West Des Moines, Iowa 50266
(515) 225-0495
Fax: (515) 225-2201
E-mail: Info@iowanurses.org or
Lgoeldner@iowanurses.org
www.iowanurses.org
Office Hours: 8:30 AM to 4:00 PM Central Time

Kansas State Nurses Association (KSNA)
Janice Jones, MN, RN, CNS, President (10/05)
Terri R. Roberts, JD, RN, Executive Director
1208 SW Tyler
Topeka, Kansas 66612-1735
(785) 233-8638
Fax: (785) 233-5222
E-mail: troberts@ksna.net
www.nursingworld.org/snas/ks
Office Hours: 8:00 AM to 4:30 PM Central Time

Kentucky Nurses Association (KNA)
Susan Pohl, BSN, RNc, CDE, President (10/05)
Sharon Mercer, MSN, RN, CNAA, BC, Executive Director
1400 South First Street
PO Box 2616
Louisville, Kentucky 40201-2616
(502) 637-2546
Fax: (502) 637-8236
E-mail: mercer@kentucky-nurses.org
www.kentucky-nurses.org
Office Hours: 8:00 AM to 4:30 PM Eastern Time

Louisiana State Nurses Association (LSNA)
Nita Greene, MSN, RN, CRRN, President (04/07)
Joe Ann Clark, EdD, MSN, RN, Executive Director
5800 One Perkins Place, Suite 2-B
Baton Rouge, Louisiana 70808
(225) 201-0993
(800) 457-6378
Fax: (225) 201-0971
E-mail: lsna@lsna.org
www.lsna.org
Office Hours: 9:00 AM to 4:00 PM Central Time

Maine: ANA-Maine (ANA-ME)
Joe Niemczura, MS, RN, President (10/05)
Executive Director (vacant)
PO Box 3000, PMB #280
York, Maine 03909
(207) 667-0260
E-mail: anamaine@prexar.com
www.anamaine.org

Maryland Nurses Association (MNA)
Denise Moore, MS, APRN,BC, President (11/05)
Kathryn V. Hall, MS, RN, CNAA, Executive Director
21 Governor's Court, Suite 195
Baltimore, Maryland 21244
(410) 944-5800
Fax: (410) 944-5802
E-mail: khall@marylandrn.org
www.marylandrn.org
Office Hours: 8:30 AM to 4:30 PM Eastern Time

Massachusetts Association of Registered Nurses (MARN)
Susan Krupnick, MSN, RN, APRN, BC, CARN, President (05/06)
Cammie Townsend, MBA, MS, RN, Director of Association Management
PO Box 70668
Worcester, Massachusetts 01607-0668
Telephone/Fax: (508) 881-8812
E-mail: info@marnonline.org
www.marnonline.org

Michigan Nurses Association (MNA)
Cheryl Johnson, BSN, RN, President (10/05)
Tom Bissonnette, MS, RN, Executive Director
2310 Jolly Oak Road
Okemos, Michigan 48864-4599
(517) 349-5640, ext. 14
Fax: (517) 349-5818
E-mail: tom.bissonnette@minurses.org
www.minurses.org
Office Hours: 9:00 AM to 5:00 PM Eastern Time

Minnesota Nurses Association (MNA)
Monica Vollmuth, RN, President (10/05)
Erin Murphy, RN, Executive Director
1625 Energy Park Drive
St. Paul, Minnesota 55108
(651) 646-4807 ext. 152 or (800) 536-4662
Fax: (651) 647-5301
E-mail: emurphy@mnnurses.org
www.mnnurses.org
Office Hours: 8:15 AM to 4:30 PM Central Time

Mississippi Nurses Association (MNA)
Janet Harris, MSN, RN, President (10/05)
Ricki R. Garrett, Executive Director
31 Woodgreen Place
Madison, Mississippi 39110
(601) 898-0670
Fax: (601) 898-0190
E-mail:rgarrett@msnurses.org
www.msnurses.org
Office Hours: 8:00 am to 4:30 pm Central Time

Missouri Nurses Association (MONA)
Dianne Schmidt, PhD, RN, President (10/05)
Belinda Heimericks, MSN, RN, Executive Director
1904 Bubba Lane, P.O. Box 105228
Jefferson City, Missouri 65110-5228
(888) 662-MONA
(573) 636-4623
Fax: (573) 636-9576
E-mail: belinda@missourinurses.org
www.missourinurses.org
Office Hours: 8:00 AM to 5:00 PM Central Time

Montana Nurses Association (MNA)
Kate Steenberg, RN, President (12/05)
Eve Franklin, Executive Director
104 Broadway, Suite G-2
Helena, Montana 59601
(406) 442-6710
Fax: (406) 442-1841
E-mail: info@mtnurses.org or evef@mtnurses.org
www.mtnurses.org
Office Hours: 8:30 AM to 4:30 pm Mountain Time

Nebraska Nurses Association (NNA)
Nancy Shirley, PhD, RN, President (10/06)
Executive Director (vacant)
715 South 14th Street
Lincoln, Nebraska 68508
(402) 475-3859
Fax: (402) 475-3961
E-mail: ne.nurses@prodigy.net
www.nursingworld.org/snas/ne/
Office Hours: 8:00 AM to 4:30 PM Central Time

Nevada Nurses Association (NNA)
Pam Johnson, BSN, RN, President (10/05)
Dawn Norris, Association Manager
PO Box 34660
Reno, Nevada 89533
(775) 747-2333
Fax: (775) 329-3334
E-mail: NNA@NVNurses.org or dnorris@nvnurses.org
www.nvnurses.org
Office Hours: 9:00 AM to 5:00 PM Pacific Time

New Hampshire Nurses Association (NHNA)
Susan Fetzer, RN, President(04/06)
Robert Best, JD, MHA, BSE, Executive Director
48 West Street
Concord, New Hampshire 03301-3595
(603) 225-3783
Fax: (603) 228-6672
E-mail: bob@nhnurses.org
www.NHnurses.org
Office Hours: 9:00 AM to 5:00 PM Eastern Time

New Jersey State Nurses Association (NJSNA)
Linda Parry Carney, MA, RN, President (08/06)
Andrea Aughenbaugh, RN, CS, CAE, Chief Executive Officer
1479 Pennington Road
Trenton, New Jersey 08618-2661
(609) 883-5335, ext. 10
Fax: (609) 883-5343
E-mail: njsna@njsna.org or andrea@njsna.org
www.njsna.org
Office Hours: 8:30 AM to 4:30 PM Eastern Time

New Mexico Nurses Association (NMNA)
Debra L. Cyphert, MSN, RN, FNP-C, President (11/05)
Carrie Roberts, MSN, RN, CNP, Executive Director
PO Box 29658
Santa Fe, New Mexico 87592-9658
Federal Express delivery only:
3018 Cielo Court, Suite C
Santa Fe, New Mexico 87507
505-471-3324
Fax: 505-471-3314
E-mail: nmnurses@hotmail.com
www.nursingworld.org/snas/nm
Office Hours: 8:00 AM to 5:00 PM Mountain Time

New York State Nurses Association (NYSNA)
Lolita Compas, MA, RN, CEN, President (10/05)
Lola Fehr, MSN, RN, CAE, FAAN, Executive Director
11 Cornell Road
Latham, New York 12110
(518) 782-9400, ext. 279
Fax: (518) 782-9530
E-mail: lola.fehr@nysna.org
www.nysna.org
Office Hours: 8:30 AM to 5:00 PM Eastern Time

North Carolina Nurses Association (NCNA)
Susan Pierce, PhD, RN, President (10/05)
Sindy Barker, CAE, Executive Director
103 Enterprise Street
PO Box 12025
Raleigh, North Carolina 27605
(919) 821-4250
Fax: (919) 829-5807
E-mail: rns@ncnurses.org or sindybarker@ncnurses.org
www.ncnurses.org
Office Hours: 8:30 AM to 4:30 PM Eastern Time

North Dakota Nurses Association (NDNA)
Jane Roggensack, MSN, BSN, RN, President (10/05)
Sharon Moos, MBA, RN, Executive Administrator
531 Airport Road, Suite D
Bismarck, North Dakota 58504-6107
(701) 223-1385
Fax: (701) 223-0575
E-mail: ndna@prodigy.net
www.ndna.org
Office Hours: 8:30 AM to 4:30 PM Central Time

Ohio Nurses Association (ONA)
Karen Budd, PhD, RN, President (10/05)
Gingy Harshey-Meade, MSN, RN, CNAA,BC, Chief Executive Officer
4000 East Main Street
Columbus, Ohio 43213-2983
(614) 237-5414, ext. 1020
Fax: (614) 237-6081
E-mail: gharsheymeade@ohnurses.org
www.ohnurses.org/
Office Hours: 8:30 AM to 4:30 PM Eastern Time

Oklahoma Nurses Association (ONA)
Karen Tomajan, MS, RNC, CRRN, President (11/06)
Jane Nelson, CAE, Executive Director
6414 North Santa Fe, Suite A
Oklahoma City, Oklahoma 73116
(405) 840-3476
Fax: (405) 840-3013
E-mail: ona.ed@oknurses.com
www.oknurses.com
Office Hours: 8:30 AM to 5:00 PM Central Time

Oregon Nurses Association (ONA)
Debra Cassell, BSN, RN, CNOR, RNFA, President (06/06)
Susan E. King, MS, RN, Executive Director
18765 SW Boones Ferry Road
Tualatin, Oregon 97062
(503) 293-0011
Fax: (503) 293-0013
E-mail: ona@oregonrn.org or king@oregonrn.org
www.oregonrn.org
Office Hours: 8:30 AM to 5:00 PM Pacific Time

Pennsylvania State Nurses Association (PSNA)
Susan Simmons, PhD, RN, President (10/06)
Michele P. Campbell, MSN, RN, Executive Administrator
2578 Interstate Drive, Suite 101
Harrisburg, Pennsylvania 17110-9601
(717) 657-1222 or (888)-707-7762
Fax: (717) 657-3796
E-mail: mcampbell@panurses.org
www.panurses.org
Office Hours: 8:30 AM to 4:30 PM Eastern Time

Rhode Island State Nurses Association (RISNA)
Sylvia Weber, MS, RN, CS, President (10/05)
Pamela L. McCue, MSN, RN, Executive Director
550 S. Water Street, Unit 540B
Providence, Rhode Island 02903-4344
(401) 421-9703
Fax: (401) 421-6793
E-mail: risna@prodigy.net
www.risnarn.org
Office Hours: Monday-Thursday 10:00 AM to 3:30 PM Eastern Time

South Carolina Nurses Association (SCNA)
Alice Wyatt, MSN, APRN-BC, President (11/06)
Judith C. Thompson, Executive Director
1821 Gadsden Street
Columbia, South Carolina 29201
(803) 252-4781
Fax: (803) 779-3870
E-mail: judith@scnurses.org www.scnurses.org
Office Hours: 8:30 AM to 4:30 PM Eastern Time

South Dakota Nurses Association (SDNA)
Darcy Sherman-Justice, MS, RNC, President (10/05)
Tobi L. Lyon, BS Executive Director
116 N. Euclid
Pierre, South Dakota 57501-1015
(605) 945-4265
Fax: (605) 945-4266
E-mail: tlyon@rap.midco.net
www.nursingworld.org/snas/sd/
Office Hours: 10:30 AM to 5:00 PM Central Time

Tennessee Nurses Association (TNA)
Maureen Nalle, PhD, RN, President (11/05)
Deanna Menesses, Executive Director
545 Mainstream Drive, Suite 405
Nashville, Tennessee 37228-1201
(615) 254-0350
Fax: (615) 254-0303
E-mail: dmenesses@tnaonline.org
www.tnaonline.org
Office Hours: 8:30 AM to 4:30 PM Central Time

Texas Nurses Association (TNA)
Kathleen Light, EdD, MSN, RN, President (06/07)
Clair B. Jordan, MSN, RN, Executive Director
7600 Burnet Road, Suite 440
Austin, Texas 78757-1292
(512) 452-0645
Fax: (512) 452-0648
E-mail: memberinfo@texasnurses.org or cjordan@texasnurses.org
www.texasnurses.org
Office Hours: 8:00 AM to 5:00 PM Central Time

Utah Nurses Association (UNA)
Marianne Craven, RN, President (01/06)
Executive Director (vacant)
4505 South Wasatch Boulevard, #290
Salt Lake City, Utah 84124
(801) 272-4510
Fax: (801) 293-8458
E-mail:una@xmission.com
www.utahnurses.org
Office Hours: 9:00 AM to 5:00 PM Mountain Time

Vermont State Nurses Association (VSNA)
Cathy Dudley, RN, President (10/06)
Margaret M. Sharpe, BSN, RN, Executive Director
100 Dorset Street, Suite 13
South Burlington, Vermont 05403-6241
(802) 651-8886
Fax: (802) 651-8998
E-mail:vtnurse@prodigy.net
www.uvm.edu/~vsna/
Office Hours: Monday-Thursday 9:00 AM to 3:00 PM Eastern Time

Virgin Islands State Nurses Association (VISNA)
Gloria Callwood, PhD, RN, President (10/05)
Tracy Prado de Zela, Executive Director
PO Box 2339
Kings Hill, U.S. Virgin Islands 00851-2339
(340) 713-0293
E-mail: tropicallady@hotmail.com

Virginia Nurses Association (VNA)
Teresa Haller, MBA, MSN,RN, President (10/06)
Jan Marshall Johnson, MS, RN, Executive Director
7113 Three Chopt Road, Suite 204
Richmond, Virginia 23226
(804) 282-1808, ext. 2373
Fax: (804) 282-4916
E-mail: vnajmj@aol.com
www.virginianurses.com
Office Hours: 8:30 AM to 5:00 PM Eastern Time

Washington State Nurses Association (WSNA)
Kim Armstrong, RN, President (06/07)
Judith A. Huntington, MN, RN, Executive Director
575 Andover Park West, Suite 101
Seattle, Washington 98188-3321
(206) 575-7979, ext. 3002
Fax: (206) 575-1908
E-mail:wsna@wsna.org or jhunting@wsna.org
www.wsna.org
Office Hours: 8:30 AM to 4:30 PM Pacific Time

West Virginia Nurses Association (WVNA)
Pam Neal, BSN, RN, President (10/06)
Cheri Heflin, Executive Director
100 Capitol Street, Suite 1009
PO Box 1946
Charleston, West Virginia 25301
(304) 342-1169 or (800) 400-1226
Fax: (304) 346-1861
(304) 346-0300 (direct)
E-mail: centraloffice@wvnurses.orgor
Cheri@chandcompany.com
www.wvnurses.org
Office Hours: 8:30 AM to 4:30 PM Eastern Time

Wisconsin Nurses Association (WNA)
Pat Keller, MSN, RN, President (10/05)
Gina Dennik-Champion, MSN, MSH, RN, Executive Administrator
6117 Monona Drive
Madison, Wisconsin 53716
(608) 221-0383
Fax: (608) 221-2788
E-mail: info@wisconsinnurses.orgor
gina@wisconsinnurses.org
www.wisconsinnurses.org
Office Hours: 7:30 AM to 4:00 PM Central Time

Wyoming Nurses Association (WNA)
Linda Mink, MN, RN, President (06/06)
Shea Ward, Executive Director
Majestic Building, Room 305
PO Box 895
Casper, Wyoming 82602-0895
(307) 266-2000
Fax: (307) 266-2010
E-mail: wyonurse@aol.com
www.wyonurse.org
Office Hours: Monday/Wednesday/Thursday 8:00 AM to 1:00 PM Mountain Time;
Tuesday/Friday 9:00 AM to 1:00 PM Mountain Time

American Nurses Association (ANA)
Barbara A. Blakeney, MS, RN, President (06/06)
Linda J. Stierle, MSN, RN, CNAA, BC, Chief Executive Officer
8515 Georgia Avenue, Suite 400
Silver Spring, Maryland 20910
(301) 628-5000
(800) 274-4ANA
Fax: (301) 628-5001
E-mail: lstierle@ana.org
www.nursingworld.org
Office Hours: 9:00 AM to 5:00 PM Eastern Time

Constituent Assembly Executive Committee

Kathy Player, EdD, RN, Chairperson (6/04-6/06)
President
Arizona Nurses Association
16426 S. Mountain Stone Trail
Phoenix, Arizona 85048
(480) 460-3376 (H)
(602) 589-2704 (W)
Fax: (602) 589-2054
E-mail: kplayer@yahoo.com

Cheryl Schmidt, PhD, RN, Vice-Chairperson (6/05-6/07)
President
Arkansas Nurses Association
320 West Cross Street
Benton, Arkansas 72015
(501) 686-8705 (W)
Fax: (501) 686-686-8350
E-mail: ckschmidt@uams.edu

Sindy Barker, CAE, Secretary (6/04-6/06)
Executive Director
North Carolina Nurses Association
103 Enterprise Street
PO Box 12025
Raleigh, North Carolina 27605
(919) 821-4250 (W)
Fax: (919) 283-5807
E-mail: sindybarker@ncnurses.org

Linda Easterly, MS, RN, BSN, COHN-S, Member-at-Large (6/05-6/07)
President
Georgia Nurses Association
121 Heather Glen Boulevard
Kathleen, Georgia 31047
(478) 988-4133 (H)
(478) 988-1858 (W)
Fax: (478) 988-1853
E-mail: leasterly@hhc.org

Judy Huntington, MN, RN, Member-at-Large (6/05-6/07)
Executive Director
Washington State Nurses Association
575 Andover Park West, Suite 101
Seattle, Washington 98188-3321
(206) 575-7979, ext. 3002 (W)
Fax: (206) 575-1908
E-mail: jhuntin@wsna.org

APPENDIX D

Canadian Nursing Organizations

Alberta Association of Registered Nurses
11620 168 Street
Edmonton, Alberta T5M 4A6
Phone: 780-451-0043
Fax: 780-452-3276
E-mail: aarn@nurses.ab.ca
Website: www.nurses.ab.ca

The Association of Nurses of Prince Edward Island
137 Queen Street, Suite 303
Charlottetown, Prince Edward Island C1A 4B3
Phone: 902-368-3764
Fax: 902-628-1430
E-mail: anpei@pei.aibn.com
Website: www.anpei.ca

Association of Registered Nurses of Newfoundland
55 Military Road, Box 6116
St. John's, Newfoundland A1C 5X8
Phone: 709-753-6040
Fax: 709-753-4940
E-mail: info@arnn.nf.ca
Website: www.arnn.nf.ca

Canadian Nurses Association
50, The Driveway
Ottawa, Ontario K2P 1E2
E-mail: international@cna-nurses.ca
Website: www.cna-nurses.ca/cna/

College of Nurses of Ontario
101 Davenport Road
Toronto, Ontario M5R 3P1
Phone: 800-387-5526 or 416-928-0900
Fax: 416-928-5607
E-mail: mrisk@cnomail.org
Website: www.cno.org

College of Registered Nurses of Manitoba
647 Broadway Avenue
Winnipeg, Manitoba R3C 0X2
Phone: 204-774-3477
Fax: 204-775-6052
E-mail: info@crnm.mb.ca
Website: www.crnm.mb.ca

College of Registered Nurses of Nova Scotia
Suite 600, Barrington Tower
Scotia Square, 1894 Barrington St.
Halifax, Nova Scotia B3J 2A8
Phone: 902-491-9744
Fax: 902-491-9510
E-mail: info@crnns.ca
Website: www.crnns.ca

Nurses Association of New Brunswick/ Association des infirmières et infirmiers du Nouveau-Brunswick
165 Regent Street
Fredericton, New Brunswick E3B 3W5
Phone: 506-458-8731
Fax: 506-459-2838
E-mail: nanb@nanb.nb.ca
Website: www.nanb.nb.ca

Ordre des infirmières et infirmiers du Québec
4200, boul. Dorchester Ouest
Montréal, Québec H3Z 1V4
Phone: 514-935-2501 or 800-363-6048
Fax: 514-935-1799
E-mail: inf@oiiq.org
Website: www.oiiq.org

Registered Nurses Association of British Columbia
2855 Arbutus Street
Vancouver, British Columbia V6J 3Y8
Phone: 604-736-7331
Fax: 604-738-2272
E-mail: info@rnabc.bc.ca
Website: www.rnabc.bc.ca

Registered Nurses Association of Ontario
1600—438 University Avenue
Toronto, Ontario M5G 2K8
Phone: 416-599-1925 or 800-268-7199
Fax: 416-599-1926
E-mail: info@rnao.org
Website: www.rnao.org

Registered Nurses Association of the Northwest Territories
Executive Director/Registrar
RNANT/NU
PO Box 2757
Yellowknife, Northwest Territory X1A 2R1
General Inquiries: admin@rnantnu.ca
Registrar: registrar@rnantnu.ca
Executive Director: ed@rnantnu.ca
Website: www.rnantnu.ca

Saskatchewan Registered Nurses' Association
2066 Retallack Street
Regina, Saskatchewan S4T 7X5
Phone: 306-359-4200
Fax: 306-525-0849
E-mail: srna@srna.org
Website: www.srna.org

Yukon Registered Nurses Association
204—4133 4th Avenue
Whitehorse, Yukon Y1A 1H8
Phone: 867-667-4062
Fax: 867-668-5123
e-mail: yrna@yknet.ca
Website: www.yrna.ca

INDEX

Page numbers followed by *b*, *t*, and *f* indicate boxes, tables, and figures, respectively.

H

M

O